A Companion to the Atlas of
Pediatric Physical Diagnosis

Common & Chronic
Symptoms in Pediatrics

A Companion to the Atlas of
Pediatric Physical Diagnosis

Common & Chronic Symptoms in Pediatrics

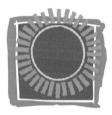

J. CARLTON GARTNER, Jr., MD

Edmund R. McCluskey Professor of Pediatrics,
University of Pittsburgh School of Medicine;
Vice Chairman, Department of Pediatrics,
Director, Diagnostic Referral Service,
Children's Hospital of Pittsburgh, Pittsburgh, Pennsylvania

BASIL J. ZITELLI, MD

Professor of Pediatrics,
University of Pittsburgh School of Medicine;
Diagnostic Referral Service,
Children's Hospital of Pittsburgh, Pittsburgh, Pennsylvania

with 339 illustrations

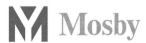 Mosby

St. Louis   Baltimore   Boston   Carlsbad   Chicago   Naples   New York   Philadelphia   Portland
London   Madrid   Mexico City   Singapore   Sydney   Tokyo   Toronto   Wiesbaden

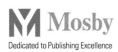

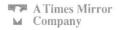

Vice President and Publisher: Anne S. Patterson
Editor: Laura DeYoung
Developmental Editor: Jennifer Byington Geistler
Editing Assistant: Karen Crutcher Copeland
Project Manager: Carol Sullivan Weis
Senior Production Editor: Christine Carroll Schwepker
Manufacturing Manager: Karen Lewis
Designer: Renee Duenow

Printed in the United States of America
Composition by Graphic World, Inc.
Printing/binding by World Color

Mosby–Year Book, Inc.
11830 Westline Industrial Drive
St. Louis, Missouri 63146

Library of Congress Cataloging-in-Publication Data
Common & chronic symptoms in pediatrics: a companion volume to the Atlas of
  pediatric physical diagnosis/(edited by) J. Carlton Gartner, Jr.,
Basil J. Zitelli.
     p.   cm.
  Includes bibliographical references and index.
  ISBN 0-8151-3407-X
  1. Children—Diseases—Diagnosis. 2. Children—Medical
  examinations. 3. Physical diagnosis. I. Gartner, J. Carlton (John
  Carlton) II. Zitelli, Basil J. (Basil John), 1946–   . III. Atlas
  of pediatric physical diagnosis.
  (DNLM: 1. Diagnosis—in infancy & childhood. 2. Physical
  Examination—in infancy & childhood.   WS   141 C734 1997)
  RJ50 A86   1997 Suppl.
  618.92'00754—dc21
  DNLM/DLC
  for Library of Congress   97-10508
                                                            CIP

97 98 99 00 01 / 9 8 7 6 5 4 3 2 1

Contributors

Miriam D. Bloom, MD
Assistant Professor of Pediatrics,
University of Pittsburgh School of Medicine;
Diagnostic Referral Service,
Children's Hospital of Pittsburgh,
Pittsburgh, Pennsylvania

John D. Farrell, MD
Former Chief Resident in Pediatrics,
Children's Hospital of Pittsburgh;
Private Practice,
South Riding, Virginia

J. Carlton Gartner, Jr., MD
Edmund R. McCluskey Professor of Pediatrics,
University of Pittsburgh School of Medicine;
Vice Chairman, Department of Pediatrics,
Director, Diagnostic Referral Service,
Children's Hospital of Pittsburgh,
Pittsburgh, Pennsylvania

Dena Hofkosh, MD
Associate Professor of Pediatrics,
University of Pittsburgh School of Medicine;
Director, Child Development Unit,
Children's Hospital of Pittsburgh,
Pittsburgh, Pennsylvania

Sara C. McIntire, MD
Associate Professor of Clinical Pediatrics,
University of Pittsburgh School of Medicine;
Diagnostic Referral Service,
Children's Hospital of Pittsburgh,
Pittsburgh, Pennsylvania

J. Jeffrey Malatack, MD
Professor of Pediatrics,
Temple University School of Medicine;
Director, Diagnostic Referral Service,
St. Christopher's Hospital for Children,
Philadelphia, Pennsylvania

Mark J. Mendelsohn, MD
Assistant Professor of Pediatrics,
University of Virginia School of Medicine,
Charlottesville, Virginia

Mary M. Moran, MD
Assistant Professor of Pediatrics,
Temple University School of Medicine;
Diagnostic Referral Service,
St. Christopher's Hospital for Children,
Philadelphia, Pennsylvania

Beth Moughan, MD
Assistant Professor of Pediatrics,
Temple University School of Medicine;
Diagnostic Referral Service,
St. Christopher's Hospital for Children,
Philadelphia, Pennsylvania

Eugene M. Mowad, MD
Assistant Professor of Clinical Pediatrics,
Northeastern Ohio University College of Medicine;
Diagnostic Referral Service,
Tod Children's Hospital,
Youngstown, Ohio

Lisa M. Nalven, MD
Clinical Assistant Professor of Pediatrics,
University of Pittsburgh School of Medicine;
Child Development Unit,
Children's Hospital of Pittsburgh,
Pittsburgh, Pennsylvania

James A. Nard, MD
Associate Professor of Clinical Pediatrics,
Northeastern Ohio University College of Medicine;
Diagnostic Referral Service,
Tod Children's Hospital,
Youngstown, Ohio

Jean M. Tersak, MD
Hematology-Oncology Fellow,
Children's Hospital of Pittsburgh,
Pittsburgh, Pennsylvania

Andrew H. Urbach, MD
Professor of Pediatrics,
University of Pittsburgh School of Medicine;
Diagnostic Referral Service,
Children's Hospital of Pittsburgh,
Pittsburgh, Pennsylvania

Basil J. Zitelli, MD
Professor of Pediatrics,
University of Pittsburgh School of Medicine;
Diagnostic Referral Service,
Children's Hospital of Pittsburgh,
Pittsburgh, Pennsylvania

To our parents, our first teachers
To our wives, Kay and Suzanne, and our children, Amy, Carlton, and Andrew;
and Matthew, Daniel, Benjamin, and Anne, who supported our effort

Especially to Paul C. Gaffney, MD,
our teacher, mentor, role model, and founder of the Diagnostic Referral Service, for his
wisdom, guidance, and good humor in difficult situations

To Thomas K. Oliver, Jr., MD,
whose strong support for education in general pediatrics created the environment
in which this book could develop

Foreword

The more usual pediatric patient requires evaluation of an acute problem that is of short duration, is often self-limited or responsive to a short course of therapy, and has only a temporary impact on the patient and family. The patient with symptoms that become chronic is at risk for long-term disability (both physical and psychologic), and the impact on the family and child may compromise their functioning.

There has been a rapid increase in laboratory, imaging, and other diagnostic techniques. The fact remains, however, that careful history and physical examination are, as in all of medicine, the basic modalities with which the physician must deal. The art is knowing how to interpret findings and knowing when and what laboratory and imaging assistance is required.

The authors have a large amount of experience in evaluating complicated patients in their diagnostic referral activities. Most of the contributors have backgrounds as chief residents in pediatric training programs and have continued to be active teachers of medical students and house officers. They have brought together under one cover a body of information that has a great deal to offer the physician who takes on the responsibility of answering the sometimes frustrating challenge of the patient with chronic symptoms.

Paul C. Gaffney, MD
Professor of Pediatrics Emeritus,
University of Pittsburgh School of Medicine;
Director Emeritus, Diagnostic Referral Service,
Children's Hospital of Pittsburgh,
Pittsburgh, Pennsylvania

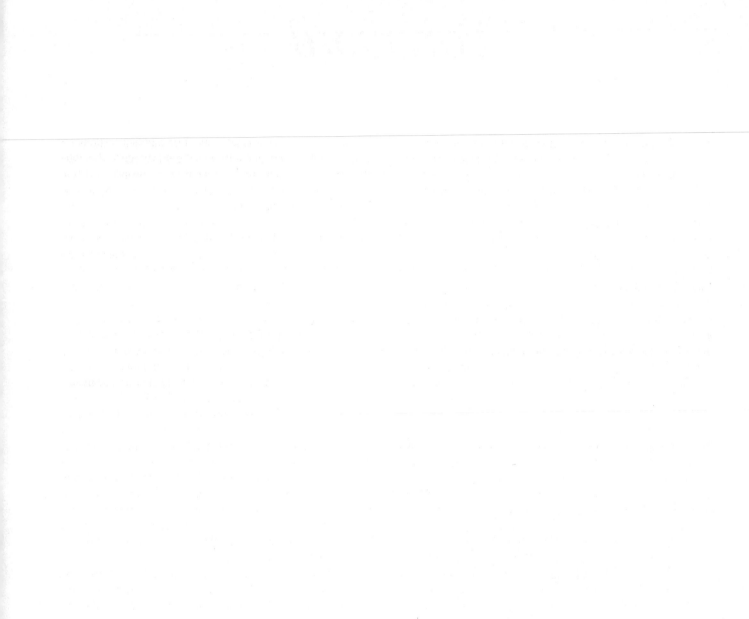

Preface

Textbooks of pediatrics are excellent sources of information for students, residents, and practicing physicians. It is reasonably easy to look up the treatment of a disorder or review the pathophysiology of a recognized condition, but how does the physician approach the patient with chronic abdominal pain, fatigue, cough, or limp? To use a standard text, the clinician is forced to look in various sections, under specific diagnoses, to find out about the key presenting signs and symptoms. The physician could also look at a book that lists differential diagnosis, but this is not particularly helpful in planning the investigation of an individual patient.

This book was conceived in an effort to organize an approach to specific subacute or chronic problems that do not fit well into body systems, such as cardiovascular disease or renal disease. Each contributor has a current or past association with the Children's Hospital of Pittsburgh, and most are or were part of the Diagnostic Referral Service. They have significant clinical experience in the diagnosis and management of a wide variety of pediatric disorders. Most of the disorders are common referral problems from our community physicians and are also frequent (and often difficult and frustrating) complaints in the resident continuity clinic. Almost all of the signs and symptoms include a wide variety of differential diagnoses and potentially costly investigations. Our discussions emphasize a meticulous history and physical examination, allowing the physician to plan a thoughtful, limited, and directed evaluation. We attempt to discuss many of the common, "cardinal" features of illness and emphasize the thought process that leads to diagnostic accuracy. In addition, we enhance the text with photographs and tables from another book that originated in our department, the *Atlas of Pediatric Physical Diagnosis*.

Each chapter has a similar structure and has sections on background or literature survey, pathophysiology, differential diagnosis, history, physical examination, and approach to the patient. Tables of differential diagnosis are included, as well as tables that emphasize key points in the history or examination, which can narrow the investigation. Each chapter closes with several cases that illustrate the approach to patients. In most of these cases a careful history is the most important factor in arriving at a diagnosis. The references are selective, with an emphasis on current reviews or initial clinical descriptions of a disorder.

How were the chapter topics selected? We arrived at the final list based on clinical problems referred to our own practice (abdominal pain, fatigue, fever of unknown origin, etc.) and included a few challenging concerns (e.g., limp and syncope) because they represent major diagnostic dilemmas. (We should admit that the first list of topics was developed in an area very conducive to thought—the confines of an airplane cabin on a return trip from Krakow and our first exposure to the eastern European healthcare system. Months later this list finally resurfaced on the back of an airline ticket envelope.) Our hope is that this book will be useful to many physicians and other healthcare workers, including those in training for their future careers. In this era of cost containment, the generalist physician must spend more time in the primary investigation of many of the problems presented in this book and refer only *selected* patients for further subspecialty evaluation. This text should be a source of key information about differential diagnosis and an aid in making decisions about further investigation and referral.

J. Carlton Gartner, Jr., MD
Basil J. Zitelli, MD

Contents in Brief

Contents

A Companion to the Atlas of
Pediatric Physical Diagnosis

Common & Chronic Symptoms in Pediatrics

I

Pain

Recurrent Abdominal Pain

J. CARLTON GARTNER, Jr.

 ## Key Points

- Recurrent abdominal pain is a common pediatric condition, affecting 10% to 15% of children.

- Organic disorders are found in a very small number of cases.

- Careful history, physical examination, and selective screening laboratory tests prevent overinvestigation and enhance management by the primary physician.

Chronic recurrent abdominal pain (RAP) is the most common pain-related complaint of the school-age child. The overall incidence is approximately 10%, with a greater frequency in girls. In one survey by Apley, almost 30% of girls between 8 and 10 years of age were affected. Apley's proposed definition—at least three episodes of pain occurring over a period of 3 months in a child at least 3 years of age (although the pain is rare before age 5 and after age 15)—is the most commonly used. The pain must be severe enough to interfere with usual daily activity. The incidence of definite organic disease as a cause of RAP is low, certainly less than the usual figure of 5% to 10%. Despite numerous investigative techniques, the etiology remains obscure, although, with rare exceptions, the pain is believed to be real by most observers. Overt psychiatric problems are rare, and a number of studies suggest that affected children are not significantly different from those with organic bowel disorders. A relentless search for all possible organic causes is unrewarding and may be harmful, but a strictly psychologic approach is rarely helpful. This chapter reviews the epidemiology, family dynamics, theories of etiology, and role of several key organic disorders that must be recognized in relationship to RAP. The goal is an organized approach that helps children, improves outcome, and avoids unnecessary investigation.

Pathophysiology/Pathogenesis

Because there is no defined etiology of RAP, it is useful to review the usual description of RAP, the sources and anatomic locations of pain in the abdomen, and finally the major current theories of pathogenesis. In a review of 119 patients, Liebman clarified the character of the pain as follows: central location in the abdomen (periumbilical 57%, lower abdomen 27%), cramping or a dull ache, occurring several times per week or per month (daily in only 16%), with episodes lasting several minutes to several hours. Most patients have associated symptoms, which range in frequency from affecting 10% to 60% of patients and include pallor, tiredness, anorexia, dizziness, headache, vomiting, enuresis, low-grade fever (<100° F), diarrhea, and constipation.

Abdominal pain receptors are located in the submucosa, muscular layer, and serosa of the intestine; the capsules of solid organs; and the parietal peritoneum. Stretching usually stimulates pain fibers; pain is not well localized and is often referred to the midline because the sensory C fibers travel to both sides of the spinal cord. The location of RAP in the periumbilical and lower abdomen suggests that the source is the small intestine or proximal colon. Pain from the stomach and duodenum is more commonly referred to the epigastric area, and pain from the parietal peritoneum is more intense and better localized, usually to one side. (Apley notes that central pain is the hallmark of RAP.)

Numerous theories regarding the etiology of RAP have been proposed. Apley's initial hypothesis was that the response was conditioned and learned from a pattern of reaction common to family members. He also felt that autonomic tone was elevated in children with RAP, citing the common finding of dilated pupils in earlier studies that measured pupillary responses. Other investigators demonstrated increased rectosigmoid motility in response to neostigmine (Prostigmin), suggesting increased parasympathetic tone. Results of studies, however, have been inconsistent and have not been confirmed by subsequent investigators.

3

Constipation and poor evacuation habits (dyskinesia) were proposed by Davidson as a cause of pain and do play a role in some patients. Several authors have cited unrecognized constipation as a major factor in etiology. The opposite bowel pattern—bloating, gas, loose stools—has been related to carbohydrate malabsorption and RAP. Barr identified that 40% of patients with RAP had lactose malabsorption, and a substantial portion (70%) responded to elimination of this carbohydrate from the diet. Better controlled studies have found a much lesser incidence of pain caused by this mechanism, but it must be considered. Other carbohydrates found in fruit juices or even in medications, as well as the sugar alcohol sorbitol, may be offending agents. Several investigators have documented abnormal peristaltic waves in the upper intestine and even abnormal intestinal permeability to substances such as ^{51}Cr-EDTA in patients with RAP. The question remains whether these findings are part of the pathogenesis or are nonspecific. Fortunately, studies of the association of RAP with *Helicobacter pylori* have shown little relationship, as opposed to the documented strong association with antral gastritis and duodenal ulcer disease.

Many pediatricians and internists have searched for a relationship between RAP and two common adult disorders—irritable bowel syndrome and nonulcerative dyspepsia. Although a small percentage of patients with RAP may be diagnosed with irritable bowel syndrome later in life, most are not. Nonulcerative dyspepsia may occur most frequently as an infectious disorder related to *H. pylori,* and further studies are in progress.

Psychodynamic theories for RAP, which have been prominent for many years, were initially documented by Apley, who found that RAP tended to "run in families" and that these same families also had substantially higher incidences of migraine, peptic ulcer disease, "nervous breakdown," and appendectomy. He described the children as "high strung," perfectionistic, sensitive, anxious overachievers. Patient and family characteristics have been further delineated in more recent controlled studies. Dependency, fearfulness, anxiety, and poor self-esteem are frequently associated with RAP, and often stressful life events and marital difficulties occur in affected families. Findings are not uniform, and in one study patients with RAP had higher depression scores than controls but were similar to those of patients with inflammatory bowel disease. Maternal depression has been statistically associated with RAP in children. Recent studies have uncovered another potential association; somatization disorder is found more frequently in family members. This disorder includes chronic symptoms of multiple different areas (pain, conversion symptoms, psychosexual dysfunction, etc.). Pain in individuals diagnosed with somatization disorder often begins in childhood.

Because treatment of specific psychologic difficulties or specific organic disorders has not led to dramatic improvement in children with RAP, a multifactorial etiology, such as that proposed by Levine and others, may be the most useful for the physician treating such patients. Patient characteristics (genetics, personality, evacuation habits, etc.), family dynamics, coping mechanisms, lifestyle, and specific life events may all play a role in producing mild to severe pain. Attention to each of these factors may be helpful in treating the patient (and the family). Another useful model proposed by Barr categorizes patients into three groups: pure organic, pure psychologic, and the largest group, "dysfunctional," in which there may be a relationship between environmental factors or stresses and physiologic variables, such as constipation and carbohydrate intolerance.

Background/Literature Survey

The literature dealing with RAP falls, with some exceptions, into three categories: (1) reviews, including more common organic causes; (2) role of behavioral or psychologic factors; and (3) specific disorders or methods of investigation for organic causes. The last category is covered in this chapter under Differential Diagnosis. Apley's book, which includes information from a previous survey of 1000 outpatients and a hospital study of 100 inpatients, remains a classic, although dated by methods of investigation. He has sufficient follow-up to review outcome: about one third of the patients continue to have abdominal pain as adults, one third develop a "replacement pain" (usually headache), and one third recover completely. His thoughtful clinical approach with an emphasis on the family is a paradigm for patient care. Many reviews of RAP are available and offer excellent overviews, emphasizing certain information such as clinical symptoms, differential diagnosis and a multifactorial model, long-term follow-up, and general diagnostic approach.

Many articles have attempted to relate abdominal pain to specific psychiatric profiles, such as depression. A valuable older paper is Schmitt's review of school phobia. School-related stress certainly may lead to gastrointestinal symptoms, and a careful school attendance record is critical information. Several studies have failed to find differences in the psychologic profile of control children and those with RAP. Another study found that patients with organic bowel disorders (e.g., ulcerative colitis) and patients with RAP were different from controls but not from each other. Anxiety scores are higher in RAP patients and their parents, and there is an increased incidence of maternal depression. Stressful life events are more frequent in the families of children with RAP, especially medical illness, hospitalization, and death. As mentioned previously, somatization disorder affects these families with increased frequency.

Differential Diagnosis

Lengthy lists of diagnostic possibilities are probably not particularly relevant to the approach to RAP, although several such lists are available. As noted previously the incidence of organic disorders is low, probably at most 5% to 10% of cases. In his survey of 100 patients, Apley found eight who may have had an organic cause, although the diagnosis was questionable in some cases. In a survey of more than 1400 patients reported in the medical literature in 1985, only 6.8% had an organic etiology. Finally the Mayo Clinic follow-up of 161 patients conducted by Stickler and Murphy detected only three patients who developed a definite disease: Crohn's disease in each. The list of possible diagnoses is extensive, but it is illogical to list all potential causes. As Apley has written, the continuous search for an organic etiology may be harmful; the physician runs the risk of becoming (quoting Weiss) "a pathologic agent in perpetuating the illness by his well-meaning but never-ending efforts to find a physical cause." It is more logical to discuss the common disorders that may require careful analysis before planning an approach to the patient. These can be divided into gastrointestinal, urinary tract, psychogenic, and finally a category of "other" causes of RAP.

Gastrointestinal Causes

Because of the Mayo Clinic survey, Crohn disease (regional enteritis) is a major consideration in children with RAP. Rarely is pain the only symptom or sign of this disorder. Clues to the diagnosis are multiple and include change in bowel movements (usually diarrhea, often accompanied by nocturnal stools); weight loss; pallor; deceleration in growth, which may precede gastrointestinal symptoms (Fig. 1-1); rashes; arthritis; perianal disease (skin tags, fistulas) (Fig. 1-2); and digital clubbing (Fig. 1-3). Occasionally, diagnosis may be difficult in the early stages of disease. Two of the "missed" patients in the Mayo Clinic series had weight loss, and one had anemia at presentation, making the diagnosis of RAP less likely.

The role of *H. pylori* in RAP is currently the subject of investigation. Certainly the relationship of this organism to antral gastritis and duodenal ulcer disease in adults has been verified. A review of these relationships in children, using 45 published studies, confirmed the association with antral gastritis and duodenal ulcer but found "weak or no association with recurrent abdominal pain." In a nonblinded study, Chong and others found *H. pylori* seropositivity and antral gastritis more frequently in a group of children with RAP. However, by strict criteria only 12 of the 218 children with RAP had a clear association with *H. pylori*. Thus this association may explain a small percentage of children with RAP. Unfortunately, antibody alone is not an effective diagnostic tool, and endoscopy with culture, urease testing, histology, and polymerase chain reaction (PCR) testing for the organism are more accurate. In this same study peptic ulcer disease was found in 14 of the 218 patients with RAP (although only 111 underwent endoscopy for severe or persistent symptoms); nine duodenal and five gastric ulcers were found, and only four of these were positive for *H. pylori*. Thus peptic disorders should be considered in the differential diagnosis of RAP but do not explain most cases. Symptoms in older children are similar to those in adults: pain at night or in the early morn-

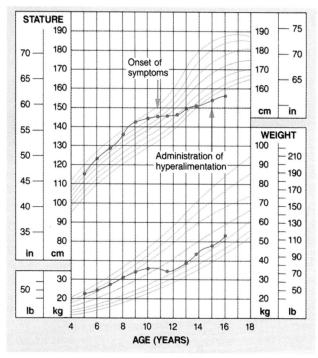

FIG. 1-1 Crohn disease. This growth curve demonstrates a fall-off before onset of disease symptoms and continued poor growth through many exacerbations requiring steroid therapy. Home hyperalimentation maintained weight gain.

ing, recurrent emesis, pain several hours after meals, and relief after eating. Infants and toddlers may have more vague symptoms: feeding difficulties, emesis, and bleeding or perforation. Nighttime pain is a clue mentioned by several authors because it is unusual in patients with nonorganic RAP.

Constipation is a common and treatable association with RAP. Numerous authors have commented on the association, which must be considered even when the initial history is inconclusive. Occasionally the child with stool retention appears to have regular bowel movements, but abdominal palpation or rectal examination reveals major stool retention. An abdominal radiograph is occasionally necessary.

Carbohydrate malabsorption may play a role in some patients with RAP. As noted previously, the initial euphoria that many patients' pain might be alleviated by the removal of carbohydrates has been tempered by later studies. Nonetheless, as pointed out by Hyams and others, carbohydrates include substances other than lactose; sorbitol, fructose, and high-fiber substances are prevalent in some diets and may be unrecognized as potential causes of malabsorption.

Pancreatitis may be overlooked as a cause of recurrent pain. Fulminant acute pancreatitis is accompanied by emesis, abdominal pain, and signs of acute illness. However, recurrent or familial forms of this disorder may be more difficult to diagnose because of a less intense presentation. Pancreatic enlargement confirmed by ultrasound, mild elevation of enzymes, and perhaps a family history may be clues. The causes of pancreatitis must be recognized; congenital abnor-

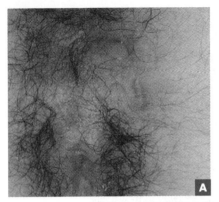 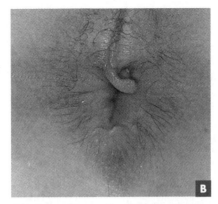 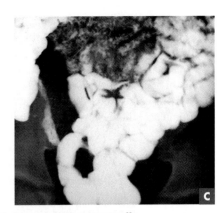

FIG. 1-2 *A,* In this patient with Crohn disease the slightly raised, erythematous lesion eventually drained and represented a fistulous opening. *B,* Note the scar from a previous incision and drainage. Perianal skin tags are common in Crohn disease and are a good clue to diagnosis. *C,* Stricture of the terminal ileum and segmental involvement of the small bowel and colon are characteristic findings on barium enema examination of a child with Crohn disease.

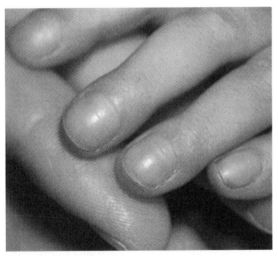

FIG. 1-3 Osteoarthropathy (clubbing). Note thickening and loss of the angle at the nailbed.

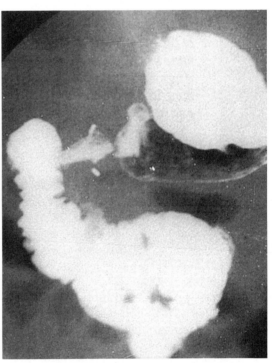

FIG. 1-4 Malrotation in biliary atresia. The duodenal "C" loop is not closed and is displaced to the right.

malities of the ducts, familial and genetic causes, and trauma are more common in children. Often dismissed as a cause of recurrent pain in children but diagnosed more frequently in adults is cholelithiasis. Hemolytic anemia with stone formation is a known cause of biliary colic, with conditions such as hereditary spherocytosis and sickle cell disease among the common causes. Patients need not have hemolytic disease, however. In infants and toddlers, total parenteral nutrition is a predisposing cause. Other conditions may lead to stone formation in older children, such as inflammatory bowel disease, vomiting, dehydration, and biliary tract abnormalities.

Recently, gallstone formation has been described in pediatric patients with apparent predisposing conditions similar to those found in adults, such as obesity, female gender, and pregnancy. Although right upper quadrant pain and jaundice are most common in patients with cholelithiasis, the occasional patient has more vague, recurrent epigastric pain. This type of presentation is more common in the school-age child.

In younger children a rare but important cause of recurring episodes of pain is malrotation with midgut volvulus. The pain is usually accompanied by emesis and intermittent diarrhea. Gastrointestinal series may need to be repeated and

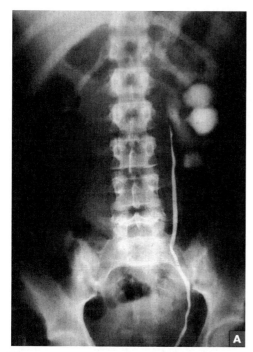 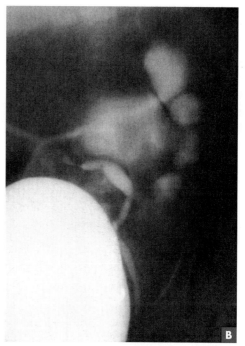

FIG. 1-5 *A,* Retrograde ureterogram defines obstruction at the ureteropelvic junction. *B,* The coexistence of vesicoureteric reflux and UPJ obstruction is seen in this voiding cystourethrogram.

performed during an episode to demonstrate the obstruction, but between episodes the duodenal "C" loop is abnormal (Fig. 1-4). At times physicians presume these patients have allergic enteritis or cyclic vomiting until the correct diagnosis is made.

Finally, several authors mention intestinal infection with parasites as a cause of RAP. Most commonly mentioned is infestation with *Giardia lamblia.* Isolated abdominal pain is unusual in this condition because most patients have diarrhea, bloating, and foul-smelling stools. Inquiry about these associated symptoms should allow appropriate investigation.

Urinary Tract Disorders

Urinary tract disorders are a possible cause of RAP, and Apley found that at least 50% of the organic causes involved the urinary tract. Recurrent or chronic infection; obstruction, especially of the ureteropelvic junction (UPJ) (Fig. 1-5); and urolithiasis are possible, but the pain is more likely to be peripheral in the abdomen. Apley's "rule" suggests that the further the pain is from the umbilicus, the more likely it is to have a defined cause. A disorder that may be overlooked is intermittent UPJ obstruction sometimes accompanied by emesis, known as *Dietl crisis.* The patient must be evaluated during an episode to detect the abnormality on physical examination or by ultrasound.

Urinary tract infection and urolithiasis are mentioned in several texts as possible causes of RAP. In these conditions the pain occurs most frequently in the flank and may be colicky in nature. A family history may be present in the patient who has suspected renal stones. In addition, caution should be exercised when interpreting abnormal urine culture results. In the absence of a history of past infection, fever, and pyuria, a more likely explanation for the abnormal culture is asymptomatic bacteriuria.

Psychogenic Causes

There are some children with recurrent pain who meet criteria for a predominantly psychogenic diagnosis. The most easily recognized of these is a conversion disorder. The predominant symptoms in this category are pain and gait disturbance, which is often manifested in adolescents as weakness or inability to stand or walk. Usually a stressful situation exists, such as school, as well as an understanding ally (parent) and a role model for symptoms. RAP may occasionally be a true conversion symptom or part of the myriad of symptoms seen in somatization. In general surveys looking for psychiatric symptoms in children, the most prevalent is anxiety. Further study may lead to a model for RAP that includes anxiety disorder as a major factor or even pharmacologically treats this symptom.

Other Causes

Causes of pain in addition to those previously mentioned are rare but should be mentioned for completeness. Pain in the back may be referred to the abdomen; patients with intervertebral disk disease or spine disease occasionally experience pain in the midabdomen (see Fig. 2-8). Careful history and

Differential Diagnosis of Recurrent Abdominal Pain

Gastrointestinal Causes
Crohn disease
Antral gastritis, peptic ulcer disease *(H. pylori)*
Constipation
Carbohydrate malabsorption
Pancreatitis
Cholelithiasis
Malrotation and volvulus
Intestinal parasitic infection *(G. lamblia)*

Urinary Tract Disorders
UPJ obstruction (Dietl crisis)
Urinary tract infection
Urolithiasis

Psychogenic Causes
Conversion reaction
Somatization disorder
Anxiety disorder

Other Causes
Intervertebral disk disease
Spine disease
Musculoskeletal trauma
Migraine or cyclic vomiting
Abdominal epilepsy

examination should lead to the correct diagnosis. Usually the pain associated with these conditions is more constant, similar to the pain caused by musculoskeletal trauma, which rarely produces abdominal discomfort in the typical pattern of RAP. Two additional potential causes are migraine and epilepsy. Although abdominal migraine (and perhaps cyclic vomiting) is mentioned in most reviews of RAP, vague recurrent pain is unlikely to be due to migraine. Abdominal epilepsy is rare and should be associated with change in consciousness. The toddler with migraine may be a challenge but rarely has nonspecific discomfort that could be mistaken for abdominal pain.

Box 1-1 presents the differential diagnosis and key findings of organic causes of RAP.

History

As with most chronic conditions, time spent on the history is the most important in reaching a correct diagnosis. Most decisions about the pursuit of an organic cause are made based on the history, which also gives the necessary support for the important decision **not** to refer the patient for further investigation. A cardinal principle exists: time spent on the history prevents a random and unhelpful approach later. For the consultant who sees children after many previous investigations have taken place, it is useful to take a complete history, unbiased by previous data that may be reviewed after the history and examination are completed.

As with any good pediatric history, it is useful to see the child and family together initially, but later some key areas should be discussed separately, such as the marital and social histories. It is important to obtain answers to some open-ended questions. What type of child is he or she? What do the parents feel is causing the pain? What worries or fears does the child have? How has the child's symptom affected the family? What activities has the child discontinued? Do the parents have any insight into the cause of the pain? (Some parents have already seen the effects of stressors on their child and know that school is a problem, for example.) In addition, talking to the child separately often yields information that was not revealed in the presence of the parents, such as marital discord, health worries, sexual activity, or possible abuse.

Specifics of the pain are important, including onset, duration, character, location, radiation, frequency, timing, relationship to meals or other daily events, triggers, and relievers of the pain. In older girls the relationship to the menstrual cycle should be discussed. Vague answers to these open-ended questions are common with nonorganic RAP. What does the patient do when the pain occurs? How does it affect activity? Key questions at this point deal with school attendance. School is one of the great stresses for children, and school phobia may be a subtle diagnosis. The examiner should be cautious here. Many parents of children with RAP are sensitive to the suggestion that their child might have a "psychologic problem," and inquiry must be matter-of-fact and without a hint of judgement. Carefully intermixing questions dealing with organic and nonorganic issues is a helpful approach so that the interview process is nonthreatening.

Once there is a clear description of the pain episodes, associated symptoms should be sought. Frequent pain associations with typical RAP were mentioned earlier (i.e., pallor, mild anorexia, etc.). A review of systems is useful at this point. Major questions related to the gastrointestinal tract should be asked with specifics about growth, weight gain, emesis, diarrhea, constipation, stool pattern, bloating, distension, hematemesis, hematochezia, and jaundice. In addition to the usual questions the physician should inquire about frequent complaints that are known to be largely functional, such as headache, limb pain, dizziness, fatigue, and weakness. Most often, patients with typical RAP have other stress- or tension-related symptoms, and the complaint of pain does not "run alone."

Family history is important. Apley noted the frequency of pain in family members. In addition, hereditary conditions or even associations, including pancreatitis, urolithiasis, migraine, peptic ulcer disease, epilepsy, inflammatory bowel disease, hemolytic anemia, and splenectomy, should be sought. Are there family members with similar symptoms? This may be a clue to either organic or functional symptoms.

In addition, inquiry about reaction patterns in the family are important (i.e., pain, irritable bowel syndrome, headache). Previous surgery and medical investigations on parents or family members may be significant. Symptoms of or treatment for depression, especially maternal depression, may have an association with RAP.

Social history may provide important information about recent travel, moves, change in schools, water and food consumption, marital discord, recent losses (grandparent, pet, etc.), and general family activity and function. If possible, a brief review of a typical day may be useful, including meals, activities, sleep pattern, daycare or school schedule, and time of bowel movements. In adolescents a brief review of key questions (HEADS: *h*ome, *e*ducation, *a*ctivities, *d*rugs/alcohol, *s*exual activity) is important. The physician should not forget to inquire about possible sexual abuse or violence. These factors may play a larger role than previously thought, and answers often depend on the manner in which questions are asked.

Past history should be reviewed for organic disorders and also for a sense of how the family sees the child. Children with previous serious illnesses or extreme prematurity may be susceptible to medical complications but also may be treated in a very protective fashion by their parents and may be vulnerable so that their symptoms are seriously exaggerated in importance.

At the end of an extensive history the physician should have a clear idea whether the child being examined has typical RAP, which usually does not have a recognized organic cause, or has symptoms of an atypical nature. Most patients (about 85%) fall into the former category.

Physical Examination

Although the physical examination is usually normal in the child with typical RAP, a meticulous evaluation is important for several reasons. There may be subtle clues to an organic disorder, and the patient and family need to be assured that the physician is thorough. A cursory approach is not likely to alleviate the intense anxiety that may accompany this chronic symptom.

As noted in several other chapters, a carefully constructed growth curve is critical. The pattern of growth over several years is important; deceleration in growth may be the earliest sign of Crohn disease or other conditions associated with malabsorption (Fig. 1-1). Weight-for-height is another important clue. Children with gastrointestinal disorders often have a low weight-for-height and a fall-off in linear growth (failure to thrive) (Fig. 1-6). Relative obesity is reassuring in a child who has chronic abdominal symptoms, although there is no systematic study of this sign and its relationship to RAP.

Vital signs should be noted. Hypertension may be a clue to the rare patient with chronic renal disease but more likely is a sign of anxiety in the older child. General appearance may be helpful. Many children with depression or anxiety

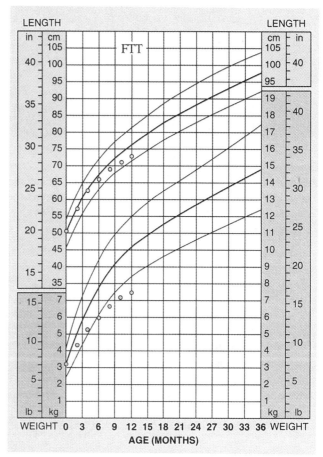

FIG. 1-6 An example of a growth curve. Typical failure to thrive with deceleration of weight gain.

make poor eye contact and seem unsure of answers to specific questions about the abdominal pain, often turning to their parents for answers. Skin examination (pallor, subcutaneous tissue, rashes, and nodules) may offer clues. Younger children should be examined, if possible, standing on the table so that abdominal protuberance or wasting of the gluteal area may be assessed. Once again this sign is found in chronic digestive disorders, especially in celiac disease. Digital clubbing may be another sign of inflammatory bowel disease, and nail examination should always be performed (Fig. 1-3). Holding the distal phalanges of the middle fingers together with the nails and distal interphalangeal joints touching may allow better evaluation of the loss of nailbed angle that occurs with osteoarthropathy. (With clubbing the nails are exactly parallel, and there is no space visible between the nailbases.)

Ear, nose, and throat; chest; and cardiac examinations should be completed. The major goal of these tests is to locate signs of a chronic illness, such as chronic infection, pulmonary disease, cardiomyopathy, and pericarditis. Careful observation of the respiratory rate and pattern, cardiac sounds and rhythm, and peripheral pulses is important.

Abdominal palpation is obviously critical. The patient's appearance and reaction should be noted. In a study of acute

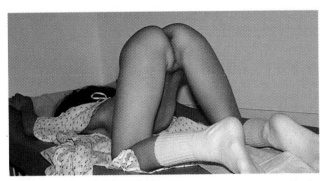

FIG. 1-7   Knee-chest position. The sway-back position with the knees widely separated facilitates examination and provides the best visualization of anatomic structures and abnormalities.

abdominal pain with meticulous hospital follow-up, the best correlation to an eventual organic diagnosis was whether the patient kept his or her eyes open during the emergency room examination. Patients who closed their eyes most frequently had a nonorganic diagnosis. (Presumably, patients who had true pain watched for the physician to palpate the tender area!) Many younger patients with typical RAP complain of pain during the examination but are easily distracted. Quality and pattern of bowel sounds should be noted. Peristaltic rushes or high-pitched bowel sounds are abnormal and suggest partial obstruction. Organomegaly and masses should be sought, and the span and texture of the liver should be noted (see Chapter 24). It is especially important to check for retained fecal material because constipation is frequently denied in the history. Palpation of the lower abdomen should detect a distended bladder, which may be a clue to obstructive uropathy.

Perianal examination should be done with attention to possible fissures, occult fistulas, hemorrhoids, and skin tags. A brief inspection of the patient's underwear may provide evidence of fecal or urinary incontinence. The question of routine rectal examination is often raised. Some younger children are extremely apprehensive about this procedure, and it occasionally may be necessary to postpone this examination until the child is more comfortable with the examiner. However, rectal examination is a very useful tool in that both occult constipation and gastrointestinal bleeding may be diagnosed. (In a recent article about constipation there was little value in obtaining a plain abdominal radiograph if both palpation and rectal examination were normal.)

Male genital examination could disclose hernias, undescended testes, or hypospadias. Female genital examination with gentle traction on the labia majora in the frog-leg position allows inspection of the hymen, urethra, and distal vagina. A much better view is obtained in the prone, knee-chest position with the buttocks elevated. In this position, with relaxation, the hymenal ring may be seen (Fig. 1-7). Children who have been sexually abused may have normal examinations, but any evidence of old trauma should be carefully noted. Photographs in several publications are very

helpful guides. In addition, girls with an imperforate hymen may complain of periodic abdominal pain until the problem is recognized. In pubertal girls, a careful pelvic examination is important. Discovery of a sexually transmitted disease may be one clue to the cause of the pain. If the physician is not skilled in this part of the examination, a colleague in adolescent medicine or gynecology may be an important consultant.

Neurologic and musculoskeletal examination complete the evaluation. It is useful to observe the patient sitting on and moving on and off of the examination table. Clues to spine and disk disease may be uncovered. Occasionally, abdominal pain is referred from the spinal area. Neurologic examination should include a brief inspection of gait (see Chapter 6).

Approach to the Patient

Completion of a meticulous history and thorough physical examination are the crucial parts of the evaluation of the patient with RAP. Although many physicians are quick to schedule tests and procedures, these are of little value and may be detrimental if the history and examination do not suggest a specific diagnosis other than typical RAP. The usual patient has episodic, centrally located, daytime pain lasting for minutes to several hours without a recognized trigger mechanism. The patient is somewhat overly dependent, anxious, or fearful, with poor self-esteem. There may be stressful life events or maternal depression. Growth, development, and general examination are normal. In such patients, only a few screening tests (discussed in the following section) are necessary before starting a therapeutic approach.

If the history or examination is not typical, as happens in perhaps 10% to 15% of cases, the examiner must decide on a specific diagnosis to be pursued before initiating therapy. Clues to an organic disease have been tabulated by several authors. These clues are listed in Box 1-2. Generally, peripheral abdominal pain, nocturnal pain that truly awakens the child from sleep, and meal-related pain are unusual in typical RAP. Recurrent and frequent emesis is unusual. Family and social histories that are unremarkable and a child who is relaxed and an average student are features more suggestive of an organic cause. Although not studied in a controlled fashion, generally children with typical RAP miss school frequently but do well academically. Changes in bowel habits, especially diarrhea, and constitutional symptoms, such as growth deceleration, fever, weight loss, and rash, are not typical. Hematochezia is abnormal. Physical examination should be truly normal; findings such as perianal skin tags, organomegaly, and digital clubbing must be pursued. Finally, screening tests should be normal.

Laboratory and Procedures

Screening tests rarely raise suspicion of an organic disease that was presumed unlikely based on information from the history and physical examination. In most patients these tests are normal and support a noninvasive approach with limitation of procedures. Generally these tests include a complete blood count, sedimentation rate, serum albumin and total protein values, pancreatic enzyme levels (lipase and amylase), urinalysis and culture, and stool examination for occult blood. Some authors include stool examination for ova and parasites and some type of screening for malabsorption, such as lactose breath hydrogen or fecal alpha$_1$-antitrypsin tests. Our feeling is that these latter tests are necessary only if the history or examination suggests parasitic disease or malabsorption. If so, a screening test, such as D-xylose absorption, may be indicated (see Chapter 18). The yield of the initial screening tests is limited, and in fact an abnormal urine culture may be more suggestive of occult bacteriuria, which is generally a benign condition unless there is a history of recurrent pyelonephritis.

The question of more diagnostic screening tests is often raised at this point in the evaluation. Should a plain abdominal radiograph be performed? What about the yield of abdominal ultrasonography in patients with RAP? As noted previously, if the history and abdominal and rectal examinations are normal, a plain film is not useful. Several studies have

evaluated ultrasound as a screening test (i.e., not used to confirm a suspicion of an organic process). In one retrospective study of 65 children with typical RAP, 12% had abnormal ultrasound studies but only four patients had findings that might explain the pain. These findings included mild unilateral UPJ obstruction, mild pelvocaliectasis, and in one patient a 1-cm loss of renal parenchymal tissue. The patient with obstruction did not have symptoms during a diuretic renal scan. The authors concluded that the findings were not related to the RAP in these patients, but they produced anxiety that worsened symptoms! Whereas ultrasound may be quite valuable in confirming certain disorders, such as pancreatitis or gallbladder disease, it is not a true screening test and should be reserved for patients with clues to a specific disorder.

Further use of laboratory procedures at this point in the evaluation is recommended only to pursue suspected organic disorders (peptic ulcer disease, Crohn disease, etc.) and often warrants consultation with a subspecialty colleague in pediatric gastroenterology. Before the family may be reassured, the physician must be assured that the child has typical RAP. Failure to complete this process at the onset leads to the cycle of doing "one more test" that might yield the "true" diagnosis and endless doctor shopping, which often happens in the evaluation of RAP.

In the child with typical abdominal pain by history, examination, and screening testing, the investigation should cease and treatment should begin. It is most important to convince the parents that further testing is not necessary. A helpful approach is to discuss RAP as a known entity that has been well studied, for example, in the long-term follow-up study by the Mayo Clinic. Acknowledgment that the pain is real is critical for parental acceptance. Real pain does not necessarily mean that surgery or medication is necessary. We often use the example of recurrent headache, which most parents understand as a real pain that requires a treatment plan. In fact, parents should be told that an overly zealous diagnostic or therapeutic approach may actually harm their child. Acceptance of the pain and a return to normal activities, especially school, is the first and most crucial part of the treatment. Reassurance with close follow-up by telephone and scheduled office visits is important. Additional parts of the plan may include dietary interventions to aid constipation, a more regular schedule for meals, and time for bowel movements. It is important to tell the child directly that the pain is real, but that it will improve with time. The school should be an ally of the physician and parents in helping the child. Instead of a daily phone call to bring the child home, for example, the school nurse may allow a brief respite period and then a return to class. The parents may try the same approach at home, essentially a "time-out" with encouragement to return to activity.

Occasionally the physician may uncover a family or situation in which RAP is only one small part of a major family disruption. In this situation, consultation with a psychiatrist may be necessary. A parent may require major help before the child's pain can be treated. Examples are depression or somatization disorder in a close family member.

SUMMARY

RAP is a frequent and vexing complaint, usually affecting children between 5 and 15 years of age, peaking in incidence in 9-year-old girls. Despite numerous studies, the cause remains obscure and largely nonorganic. At most, 5% to 10% of children are found to have a specific diagnosis. Both uncontrolled and controlled studies support the relationship of RAP to familial, social, and personal characteristics of the patients, although specific predictors are lacking. The search for organic disorders should be specific and not random, using clues from a careful history and physical examination. On the other hand, typical RAP is not a diagnosis of exclusion. Few tests except those suggested for screening should be necessary in the typical patient. By limiting extensive investigation to those patients who do not have classic RAP, a large group of children can be spared needless and expensive testing. It is hoped that this type of approach will improve the long-term outlook of this disorder.

ILLUSTRATIVE CASES

Case 1. R.L. is a 14-year-old girl first seen with intermittent abdominal pain lasting for 3 months. Onset of symptoms accompanied fever and pneumonia in the left lower lobe. After this improved, she continued to complain of upper abdominal pain in the epigastric area several times per week lasting for about an hour. Evaluation 1 month into her illness revealed mildly elevated transaminase values, and detailed investigation procedures, including hepatitis screening, hepatic and gallbladder ultrasound, ceruloplasmin, 24-hour urine copper, alpha₁-antitrypsin level, and markers for chronic active hepatitis, were normal. Hepatic enzymes returned to normal. She developed vague leg pain and missed school excessively. Family history revealed irritable bowel disease in the mother. Both parents were anxious. Office examination was entirely normal. Repeat liver function testing was completely normal.

This adolescent had mild transaminase elevation but a clinical history more suggestive of typical RAP. She was followed-up with office visits and telephone calls and slowly returned to school, despite occasional episodes of pain with rare emesis. Subsequently a second rise in hepatic enzymes led to repeat abdominal ultrasound that revealed numerous gallstones. She has remained asymptomatic since surgical therapy. Review of the original ultrasound confirmed the normal findings at the time.

This case illustrates the difficulty of establishing a typical personality for children with RAP. All other features of the illness suggested a nonorganic problem, but the "hepatitis" was troublesome and led to repeat investigation. The physician must keep an open mind in difficult clinical situations, but the initial decision to follow the patient and send her back to school was, we believe, good clinical judgment. The recurrence of hepatic enzyme elevation was the clue that led to the correct diagnosis.

Case 2. K.B. was examined for the first time at age 8 years with complaints of stomach pain, headaches, and dizzy spells. Her abdominal pain began 2 years earlier, was epigastric, lasted for several hours, and was unrelated to any activity. During the pain episodes she felt light-headed and weak, complained of leg pain, and appeared pale. The pain waxed and waned in frequency from daily to several times per week. She missed school frequently because of pain, about 2 weeks each semester, but continued to do well academically. Her appetite and growth were normal, as were bowel movements.

Review of systems was positive for nonspecific headaches and difficulty falling asleep. She had occasional hyperventilation episodes and frequent low-grade fevers.

Family and social histories were very complicated and included a recent divorce, financial trouble, and a pregnancy for the biologic father's new wife. A grandfather had peptic ulcer disease, and the mother was seeing a psychiatrist for panic attacks.

Physical examination was normal with growth at the 50th percentile. Screening laboratory tests were all normal.

This child is fairly typical of many children with RAP; she has many stresses with significant findings in the family and social histories. In addition she has other vague complaints, misses school frequently, yet is healthy on examination. She did not appear depressed, but the diagnosis was considered. Her mother suspected that the pain was related to life events and, with reassurance and support, the child improved steadily.

Case 3. E.D. is a 10-year-old boy first seen with a 9-month history of episodic abdominal pain and emesis. Pain was sudden in onset and epigastric. It lasted for several days and was accompanied by emesis of gastric contents. During a recent admission to his local hospital, plain abdominal x-ray studies, upper gastrointestinal series, and abdominal ultrasound were normal, as were a complete blood count, electrolytes, urinalysis, sedimentation rate, serum amylase levels, liver function tests, and stool tests for occult blood.

Family history was positive for peptic ulcer disease in the father and grandfather. Social history was not remarkable. The patient had difficulty getting back to school after episodes and usually missed about 1 week each time. There was some mild weight loss during episodes, but this was quickly regained. Physical examination was normal. Later laboratory evaluation after the recent hospitalization revealed a mildly elevated sedimentation rate of 41 mm/hr, which rapidly returned to normal.

E.D.'s normal evaluation and his difficulty going back to school were reassuring that this was typical RAP. He really did not fit the usual stereotype in personality and ancillary complaints. The physician elected to follow his case. Endoscopy was considered, but the lengthy stretches between episodes made peptic ulcer disease unlikely. He *slowly improved and completed the school year. During a subsequent severe episode, he had both epigastric and shoulder pain for the first time and a mildy tender abdomen. Routine labwork was once again essentially normal except for a slightly elevated amylase level (212 IU). Lipase, however was strikingly elevated at >24,000 IU! He required long-term management for pancreatitis, including pancreatectomy. He is now free of pain but requires insulin therapy.*

This case, as does Case 1, illustrates the occasional subtle presentation of organic causes of abdominal pain. Review of all studies failed to demonstrate abnormalities of the pancreas, although there was no record of a previous lipase value. With the exception of some unwillingness to return to school, this boy evidenced no difficulties. He had a solid family and related well to peers and adults. Careful follow-up was the key. Parents acted as allies; they were willing to push him back to regular activity when he felt better. They, like the physicians, were willing to tolerate uncertainty for a time.

ANNOTATED BIBLIOGRAPHY

Apley J: *The child with abdominal pain,* ed 2, Oxford, 1975, Blackwell Scientific.

This text provides an excellent overview of RAP, including definition, epidemiology, and a survey of 1000 school children. Although the medical investigations are "dated" by today's standards, the information provides a sound background for an understanding of the problem.

Levine MD, Rappaport LA: Recurrent abdominal pain in school children: the loneliness of the long-distance physician, *Pediatr Clin North Am* 31:969-991, 1984.

The approach to pathogenesis developed in this article is perhaps the most useful one for the practicing physician. A combination of factors, including genetic predisposition, lifestyle, personality, and organic factors (such as constipation), may all play a role in RAP. This model allows the physician to develop an individual therapeutic approach.

Stickler GB, Murphy DB: Recurrent abdominal pain, *Am J Dis Child* 133:486-489, 1979.

This is the most thorough long-term follow-up of children with RAP. The minimum review period is 5 years, and many of the patients are reviewed 10 years after their visit to the Mayo Clinic. The paucity of organic disease is reassuring to physicians. This information can be shared with parents after the initial history and physical examination.

BIBLIOGRAPHY

Apley J: The child with abdominal pain, *Pediatr Clin North Am* 14:63-72, 1967.

Barr RG: Recurrent abdominal pain. In: Levine MD, Carey WP, Crocker AC, Gross RT, eds: *Developmental-behavioral pediatrics,* Philadelphia, 1983, WB Saunders.

Barr RG, Levine MD, Watkins JB: Recurrent abdominal pain of childhood due to lactose intolerance: a prospective study, *N Engl J Med* 300:1449-1452, 1979.

Byrne WJ, Arnold WC, Stannard MW, Redman JF: Ureteropelvic junction obstruction presenting with recurrent abdominal pain: diagnosis by ultrasound, *Pediatrics* 76:934-937, 1985.

Chong SKF, Lou Q, Asnicar MA, et al: *Helicobacter pylori* infection in recurrent abdominal pain in childhood: comparison of diagnostic tests and therapy, *Pediatrics* 96:211-215, 1995.

Davidson M: Recurrent abdominal pain: look to dyskinesia as the culprit, *Contemp Pediatr* 3:16-42, 1986.

Gartner JC, Jr.: Recurrent abdominal pain: who needs a workup? *Contemp Pediatr* 6:62-82, 1989.

Green M, Solnit AJ: Reactions to the threatened loss of a child: a vulnerable child syndrome, *Pediatrics* 34:58-66, 1964.

Holcomb GW, Holcomb GW III: Cholelithiasis in infants, children, and adolescents, *Pediatr Rev* 11:268-274, 1990.

Hyams JS: A simple explanation for chronic abdominal distress, *Contemp Pediatr* 8:88-104, 1991.

Liebman WM: Recurrent abdominal pain in children: a retrospective survey of 119 patients, *Clin Pediatr* 17:149-153, 1978.

Macarthur C, Saunders N, Feldman W: *Helicobacter pylori,* gastroduodenal disease, and recurrent abdominal pain in children, *JAMA* 273:729-734, 1995.

McCann J, Voris J, Simon M: Genital injuries resulting from sexual abuse: a longitudinal study, *Pediatrics* 89:307-317, 1992.

Oberlander TF, Rappaport LA: Recurrent abdominal pain during childhood, *Pediatr Rev* 8:313-319, 1993.

Raymer D, Weininger O, Hamilton JR: Psychological problems in children with abdominal pain, *Lancet* 1:439-440, 1984.

Rockney RM, McQuade WH, Days AL: The plain abdominal roentgenogram in the management of encopresis, *Arch Pediatr Adoles Med* 149:623-627, 1995.

Routh DK, Ernst AR: Somatization disorder in relatives of children and adolescents with functional abdominal pain, *J Pediatr Psychol* 9:427-437, 1984.

Schmitt BD: School phobia—the great imitator: a pediatrician's viewpoint, *Pediatrics* 48:433-441, 1971.

Shanon A, Martin DJ, Feldman W: Ultrasonographic studies in the management of recurrent abdominal pain, *Pediatrics* 86:35-38, 1990.

Wald A, Chandra R, Fisher SE, et al: Lactose malabsorption in recurrent abdominal pain of childhood, *J Pediatr* 100:65-68, 1982.

2

Back Pain

SARA C. McINTIRE

 ## Key Points

- Back pain in pediatric patients is uncommon and is often associated with serious organic pathology.

- Back pain associated with neurologic symptoms or signs requires immediate investigation.

- Painful scoliosis usually signifies an underlying structural, neoplastic, or inflammatory process.

*B*ack pain in infancy, childhood, and adolescence is uncommon and important to address because of the prospect of serious organic pathology. Precise data on the incidence and causes of back pain are lacking. However, acute or chronic back pain in a child of any age demands prompt evaluation for organic causes; back pain associated with neurologic symptoms or signs requires immediate investigation. Unlike the adult population, pediatric patients rarely experience back pain as a result of psychologic causes, such as conversion disorders. This chapter concerns the initial clinical, laboratory, and radiologic evaluation of patients with back pain by primary care physicians. Consultation with colleagues from orthopedics, neurology, neurosurgery, and radiology is essential in the diagnosis and treatment of many disorders that cause back pain.

Pathophysiology

A comprehensive review of the anatomy of the spine and its associated elements is beyond the scope of this chapter, and the reader is referred to the references. However, there are some key general principles to consider when evaluating the patient with back pain and a potential disorder of the spinal column:

1. Serious causes of back pain, such as spinal cord tumors, may be associated with only minimal neurologic symptoms and mild pain.

2. Painful scoliosis usually implies a structural, neoplastic, or inflammatory process as the underlying mechanism. Juvenile idiopathic scoliosis in general is not painful.

3. Spinal deformities caused by poor posture alone (i.e., kyphosis or lordosis) usually are not painful; anything other than mild aching or discomfort with postural deformities, typically experienced after long periods of activity, indicates organic disease.

4. The immature spine is more flexible than the adult spine, thus extremes of bending lead to overuse injuries rather than fractures.

5. A history of a minor injury to the neck or back followed by disproportionate symptoms or signs may indicate the presence of a significant structural abnormality or mass lesion.

6. Psychogenic origin of back pain in children occurs but is uncommon and is a diagnosis of exclusion.

Literature Survey

Many major pediatrics textbooks review common disorders associated with back pain but lack an inclusive approach to the symptom of back pain. Textbooks in pediatric orthopedics are more helpful, offering extensive reviews of back pain that emphasize structural and traumatic causes. However, for the busy pediatrician or family practitioner whose office library does not include subspecialty literature, a few key reviews of back pain in pediatric patients are truly useful. These reviews emphasize the significant proportion of patients with organic disease and the importance of early laboratory and radiographic evaluation. Low back pain (LBP) without gross structural disease, which is very common in adults, now receives more attention in the pediatric literature and is an important area of knowledge for the physician who sees adolescents. Finally, sports-related back injuries are a significant cause of LBP in adolescents.

BOX 2-1

Differential Diagnosis of Back Pain

Structural
Spondylolysis
Spondylolisthesis
Scheuermann disease
Scoliosis
Diastematomyelia
Tethered cord

Trauma
Low back pain
Intervertebral disk herniation
Fractures: compression, apophyseal ring

Infectious or Parainfectious
Osteomyelitis
Tuberculous spondylitis
Epidural abscess
Diskitis
Transverse myelitis

Inflammation
Juvenile ankylosing spondylitis
Reiter syndrome
Disk space calcification

Mass Lesions
Bone tumors
Osteoid osteoma
Benign osteoblastoma
Aneurysmal bone cyst
Eosinophilic granuloma
Ewing sarcoma
Neuroblastoma
Leukemia or lymphoma

Intraspinal tumors
Neurenteric cysts
AVM
Lipomas, dermoid cysts
Arachnoid cyst
Gliomas

Mass Lesions—cont'd
Intraspinal tumors—cont'd
Neurofibroma
Teratoma

Systemic or Metabolic
Hemolytic anemia
Storage diseases
Osteoporosis

Referred Pain
Pneumonia
Appendicitis
Pancreatitis
Cholecystitis
Pyelonephritis
UPJ obstruction
Psoas abscess
Endometriosis
Hydrometrocolpos

Psychogenic

AVM, Arteriovenous malformation; *UPJ*, ureteropelvic junction.

Differential Diagnosis

Although the general pediatric literature emphasizes a few major causes of back pain, an expanded differential diagnosis is offered to inform pediatricians and family practitioners about common and uncommon causes (Box 2-1). The basic etiologic categories are structural, trauma, infectious or parainfectious, inflammatory, mass lesions, metabolic, referred pain, and psychogenic.

Structural

Spondylolysis

Spondylolysis is a fracture of the pars interarticularis of the vertebral arch that may be unilateral or bilateral. The location of the defect is typically in the lumbar spine but occasionally occurs in the thoracic region. It is believed to be the result of repetitive trauma. It occurs primarily in older children and adolescents. Female gymnasts in particular may be at high risk for this lesion. In a recent paper by Micheli and Wood, spondylolysis was the most common cause of back pain in adolescent athletes.

The onset of the pain may be acute in association with a discrete trauma, such as a fall onto the buttocks, or may arise gradually in the context of repetitive flexion-extension movements, such as in gymnastics, football, or rowing. Patients describe an aching pain over the lower spine that is aggra-

vated by movement and relieved by rest. The pain may radiate into the buttocks and posterior thighs.

The physical examination may disclose exaggeration or loss of the normal lumbar lordosis. Palpation of the lower paraspinous area often reveals tenderness and mild muscle spasm. Forward and lateral flexion and extension may be limited by pain. Tightness of the hamstring muscles limits forward flexion of the hips. Scoliosis may be present in the acutely symptomatic patient as well. The neurologic examination, which must be thorough, is normal unless there is an associated lesion, such as a herniated disk.

Plain radiographs in the anteroposterior, lateral, and oblique views demonstrate the defect if it is large. However, if the defect is small, radiographs may be normal. In this case a bone scan is helpful in localizing the site of the pain but is not specific for spondylolysis. A newer technique, single photon emission computed tomographic (SPECT) bone scintigraphy, is more specific for spondylolysis than conventional radionuclide imaging. More importantly, SPECT imaging identifies defects before they are evident on plain films and permits exclusion of spondylolysis as the source of pain in a symptomatic patient with an incidental defect found on plain radiographs.

Spondylolisthesis

Spondylolisthesis is the forward slippage of one vertebral body upon another, often in the presence of spondylolysis.

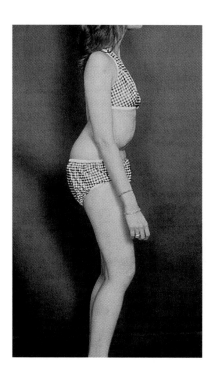

FIG. 2-1 Spondyloptosis (severe spondylolisthesis) in a 16-year-old girl. In the lateral view the torso is thrust forward, the buttocks are flattened, and there are flexion deformities of the hips and knees.

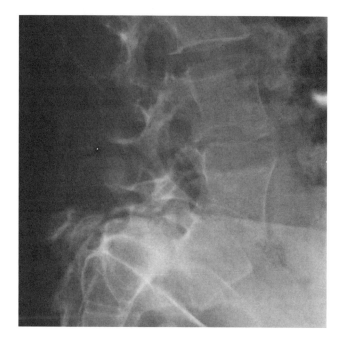

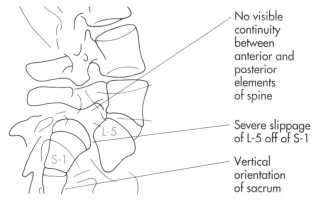

No visible continuity between anterior and posterior elements of spine

Severe slippage of L-5 off of S-1

Vertical orientation of sacrum

FIG. 2-2 Spondyloptosis in a 16-year-old girl. The L5 vertebra has completely translocated off the sacrum because of a congenital insufficiency of the posterior elements. The lumbar spine has essentially migrated anteriorly and into the pelvis.

The usual pattern is slippage of the L5 vertebral body upon S1. As expected, this disorder affects older children and adolescents and occurs during activities with repetitive flexion-extension movements.

Patients may initially complain of abnormal posture, either increased or absent lumbar lordosis. When present, the back pain is dull, aching, brought on by motion, and relieved by rest. The pain may radiate into the sacroiliac joints or lower extremities, and paresthesias may occur from sciatic nerve traction. Other neurologic symptoms are missing in isolated spondylolisthesis, and their presence signifies another lesion.

Visual inspection of the patient with spondylolisthesis reveals increased (Fig. 2-1) or absent lumbar lordosis. Palpation may uncover a shelf (or "step-off") of the lumbar spine; pressure over the spinous processes of the lower lumbar spine elicits tenderness. Impaired forward flexion and hamstring tightness may be discernible as well. In isolated spondylolisthesis the neurologic examination is unremarkable.

Anteroposterior and lateral radiographs are the imaging studies of choice to confirm the diagnosis of spondylolisthesis. Forward slippage of the L5 upon the S1 vertebral body is the usual finding in the lateral projection (Fig. 2-2).

Scheuermann Disease

Back pain is a frequent complaint in patients with Scheuermann disease. It is defined as a fixed kyphotic deformity characterized radiographically by vertebral endplate irregularities, Schmorl nodes, and wedging of at least three adjacent vertebrae. Although the exact cause of this disease is unknown, it is recognized as a disorder with a hereditary component that begins in adolescence and progresses until the skeleton is mature. Patients have kyphosis or kyphoscoliosis, usually of the thoracic spine, that does not correct with changes in posture. The pain is worsened by activity and may be greatest at the apex of the deformity. The deformity is best appreciated by viewing the patient from the side. Maximal hyperextension of the back reveals the fixed nature of the deformity and distinguishes the patient with Scheuermann disease from the patient with poor posture alone. Anteroposterior and lateral radiographs are diagnostic of this condition (Fig. 2-3).

Scoliosis

Although idiopathic juvenile scoliosis may be associated with dull or aching discomfort, primarily after long periods of activity, the acute onset of scoliosis with any degree of pain or progressive scoliosis with more than mild pain is an indication for a prompt evaluation for structural disorders. Disor-

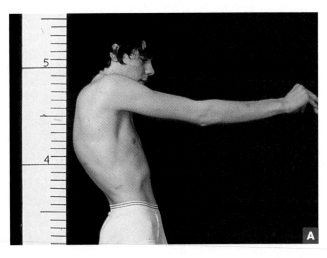

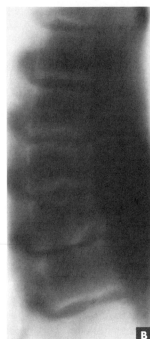

FIG. 2-3   Moderate thoracic kyphosis secondary to Scheuermann disease. *A,* The patient is attempting to correct the deformity, but because of its fixed nature, he cannot and must compensate for this with an increased lumbar lordosis. *B,* This tomographic cut demonstrates the anterior wedging of three consecutive vertebral bodies and clearly shows the associated erosion of the vertebral endplates and Schmorl nodes.

BOX 2-2

Painful Scoliosis: Differential Diagnosis

Structural
Spondylolysis
Spondylolisthesis
Intraspinal anomalies

Infectious
Osteomyelitis
Tuberculous spondylitis
Diskitis

Trauma
Low back pain
Disk herniation

Mass Lesions
Osteoid osteoma
Osteoblastoma

Referred Pain
Appendicitis
Pneumonia
Pyelonephritis
Psoas abscess
Ureteropelvic junction
   obstruction

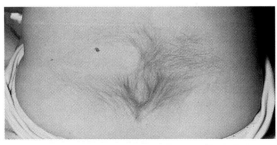

FIG. 2-4   Occult spinal dysraphism. Note hairy patch over the lumbar region, here associated with diastematomyelia. (Courtesy Dr. Michael J. Painter, Pittsburgh.)

ders associated with painful scoliosis, such as infection, disk herniation, spondylolysis or spondylolisthesis, intraspinal anomalies, malignant spinal cord tumors, and osteoid osteoma, are discussed elsewhere in the chapter (Box 2-2).

Diastematomyelia

Diastematomyelia is a rare congenital malformation of the spinal cord in which the cord is fully or partially divided by a septum or spur that tethers the cord (see following section); other associated malformations include spina bifida and hemivertebrae. It usually involves the lumbar spine, and it is more common in girls than in boys. The cause is unknown.

This is a rare cause of back pain and usually presents with other more prominent neurologic signs and symptoms. The presence of midline cutaneous defects of the lower spine at birth are clues to the existence of this and other congenital spinal lesions (Fig. 2-4). In the absence of such defects this condition is also suspected in the presence of congenital scoliosis, delayed onset of walking, gait abnormalities, muscle involvement of the lower limbs, foot deformities, and sphincter dysfunction. However, on rare occasions, neurologic function may be preserved for years, until school-age or adolescence; the gradual and insidious development of subtle signs of involvement, particularly weakness of the legs and rectal or urinary sphincter dysfunction, may go unnoticed until function is more obviously compromised. Clearly, conditions such as this mandate a meticulous history and detailed neurologic examination in children with complaints of mild but persistent back pain.

The initial evaluation includes anteroposterior and lateral radiographs of the spine, which identify a bony spur or septum in some cases and associated bony abnormalities, such as spina bifida or hemivertebrae. Magnetic resonance imaging (MRI) is necessary to delineate the entire defect in all patients with known or suspected diastematomyelia.

Tethered Cord

A tethered cord exists when there is restriction of movement of the distal end of the spinal cord, or cauda equina. In addition to diastematomyelia, a number of other lesions may produce a tethered cord, such as lipomyelomeningoceles, lipomas of the filum terminale, fibrous bands, anomalous posterior spinal nerve roots, and adhesions after surgical repair of these conditions. Progressive neurologic dysfunction of the lower extremities, bowel, and bladder result when tethering is untreated.

Back pain may occur secondary to a tethered cord, regardless of the causative anomaly. The onset or worsening of back pain during exercise or a period of rapid growth is a common feature of patients with an occult tethered cord. The pain may radiate into the legs, mimicking disk herniation. However, there are often other symptoms or signs that are more conspicuous, such as cutaneous lesions of the lower back and progressive orthopedic foot deformities. Subtle changes in muscle bulk and strength make the occult causes of a tethered cord difficult to detect. MRI is the imaging study of choice for the initial diagnosis of a tethered cord. Plain radiographs are obtained for information regarding associated bony abnormalities.

Trauma

This section pertains to the evaluation of patients physicians might expect to see in the office but does not address those patients with back pain caused by a car accident or other major trauma.

Low Back Pain

Lumbar low back pain (LBP) related to mechanical strain without gross structural change (i.e., spondylolysis or spondylolisthesis, tumors, disk herniation, anomalies) is a condition that affects adolescents, especially those involved in weight lifting and athletic activities such as gymnastics. The pain is presumably the result of microscopic trauma from overuse. Although the differential diagnosis of the symptom of LBP includes most of the disorders discussed in this chapter, in some patients, the term *low back pain* may be properly used as a diagnosis, provided all other ailments have been excluded in an appropriate manner.

LBP is extremely common in adults and receives a great deal of attention in the medical literature. However, this diagnosis is absent from most general pediatric references until the discussion of adolescence, and the incidence is low even in this age group. However, in Olsen and others' recent prospective survey of more than 1200 adolescents ages 11 to 17 years, 30% reported that they had experienced the symptom of LBP; one third of those patients limited activity as a result of the pain. This study signifies a more widespread problem, with greater morbidity in the pediatric population than the general literature indicates.

The evaluation of the adolescent with LBP begins with a careful history of the onset of the complaint, noting whether it was related to lifting, twisting, work, or athletic activity. Pain related to muscular strain or overuse is usually dull, aching, of mild to moderate intensity, worse with activity, and corrected with rest. Constitutional and neurologic symptoms are absent. The examination, which must be thorough, generally reveals limited range of lumbar spinal motion, paraspinous muscle spasm and tenderness, and a completely normal neurologic examination.

If the history and physical examination are consistent with LBP and there are no features suggestive of serious pathology, radiologic studies may be deferred while symptomatic measures, such as rest and analgesics, are initiated. Atypical features, such as weakness, sensory loss, or bladder dysfunction, imply a more serious cause and demand prompt radiologic investigation.

Intervertebral Disk Herniation

Intervertebral disk herniation is a rare lesion in young children and is diagnosed more often in adolescents. As in adults, it typically occurs in the lumbar spine, although cervical disk herniation has been reported as a complication of antecedent intervertebral disk calcification (an inflammatory disorder of unknown etiology). Some authors have noted a high incidence of associated congenital structural anomalies. LBP or ache, with or without radiation into the legs, is the principal symptom. The pain improves with rest and is exacerbated by sneezing, coughing, passing of stools, and exercising. Inquiry regarding neurologic symptoms, such as numbness and weakness, is indispensable, but these symptoms are generally absent.

On examination, patients with a symptomatic disk herniation walk slowly to avoid pain or with a stiff gait because of hamstring spasm. The normal lumbar curve may be flattened. Acute scoliosis often occurs and may be quite pronounced because of the greater flexibility of the pediatric spine (Fig. 2-5). Diffuse tenderness over the lumbar spine, paraspinous muscle spasm, and pain along the sciatic nerve may be elicited by palpation. Mobility of lumbar flexion may be limited by pain or muscle spasm. The straight-leg raising sign is usually positive and correlates well with disk herniation. Muscle bulk and strength, deep tendon reflexes, sensation, and sphincter function must be assessed; abnormal

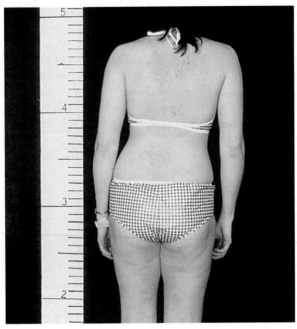

FIG. 2-5 Herniated intervertebral disk. Diskogenic scoliosis in a 16-year-old girl with a herniated disk at L4-5. The trunk is shifted away from the affected side. The normal lumbar lordosis is absent, and spinal motion is severely limited.

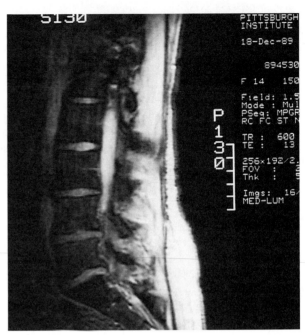

FIG. 2-6 On this sagittal MRI view, the L4-5 disk bulges posteriorly, compressing the cauda equina. (Courtesy the Department of Pediatric Radiology, Children's Hospital of Pittsburgh.)

findings are highly significant, but their absence does not exclude disk herniation.

Radiographic studies indicated in cases of suspected disk herniation include plain anteroposterior and lateral radiographs and another study, such as computed tomography (CT) or magnetic resonance imaging (MRI). Plain films are usually normal in adolescents with disk herniation because the age-related changes associated with herniation in adults are absent. MRI offers the advantages of clear delineation of the location and size of the herniation and differentiation of this disk disease from mass lesions (Fig. 2-6).

Lumbar Apophyseal Ring Fracture

In this disorder there are both an avulsion (fracture) of the posterior portion of the lumbar apophysis and partial disk herniation posteriorly into the spinal canal. Lumbar apophyseal ring fracture is an uncommon cause of LBP but an important one to consider in adolescent athletes, especially gymnasts and weight lifters. Importantly this lesion may be overlooked in the presence of a coexistent and more common lesion, such as Scheuermann disease, or confused with an isolated intervertebral disk herniation.

Patients complain of LBP, often associated with recent trauma, but in all other regards the history and physical examination are nearly identical to those of a patient with a herniated intervertebral disk. This is a vital injury to recognize because it may lead to spinal canal stenosis if the avulsed fragment is not excised.

Anteroposterior and lateral radiographs of the spine should be obtained to locate the avulsed fragment of bone. However, the films may not reveal this finding, in which case a CT scan is indicated to survey for the fragment and the degree of disk herniation.

Compression Fractures

Compression fractures of the vertebral bodies of the spine are highly unusual in normal children and adolescents. On rare occasions, acute trauma produces such fractures in pediatric patients with no risk factors for increased bone fragility. However, compression fractures occur spontaneously or after minor trauma in children with conditions such as osteoporosis (of any etiology), chronic hemolytic anemia, osteogenesis imperfecta, eosinophilic granuloma of bone, primary or metastatic malignancies, vertebral osteomyelitis, and chronic steroid use. Patients with symptomatic compression fractures experience localized or diffuse back pain, depending on the number of vertebral bodies involved. Paraspinous muscle spasm and tenderness to palpation are evident on examination.

Plain radiographs detect compression fractures and survey for evidence of generalized osteoporosis.

Infectious or Parainfectious

The vertebrae and intervertebral disks may be primarily infected with specific organisms, as in bacterial osteomyelitis, or may be affected secondarily after a viral illness, as in transverse myelitis.

Pyogenic Osteomyelitis

Pyogenic infection of the vertebral bodies of the spine is rare in pediatric patients. In the older child or adolescent with acute onset of fever and well-localized back pain, the diagnosis is easily suspected and investigated. However, the infant or very young child may not localize pain precisely enough to suggest osteomyelitis, and in any age patient, indolent infections may cause only chronic vague symptoms without impressive fever or well-localized pain. In a retrospective review by Correa and others, of eight children with vertebral osteomyelitis, one third had symptoms consistent with bone infection for 3 or more weeks before diagnosis.

The cardinal symptoms of vertebral osteomyelitis are neck or back pain and stiffness. Fever, albeit an important and helpful sign of an inflammatory process, is absent in up to 50% of patients. In patients with cervical spine involvement, prominent complaints of sore throat, difficulty swallowing, and pain upon swallowing may obscure associated features, such as neck pain, paraspinous muscle spasm, or limitation of neck motion. A painful torticollis may accompany cervical spine infection just as a painful scoliosis may attend infection of the thoracic or lumbar spine.

Patients may complain of relatively acute or chronic back pain. The pain may be dull or aching and is usually moderate to severe. Diffuse abdominal pain is a common and sometimes misleading complaint. Radicular pain from nerve root compression leads to hip and leg pain. Infants may cry with positional changes or diapering, and young children may refuse to sit or walk to guard against pain. Older children and adolescents may attempt to walk but avoid sudden, rapid, jarring, bending, or twisting motions. Although worsened by motion, the pain generally is not completely relieved by rest and frequently wakes patients from sleep. Even older children and adolescents may or may not localize the pain when asked where their back hurts.

Risk factors for osteomyelitis in children include trauma, varicella infection, sickle cell anemia, and immunosuppression, but most cases arise from hematogenous spread of bacteria in otherwise healthy children. The usual organism is *Staphylococcus aureus,* followed by group A streptococci. Infection with *Salmonella* species is rare but is an appropriate concern in patients with sickle cell anemia and osteomyelitis of any bone. *Aspergillus* osteomyelitis occurs in children with acquired or congenital immunodeficiencies, such as AIDS or chronic granulomatous disease. *Brucella* species and *Bartonella henselae* (the agent of cat-scratch disease) are unusual but well described as causes of pediatric spinal osteomyelitis.

On physical examination, patients may have fever and generally appear ill. Localized back tenderness is usually present and may be associated with stiffness, decreased range of spinal motion, paraspinous muscle spasm, scoliosis,

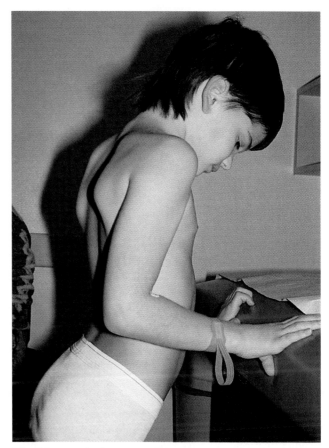

FIG. 2-7 Vertebral osteomyelitis. This 10-year-old boy had a 2-week history of intermittent fever, malaise, and steadily worsening lower back and left hip pain, exacerbated by movement. He had an exaggerated lumbar lordosis and extreme limitation of flexion both when standing and sitting. The straight-leg raising test also accentuated his pain.

and a positive straight-leg raising test (Fig. 2-7). A positive Gowers sign generally reflects pain rather than true muscular weakness. Although neurologic impairment can occur in pyogenic vertebral osteomyelitis, rapid emergence of abnormal function raises the possibility of an epidural abscess.

Patients with suspected osteomyelitis should have a complete blood count (CBC), erythrocyte sedimentation rate (ESR), and blood cultures drawn before initiation of antimicrobial therapy. A purified protein derivative tuberculin test (PPD) and chest radiograph are indicated if tuberculosis is a possibility. Plain anteroposterior and lateral radiographs of the spine may be normal early in the course of the illness but should not dissuade the physician from pursuing the diagnosis of osteomyelitis. When present, disk space narrowing and erosion of vertebral endplates are hallmarks of vertebral osteomyelitis on plain radiographs. A bone scan is usually positive and is a useful test for localization of the infection (Fig. 2-8). MRI is an extremely sensitive study for the detection of osteomyelitis. Consultation with colleagues from radiology

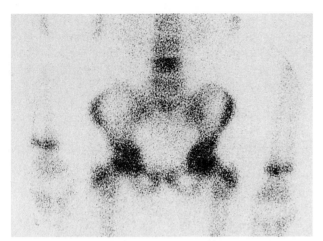

FIG. 2-8   Vertebral osteomyelitis. Bone scan of patient in Fig. 2-7 revealed selectively increased uptake in the L4 vertebral body. (Courtesy the Department of Pediatric Radiology, Children's Hospital of Pittsburgh.)

and orthopedic surgery is advisable when selecting studies and methods to recover material for appropriate cultures, stains, and pathologic review.

Sacroiliac Joint Infection

The sacroiliac joint is another site of infection in older children that can cause back pain, although pyogenic infection is rare in pediatric patients. Pelvic trauma may be a risk factor in a small number of cases. A typical presentation is of an acute or subacute illness with fever, LBP, hip and sacroiliac joint pain, and limp or refusal to bear weight. On examination, patients have fever, tenderness localized to the involved joint, and a positive straight-leg raising test. A FABERE (*f*lexion, *ab*duction, *e*xternal *r*otation, and *e*xtension) maneuver of the hip is positive but is not specific for sacroiliac joint infection.

Pertinent laboratory studies include a CBC, ESR, and blood cultures. Plain radiographs of the sacroiliac joints are normal early in the course of the illness and demonstrate sclerosis and lytic areas only later. Bone scans are positive early in the illness and thus are extremely valuable in early diagnosis. Identification of the bacterial cause is essential to determine therapy; therefore consultation with an orthopedic surgeon for joint aspiration and/or drainage is appropriate.

Tuberculous Spondylitis

Given the recent rise in primary pulmonary tuberculosis cases in the United States, it is reasonable to anticipate a concomitant increase in the incidence of tuberculous spondylitis, once a rare disorder. Therefore pediatricians and family practitioners must consider this disease in children with evidence of inflammation and back pain, especially if the pain is subacute or chronic.

Bone disease caused by *Mycobacterium tuberculosis* most commonly involves the vertebral bodies of the spine and fol-

lows the initial lung disease, if untreated, by lymphohematogenous spread. Dissemination of the tubercle bacilli may be silent, without evidence of spondylitis or other foci of disease appearing until months to years after the primary pulmonary infection. Because the blood supply to bone is greatest in young children, they are at greater risk for skeletal tuberculosis. Therefore a careful medical history of risk factors, exposures, and symptoms of pulmonary tuberculosis is indicated in patients with known or suspected vertebral infection. Children at high risk include immigrants from countries with a high prevalence of tuberculosis, immunocompromised children, and children who have been exposed to adults with known infectious tuberculosis or adults who have been incarcerated.

The symptoms and signs of tuberculous spondylitis include low-grade fever, back pain, pain at night that disturbs sleep, and changes in the spinal contour or mobility, depending on the portion of the spine affected. Thoracic vertebrae are the most commonly involved; it is not unusual for more than one vertebral body to be affected, eventually leading to marked kyphosis. Unilateral paraspinous muscle spasm or tenderness suggests the presence of a paravertebral abscess, which is a frequent finding in tuberculous spondylitis. Evidence of chest and visceral involvement must be sought through thorough lung and abdominal examination.

General laboratory studies and radiographs in patients with suspected tuberculous spondylitis include a CBC, ESR, urinalysis, hepatocellular enzymes, and anteroposterior and lateral views of the chest and spine. Early changes on spine films include subtle disk space narrowing and wedging of the vertebrae. These changes magnify as the disease progresses and more classic changes of gibbous deformity and severe kyphosis appear. Abdominal ultrasound, CT, or MRI can locate paravertebral abscesses. Aspiration of the abscess can be performed under CT guidance.

Although the results of these measures may strongly suggest tubercular disease, they are not diagnostic and more specific means are necessary to document disease from *M. tuberculosis* and to plan therapy. A positive Mantoux test or PPD is the definitive skin test. Interpretation of any induration measured 48 to 72 hours after the test is performed depends on the child's clinical status and history. For example, 5 mm of induration is positive in a child at high risk for tuberculosis, and greater than 15 mm of induration is a positive test even in the absence of any risk factors. Also, culture of organisms recovered from gastric aspirates, sputum, bone, and other tissues allows antimicrobial sensitivity testing, which is essential to guide therapy. Consultation with subspecialists experienced in diagnosis and management of tuberculosis is especially advisable in the era of multiple-drug–resistant organisms.

Diskitis

Diskitis is an inflammatory condition of the intervertebral disk space that usually affects the lumbar spine. Controversy exists regarding the cause of this disorder. A proportion of cases are associated with *S. aureus* infection of the disk space and adjacent bone. However, other cases have negative cultures of the disk, do not involve bone, and resolve without antimicrobial therapy. Both viral upper respiratory tract infection and trauma preceding the onset of diskitis are common, but neither is firmly established as causative. Regardless of the inciting event, necrosis of the epiphyseal endplates and disks appears to lead to the clinical syndrome of diskitis.

As noted by Wenger, different age groups have a characteristic chief complaint, typically sudden in onset. Although back pain occurs in all groups, infants and toddlers resist diaper changes and/or refuse to sit, crawl, stand, or walk; children over 3 years of age complain of abdominal pain in addition to LBP and gait changes; and older children and adolescents complain of LBP and stiffness but do not refuse to walk. The pain is milder and less localized than the severe and focal pain of vertebral osteomyelitis and epidural abscess. Low-grade fever, irritability, anorexia, and nausea are other common complaints of patients with diskitis. Because of the nonspecific nature of these symptoms, patients are regularly evaluated for other conditions before the correct diagnosis is made. Diskitis mimics more common conditions, such as urinary tract infection, appendicitis, toxic synovitis, and septic arthritis. The differential diagnosis also includes uncommon but serious causes of back pain, such as meningitis, psoas abscess, bacterial osteomyelitis, and tuberculous spondylitis.

On physical examination, patients are not toxic and the general inspection is normal. Febrile patients have temperatures less than 39°C. They are uncomfortable or inconsolable with any manipulation of the spine or hips and become calm in a prone position. The lumbar spine is tender to palpation. A Gowers sign may be evident when the patient rises from the prone position. Unlike other inflammatory or neoplastic processes of the spinal column, scoliosis is absent. Either increased or decreased lumbar lordosis is observed in older children and adolescents who will stand and walk. Decreased range of motion and tenderness of the lumbar spine, as well as paraspinous muscle spasm, are evident on palpation. Hamstring spasm, when present, limits forward flexion. The straight-leg raising test may be positive. The neurologic examination is normal, although patients with cervical or thoracic diskitis may have a positive Kernig sign.

Appropriate laboratory studies include a CBC with differential and platelets and an ESR. The white blood cell count is either normal or slightly increased, and the other hematologic parameters are normal. The ESR is elevated but generally less than 50 mm/hr. A blood culture is indicated in all febrile patients with back pain, but positive cultures are exceptional in diskitis.

Radiologic studies are essential to diagnose diskitis. Early in the disease, plain radiographs of the involved spine are normal, whereas technetium 99 bone scanning shows localization of the isotope to the intervertebral disk space. After 2 to 4 weeks, plain radiographs show characteristic changes of disk space narrowing and irregularity of vertebral margins and the bone scan becomes normal. SPECT imaging is another tool for the detection of diskitis but is not widely used for this purpose in pediatric patients. MRI is an excellent modality for imaging soft tissues of the spinal column and can distinguish diskitis from abscesses and tumors.

The most challenging issue in the evaluation of patients with suspected diskitis is determining which patients require needle aspiration of the disk space for bacterial culture and antimicrobial sensitivity testing. This issue is addressed later in this chapter.

Transverse Myelitis

Transverse myelitis is an inflammatory disorder of unknown etiology that affects the spinal cord, often after a benign viral infection in children. Other disorders associated with transverse myelitis include Lyme disease, mycoplasmal infection, spinal cord irradiation, trauma or compression by mass lesions, systemic lupus erythematosus, multiple sclerosis, and meningovascular syphilis. Regardless of the cause, asymmetric destruction of white and gray matter occurs.

Transverse myelitis is rapid in onset and progression of symptoms and signs. The constellation of acute onset of back pain, rapidly progressive lower extremity weakness, loss of sensation, and bladder or bowel dysfunction is highly suggestive of this disorder. Before making a diagnosis of transverse myelitis, however, the physician must exclude spinal epidural abscess and mass lesions of the spinal column. MRI with gadolinium enhancement and contrast myelography are the procedures of choice in this circumstance.

Epidural Abscess

Epidural abscess is another rare cause of acute back pain in pediatric patients but has devastating effects on neurologic function if not promptly diagnosed. The hallmarks of this infection include prominent constitutional symptoms (fever, malaise, headache), localized and exquisite back pain, refusal to lie prone because of pain, and abnormal neurologic function. Abnormal neurologic function ranges from paresthesias in the distal extremities to weakness, inability to walk, absent deep tendon reflexes and sensation, and impaired sphincter function. Hematogenous spread of bacteria, usually *S. aureus,* is the pathologic mechanism.

Epidural abscess is a true neurologic emergency with devastating consequences if the diagnosis is delayed. MRI with gadolinium enhancement or contrast myelography and early consultation with a neurosurgeon are imperative.

Inflammation

Inflammatory conditions unrelated to infections account for a small number of pediatric patients who have back pain. Recognition of rheumatologic conditions is especially important because of the potential for permanent joint destruction and significant extraarticular involvement.

Juvenile Ankylosing Spondylitis

Juvenile ankylosing spondylitis (JAS) is a chronic inflammatory disorder of the spine and sacroiliac joints. Onset in the second decade of life is characteristic. It is more common in boys; has important extraarticular manifestations, such as iridocyclitis and aortic insufficiency; and is usually associated with a positive test for HLA-B27.

In the older child and adolescent, chronic LBP or stiffness may be the first symptom of JAS. Sacroiliitis often presents as hip pain or sciatica that is made worse by standing on one leg. Other prominent historic features include insidious onset, a remittent course, morning stiffness, pain in the heels and ankles, lack of relief with rest, and improvement of symptoms with exercise. A family history may reveal other relatives affected with AS or other rheumatologic conditions, such as Reiter syndrome.

Early in the course of the disease the physical examination may be normal or show only a subtle loss of the normal lumbar lordotic curve, a decrease in lumbar flexion, or paraspinous muscle spasm. As the disease progresses these changes become more evident. Fever may be a part of the presentation, but the absence of an elevated temperature does not exclude JAS. Careful examination of the spine and sacroiliac joints is mandatory.

Laboratory studies should include a CBC, ESR, urinalysis, liver enzyme tests, an antinuclear antibody (ANA), and a rheumatoid factor. A positive HLA-B27 test does not alone make the diagnosis, nor is it a measure of response to therapy; thus it is not mandatory to obtain this test at the initial evaluation. Plain radiographs of the spine and sacroiliac joints should be obtained, although in most patients the films are normal early in the course of the disease. Slit-lamp examination by an experienced ophthalmologist is indicated in all patients. Consultation with a pediatric rheumatologist for confirmation of the diagnosis and management is advised.

Reiter Syndrome

In its classic form, Reiter syndrome is an illness comprised of arthritis, conjunctivitis, and urethritis, which often presents after an enteric or a venereal infection. It is included in this chapter because LBP occurs as part of the syndrome and may precede more typical symptoms. As in the adult population, in pediatrics the disease is largely confined to male patients. It is rarely seen in young children; patients are usually adolescents. HLA-B27 is present in nearly 80% of patients with Reiter syndrome but is insufficient alone to certify the diagnosis.

Difficulties in diagnosing Reiter syndrome arise because the classic triad is seldom encountered in pediatric patients. Also, patients and families may not remember the instigating infection because symptoms of Reiter syndrome usually occur weeks later; thus specific inquiry about symptoms occurring weeks to months before presentation is indispensable. Patients complain of lumbar pain and stiffness that worsens with bed rest or sitting. The spinal examination may reveal pain on palpation, limited lumbar flexion, and paraspinous muscle spasm. A search for other clinical features of Reiter syndrome is indicated if the history suggests this diagnosis. Suspicious findings include nonpurulent conjunctivitis; urethral erythema; sacroiliitis; asymmetric arthritis of the knees, elbows, and wrists; and enthesitis.

As with JAS the diagnosis of Reiter syndrome is made on clinical evidence supported by selected laboratory studies and radiologic images. Of paramount importance is the evaluation for infectious causes of Reiter syndrome, such as chlamydial infection, because therapy with antibiotics is essential.

Disk Space Calcification

Disk space calcification is a rare cause of back pain in children, and the cause is unknown. Boys are affected more often than girls. A history of trauma or an upper respiratory tract infection precedes the inflammation in many cases. The principal manifestations are neck or back pain and stiffness, torticollis, and fever, and the examination reveals tenderness to palpation over the spine and paraspinous muscle spasm. The symptoms subside spontaneously over several days to weeks with supportive care alone. Involvement of both the cervical and thoracic disk spaces with herniation into the spinal canal has been reported as a complication of this disorder. Plain radiographs reveal calcification of the intervertebral disk space. CT allows discovery of protrusion of the nucleus pulposus if present.

Mass Lesions

Benign and malignant disorders affect the bony elements of the spine, spinal cord, meninges, and nerves. Mass lesions involving these structures are rare yet essential to recognize because of the devastating consequences of delayed diagnosis and treatment. Unfortunately, delayed recognition of these lesions is common because their initial signs may be minimal. Therefore careful scrutiny of all patients with back pain, especially those with an accompanying scoliosis, is essential to detect subtle findings that prompt rapid diagnostic measures. This section emphasizes bone and intraspinal tumors.

Bone Tumors

Benign tumors of the bones of the spine include osteoid osteomas, benign osteoblastomas, aneurysmal bone cysts, and eosinophilic granulomas of bone. Primary and metastatic malignancies affect the bones of the spine as well. Ewing and osteogenic sarcomas are the most common primary vertebral tumors, and neuroblastomas, Wilms tumors, leukemias, and lymphomas may all spread to involve the spine. Common clinical features of bone tumors are back pain, nighttime back pain, pain that is not appreciably relieved by rest, and scoliosis. Malignant tumors of bone cause symptoms and signs referable to the nervous system when intraspinal spread occurs. Constitutional manifestations of fever, lassitude, weight loss, pallor, and easy bruising are clues to the diagnosis of lymphoreticular and other malignancies. However, bone and joint pain from leukemic infiltrates is well known to develop before more obvious signs of pallor and petechiae.

Osteoid osteoma is a fascinating disorder. Although the pathology of the tumor is well described, the precise cause is unknown. Back pain is the chief complaint of patients with vertebral lesions and typically occurs at night. The pain is intensified by rest, awakens patients from sleep, and responds dramatically to aspirin. Painful scoliosis is frequently present. On examination the involved area of the spine is tender to palpation and the range of spinal motion is decreased; paraspinous and hamstring muscle spasms are also present. Otherwise, patients appear well and lack constitutional symptoms.

Intraspinal Tumors

Benign and malignant intraspinal tumors present an onerous diagnostic challenge because they may cause a paucity of symptoms. Also, they often occur in young children who may be unable to articulate their complaints specifically. In the early stages, back pain may be the only indication of a tumor. Therefore careful consideration of the possibility of an intraspinal tumor is always appropriate in pediatric patients with back pain. Congenital intraspinal lesions include solid, cystic, and vascular malformations, such as lipomas, teratomas, neurenteric and dermoid cysts, and arteriovenous malformations. Arachnoid cysts are a common malformation of the meninges. Gliomas are the most common malignant intraspinal tumors. Neurofibromas are lesions of the nerve roots exiting the spinal cord. Neurofibromas are seen in patients with neurofibromatosis but only very rarely affect children. Epidermoid tumors occurring after lumbar puncture are less frequent in the era of stylet use but still occur.

Back pain caused by tumors is often poorly localized, unlike the pain of vertebral osteomyelitis. The pain is sharpened by Valsalva maneuvers—sneezing, coughing, and straining—and by back flexion. Although the pain improves with rest, nighttime pain or pain that arouses the child from sleep raises suspicions of a tumor. It is critical to inquire about other neurologic symptoms, such as weakness, sensory disturbances, bowel or bladder dysfunction, and foot deformities. On rare occasions, intermittent headache and vomiting occur when lesions cause cerebrospinal fluid obstruction.

The importance of the association of back pain and scoliosis upon physical examination cannot be overemphasized; tumors cause paraspinous muscle spasm, which in turn leads to scoliosis (or torticollis if the cervical spine is involved). Similarly, muscular atrophy and weakness, pathologic reflexes, diminished sensation, laxity of the anal sphincter, and foot deformities point to intraspinal pathology. A positive straight-leg raising test is common in patients with intraspinal tumors. Inspection of the skin overlying the back is important as well.

Plain radiographs should be obtained first in all patients with suspected mass lesions and may be diagnostic in some cases, such as aneurysmal bone cyst, or suggestive of an oc-

cult intraspinal process. On plain radiographs an osteoid osteoma appears as a radiolucent area, or nidus, surrounded by sclerotic tissue, although CT scanning may be necessary to locate nidus more precisely. Primary malignancies of bone, such as Ewing sarcoma, are apparent as vertebral collapse on plain radiographs; MRI delineates the tumorous involvement of other structures. MRI is also the study of choice for the diagnosis of intraspinal mass lesions.

Systemic or Metabolic

There are a number of systemic and metabolic diseases, such as chronic hemolytic anemia, storage diseases, and osteoporosis of any cause, that affect the spinal column in children. In general these conditions involve the vertebrae and cause back pain when compression fractures occur spontaneously or even after trivial injuries.

Chronic Hemolytic Anemia

Patients with long-standing sickle cell anemia or thalassemia are susceptible to compression fractures that may occur spontaneously or after insignificant trauma. Extramedullary hematopoiesis in the vertebral marrow spaces predisposes the bones of the spine to fractures. Plain radiographs are diagnostic of compression fractures.

Storage Diseases

Storage diseases are a heterogeneous group of disorders in which enzyme deficiencies lead to the accumulation of metabolic products. Gaucher disease is the classic storage disorder associated with painful involvement of the spine. In this rare disorder the absence of an enzyme, beta-glucocerebrosidase, leads to the accretion of glucocerebroside in the central nervous system, liver, spleen, and other reticuloendothelial tissues. Of the three forms of Gaucher disease, types 1 and 3 have pronounced skeletal involvement. Type 2, also called *acute infantile neuropathic Gaucher disease,* is fulminant, causes death in infancy, and does not involve the bones to the same extent as the others. Common manifestations of painful spinal involvement in Gaucher disease include nonspecific bone pain, acute "bone crises" mimicking acute osteomyelitis, and pathologic compression fractures.

Osteoporosis

Osteoporosis is present in a number of rare pediatric disorders and is a risk factor for back pain from compression fractures. Examples include osteogenesis imperfecta, homocystinuria, and Cushing syndrome. Idiopathic juvenile osteoporosis is characterized by the onset of profound osteoporosis in children between the ages of 8 and 15 years, leading to recurrent fractures of long bones and vertebrae. The cause is unknown, and the condition remits spontaneously after several years. A more common risk factor for osteoporosis is chronic steroid use; patients with steroid-dependent asthma or systemic lupus erythematosus, for example, are vulnerable to osteoporosis and fractures.

Referred Pain

Back pain also arises in children as a result of disorders of thoracic, abdominal, retroperitoneal, and pelvic viscera. In general, location of the pain away from the midline and other symptoms more typical of the primary illness readily distinguish these disorders from those affecting the spine and its contents. The location of the pain is particularly important to determine, and a careful review of the history and associated symptoms is essential.

Pneumonia is a well-known cause of back pain in children. Also, irritation of the diaphragm from a pleural effusion may result in shoulder pain. The diagnosis is straightforward when the pain is accompanied by fever, malaise, cough, increased pain upon inspiration, tachypnea, and typical auscultatory findings. However, patients or parents may not report cough if it is minimal, and the chest examination may be unrevealing in young children. Plain radiographs of the chest are usually diagnostic.

Appendicitis is extremely common in children and is quickly suspected in the presence of classic features, such as fever, anorexia, nausea, periumbilical pain that shifts to the right lower abdominal quadrant, and localized tenderness at McBurney's point. However, patients may complain of back or flank pain instead of abdominal pain, especially if the appendix is retrocecal. Although uncommon in children, pancreatitis and cholecystitis are frequently associated with back pain. The presence of fever, vomiting, nausea, and anterior abdominal tenderness in classic locations suggests these ailments in the patient also complaining of back pain.

Pyelonephritis is often accompanied by flank pain. Patients complain of back pain, but when asked to locate the area they point to the flank or costovertebral angle. Fever, nausea, and vomiting are prominent in renal infections but are nonspecific; unusual urinary frequency or urgency, dysuria, hematuria, and malodorous urine, when present, are more suggestive findings. Intermittent ureteropelvic junction (UPJ) obstruction presents with acute onset of flank or anterior upper abdominal pain, nausea, and vomiting that lasts several hours and then subsides gradually. Unless a careful review of symptoms is addressed and the patient is examined while ill clinically, episodic back or flank pain from UPJ obstruction may go undiagnosed because the physical examination and imaging study (in this case an abdominal ultrasound) are normal if performed when the patient is well.

The psoas muscle is another retroperitoneal structure that causes back pain when infected with pyogenic organisms. Fever, abdominal and/or hip pain, and limp or refusal to walk are the most common presenting complaints. The abdominal examination can be relatively benign in some patients. In these cases the hip pain and the gait disturbance lead to an investigation for septic arthritis or osteomyelitis before the correct diagnosis is entertained.

Finally, back pain occurs in disorders of pelvic structures. Although back pain is common in girls with dysmenorrhea, endometriosis ought to be considered in a girl with a family history of endometriosis, escalating dysmenorrhea, and moderate to severe back pain during menstruation. An imperforate hymen in postpubertal girls leads to hydrometrocolpos, which can cause severe episodic back pain. The findings of an abdominal mass and a bulging, closed hymen are diagnostic.

Psychogenic

Back pain of psychogenic origin does occur in pediatric patients but is very uncommon. Although practitioners must consider functional causes of chronic symptoms, especially in patients who are missing school, an inclusive search for organic pathology is prudent in patients with back pain. Also, preexisting psychologic disturbances may amplify complaints in patients with medical disorders. Clinical features associated with psychosomatic musculoskeletal pain include female gender, adolescent age, more than 6 months of symptoms, and a bright affect that is incongruent with the complaint of pain.

History

A medical history in patients with back pain begins with a thorough exploration of the current complaint and includes a review of symptoms, past illnesses and injuries, family history, and social circumstances. The age at onset of the pain is important because some disorders are more common in particular age groups. For example, diskitis is generally a problem in young children, whereas LBP, spondylolisthesis, and Scheuermann kyphosis are seen most often in adolescents. Tumors can affect patients of any age. Although most organic disorders that cause back pain in pediatric patients have no predilection for a particular gender, ankylosing spondylitis is far more common in boys than in girls.

It is important to determine the date of onset of the pain, athletic and occupational risk factors for structural disorders, and whether any trauma preceded the onset of the pain. For example, did the pain begin after falling, twisting, weight lifting, or participating in gymnastics? If so, the patient is more likely to have a structural or mechanical cause of back pain, such as spondylolysis or LBP. Although minor episodes of trauma may precipitate pain caused by relatively benign disorders, such as spondylolisthesis, practitioners must be suspicious of more serious disorders, such as intraspinal anomalies or masses, if the complaint is out of proportion to the aggravation.

If the pain occurs at night or at rest, infectious, malignant, and inflammatory causes of back pain should be considered. Osteomyelitis and osteoid osteoma are especially likely to cause pain at night and wake the patient from sleep. The association of night pain, morning stiffness, and improvement with activity suggests an inflammatory process. The location of the pain may suggest the cause as well; lumbar pain, for example, is characteristic of structural, inflammatory, and traumatic disorders. If the patient complains of back pain but shows the examiner a location away from the midline, such as the flank, a source of referred pain, such as urinary tract pathology, should be considered. The severity of the pain should be assessed. If the patient complains of intense pain, infection is the likely source. Also, the physician should ask what makes the pain better or worse to help categorize the problem. LBP, intervertebral disk herniation, spondylolysis or spondylolisthesis, and compression fractures improve with rest and escalate with activity; in contrast, leukemia and osteoid osteoma do not improve with rest and wake the patient from a deep sleep. Inflammatory conditions, such as ankylosing spondylitis, are notable for improvement with activity. Valsalva maneuvers—coughing, sneezing, laughing, and straining—intensify pain in patients with diastematomyelia, other intraspinal disorders, and intervertebral disk herniation. The practitioner should ask whether the patient worsened after chiropractic manipulation. Finally, it should be determined whether the pain radiates or travels in a pattern that suggests impingement upon nerve roots.

It is critical that the physician ask whether the patient or parents have noticed changes in the spinal curvature and/or foot deformities. Idiopathic juvenile scoliosis is not a painful disorder; the simultaneous onset of scoliosis and back pain is a cardinal symptom of a serious disorder affecting the spinal column (Box 2-2). The physician should ask whether rounding or flattening of the back has occurred. The new appearance of a foot deformity, such as a cavus, is equally serious and may be the only other indication of an intraspinal glioma, for example, in a patient with mild complaints of back ache.

In addition, careful inquiry regarding neurologic symptoms is necessary in all patients. The history must be explored for evidence of muscular weakness, gait changes, poor balance, sensory disturbances, and bowel or bladder dysfunction. Weakness may not be readily apparent even to the patient, who might complain only of being tired; parents might observe that the child must be carried up stairs and misinterpret this as fatigue rather than weakness. Gait changes may be reported as clumsiness. New onset of toe walking should be noted. Is there numbness or tingling or burning to imply sensory changes? Urinary retention or incontinence, dribbling, and constipation are evidence of bladder and bowel involvement respectively.

A thorough review of symptoms is helpful. Constitutional symptoms, such as fever, chills, weight loss, fatigue, night sweats, and pallor, suggest infectious, inflammatory, or malignant processes. Earlier illnesses should be surveyed. A history of a benign, self-limited, upper respiratory tract infection followed by back pain and gait refusal in a young child is given in diskitis and transverse myelitis. The same scenario followed by neck pain and stiffness suggests disk space calcification. Are other joints painful or swollen? Is the patient stiff in the morning or after naps? If so, ankylosing spondylitis or Reiter syndrome are likely, especially if the patient is an adolescent and the family history is positive. If the history points to infection, this should be pursued with detailed questions regarding pneumonia, cough, travel, exposures to adults with known or suspected tuberculosis, and contact with animals.

A complete review of symptoms includes questions about sources of pain referred to the back. Is there chest pain or cough indicative of a respiratory disorder? Biliary tract or pancreatic disease are considered if the patient has anorexia, weight loss, nausea, vomiting, or abdominal pain. The clinical diagnosis of back pain from pyelonephritis is usually simple; the pain is in the flank, and the patient has fever, vomiting, dysuria, frequency, and changes in the urinary color and odor. The pattern of pain is important; for example, the hallmark of UPJ obstruction is its episodic nature. Symptoms from endometriosis and hydrometrocolpos occur during menses, thus pain recurring monthly is typical of these disorders.

One should also obtain information regarding medications and family history of inherited illness, such as sickle cell anemia, mechanical back disorders, and rheumatic conditions. Knowledge of the social circumstances, with particular attention to school attendance and performance, is essential to identify patients with possible psychogenic back pain.

Physical Examination

Complete examination of the spinal column is compulsory in patients with back pain, as is a conscientious survey of the entire patient. Does the patient look well or as if there is a systemic disease? Growth parameters convey vital information about general health, and temperature measurement is important in all patients. The skin, lymph nodes, liver, and spleen should be examined for signs of malignancy. Pallor, petechiae, ecchymoses, hepatosplenomegaly, and large, firm, matted lymph nodes point to leukemia and lymphoma. Diminished or adventitious breath sounds are clues that pneumonia is causing the back pain. The abdominal examination is crucial because a number of more common pediatric disorders associated with back pain originate in the abdomen; appendicitis, psoas abscess, and pancreatitis are good examples. Hepatosplenomegaly is present in certain malignancies and storage diseases, such as Gaucher disease. Evidence of rash, eye inflammation, peripheral joint arthritis, and enthesopathy (pain resulting from inflammation at the point of insertion of ligaments and tendons into bone) are associated with Reiter syndrome and ankylosing spondylitis.

Visual inspection of the spine and extremities is very important. The skin over the back must be examined for midline lesions, such as vascular masses, nevi, tufts of hair, and dimples. These lesions are associated with spinal anomalies, such as diastematomyelia and other causes of a tethered cord. The physician should observe posture from the side to assess the spine for scoliosis, kyphosis, hyperlordosis, or flattening of the normal lumbar lordotic curve, as well as check for scoliosis in forward bending. The mobility of the spine in flexion, extension, and lateral bending should be ascertained. Is there a fixed thoracic kyphosis implying Scheuermann disease? Is the lumbar spine stiff, with decreased flexion and lateral bending typical of disk herniation or spondylolysis? The extremities are observed while the patient is at rest and while he or she is walking. Is there a foot deformity or obvious atrophy? The examiner should instruct the patient to stand on one leg at a time; pain from sacroiliitis increases on the weight-bearing side with this maneuver. The patient's gait is observed for evidence of pain, poor balance, or weakness. The practitioner should watch how the patient transfers from the prone to a sitting or standing position. Does he or she move in a way that suggests avoidance of pain or implies weakness?

The patient should identify the painful area. The examiner notes the degree of tenderness; mild pain is typically elicited with structural disorders, whereas moderate to severe pain is produced in examination of patients with osteomyelitis and diskitis. The paraspinous and hamstring muscles are palpated for evidence of spasm and tenderness. The physician should locate the pelvic brims and note whether they are level.

Two particular examination techniques are useful in patients with back complaints—the straight-leg raising test and the FABERE maneuver. The straight-leg raising test is performed with the patient supine. The examiner lifts the leg slowly by cupping the heel with one hand and keeping the knee extended with the other hand. Pain felt between 30 and 60 degrees of flexion is considered a positive sign. Although this test is best known for its association with disk herniation, it is also positive in patients with sacroiliac joint infection, diskitis, lumbar apophyseal ring fracture, and intraspinal tumors. Unlike the knee or elbow joint, the sacroiliac joint is difficult to examine. As mentioned earlier in the text, the *FABERE* test is an acronym for *f*lexion, *ab*duction, *e*xternal *r*otation, and *e*xtension of the hip. This test is also performed with the patient in a supine position. The patient flexes the knee and places the lateral malleolus on the opposite knee. Next, downward pressure is applied to the flexed knee. Pain caused by these actions indicates sacroiliac joint disease. All other joints should be surveyed for tenderness, swelling, warmth, erythema, and decreased range of motion.

Finally, a careful neurologic examination is of paramount importance. This aspect of diagnosis should include assessment of strength, reflexes, and sensory function. True muscular weakness, abnormal deep tendon reflexes, and loss of sensation are significant findings that mandate a comprehensive search for their cause. A rectal examination, although not absolutely essential for all patients, evaluates anal sphincter function; diminished tone may indicate an intraspinal tumor. Measurement of leg circumference at the thigh and calf may reveal atrophy, which is an important clue to the presence of long-standing organic disease.

Approach to the Patient

The cardinal issue in evaluation of the patient with back pain is whether there is neurologic involvement. If the history or physical examination reveals any evidence of neurologic involvement, immediate imaging studies and consultation with appropriate subspecialists are warranted. For example, a child with back pain, lower extremity weakness, and diminished deep tendon reflexes has spinal cord involvement and evaluation is indicated on an emergent basis to identify treatable disorders. Even subtle findings, such as the new onset of back pain and scoliosis or a mild foot deformity, demand prompt investigation (Box 2-2). Although plain films may reveal abnormal findings, such as spina bifida occulta or the spur of diastematomyelia, MRI is currently the best imaging modality for the detection of spinal cord lesions. Consultation with colleagues in neurology, neurosurgery, and/or hematology or oncology is appropriate in these situations.

In the absence of neurologic involvement, a thorough history and physical examination usually allow the clinician to make a diagnosis and confirm it with the appropriate radiographic and laboratory studies in a timely fashion. Certain key clinical associations permit the clinician to focus quickly on the likely cause (Box 2-3).

Because structural disorders are common causes of back pain in children, plain radiographs of the spine are appropriate as the initial imaging study in most patients and often prove the diagnosis. For example, a healthy adolescent with upper back pain and a fixed thoracic kyphosis is likely to have Scheuermann disease, and plain radiographs are indicated to verify the diagnosis. In other cases the history and physical examination are insufficient to permit a precise diagnosis but instead suggest the most likely problem. A teenage gymnast with chronic and recurrent LBP exacerbated by motion who has a normal physical examination except for limited lumbar range of motion and paraspinous or hamstring muscle spasm is likely to have a structural cause of pain, such as spondylolysis and/or spondylolisthesis. In this setting, plain radiographs of the spine, including oblique views, are essential; other studies, such as conventional bone scanning, SPECT scanning, or MRI, are valuable if the plain radiographs are normal, and consultation with an orthopedic surgeon or sports medicine specialist helps select the best modality.

A traumatic cause of back pain is likely when the history is suggestive. A patient with steroid-dependent asthma who falls onto his or her buttocks, complains immediately of back pain, and has a normal examination except for localized tenderness over the spine presumably has a compression fracture that will be evident on spine radiographs. Compression fractures also occur spontaneously or after minor trauma in patients with metabolic diseases. Weight lifting or other vertical loading trauma associated with the acute onset of back pain with radiation, scoliosis, and signs of nerve root compression on physical examination points to intervertebral disk herniation. In this setting, plain radiographs are usually normal but identify associated problems, such as spondylolysis; MRI is preferred to confirm the diagnosis of disk herniation.

Children with back pain, fever, and other constitutional symptoms and signs are more likely to have an infectious, in-

Back Pain: Key Associations

History

Gymnastics, rowing—spondylolysis or spondlolisthesis

Trauma—disk herniation, compression fracture

Pain worse with motion—spondylolisthesis, disk herniation, compression fractures

Pain better with rest—intervertebral disk herniation and other structural disorders

Nighttime pain, pain at rest—osteomyelitis, leukemia, osteoid osteoma

Severe pain—osteomyelitis, epidural abscess

Back stiffness—osteomyelitis, diskitis, sacroiliac inflammation

Increased pain with cough, strain—mass lesions of the spinal cord

Weakness, sensory loss, bowel or bladder dysfunction—spinal cord neoplasms, tethered cord

Physical Examination

Nevi, hair tufts, vascular lesions over spine—tethered cord, diastematomyelia, spina bifida occulta

Increased lumbar curve—spondylolisthesis, proximal muscle weakness

Fixed kyphosis—Scheuermann disease

Impaired spinal range of motion—diskitis, sacroiliac inflammation, osteomyelitis, disk herniation, spondylolysis, spondololisthesis

Positive straight-leg raising test—disk herniation, sacroiliac inflammation, spinal tumors

Weakness, sensory loss, abnormal deep tendon reflexes, depressed anal sphincter tone—intraspinal tumor, epidural abscess, disk herniation

---

flammatory, or neoplastic disorder. Again, those patients with a history or physical examination suspicious for involvement of the spinal cord must be evaluated on an emergent basis. The older child with high fever, severe and localized back pain, and serologic evidence of inflammation may have osteomyelitis; even subtle changes on the neurologic examination in this case should prompt consideration of epidural abscess or transverse myelitis. Although it is important to obtain plain radiographs of the involved area, there should be no delay in obtaining detailed imaging of the spinal column and its contents.

The toddler with back pain, low-grade fever, and refusal to walk warrants an evaluation for diskitis, including a CBC, blood culture, ESR, urinalysis, plain radiographs of the spine, and either a bone scan or an MRI. Early in the illness, radiographs are normal, bone scan shows increased radionuclide uptake in the affected disk space, and MRI reveals typical inflammatory signal changes in the disk space. Aspiration of the disk space is generally reserved for patients who do not respond to conservative management or who are at risk for unusual infections. Consultation with a pediatric orthopedic surgeon and/or infectious disease specialist may be necessary.

An adolescent boy with lumbar pain, stiffness, enthesopathy, and a family history of ankylosing spondylitis merits evaluation for rheumatologic conditions. Consider the prospect of malignancy in patients with painful scoliosis, nighttime pain and constitutional symptoms. Keep in mind that referred pain from common pediatric disorders—pneumonia and pyelonephritis—occurs far more often than rheumatologic or malignant disorders!

SUMMARY

In conclusion, back pain in children is uncommon but the high incidence of serious organic disease makes thorough investigation mandatory. In many patients a thorough history and physical examination combined with plain radiographs of the spine provide an adequate foundation for the correct diagnosis. Other patients require additional laboratory studies, radiographic images, and consultation with subspecialists for evaluation and subsequent management. Although back pain is infrequent in pediatric patients, primary care practitioners can start the investigation of this complaint with confidence.

ILLUSTRATIVE CASES

Case 1. A 13-year-old previously healthy girl has a 7-month history of intermittent back pain. Her first episode of pain began after twisting her back during a volleyball game. The pain (which was mild) was located in the lumbar region, relieved with rest and use of ibuprofen, and resolved after 1 week. Several weeks later, she had a similar episode of pain that resolved after a few days. Over the next few months, she continued to have intermittent episodes of lower back pain, which began to limit her participation as a flag-bearer for the school marching band. She denies having fevers, weight loss, joint symptoms, unusual urinary frequency, dysuria, weakness, or changes in bowel or bladder function. Family history is remarkable for rheumatic fever in the mother as a child.

On examination she appears well, with normal vital signs. Her general physical examination is unremarkable, and a complete neurologic examination is normal. The inspection of her spine reveals a flattened lumbar curve. On palpation she has moderate tenderness and spasm of the lumbar paraspinous muscles. Flexion and extension of the lumbar spine are decreased.

Before her visit the patient had an intravenous pyelogram (IVP) performed to evaluate her back pain. Her parents brought those films and other medical records for review. Bilateral spondylolysis at L2-3 is evident on the scout film for the IVP. No other studies were obtained. A back brace is recommended by the orthopedic consultant. Her condition greatly improves after 1 month and continues to be well.

This case illustrates the chief historic features of a symptomatic spondylolysis: an onset after trauma, then months of intermittent pain relieved by rest and exacerbated by physical activity.

Case 2. A 9-year-old boy previously in good health is referred for evaluation of bilateral hip pain, LBP, and stiffness that began 6 weeks before presentation. He has no fever but is tired, complains of a poor appetite, has lost 4 pounds, and has night sweats. The pain does not improve with rest and is worse with walking. Aspirin does not relieve his pain. He recalls no recent injury and is not involved in sports of any kind. He denies cough, rash, heel pain, other joint complaints, weakness, gait changes, loss of sensation in his extremities, and bowel or bladder dysfunction. There is no family history of rheumatoid arthritis or ankylosing spondylitis. He has no known risk factors for tuberculosis, and he is not exposed to cats.

On physical examination he is thin but looks well. The musculoskeletal examination is remarkable only for a flattened curve of the lower spine, pain in the lumbar region with flexion and palpation, and decreased spinal mobility. He has a normal neurologic examination, including testing of reflexes, gait, strength, and sensation.

Plain radiographs of the spine were obtained by the referring physician. The films show unequivocal evidence of disk space narrowing between L2 and L3 and loss of cortex at the anterior margin of the L3 vertebra. A bone scan shows increased uptake of the isotope at L3.

At this point, chronic osteomyelitis is suspected. A CBC and chemistries are normal, and a PPD is nonreactive. The ESR is 55 mm/hr. A myelogram under CT guidance shows normal intraspinal contents, changes in the L3 vertebral body consistent with osteomyelitis, and an abscess in the superior aspect of the left psoas muscle. The disk space and abscess are both aspirated. Polymorphonuclear cells are present, but bacteria and acid-fast organisms are absent, and all cultures are negative. He is treated with a back brace and parenteral antibiotics for 4 months, which results in complete resolution of symptoms and signs.

This case illuminates several important features of vertebral osteomyelitis. First, fever was never present, unlike other infectious diseases in which fever is a reliable indi-

cator. Second, it may present as a chronic and indolent process with hip pain and stiffness, thus mimicking a rheumatologic disorder, such as ankylosing spondylitis. Third, a prominent symptom in this patient was hip pain, a frequent feature of inflammation in the spine. Finally, his symptoms and signs, although clearly denoting an abnormality of the lower spine, were also consistent with LBP without structural disease. The referring physician recognized that this patient had no risk factors for mechanical strain and felt further investigation was indicated.

Case 3. A 4-year-old girl complains of back pain 2 weeks after an upper respiratory tract infection. Her parents brought her in for evaluation when they noticed she was having difficulty climbing stairs and getting out of chairs. There is no history of fever or trauma, and she is not involved in sports. Her review of systems is entirely normal except for back pain.

On physical examination she is a well-appearing child with an oral temperature of 37.7° C. Her other vital signs are normal. Her general physical examination is normal. Her gait is slow and stiff. Her lumbar spine is flattened, and she refuses to bend in any direction. She is unable to climb onto the examination table without help. A Gowers sign is present, but her muscle strength, sensation, and deep tendon reflexes are normal. Her lumbar spine is mildly tender to palpation.

A CBC is normal. An ESR is 25 mm/hr. Plain radiographs of the spine are normal. A technetium 99 bone scan shows uptake in the L2-3 disk space. A blood culture is obtained and is sterile after 72 hours. After 3 days of bed rest and the use of acetaminophen for pain control, her symptoms begin to improve. Her condition is normal 10 days after the onset of her symptoms. Three weeks after her original presentation, repeat radiographs of the lumbar spine reveal changes typical of the later stage of diskitis.

This case illustrates the mild symptoms typical of diskitis. It also serves to remind us that plain radiographs of the lumbar spine may be entirely normal if taken early in the course of an infectious or inflammatory process.

ANNOTATED BIBLIOGRAPHY

Bunnell WP: Back pain in children, *Pediatr Rev* 6:183-189, 1984.
  Although this article is more than 10 years old, the discussion of the differential diagnosis of back pain is extremely useful.

Dyment PG: Low back pain in adolescents, *Pediatr Ann* 20:170-178, 1991.
  An excellent review of common causes of back pain in teenagers, this article emphasizes mechanical low back pain.

Micheli LJ, Wood R: Back pain in young athletes, *Arch Pediatr Adolesc Med* 149:15-18, 1995.
  This article is an excellent review of causes of low back pain in adolescent athletes. The comparison with adults is especially helpful.

BIBLIOGRAPHY

Bellah RD, Summerville DA, Treves ST, et al: Low-back pain in adolescent athletes: detection of stress injury to the pars interarticularis with SPECT, *Radiology* 180:509-512, 1991.

Correa AG, Morven SE, Baker CJ: Vertebral osteomyelitis in children, *Pediatr Infect Dis J* 12:228-233, 1993.

Crawford AH, Kucharzyk DW, Ruda R, et al: Diskitis in children, *Clin Orthop* 206:70-79, 1991.

duLac P, Panuel M, Devred P, et al: MRI of disc space infection in infants and children, *Pediatr Radiol* 20:175-178, 1990.

Epstein JA, Epstein NE, Marc J, et al: Lumbar intervertebral disc herniation in teenage children: recognition and management of associated anomalies, *Spine* 9:427-432, 1984.

Heinrich SD, Zembo MM, King AG, et al: Calcific cervical intervertebral disc herniation in children, *Spine* 16:228-231, 1991.

Hensinger RN: *The pediatric spine,* New York, 1985, Thieme.

Inselman LS: Tuberculosis in children: an unsettling forecast, *Contemp Pediatr* 7:110-130, 1990.

Jackson DW, Wiltse LL, Cirincione RJ: Spondylolysis in female gymnasts, *Clin Orthop* 118:68-73, 1976.

Jonsson OG, Sartain P, Ducore JM, et al: Bone pain as an initial symptom of childhood acute lymphoblastic leukemia: association with nearly normal hematologic indices, *J Pediatr* 117:233-237, 1990.

King HA: Back pain in children, *Pediatr Clin North Am* 31:1083-1095, 1984.

Koranyi K: Fever, back pain, and pleural effusion in a 4-year-old boy, *Pediatr Infect Dis J* 13:657, 672-673, 1994.

MacCartee CC, Griffin PP, Byrd EB: Ruptured calcified thoracic disc in a child, *J Bone Joint Surg Am* 54A:1272-1274, 1972.

Ogden JA: *Skeletal injury in the child.* Philadelphia, 1990, WB Saunders.

Olsen TL, Anderson RL, Dearwater SR, et al: The epidemiology of low back pain in an adolescent population, *Am J Public Health* 82:606-608, 1992.

Orlowski JP, Mercer RD: Osteoid osteoma in children and young adults, *Pediatrics* 59:526-532, 1977.

Sherry DD, McGuire T, Mellins E, et al: Psychosomatic musculoskeletal pain in childhood: clinical and psychological analyses of 100 children, *Pediatrics* 6:1093-1099, 1991.

Sills EM: What's causing the back pain? *Contemp Pediatr* 5:85-96, 1988.

Tachdjian MO: *Pediatric orthopedics,* vol 3, ed 2, Philadelphia, 1990, WB Saunders.

Vyskocil JJ, McIlroy MA, Brennan TA, et al: Pyogenic infection of the sacroiliac joint: case reports and review of the literature, *Medicine* 70:188-197, 1991.

Wenger DR, Bobechko WP, Gilday DL: The spectrum of intervertebral disc space infection in children, *J Bone Joint Surg* 60A:100-108, 1978.

Zsolway KM, Pasquariello PS, Tunnessen WW: The tip of the iceberg, *Contemp Pediatr* 11:81-83, 1994.

Chest Pain

J. CARLTON GARTNER, Jr.

Key Points

- Chest pain is usually a benign problem in childhood and is rarely due to cardiac causes.

- Exercise-induced asthma and esophagitis should be considered in the differential diagnosis.

- In older children a psychogenic cause must be recognized, including unrecognized hyperventilation.

Recurrent chest pain is a common symptom during childhood. For older children, chest pain ranks behind only headache and abdominal pain in frequency of complaints. For younger children, chest pain is similar in frequency to limb pains. In patients between 10 and 21 years of age, chest pain accounts for 650,000 physician visits annually. It was the seventh most common concern in a survey of urban African-American adolescents. In a 1-year prospective study conducted in an urban pediatric emergency room, more than 400 of the estimated 70,000 visits were for a complaint of chest pain. Children of all ages may experience chest pain, and approximately 40% of them have recurring episodes. Follow-up studies suggest that over time preliminary organic diagnoses are recategorized as nonorganic or idiopathic. The focus of this chapter is those patients who have continued or recurring chest pain over weeks or months.

Pathophysiology

A detailed discussion of the neuroanatomic and neurohumoral transmission of pain is beyond the scope of this text. Some anatomic principles may be helpful in approaching the patient. Pain "in the chest" may arise from the chest wall, deep thoracic viscera, parietal pleura, diaphragm, and upper abdominal viscera. Thoracic dermatomes T1-4 include the central thoracic structures (heart, great vessels, mediastinum,

and esophagus), and T5-8 include the lower structures (thorax, diaphragm, and abdominal viscera). The pain is usually substernal or precordial in location for upper dermatomes and near the xiphoid or midback for lower dermatomes. Pain from the diaphragm may be referred to the neck and ipsilateral shoulder because of phrenic innervation. Careful examination with attention to dermatomal distribution of pain may at times help in diagnosis of unusual conditions, such as radiculitis.

Literature Survey

There are several prospective and retrospective reviews of patients with chest pain. Unfortunately, comparisons are difficult because of inconsistency in the patient populations studied. Several reports include only emergency room patients, and others include outpatient or even cardiac clinic patients. Duration of symptoms ranges from hours to months or even years. Also, the largest diagnostic group in most series is musculoskeletal or idiopathic causes. Emphasis generally has been placed on excluding serious underlying cardiac disorders (with electrocardiogram [ECG] or echocardiogram), but these disorders make up only a very small fraction of final diagnoses. The largest prospective follow-up study of emergency room patients demonstrated that more than 40% of the patients had persistent symptoms (lasting 6 months to 2 years) and that disorders initially thought to be organic were later considered idiopathic. (The category of idiopathic disorders increased from 13% to 34% over time.) There is no carefully conducted prospective study that looks at two recently proposed causes of recurrent chest pain—exercise-induced reactive airway disease and gastrointestinal disease, especially esophagitis. At best only some general principles can be derived from currently published literature.

Surprisingly, younger children suffer chest pain almost as frequently as adolescents; rates of presentation before and after age 12 years are similar in published reports. Girls somewhat outnumber boys, especially in the adolescent category

(60% girls). Most patients are diagnosed with musculoskeletal (chest wall syndrome, costochondritis, and traumatic) or idiopathic categories. Few serious organic disorders are discovered, and those that are uncovered may be unrelated to the pain (i.e., mitral valve prolapse). Chest x-ray films are helpful only in acute, recent-onset pain (such as pneumonia) or when physical examination is abnormal (i.e., murmur, rub). Psychogenic pain is a true entity but is difficult to diagnose with certainty on many occasions. Pain of longer duration is more likely to remain idiopathic and is less likely to disappear. Most patients are concerned about their heart as the source of pain. Unless there are fingings on examination, laboratory tests and procedures are unlikely to be helpful. A review of differential diagnosis in more detail may be valuable. The emphasis is on the cause of recurrent and more chronic symptoms.

Differential Diagnosis

Idiopathic or Psychogenic Disorders

Why is idiopathic chest pain the initial category of discussion? It is clear that this represents the largest diagnostic category over time. A significant portion of patients initially labeled as idiopathic have psychogenic pain. Asnes and others found definite evidence of pain related to recent stressful life events in 36 of 123 patients seen in their pediatric clinic. They point out that more than 50% of the children had other complaints frequently associated with stress (e.g., headache, abdominal pain, limb pain). Unfortunately, long-term follow-up was not available. In a study of 100 consecutive children referred for cardiologic evaluation, 13 met criteria for a major depressive disorder. All four children who had chest pain as their primary symptom were depressed and had normal cardiac examinations. Although it is repeatedly stated that adults have a much higher incidence of organic causes for chest pain, Katon and others interviewed adults after coronary arteriography. Patients with normal arteriography more frequently had atypical chest pain, had more autonomic symptoms (i.e., tachycardia, dizziness, etc.), had higher scores for anxiety and depression, and more frequently met criteria for panic disorder, depression, and phobias.

In a prospective study of adolescents with chest pain, Pantell and Goodman found 43% to be idiopathic, and by inference from their text many of these patients had recent stressful life events. Of note is a separate category of hyperventilation (13%). Several articles describe this as a cause of chest pain. Symptoms usually ascribed to acute hyperventilation may be absent. Lum describes multiple symptoms associated with hyperventilation, ranging from more usual (shortness of breath, tetany, yawning, and light-headedness) to uncommon (epigastric pains, cramps, and tremors). There is usually underlying anxiety notable upon closer questioning. Psychogenic pain should not be a diagnosis of exclusion. It may be the best explanation after a thorough history and examination.

Two more areas warrant potential investigation in the category of idiopathic disorders—esophagitis and reactive airway disease. These entities have been discovered in patients who had no obvious cause of chest pain on initial evaluation. Each is described separately in later sections of this chapter.

Musculoskeletal Disorders

In most series, pain (which may be reproducible) is evident somewhere on the thorax. Costochondritis may occur after a respiratory tract infection, may be localized (usually to the left fourth to sixth costrochondral junctions), or may radiate to the back or abdomen. Chest wall syndrome is a more generalized form of this disorder, usually diagnosed by careful palpation of the chest. Maneuvers such as flexion of the arms across the chest with traction or neck extension with backward arm pressure may reproduce the pain. Tietze syndrome is accompanied by swelling visible at the right sternoclavicular or second sternochondral junction. Pain is present for weeks, and swelling may last for years. Xiphoid cartilage syndrome may be accompanied by aching pain lasting for minutes to hours, and pain in the xiphoid area may sometimes be a component of a "stitch." A stitch is a sharp, crampy pain in the right upper quadrant and under the right costal margin, which usually occurs while running or walking.

Many individuals have experienced precordial catch syndrome as originally described by Miller and Texidor (Texidor twinge). This twinge is a sudden, sharp, stabbing pain, usually occuring during rest; localized to the area of the cardiac apex; and aggravated by deep inspiration so that most patients breathe shallowly. The pain is brief (lasting only seconds to a few minutes), and the cause is unknown. Slipping rib syndrome is thought to result from the tip of the eighth, ninth, or tenth rib overriding the one above. The pain may be reproduced by bending over, breathing deeply, or grasping the costal margin and pulling anteriorly (hooking maneuver). Trauma to the chest may be a cause of pain and may go unrecognized during initial questioning.

Breast Disorders

At first glance, breast disorders may not seem to warrant a separate category. However, breast tissue in adolescent boys is a great source of anxiety. Although some minor, often tender, enlargement occurs in 50% of boys during pubertal development, visible changes may lead to a complaint of chest pain, resulting in an office or clinic visit. Reassurance and understanding are the keys to management in the majority of patients.

Pulmonary Disorders

Pneumonia, pleural effusion, pneumothorax, and other acute illness are unlikely sources of chronic, recurrent chest pain. The patient with cancer or tuberculosis may have chest pain, but it should be accompanied by other systemic

TABLE 3-1

Differential Diagnosis of Chest Pain

Diagnosis	Characteristics
Idiopathic Disorders	Largest category, includes psychogenic disorders and some patients later found to have esophagitis or reactive airway disease
Psychogenic	Multiple complaints, life stresses, school absence, vulnerable child
Hyperventilation	Lightheadedness, yawning, cramps, reproducibility
Musculoskeletal Disorders	Be certain to inquire about trauma
Costochondritis	Usually left 4th to 6th costochondral junctions
Chest wall syndrome	Generalized pain induced by several office maneuvers (see text)
Tietze syndrome	Localized swelling of sternoclavicular or sternochondral junction
Xiphoid cartilage syndrome	Localized, may last for hours
Stitch	Right costal margin while exercising
Precordial catch syndrome (Texidor twinge)	Stabbing, at apex, brief duration, shallow breaths
Slipping rib syndrome	Aggravated by bending or jarring, "hooking maneuver" stimulates
Breast Disorders	Usually gynecomastia
Pulmonary Disorders	Pneumonia, pneumothorax rare (acute), excercise-induced reactive airway disease possible if pain is exertional
Cardiovascular Disease	Rare but potentially serious; syncope, dyspnea, exertional symptoms
Myopericardial	Most common; viral prodrome, fever, malaise, rub, murmur
Structural	Left ventricular outflow obstruction, aortic/subaortic, murmur; mitral valve prolapse probably not a cause
Dysrythmia	Supraventricular, palpitations, peculiar feeling in chest
Gastrointestinal Disorders	Esophagitis, reflux, may have dyspepsia, consider further evaluation in severe and persistent cases
Vertebral/Radicular Disorders	Always examine spine and dermatomes

symptoms, such as fever, weight loss, and dyspnea. An entity that is listed in several reviews of chest pain is asthma or reactive airway disease. Patients with recognized recurrent wheezing episodes rarely present primarily with chest pain. However, a recent report describes 88 patients who were referred for exercise testing after normal cardiac evaluations. The majority (93%) had exertional chest pain. Sixty-four children experienced a fall in forced expiratory volume in 1 second (FEV1) or peak expiratory flow rate (PEFR) of at least 15% during exercise without a warm-up period. The majority experienced subjective and objective improvement after inhalational albuterol therapy. This study at least suggests that some children with chest pain on exertion may have reactive airway disease. Further studies (perhaps using blinded investigators and better controls) may help define the true prevalence of this entity.

Cardiovascular Disorders

The cardiovascular system receives much attention as a potentially serious cause of chest pain. In fact, congenital or acquired heart disease is very rarely discovered in patients with only chest pain as a complaint. In the study by Selbst

and others, 4% of children were found to have cardiac disorders. Categories of illness include acquired myopericardial disease, structural defects, and dysrhythmias. Thoughtful reviews call attention to associated symptoms that should make more detailed cardiac evaluation mandatory, including exertional pain, especially if accompanied by syncope or dizziness; anginal-type pain with exertion; recent or current viral illness with fever and malaise; significant findings on examination (e.g., murmur, rub, gallop); suspicion of dysrhythmia raised by history or examination; and abnormality of ECG or chest x-ray films (which may not be warranted on all patients). Myopericardial disease is usually accompanied by malaise and fatigue. Pain in pericarditis is often relieved or improved by sitting erect and leaning forward. The most common structural defects are left ventricular outflow obstruction from aortic valve or subvalvular stenosis and idiopathic hypertrophic subaortic stenosis (IHSS). Pain is usually exercise-induced in these conditions. The murmur of IHSS is accentuated by maneuvers that decrease left ventricular volume (such as Valsalva maneuver or standing). Frequently mentioned as a cause of chest pain, mitral valve prolapse is present in the normal, asymptomatic population. In one study the incidence of mitral valve prolapse in patients with chest pain was no higher than that of the normal population. Thus this finding on examination probably cannot explain the symptom. Supraventricular dysrhythmias are those most commonly found in the pediatric population. If exertional syncope, palpitations, or other suggestive information is uncovered in the history, a lengthy period of ECG recording may be indicated, such as 24 hour Holter monitoring.

Gastrointestinal Disorders

A number of studies in both adults and children have suggested that the gastrointestinal tract, especially the esophagus, may be the cause of nonspecific chest pain. De Caestecker used endoscopy, manometry, and later acid perfusion to study a group of patients with "noncardiac" chest pain, most of whom did not describe true dyspepsia or regurgitation. About two thirds of the patients had organic disorders, most frequently reflux and diffuse esophageal spasm. Unfortunately, during the study, pain was not reproducible in most of the patients. In a study involving children, Berezin used intraesophageal acid perfusion (Bernstein test) to evaluate nonspecific chest pain. Again, 45 of 60 had esophagitis, and in 18 pain was reproduced during the test. Patients without esophagitis did not have pain during acid perfusion. Chest pain and histologic findings resolved after antacid treatment, and follow-up acid perfusion tests were normal. This study certainly suggests that some patients have an esophageal cause of their chest pain. The study would be stronger if the patients had been studied by investigators unfamiliar with the histology or pain history.

Vertebral Column Disorders or Radiculitis

Although rare, vertebral column disorders should be listed for completeness. Any process that impinges on nerve roots can produce chest pain. Examples include vertebral collapse or infiltrative processes. It should be remembered that herpes zoster may produce pain in a dermatomal distribution before vesicles develop, and the pain may persist for prolonged periods, usually in adults. Occasional patients, usually those with recurrent herpes zoster, may have pain without rash.

Table 3-1 presents the differential diagnosis of persistent chest pain. Features that are helpful in initial history and physical examination are presented in the following sections.

History

As with most chronic complaints, time spent in obtaining a good history is often the most helpful in arriving at a diagnosis. Manner of onset, pain description, frequency, aggravating and relieving factors, and systemic symptoms, such as weight loss, fever, and cough, are important. Although there are several classic histories, such as that for the precordial catch syndrome, episodic worsening of chest pain is most

TABLE 3-2

Key Questions

Question	Value
Acute pain? First time?	Infection
Systemic symptoms?	Infection, malignancy
Duration of complaints?	Months or years— more likely psychogenic or GI
Exertional?	RAD, stitch, CWS, cardiac, slipping rib syndrome
Syncope? Palpitations?	Cardiac
Cough?	RAD
Localized?	CWS, precordial catch syndrome, breast, xyphoid
Reproducible? How?	CWS, slipping rib syndrome
Visible?	Tietze syndrome, breast, trauma
Cardiac apex, pleuritic?	Precordial catch syndrome
Associated symptoms?	Functional, HV
Abdominal pain, limb pain, headaches?	Psychogenic
Light-headedness, tetany, cramps, dizziness?	HV
Dermatomal distribution?	Herpes zoster, nerve root
Aggravated by rising from supine position?	Vertebral
Poor school attendance? Stressful life events?	Psychogenic, HV

CWS, Chest wall syndrome; *GI*, gastrointestinal; *HV*, hyperventilation; *RAD*, reactive airway disease.

common and pain is seldom constantly present. Nighttime pain is mentioned as a valuable clue to an organic diagnosis by several authors, but in the largest follow-up series, 46% of children awoke from sleep at some point with pain. This same series emphasizes the increase in idiopathic pain diagnoses over time; thus suggesting, unfortunately, that nocturnal pain may not be a sign of an organic disorder. Sometimes the patient may give clues by describing the pain in his or her own words. It is very helpful to know what diagnoses the patient and family have considered. When questioned, adolescents are most frequently concerned about cardiac-related pain. If the pain is chronic, what prompted the visit at this particular time? School function and attendance are critically important. Patients who miss school and have vague symptoms are more likely to have a functional diagnosis. Other symptoms of a nonorganic nature should be reviewed, such as abdominal pain, headache, limb pains, fatigue, and dizziness.

Family history may be relevant if there has been significant chest pain, heart disease, myocardial infarction, or sudden death. Although this information may not be genetically important, it does give some background to the complaint. A family history of asthma was not helpful in separating those with and without reactive airway disease in one study. Life events, stresses, or recent losses or separations may be of importance. Both organic and nonorganic factors may be related to the pain; minor trauma or inflammation may be accentuated by the recent hospitalization of a relative for myocardial infarction.

Separate histories from the parent(s) and the patient often yield valuable information; each may have totally unrelated concerns. The adolescent boy with gynecomastia may reveal his major concern only when alone with the examiner. Psychosexual information may be obtained in this fashion if the examiner has developed a trusting relationship. In adults, smoking has been related to an increased incidence of chest pain and may be important in older children as well.

Parents may be able to give a good overview of the problem. How much does the pain interfere with the patient's daily life? Have favorite sports or other activities continued? Can they tell when the pain is present? Also, the practitioner should get a sense of the family's overall function. Is the patient a vulnerable child? Do other family members have multiple somatic complaints? Previous evaluations and reports should be reviewed during the same visit. Once again, multiple physician involvement may be a clue to family functioning. Questions that are most helpful in establishing a diagnosis are presented in Table 3-2.

After completing a thorough history, the examiner should be able to decide if the pain warrants major investigation. Key features that suggest rare serious organic disorders are as follows: shorter duration of the complaint; exertional pain, especially if associated with syncope or dizziness; dyspnea; systemic symptoms; absence of other complaints; positive life events; and excellent school attendance.

Physical Examination

A number of diagnostic possibilities suggested by the history may be confirmed by examination. Most frequently the examination is normal, but this is important as well. General appearance and growth should be noted and compared with previous data if possible. Vital signs, including pulse regularity, should be recorded. The examiner should then locate the pain on the chest wall and try to reproduce it gently if possible. Palpation of the costal margins and xiphoid process and use of the hooking maneuver are important. In this technique the examiner puts his or her fingers around the inferior anterior rib margins and pulls anteriorly. Positions that accentuate or relieve the pain should be sought. In their description of chest wall syndrome, Epstein and colleagues describe techniques that reproduce pain, including downward pressure on the top of the head, horizontal arm traction across the chest

wall, and the "crowing rooster maneuver" in which the physician stands behind the patient and exerts backward and slightly superior traction on the arms while the patient looks up toward the ceiling. These methods may accentuate chest tenderness. The practitioner should not omit careful inspection for swelling, old trauma, dermatomal lesions, or breast development.

Careful auscultation of the heart and lungs is next. Changes in breath sounds or adventitious sounds should be noted. It is useful, if clinically suspected, to have the patient hyperventilate while seated. A parent or family member should be present. Several authors have commented on the reproducibility of symptoms in the office during hyperventilation, making this the primary diagnosis. Cardiac examination, using standing and/or the Valsalva maneuver, may accentuate the murmur of subaortic stenosis, and the murmur of mitral valve prolapse may be heard only with the patient in the sitting position. The vertebral column should be inspected and palpated. It is always helpful to ask patients to rise from a supine position and get down from the examining table. This gives valuable information about flexibility and comfort and may point to the back or spine as the source of anterior chest (or abdominal) pain. The abdomen should be inspected and palpated. At this time it may be evident that the pain is actually located in the abdomen rather than the chest, which certainly may change the clinical approach!

Completion of a careful history and examination forms the major foundation for planning any further evaluation. Time spent performing these tasks actually saves time (and money) later. Too often a brief history and cursory examination are followed by long lists of laboratory and radiographic procedures performed rather randomly. The astute clinician is often reasonably certain of a diagnosis without any further tests.

Approach to the Patient

Clues uncovered in the initial history and examination are the basis for the next steps in the evaluation and management of the patient. One might suppose that at least some "screening tests" might be helpful, but review of the literature suggests the opposite. In Selbst's large prospective series, chest x-ray films and ECGs were occasionally abnormal but did not reveal dramatic new findings not suggested by the initial work-up. Also, some patients in the series had acute chest pain, fever, and other findings suggestive of infection, making a chest x-ray film far from a screening test. Several key features seem to warrant further tests, such as exertional chest pain, especially if accompanied by syncope; tightness in the chest or palpitations; malaise; prodromal viral illness; fever; nonfunctional sounding murmur; or rub. If there is uncertainty about normal findings, chest x-ray films and an ECG may be obtained and followed by echocardiography if indicated. Although myopericardial diseases are uncommon, as a group they represent the most common cardiac cause of chest pain.

If reproducible chest wall or xiphoid pain is evident, reassurance and mild analgesia are indicated. Slipping rib syndrome is a more chronic complaint, usually seen in adults, and may require surgery. Precordial catch syndrome is a diagnosis made by history. Anxiety, paresthesia, multiple complaints, and depressive symptoms suggest hyperventilation or psychogenic pain.

Failure to make a reasonable diagnosis at this point should lead to evaluation over time. Unfortunately, most patients fall into the category of nonspecific pain of a recurrent nature with initially unrevealing history and normal examination. Further history may uncover previously unsuspected stress or conflicts, described at a later visit when the patient and family are more comfortable with the physician. Patients who have continued exertional pain despite a normal examination may benefit from pulmonary function testing and use of a bronchodilator, such as albuterol. Patients who have continued pain for prolonged periods of time without clues to suggest psychogenic origins may be candidates for acid-reflux–induced symptoms. Antacids may be dramatically effective in this condition.

Consultation can be used sparingly in evaluating patients with chest pain. At the initial visit the examiner should decide whether the symptoms or examination warrant referral to a pediatric cardiologist. Most patients do not need this referral. Only a few patients with severe and persistent symptoms require the expertise of a pulmonologist (for obtaining pulmonary function tests) or a gastroenterologist (for evaluating esophageal causes of pain).

Most primary care practitioners reluctantly refer children to a child psychiatrist or psychologist. If anxiety, depression, and dysfunctional family situations persist, referral may be extremely helpful. As with other specialists the opinion of a colleague in psychiatry about the role of emotional factors in the patient's symptoms may be valuable.

SUMMARY

Chronic chest pain is a common symptom in children, and the cause is frequently unclear. Serious organic disorders rarely present with only vague chest pain. Because a cause is often not discovered, the majority of patients carry a diagnosis of idiopathic chest pain. Many of these children have psychogenic pain after a careful history and examination are completed, but a few who are followed carefully over time may have underlying organic causes. The astute clinician can evaluate and manage the majority of these children without invasive testing or subspecialty consultation. Developments over the next few years should clarify the frequency of certain disorders, such as reactive airway disease and esophagitis, in the cause of recurrent chest pain.

ILLUSTRATIVE CASES

Case 1. *The patient is a 13-year-old boy seen in the pediatric resident clinic for further evaluation of chest pain. The pain is described as sharp and precordial and is not associated with exercise. Pain episodes last for several minutes and seem unrelated to any particular activity. General health is excellent, and the patient is an active athlete. Previously performed chest x-ray films and ECGs are normal. The resident's examination is normal.*

While examining this patient, the examiner is struck by the obvious gynecomastia. The examination is normal, and male adolescent development is normal. During gentle questioning it becomes clear that the chest pain is related to concerns about the breast tissue. With reassurance the pain complaint rapidly disappears.

This case illustrates the importance of careful questioning, especially in the adolescent, about the "hidden agenda" leading to an office visit. In this patient a history could have eliminated the need for even the basic chest x-ray film and ECG.

Case 2. *The patient is a 14-year-old girl who is referred for left-sided chest pain and anxiety about cardiac disease. The pain is sudden, left-sided, below the cardiac apex, and pleuritic. It is not exercise-induced but does seem to be related to bending forward and straightening up suddenly. She has had several episodes, each less than 1 minute in duration. She is unable to take a deep breath during the event because the pain worsens. Further questioning reveals that her grandfather recently suffered a heart attack, but her episodes preceded his illness.*

Preliminary chest x-ray films and ECGs are reviewed and are normal. Physical examination, with careful attention to the chest wall, is completely normal. This history is typical of precordial catch syndrome (Texidor twinge). The patient admits that she ignored the symptoms before her grandfather's illness, but was quite anxious after he suffered chest pain. Reassurance is effective in alleviating her worry.

It is important to recognize this cause of pain because it is relatively common and can be mistaken for cardiac or pulmonary disease. Further investigation is unnecessary.

Case 3. *A.G. is a 12-year-old boy referred for chest discomfort experienced while competing in ice hockey. He was previously well and without chronic illness. Episodes are associated with exertion and consist of a feeling of pain and tightness bilaterally. There is improvement with rest. The pain does not radiate. He has developed a mild chronic cough, which is worse at night and after exercise. There are no other systemic symptoms, such as fever, weight loss, and rash. The patient has not fainted.*

Physical examination is normal. The lungs and heart are normal. The patient is thin and muscular.

This is a somewhat vexing case. The exercise nature of the pain suggests myopericardial disease, but the cough and tightness are more consistent with reactive airway disease, although the patient never had wheezing episodes. Peak flow reading is normal, but after exercise in the office, peak flow is substantially reduced for age and wheezing is audible on chest auscultation. Peak flow returns to normal after use of a beta₂-agonist (albuterol) by metered dose inhaler.

This patient is diagnosed with exercise-induced asthma and improves with use of appropriate brochodilator therapy. With a less thoughtful approach, detailed cardiac evaluation may have been initiated. A more simple office test elicited symptoms, and then therapy was initiated quickly.

ANNOTATED BIBLIOGRAPHY

Selbst SM, Ruddy R, Clark BJ: Chest pain in children: follow-up of patients previously reported, *Clin Pediatr* 29:374-377, 1990.
More than one third of the initial diagnoses in the original study were altered with longer follow-up. Most frequently the diagnosis was changed to a nonorganic one. Only one new diagnosis of cardiac disease was made.

Selbst SM, Ruddy RM, Clark BJ, et al: Pediatric chest pain: a prospective study, *Pediatrics* 82:319-323, 1988.
This is the largest prospective study. It gives an overview of the problem, emphasizing the infrequency of a cardiac cause and the prevalence of idiopathic and musculoskeletal causes.

Wiens L, Sabath R, Ewing L, et al: Chest pain in otherwise healthy children and adolescents is frequently caused by exercise-induced asthma, *Pediatrics* 90:350-353, 1992.
This report demonstrates the role of reactive airway disease in the etiology of exertional chest pain. Unfortunately, the investigators were not blinded, but asthma may well be a much more frequent cause of chest pain than is heart disease.

BIBLIOGRAPHY

Asnes RS, Santulli R, Bemporad JR: Psychogenic chest pain in children, *Clin Pediatr* 20:788-791, 1981.

Berezin S, Meadow MS, Glassman MS, Newman LJ: Chest pain of gastrointestinal origin, *Arch Dis Child* 63:1457-1460, 1988.

Berezin S, Meadow MS, Glassman M, et al: Use of the intra-esophageal acid perfusion test in provoking nonspecific chest pain in children, *J Pediatr* 115:709-712, 1989.

Calabro J, Marchesano J: Tietze's syndrome: report of a case with juvenile onset, *J Pediatr* 68:985-987, 1966.

de Caestecker JS, Blackwell JN, Brown J, et al: The esophagus as a cause of recurrent chest pain: which patients should be investigated and which tests should be used? *Lancet* 2:1143-1146, 1985.

de Caestecker JS, Pryde A, Heading RC: Comparison of intravenous edrophonium and esophageal acid perfusion during esophageal manometry in patients with noncardiac chest pain, *Gut* 29:1029-1034, 1988.

Epstein SE, Gerber LH, Borer JS: Chest wall syndrome: a common cause of unexplained cardiac pain, *JAMA* 241:2793-2797, 1979.

Feinstein RA, Daniel WA: Chronic chest pain in children and adolescents, *Pediatr Ann* 15:685-694, 1986.

Friedman GD, Siegelaub AB, Dales LG: Cigarette smoking and chest pain, *Ann Intern Med* 83:1-7, 1975.

Heinz GJ, Zavaia DC: Slipping rib syndrome: diagnosis using the "hooking maneuver," *JAMA* 237:794-795, 1977.

Kashani JH, Lababidi Z, Jones RS: Depression in children and adolescents with cardiovascular symptomatology: the significance of chest pain, *J Am Acad Child Psychiatry* 21:187-189, 1982.

Katon W, Hall ML, Russo J, et al: Chest pain: relationship of psychiatric illness to coronary arteriographic results, *Am J Med* 84:1-9, 1988.

Lum L: Hyperventilation: the tip of the iceberg, *J Psychosom Res* 19:375-383, 1975.

Miller AJ, Texidor TA: "Precordial catch," a neglected syndrome of precordial pain, *JAMA* 159:1364-1365, 1955.

Pantell RH, Goodman BW: Adolescent chest pain: a prospective study, *Pediatrics* 71:881-886, 1983.

Savage DD, Devereux RB, Garrison RJ, et al: Mitral valve prolapse in the general population. Part 2, Clinical features: the Framingham Study, *Am Heart J* 106:577-581, 1983.

Selbst SM: Evaluation of chest pain in children, *Pediatr Rev* 8:56-62, 1986.

Sharkey AM, Clark BJ: Common complaints with cardiac implications in children, *Pediatr Clin North Am* 38:657-666, 1991.

4

Persistent Crying and Colic

MARK J. MENDELSOHN

Key Points

- Persistent crying or colic is common, affecting up to 20% of healthy infants, beginning after the first 3 weeks postnatally, lasting longer than 3 hours per day, and occurring at least 3 days per week up to 3 months of age.

- Although food allergy, particularly milk or formula intolerance, is commonly blamed for causing colic, few children actually benefit from eliminating milk from the diet.

- A calm but thorough approach and physical examination usually allow the physician to determine if serious medical disorders are causing irritability and permit reassurance when appropriate.

Persistent crying or colic in infancy is a common problem estimated to occur in 10% to 20% of healthy infants. The definition of colic is probably best illustrated in the classic article by Wessel and associates. They defined paroxysmal fussing (colic) as spells of unexplained fussiness or crying, beginning in the first 3 weeks postnatally, lasting longer than 3 hours per day, 3 days per week, and continuing for more than 3 weeks in infants younger than 3 months old. In this chapter the terms *colic* and *persistent crying* are used interchangeably because they are comparable in the literature. Acute, unexplained crying is also discussed because colic is only one of many explanations for the crying infant. The cause of colic has not been determined, despite fairly extensive investigation. Most likely, infants cry for a multitude of reasons. Crying is an early means of communication, but it may be prolonged by inappropriate parental responses to an infant, who by temperament becomes agitated when his or her needs are not met. Many early observers proposed that the gastrointestinal tract was the primary source of colic. Anyone who deals with infants on a regular basis has seen them draw up their knees

against a tense abdomen, cry, and expel flatus; occasionally the abdomen appears mildly distended. The term *colic* comes from the Greek *kōlikos*, meaning colon, so the term has an inherent bias. Allergic reactions to cow's milk protein have been implicated as a cause of colic. However, it appears that only a minority of infants benefit from a formula change. Finally, crying may be a developmental or maturational stage, and as infants reach 3 to 4 months of age, crying becomes more differentiated and more easily understood by parents. In this chapter the pathophysiology, background, and approach to the crying infant are explored fully.

Pathophysiology

It is important to emphasize that colic is *unexplained* crying, and the clinician must consider a wide differential diagnosis before labeling an infant as having colic (Table 4-1). Infant crying is generally considered to signal an unmet need. It may signal that an infant is hungry, needs attention, or is in distress. Numerous studies have found two crying peaks. The first, a daily peak, reaches a maximum in the late afternoon and evening. The second, a developmental peak, relates to a gradual increase in crying from birth to approximately 6 weeks of age. Beyond 3 months of age both the quantity and pattern of crying change. There is a decrease in the evening peak and a reduction in the overall quantity of crying. Crying appears to change its function because it becomes more intentional and less reflexive.

The infant's temperament may be an inherently important feature of colic. Infants also may exhibit other responses to their environment that demonstrate their uniqueness. Such responses include poor adaptability, withdrawal, and irregularity of their biologic functions. It is also possible that postpartum disturbances in maternal mood are associated with changes in infant behavior. In one study, maternal mood was related to the quantity and intensity of infant crying. Mothers who report excessive crying are also likely to perceive a lack of positive reinforcement from the infant. Colicky infants may

TABLE 4-1

Differential Diagnosis of Persistent Crying

Causes of chronic, persistent crying	Clues to the diagnosis
Milk-protein allergy	Vomiting, diarrhea, family history
Increased intracranial pressure	Full fontanelle, papilledema
Child abuse	Bruising, unsupported history, fractures
Metabolic	Intermittent lethargy, emesis
Colic	Pattern/timing of cry
Cardiac	
Supraventricular tachycardia	Diaphoresis, poor feeding
Central Nervous System	
Arnold-Chiari type 1 malformation	Posturing, abnormal neurologic examination
Brain or spinal cord tumor	Neurologic examination
Malformations	Dysmorphic appearance, delayed development

be temperamentally more difficult and less adaptable. Parents may have difficulty recognizing the infant's needs, resulting in interventions that do not soothe but may actually enhance the crying behavior.

Several organic causes to explain persistent crying have been proposed, most prominently an adverse reaction to cow's milk protein in a variable percentage of infants. Numerous studies have examined this hypothesis but have produced contradictory results.

Investigators from Malmo, Sweden, implicated cow's milk protein as a significant cause of colic in bottle-fed and breast-fed infants. Of the colicky infants, 71% improved when given a cow's milk–free formula, and 51% had an adverse reaction to soy formula. Furthermore, 36% of the infants reacted with colic at the reintroduction of cow's milk formula. In a separate study, 66 breast-feeding mothers were placed on a diet free of cow's milk and the colic disappeared in 35 infants; it reappeared in 35% of the infants when cow's milk was reintroduced into the mothers' diets. Forsythe investigated the effect of formula changes in colicky infants. He used a double-blind, multiple-crossover design and showed that in some instances colic improves with formula changes. However, the effect diminishes with time and is rarely reproducible. Sampson criticized many of the studies that examined cow's milk protein as a cause of colic, describing several design flaws, including insufficient blinding of the investigators, an inadequate number of patients enrolled, and inappropriate washout times and repeated challenges to control for spontaneous resolution. He concluded that food allergy or intolerance may cause increased crying in some (12% to 15%) colicky infants. A 2- to 3-month trial of a hypoallergenic formula may be warranted in some colicky infants, but parents should not be given the idea that their infant will have long-term food allergies. Other studies showed that parental counseling was more effective than dietary change in improving infant colic.

Other dietary sources of infant colic are possible, such as carbohydrate malabsorption. Moore and others found that colicky infants had increased breath hydrogen responses to lactose-containing milk. Possible explanations included increased lactose malabsorption or a difference in the colonic gas.

Review of the available studies suggests that food allergy or intolerance may cause increased crying in a minority of colicky infants. Changing formulas may serve only to further confuse and frustrate parents as their infant continues to exhibit excessive crying. A single change to a lactose-free, hydrolyzed protein formula may be helpful in a small minority of cases.

Background

In the classic 1954 article by Wessel and associates, four main theories of colic were espoused: congenital hypertonicity of the intestinal tract, allergy, immaturity of the intestinal tract, and transfer of tension from adults to the infant. Treatments recommended included motion, drugs (alcohol, phenobarbital, antihistamines), change of diet, warmth and pressure to the abdomen, monotonous noise, increased caloric intake, and enemas. Obviously, not much has changed in 40 years. In addition to their classic definition of colic, they note the possible presence of family tension in some cases. Brazelton's 1962 study of crying infants included 80 mothers and their newborns. He noted an average of $2\frac{1}{2}$ hours of crying per day during the first 7 weeks, most commonly in the early evening, with gradual reduction in each subsequent week. Brazelton hypothesized that a certain amount of crying is necessary, and the pediatrician's role is to reassure parents. An infant's early cry has physiologic significance. It expands pulmonary capacity and may discharge accumulated tension, which is stored from internal and external stimuli acting on the newborn. As the infant matures and uses other means to respond to the environment, crying represents a more specific need (i.e., hunger, fatigue, boredom, etc.). At this point, usually around 3 months of age, crying decreases as the infant and parent more easily respond to each other's cues.

In his 1966 prospective study, Paradise studied 146 newborns and demonstrated that there was no evidence to support the assertion that colic results from an "unfavorable emotional climate," a common belief held at the time. Paradise used the Minnesota Multiphasic Personality Inventory and showed that mothers of colicky infants did not exhibit higher ratings for anxiety, depression, or other emotional factors.

Recent researchers have emphasized normal crying curves for infants. Barr has proposed five featurees of normal crying. First, there is a progressive increase in crying that peaks in the second month. Second, there is a clustering of crying in the evening hours, peaking in the second month. Third, there is much individual variability during the crying peak. Fourth, there is a large degree of individual variability from day to day, and finally, early crying is usually not modifiable by differences in caretaking style.

As more researchers studied the problem of persistent crying, it became evident that a tool was necessary for accurate verification of crying behavior. The literature on colic has been difficult to interpret because of the variable definitions of excessive crying. More recent definitions have further defined excessive crying as follows: lasting longer than 3 hours per day, resulting in parental concern, and expressing distress that parents report as inconsolable. Barr examined a 24-hour diary versus an audiotape for reliability. The results validate parental diaries of crying. These findings have been supported by other investigators. Hill and others demonstrated the utility of a distress diary in the identification of infants with colic. The diary had a sensitivity of 77% and a specificity of 87%. This allows greater reproducibility in research on infant crying.

The role of allergy has also been studied. In a double-blind, multiple-crossover study, Forsythe demonstrated that in some instances colic improves with elimination of cow's milk formula. However, the effect diminishes over time and is rarely reproducible. Others have also looked at formula changes but found that modification of the parent-infant interaction was more important than formulary changes. The role of allergy in infantile colic is explored further in the section on pathophysiology.

Recently, investigators have stressed that crying behavior is an infant's first attempt at verbal communication. Colic may represent an infant's increasingly inconsolable response to a parent's inappropriate reaction to initial crying. Some cases of persistent crying may represent a stressed parent-infant relationship, and maternal emotional distress may correlate with infant crying behavior. As mentioned previously, mothers who report excessive infant crying are more likely than other mothers to perceive lack of positive reinforcement from their infants.

Differential Diagnosis

The differential diagnosis of persistent crying is best split into chronic, persistent crying (Table 4-1) and acute, unexplained crying (Table 4-2). Before labeling an infant as colicky, it is crucial for the clinician to consider a wide range of causes so that a serious, treatable cause is not overlooked. The following discussion concentrates on the treatable causes of acute, unexplained crying, which is best defined

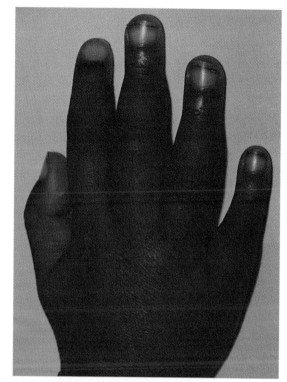

FIG. 4-1 Dactylitis (hand-foot syndrome) in a 3-year-old girl with sickle-cell disease. This syndrome, which affects primarily toddlers, is seen less frequently in older children after the bone marrow of the small bones of the hands loses hematopoietic activity. This loss of marrow activity is due to cortical thickening from increased use of hands and weight bearing by the feet.

as an episode lasting longer than any previous crying episode or more than 2 hours. Because first episodes of prolonged crying behavior may be truly acute (or become chronic), a broad initial differential diagnosis is critical. The following section concentrates on single, prolonged episodes of crying.

Infectious Diseases

Infectious disease appears to be the most common cause of unexplained crying behavior. A recent prospective study from Denver describes 56 infants who were brought to an emergency department during a 1-year period because of an episode of excessive crying without fever. Otitis media was the most common diagnosis, but other causes were also noted. Two infants had excessive crying early in the course of a viral illness. One infant's crying preceded the development of an episode of gastroenteritis by several hours. Cases of herpangina and herpetic stomatitis were also seen. Urinary tract infection without fever was diagnosed, demonstrating the importance of a urinalysis in the evaluation of unexplained crying. Osteomyelitis may cause crying without other constitutional symptoms, as can vasoocclusive crisis in an infant with sickle-cell disease (Fig. 4-1).

TABLE 4-2

Differential Diagnosis of Acute, Unexplained Crying

Causes of acute, unexplained crying	Clues to the diagnosis	Causes of acute, unexplained crying	Clues to the diagnosis
Infectious Disease		**Central Nervous System—cont'd**	
Otitis media	Pneumatic otoscopy	Meningitis/encephalitis	Altered mental status
Viral illness	History and examination	Pseudotumor cerebri	Papilledema, other causes of increased ICP
Gastroenteritis	History and examination		
Herpangina	Examination	Arnold-Chiari type 1 malformation	Neck arching, posturing
Herpetic stomatitis	Examination		
Urinary tract infection	Enhanced urinalysis (Gram stain and WBC)	**Medications**	
		Antihistamines	Paradoxical irritability
Osteomyelitis	Point tenderness to palpation	Pseudoephedrine	High blood pressure
		Phenobarbital	Behavioral changes
		Ethanol withdrawal	Irritability
Trauma		Neonatal narcotic withdrawal	Irritability, diaphoresis, restlessness
Subdural hematoma	Abnormal examination, retinal hemorrhages	DTP reaction	Temporal association
Fracture	Swelling, tenderness, pseudoparalysis	**Metabolic**	
Burn/bite	Examination	Glutaric aciduria type 1	Dystonia
Ocular or oral foreign body	Everted eyelids, oral inspection	Partial OTC deficiency	Intermittent behavioral changes, emesis
Corneal abrasion	Tearing, photophobia	Sickle-cell disease, vasoocclusive crisis	Dactylitis
Hair tourniquet syndrome	Close digital inspection		
Gastrointestinal Tract		**Cardiac**	
Constipation	Rectal examination	Supraventricular tachycardia	Poor feeding, diaphoresis
Intussusception	Intermittent irritability, lethargy, abdominal mass	Congestive heart failure	Poor feeding, diaphoresis, tachypnea
Gastroesophageal reflux	Posturing during feeding		
Gastric rupture	Peritoneal signs	**Behavioral**	
		Night terrors	Unaware of surroundings
Central Nervous System		Overstimulation	History
Subdural hematoma	Abnormal neurologic examination, check retinas	Night awakenings	Frequent in second half of the first year of life
Brain tumor	ICP signs, vomiting, behavioral changes		

CBC, Complete blood count; *DTP*, diphtheria-tetanus-pertussis vaccine; *ICP*, intracranial pressure; *OTC*, ornithine transcarbamylase; *WBC*, white blood cell.

Trauma

The examiner should always consider trauma in the differential diagnosis of the crying infant, whether it is accidental or more ominously nonaccidental. Infants with subdural hematomas may present to a physician's office with only persistent crying and may not have an altered mental status or seizures. Clues to the diagnosis include a history that does not adequately explain injuries and evidence of a chaotic social situation. A thorough neurologic examination, including a retinal examination, is mandatory (Fig. 4-2).

Crying may be the only clue to a long bone fracture (Figs. 4-3 and 4-4). Other diagnoses to consider under the category of trauma include burns, ocular or oral foreign bodies, corneal abrasions, bites, and hair tourniquet syndrome (Fig. 4-5).

Gastrointestinal Tract

In the Denver study, three infants with previously undiagnosed constipation improved after a diagnostic and therapeu-

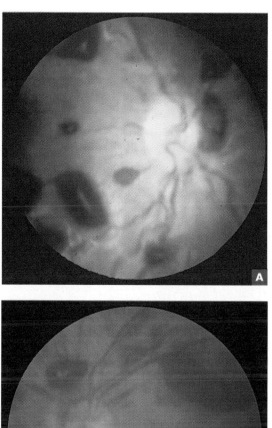

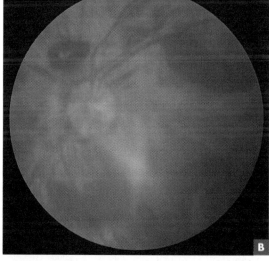

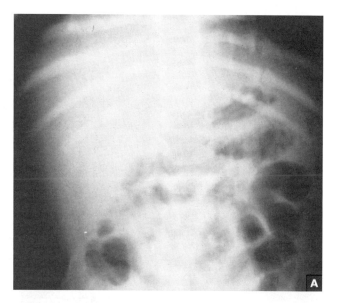

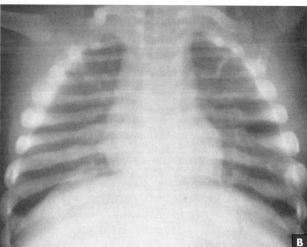

FIG. 4-2 *A,* Multiple retinal hemorrhages are seen on fundu-scopic examination of this infant who was a victim of shaken baby syndrome. Subdural hematoma and multiple metaphyseal "shake" fractures are typical associated findings. *B,* Shaken baby syndrome. Multiple retinal hemorrhages are present in the posterior fundus. There are small flame-shaped hemorrhages within the nerve fiber layer that follow the pattern of the retinal vessels. More extensive areas of hemorrhage have broken through to the preretinal space and are seen as areas of blood that obscure the retina. A Roth spot, a hemorrhage with a white center, is visible just above the optic disc. The white re-flection from the camera flash is visible because of dispersed RBCs within the vitreous. (*A* Courtesy Dr. Stephen Ludwig, Chil-dren's Hospital of Philadelphia.)

FIG. 4-3 Rib fractures. *A,* This infant was seen because of a his-tory of vomiting and irritability. An abdominal film obtained to rule out intestinal obstruction showed a normal bowel gas pat-tern but revealed multiple posterior rib fractures in various stages of healing, which were missed. *B,* When the infant was finally tracked down 2 months later, her chest x-ray film showed in excess of 20 healing rib fractures, some posterior and others anterolateral. (Courtesy the Department of Radiology, Children's Hospital of Pittsburgh.)

tic rectal examination was performed. Intussusception may present early without vomiting or diarrhea, and an infant may exhibit only intermittent irritability (Fig. 4-6). Gastro-esophageal reflux with esophagitis may cause excessive cry-ing, but there should be other clues to this diagnosis (Box 4-1).

For example, an infant without vomiting may demonstrate pos-tural changes during feedings or primary respiratory symp-toms (stridor, reflex-mediated apnea, or intermittent wheez-ing). Spontaneous gastric rupture may occur after excessive, vigorous crying.

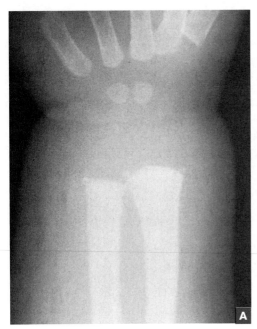
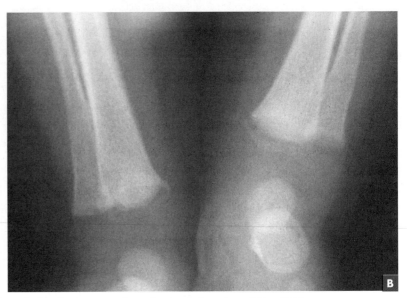

FIG. 4-4 What appear to be metaphyseal chip fractures on the anteroposterior view of the distal radius and ulna *(A)* are actually bucket-handle fractures as shown in this oblique view of both distal tibias *(B)*. The fracture lines traverse the entire width of the distal metaphyses and are a result of violent shaking. (*A* Courtesy the Department of Radiology, Children's Hospital of Pittsburgh; *B* courtesy Dr. Bruce Rosenthal, The Mercy Hospital of Pittsburgh.)

Central Nervous System

Again, it is important to emphasize that nonaccidental trauma can result in serious central nervous system pathology. Subdural hematoma should be considered, as should causes of increased intracranial pressure (ICP) (Fig. 4-7). The anterior fontanelle is usually open in infancy and can be a "window" to the diagnosis. Increased ICP can occur with trauma, tumor, or infection. Pseudotumor cerebri was diagnosed in the Denver study but can be considered only after imaging studies and lumbar puncture rule out other causes of increased ICP. An interesting case report describes an infant who had persistent crying; an extensive evaluation revealed an Arnold-Chiari type 1 malformation. In retrospect the history revealed intermittent episodes of neck arching, probably representing pain originating in the posterior fossa.

Medications

Side effects of common over-the-counter (OTC) medications may result in excessive crying, and only a careful history may illuminate the cause of the behavior. Antihistamines and many OTC cough preparations may cause irritability and hyperkinesis. Pseudoephedrine overdose has been reported, and anticonvulsants, such as phenobarbital, are associated with behavioral changes. Other medications may cause idiosyncratic reactions; thus it is crucial to question the family regarding the presence of any prescription or OTC preparations in the household. The pertussis compo-

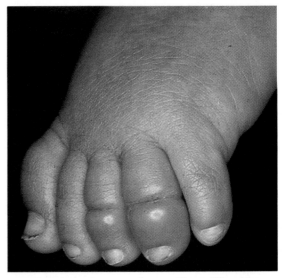

FIG. 4-5 Hair tourniquet syndrome. The mild erythema and edema of the third and fourth toes are the result of constriction by hairs that accidentally became wrapped around them. (Courtesy Dr. Thomas J. Daley, Bronx-Lebanon Hospital.)

nent of the diphtheria-pertussis-tetanus (DPT) vaccine has been implicated in rare cases of persistent crying. In a recent Institute of Medicine report, unusual, prolonged crying was judged to be temporarily related with DPT injection, but the incidence was extremely low.

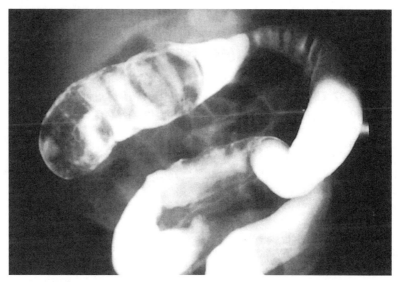

FIG. 4-6 Intussusception. Barium outlines the intussuscepted segment. Unfortunately, this lesion required laparotomy because reduction did not occur during the barium enema.

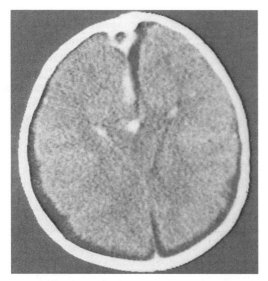

FIG. 4-7 Subdural hematomas in the shaken baby syndrome. This CT scan reveals subdural hematomas along the falx and over the cerebral convexities. These are seen as a dark rim along the falx and between the bony calvarium and the brain substance. (Courtesy the Division of Neuroradiology, University Health Center of Pittsburgh.)

BOX 4-1

Presentations of Gastroesophageal Reflux

Regurgitation
"Spitting," rumination
Emesis
Failure to thrive

Esophagitis
Irritability
Colic
Hiccups
Anemia
Hematemesis
Stricture
Protein-losing enteropathy
Melena, occult blood loss

Behavioral
Dystonic posturing
Sandifer syndrome

Respiratory
Wheezing, asthma
Recurrent pneumonia
Aspiration
Laryngospasm
Apnea

Neurologic
Seizure-like episodes

Other
Clubbing of digits
Sudden infant death syndrome or apparent life-threatening event

Other

Rare metabolic causes of persistent crying have been reported. An infant with partial ornithine transcarbamylase deficiency had excessive crying. Infants with glutaricaciduria type 1 may be irritable but also exhibit other neurologic signs, such as dystonia, that should lead to further evaluation. Infants with cardiac disease may exhibit crying behavior. Supraventricular tachycardia may be associated with irritability, poor feeding, and diaphoresis. Congestive heart failure in infancy usually produces signs or symptoms in addition to fussiness, such as failure to thrive, poor feeding, tachycardia, diaphoresis, cough, or tachypnea. Finally, infants with certain behavioral responses may cry excessively as an adaptation to their environment. Night awakenings are more common in the second half of the first year. Occasionally, overstimulation of an infant may result in persistent crying.

Table 4-2 summarizes the differential diagnosis of acute, unexplained crying.

History

As with most clinical encounters the history is vital to understanding the potential cause(s) of infant crying. Parents caring for an infant who cries excessively are usually distraught and anxious. A calm but concerned demeanor by the clinician does much to help obtain a thorough history. The quality and duration of the cry are important because some parents' tolerance is very low, thus any amount of crying is considered alarming. As stated earlier, colic usually does not become evident until 2 to 3 weeks of age, so the physician should be especially cautious in the evaluation of a crying infant before this age. It is vital to understand the pattern and timing of the cry. Does the infant cry more in the evening? Is the cry associated with other symptoms? How have the caretakers tried to quiet the infant? Have they overstimulated the baby? The amount of time spent crying can be useful information. Has a diary documented the number of hours the infant cries? When does the baby cry most? How do the parents intervene? Do they respond to the cry immediately or allow the infant time to expend energy? Temporal associations with feeding, sleep, activity, and stool and urine output may suggest a plan of intervention.

Inquiry about weight gain, feeding practices, such as overfeeding and underfeeding, and the stability of the social situation should be made. What is the infant's diet? Have other foods been introduced? Is there a change in posture, such as back or neck arching, that could indicate the pain associated with esophagitis?

A thorough review of systems should be obtained, with special emphasis on constitutional symptoms. Questions should be asked about fever, rash, vomiting, diarrhea, constipation, cough, choking or gagging, and color changes. A pregnancy history can be helpful, checking for any risk factors for infection, such as premature rupture of the membranes, maternal fever, or prematurity. The practitioner may need to inquire about illicit drug use or alcohol intake because withdrawal reactions may be expressed as persistent crying.

Are there any problems at home that may be masked by the persistent crying? Is the relationship between the parents being affected, or is it contributory to the infant's behavior? After probing for possible factors that may be involved in ongoing excessive crying, the examiner can then address issues that may alter the behavior and improve the parent-infant interactions.

Because child abuse is so prevalent in our society, it may be insightful to explore the parents' histories. Do they have histories of abuse or neglect? What support systems are available? Families exposed to abusive caretakers may not have the appropriate tools available to attempt different intervention strategies. They may have only impulsive reactions to the incessantly crying infant. Asking how the crying makes the caretaker feel may allow an opportunity to explore potential abusive behavior.

The history should either assure the clinician that the crying behavior is chronic or recurrent or alert him or her that a more detailed examination is prudent. In 20% of the infants in the Denver study the history provided useful clues to the diagnosis, although additional evaluation and/or follow-up were essential.

Physical Examination

Observation and inspection of the infant and caretakers may offer many clues as to the cause of the crying. The interactions between the parents and the infant may offer information regarding their coping mechanisms. Growth measurements demonstrate adequate nutrition and may offer a clue to organic disease. Inspection of the infant's skin may demonstrate unusual bruises, or how the infant flexes or extends an extremity may signify possible trauma.

If a thorough physical examination is not revealing, certain directed procedures should be performed. Careful examination of all extremities for tenderness or a hair tourniquet may be diagnostic (Fig. 4-5). It is important to examine the infant with all of his or her clothes removed because subtle bruises, burns, or bites are more apparent. Any bruise is abnormal in an infant, and patterns of bruising must be defined in toddlers. Otoscopic examination demonstrates an inflamed tympanic membrane if an infant is crying because of otitis media. The examiner should document landmarks, colors, and mobility of the tympanic membrane when evaluating for an abnormality.

Inspection of the eyes should also include eversion of the eyelids because a foreign body may be present. Retinal examination by indirect ophthalmoscopy helps diagnose shaken baby syndrome if retinal hemorrhages are noted. Again, careful inspection of the oropharynx may demonstrate a foreign body. Occasionally, laryngoscopy may be necessary to diagnose a hypopharyngeal foreign body if an infant winces when swallowing. Fluorescein staining of the corneas demonstrates corneal abrasions if present, even if the infant has no symptoms referable to the eyes.

A careful neurologic examination may provide a clue to the cause of the crying. A tense anterior fontanelle may signify increased intracranial pressure, which may be seen in pseudotumor cerebri, meningitis, or an intracranial mass. Increased muscle tone and hyperreflexia may be noted if there is an abnormality in the spinal cord or lower brainstem. The infant's mental status and degree of consolability are important indicators. Again, it is always vital to consider nonaccidental trauma because a life-threatening intracranial injury may present with focal neurologic findings.

Approach to the Patient

A careful history, physical examination, and a limited number of diagnostic studies are the primary requirements in the evaluation of the crying infant. It is crucial to separate acute versus chronic crying and to have a clear understanding of the age when the infant develops the symptoms.

The syndrome of colic does not usually become evident until 2 to 3 weeks of age, so persistent crying in the neonate less than 2 weeks of age should prepare the clinician to search for other causes. Again, colic tends to have two peaks—a daily peak and a developmental peak, which relates to an increased amount of crying in the second month of life. It is crucial to question the parents' response to the crying because their attempts may inadvertently increase the severity of the crying. Many parents switch formulas frequently as they search for a way to decrease the undesired behavior. As discussed in the pathophysiology section a small minority of colicky infants actually have a true protein allergy or formula intolerance, and the examiner should look for clues to this possibility. Helpful hints include a family history of allergy, vomiting or diarrhea, eczema, or eosinophilia. Occasionally a formula change may be indicated, though it rarely results in a long-lasting positive response. Some experts recommend a casein-hydrolysate formula if a change is indicated. If it appears that a breast-feeding infant is reacting to the milk protein in the maternal diet, a dairy-free maternal diet may be indicated.

A number of studies have shown the benefit of modifying the parent-infant interaction. An important first step is to have the parents keep a behavior diary, which allows the clinician to quantitate the crying and evaluate the pattern and parental responses to the crying infant. Parents should be asked to record how much time the infant spends sleeping alone; sleeping in the arms of an adult; awake, alone, and happy; awake, held, and happy; awake, alone, and crying; and awake, held, and crying. Parents should also record how much time the infant spends in each of these states and their response to each crying episode. The diary is analyzed, and the parents are then counseled to initiate one of the five following actions: (1) attempt to feed the infant, (2) allow the infant to suck on a pacifier, (3) hold the infant, (4) stimulate and play with the baby, or (5) see if the infant is tired and wants to sleep. If the crying continues for more than 5 minutes after one attempt, then another is tried. A recent study demonstrated the effectiveness of a behavioral approach supervised by trained lay personnel in counseling parents of colicky infants.

If after a thorough history and physical examination the clinician has been unable to discover the cause of the crying, additional testing may be necessary. Urinalysis and urine culture may demonstrate an occult urinary tract infection. An enhanced urinalysis has a high positive predictive value, and if dysuria and bacteriuria are present, a catheterized urine sample should be sent for culture. Laboratory studies, such as a serum glucose, electrolyte measurements, complete blood count, and blood urea nitrogen levels, are not helpful unless the clinician suspects abnormalities based on the history and physical examination.

Other studies are indicated when supported by the initial history and examination. Roentgenograms may reveal a fracture suspected during palpation of a tender extremity. A computed tomographic (CAT) scan of the head, barium enema, ECG, or metabolic study occasionally may be indicated to uncover the correct diagnosis. It is important to be specific; only those tests that confirm a diagnosis suggested by history or examination should be performed.

SUMMARY

Causes of infant crying can best be divided into acute, unexplained crying and chronic, persistent crying. This allows the clinician to consider a wide range of conditions when faced with a crying infant.

A complete history and careful examination should suggest the proper diagnosis in most cases.

Occasionally a small number of infants require an extended period of observation. This may occur during hospitalization or close follow-up for families known to be reliable. In some cases the crying may improve during the observation period, and no further evaluation is required. However, the thoughtful clinician usually discovers the cause of the persistent crying and offers specific recommendations to treat the underlying disorder.

ILLUSTRATIVE CASES

Case 1. S.N. is a 3-month-old infant first seen for fussiness and abdominal discomfort. There were no perinatal complications. She was breast-fed for the first month. She has been on a cow's milk–based formula since 1 month of age. S.N. cries frequently, with an evening peak. There is no emesis, and stools occur once a day. Good weight gain is present. The family history is unrevealing. Mild seborrhea is noted on the examination; otherwise the baby appears healthy. An elemental formula is initiated, and the family notes a significant improvement in her fussiness.

This case reflects the typical presentation of an infant with colic. She is 3 months of age, a time when persistent crying tends to improve regardless of the mode of intervention. An elemental formula is introduced, significantly decreasing the infant's crying. However, if an elemental formula is used to treat colic, it is good practice to return the infant to a cow's milk–based formula later in the first year of life, unless other signs or symptoms of protein intolerance are noted.

Case 2. At 8 weeks of age, J.L. has frequent episodes of fussiness and crying spells. He was a full-term infant who was noted to be "cranky" beginning at 1 week of age. He *also had frequent episodes of emesis and would draw his legs up to his abdomen and cry. Frequent formula changes were attempted. Some improvement was noted with decreased episodes of emesis when placed on an elemental formula. The crying persisted, and the infant was begun on an H_2 receptor antagonist and a prokinetic agent for presumed gastroesophageal reflux. The infant's crying persisted, and by the family's estimation, he cried 75% of the day. Growth rate and physical examination are normal. A parental diary is initiated, and parents are counseled to help decrease the infant's excessive crying. The family documents improvement in behavior and is able to intervene more successfully and decrease the frequency of the excessive crying.*

This case demonstrates that crying and fussiness in an infant require that the clinician complete a full assessment because other problems, such as gastroesophageal reflux, may contribute to the infant's symptoms. The parents still benefited from the advice on active intervention and were able to decrease the frequency and intensity of the crying to a more manageable level.

Case 3. *J.S. presented at 2 months of age with a 3-hour history of inconsolability. She has never cried for such a prolonged period of time. There is no history of fever, rash, vomiting, change in stool pattern, or exposure to illness. Previous growth and development had been normal. An initial general examination revealed an irritable baby, but no focal abnormalities were evident. On closer inspection there is swelling and subtle erythema of the third finger of the left hand. A hair tourniquet is removed, and by the next day the infant's finger is without swelling or tenderness.*

This case is an example of an infant with an acute, initially unexplained episode of persistent crying. On cursory examination the hair tourniquet was not noted. After a second, more detailed inspection, the hair was found and removed, resulting in cessation of J.S.'s irritability.

ANNOTATED BIBLIOGRAPHY

Brazelton BT: Crying in infancy, *Pediatrics* 29:579-588, 1962.
  This is a classic study of 80 mother-infant pairs.

Forsythe BWC: Colic and the effect of changing formulas: a double-blind, multiple-crossover study, *J Pediatr* 115:521-525, 1989.
  In some instances colic improves with elimination of cow's milk formula, but the effect diminishes over time and is rarely reproducible.

Poole SR: The infant with acute, unexplained, excessive crying, *Pediatrics* 88:450-455, 1991.
  A prospective study of 56 infants who were treated at an emergency department over a 1-year period. Of the infants, 75% could be diagnosed after a careful history and physical examination. A limited number of diagnostic studies were necessary for the remainder of the infants.

BIBLIOGRAPHY

Barr RG: The normal crying curve: what do we really know? *Dev Med Child Neurol* 32:356-362, 1990.

Barr RG, Kramer MS, Boisjoly C, et al: Parental diary of infant cry and fuss behavior, *Arch Dis Child* 63:380-387, 1988.

Daniellsson B, Hwang CP: Treatment of infantile colic with surface active substance (simethicone), *Acta Paediatr Scand* 74:446-450, 1985.

Hill DJ, Menahem S, Hudson I, et al: Charting infant distress: an aid to defining colic, *J Pediatr* 121:755-758, 1992.

Hoberman A, Wald ER, Penchansky L, et al: Enhanced urinalysis as a screening test for urinary tract infection, *Pediatrics* 91(6):1196-1199, 1993.

Jakobsson I, Lindberg T: Cow's milk proteins cause infantile colic in breast-fed infants: a double-blind crossover study, *Pediatrics* 71:268-271, 1983.

Listernick R, Tornita T: Persistent crying in infancy as a presentation of Chiari type I malformation, *J Pediatr* 118:567-569, 1991.

Lothe L, Lindberg T, Jakobsson I: Cow's milk formula as a cause of infantile colic: a double-blind study, *Pediatrics* 70:7-10, 1982.

Moore DJ, Robb TA, Davidson GP: Breath hydrogen response to milk containing lactose in colicky and noncolicky infants, *J Pediatr* 113:979-984, 1988.

Paradise JL: Maternal and other factors in the etiology of infantile colic: report of a prospective study of 146 infants, *JAMA* 197:191-199, 1966.

Sampson HA: Infantile colic and food allergy: fact or fiction? *J Pediatr* 115:583-584, 1989.

St James-Roberts I: Annotation: persistent crying in infancy, *J Child Psychiatry* 30:189-195, 1989.

Taubman B: A new answer to the old question of colic, *Contemp Pediatr* 8:44-63, 1991.

Taubman B: Clinical trial of the treatment of colic by modification of parent-infant interaction, *Pediatrics* 998-1003, 1984.

Taubman B: Parental counseling compared with elimination of cow's milk or soy milk protein for the treatment of infant colic syndrome: a randomized trial, *Pediatrics* 81:756-761, 1988.

Wessel MA, Cobb JC, Jackson EB: Paroxysmal fussing in infancy, sometimes called 'colic,' *Pediatrics* 14:421-433, 1954.

Wolke D, Gray P, Meyer R: Excessive infant crying: a controlled study of mothers helping mothers, *Pediatrics* 94:322-332, 1994.

5

Recurrent and Chronic Headaches

SARA C. McINTIRE

 ## Key Points

- Migraine and tension-type headaches account for the majority of recurrent and chronic headaches in pediatric patients.

- Patients with chronic and progressive headaches who have neurologic signs or symptoms need immediate evaluation for serious intracranial pathology.

- Imaging studies of the brain are least useful in patients with chronic nonprogressive headache and are most useful in patients with certain types of acute recurrent headache and in all patients with chronic progressive headache.

Headache is a demanding symptom often reported to physicians. Recurrent and chronic headaches disturb patients and their families, who may insist that physicians evaluate the complaint with laboratory tests and imaging studies. However, migraine and tension-type headaches account for most recurrent and chronic headaches. An accurate diagnosis follows from a detailed history and physical examination. Indiscriminate use of tests is never justified and invites frustration when all studies are normal and no "cause" of the headache surfaces. These points are central to most major studies and reviews of pediatric headache and are the fundamental tenets of this chapter.

Literature Survey

According to the classic study by Bille, who published data from nearly 9000 Swedish school children in 1962, headache is a common complaint, occurring in up to 40% of children by age 7 years and up to 70% by age 15 years. More recent

data by Linet and others confirm the accuracy of these figures. With respect to recurrent headache in pediatric patients, migraine is common and well described in the pediatric literature. Headache from mass lesions is uncommon but well represented in the literature because of its serious nature and the repercussions of a delayed diagnosis. Tension-type headache (also called *muscle contraction headache*) predominantly affects adolescents and has recently emerged in the pediatric headache literature as an important entity.

Differential Diagnosis

A complete list of causes of recurrent and chronic headaches is long and cumbersome to organize. Rothner proposes a more useful and practical headache classification, using the temporal pattern of a headache. The patterns are (1) acute single headache, (2) acute recurrent headache, (3) chronic nonprogressive headache, and (4) chronic progressive headache. This chapter addresses only the last three patterns. Box 5-1 lists causes of recurrent and chronic headaches arranged by temporal pattern.

In the pediatric population, most acute recurrent headaches are migraines, most chronic nonprogressive headaches are tension-type, and most chronic progressive headaches result from traction on pain-sensitive elements in the central nervous system and accompany serious neurologic disorders. Some patients have more than one type of headache; for example, Rothner denotes patients with migraine superimposed upon tension-type headache as having a "mixed headache syndrome."

Acute Recurrent Headache

Most children and adolescents with headaches that recur episodically have migraine. Other common recurrent condi-

Recurrent and Chronic Headaches: Temporal Patterns

Acute Recurrent Headache

Migraine
Cluster headache
Acute sinusitis
Postictal headache
Hypertension
Intermittent hydrocephalus
Vascular malformation
Subarachnoid hemorrhage
Carbon monoxide poisoning

Chronic Nonprogressive Headache

Tension-type headache
Chronic sinusitis
Ocular disorder
Disorders of teeth and temporomandibular joint
Postlumbar puncture
Posttraumatic headache

Chronic Progressive Headache

Brain tumor
Hydrocephalus
Pseudotumor cerebri
Central nervous system infection
Vascular malformation
Subdural hematoma
Arnold-Chiari malformation
Lead poisoning

Modified from Rothner AD: Headaches in children: a review, *Headache* 18(3):169-175, 1978.

Forms of Migraine

Migraine Without Aura (Common Migraine)
Migraine With Aura (Classic Migraine)
Migraine With Neurologic Deficits (Complicated Migraine)
Ophthalmoplegic migraine
Hemiplegic migraine
Basilar artery migraine
Acute confusional migraine
"Alice in Wonderland" syndrome

Migraine Variants
Cyclic vomiting
Paroxysmal vertigo
Benign infantile torticollis

tions accompanied by headache, such as sinusitis, usually pose no dilemma in diagnosis. Hypertension, structural causes of recurrent headache (e.g., vascular malformations), and carbon monoxide poisoning are very uncommon in pediatric patients. They are important to detect because early treatment may be lifesaving.

Migraine

Migraine is the most common cause of acute recurrent headache in children and adolescents. It is a familial neurovascular disorder consisting of recurrent attacks of headache separated by pain-free intervals. The pathophysiology of migraine is unknown. The vascular theory of migraine ascribes the aura to vasoconstriction of cerebral arteries and the headache to subsequent vasodilation of the same vessels. However, Oleson and colleagues' recent studies of changes in cerebral blood flow during migraine have challenged this view. Currently, some propose that migraine re-

sults from a primary neuronal event, mediated by neurotransmitters, such as serotonin and substance P, with secondary vascular changes of inflammation and swelling. More details on the hypotheses of migraine pathogenesis are available in the references.

Prensky's criteria for the diagnosis of childhood migraine are recurrent headache, with no symptoms between attacks, accompanied by at least three of the following symptoms: recurrent abdominal pain, nausea or vomiting, presence of an aura, throbbing headache pain, unilateral pain, relief of headache by sleep, and a family history of migraine in close relatives. Motion sickness is common in childhood migraine and often precedes the onset of the headache. Recurrence is a requisite feature of migraine. When a patient suffers a severe headache with typical migraine features, the physician should exercise caution in diagnosis because other serious causes of an acute severe headache, such as hemorrhage or vascular malformation, may mimic migraine.

There are several forms of migraine: migraine without aura (common migraine); migraine with aura (classic migraine); migraine with neurologic deficits (complicated migraine); and migraine variants (cyclic vomiting, paroxysmal vertigo, and benign infantile torticollis) (Box 5-2).

Migraine without aura accounts for the majority of migraine headaches in children and adolescents. Although typical auras are absent, prodromal symptoms of fatigue, irritability, dizziness, tinnitus, or pallor occur. The location of the pain may be frontal, bifrontal, occipital, or unilateral parietotemporal. Patients with unilateral pain report that the pain changes sides. A fixed pain location raises concern for a structural lesion. The pain at the onset of the headache is mild but becomes severe within minutes to hours. The quality of the pain may be throbbing, pounding, aching, or constant. Nausea, vomiting, and abdominal pain are common features, and their severity may obscure the headache. The headache usually lasts for several hours, but on rare occasions it may last for several days. Although migraine may wake a patient from sleep, nocturnal or early morning headache is more typically associated with increased intracranial pressure, stemming from mass lesions of the central nervous system.

Migraine is worsened by sound, light, odors, or exercise and improved after rest or sleep in a dark room. Some patients feel better after vomiting. Triggers of migraine include fatigue, upper respiratory tract infection, caffeine consumption or withdrawal, alcohol intake, inadequate or excessive sleep, chocolate consumption, menstruation, birth control pills, pregnancy, head trauma, sunlight, and emotional stress. Some patients with migraine suffer their headache *after* a stressful event has ended. Once the headache subsides, however, many patients feel ill and tired—the "postdrome" of migraine. The physical and neurologic examinations are normal in patients with uncomplicated migraine.

Migraine with aura is a biphasic disorder in which the patient first receives a warning signal—the aura. The aura may be a visual, sensory, or motor phenomenon. Examples include blurred vision, scotomata, tunnel vision, dysesthesia, and weakness. The headache follows the aura and has the same features as migraine without aura.

Migraine with neurologic deficits is uncommon but important to recognize. This category includes ophthalmoplegic and hemiplegic migraine, basilar artery migraine, acute confusional migraine, and the "Alice in Wonderland" syndrome. Ophthalmoplegic migraine consists of severe ipsilateral headache or orbital pain, diplopia, blurred vision, and dysfunction of the third cranial nerve; outward eye deviation, ptosis, and sluggish reaction of the pupil to light are present on physical examination. Hemiplegic migraine presents as recurrent attacks of hemiplegia and headache, which is contralateral to the side of the weakness. Aphasia and numbness often accompany this type of migraine, and alternation of the affected side is expected. Basilar artery migraine consists of recurrent attacks of occipital headache associated with a variety of transient symptoms, such as nausea, vomiting, visual dimming, tinnitus, cranial nerve dysfunction, vertigo, ataxia, weakness, and syncope, that often precede the headache. Acute confusional migraine consists of recurrent attacks of abrupt-onset confusion, with or without headache, in which the confusion lasts for several hours and resolves without sequelae. Organic causes of headache, such as congenital berry aneurysm, arteriovenous malformation (AVM), brain tumor, seizure, inborn errors of metabolism, disorders of coagulation, or drug ingestion, must be excluded before making a diagnosis of complicated migraine.

There are several rare but well-described variants of migraine, including cyclic abdominal pain and vomiting, paroxysmal vertigo, and benign paroxysmal torticollis. Headache is often absent or a minor symptom at the onset of these variants. These clinical syndromes have been observed in patients previously diagnosed with migraine, in patients who subsequently developed migraine, and in patients with a family history of migraine.

Acute Sinusitis

Even though headache and facial pain may accompany bacterial infection of the paranasal sinuses, sinusitis is an uncommon cause of acute recurrent or chronic headache. The patient with acute onset of facial pain, frontal or maxillary headache, fever, nasal congestion, purulent rhinorrhea, and percussion tenderness over one or more sinuses has acute sinusitis. The diagnosis is straightforward and may be confirmed by plain radiographs or computed tomography scans of the paranasal sinuses.

Headache and Seizure

Headache after a seizure is common. It does not always indicate underlying structural lesions. However, headache preceding a seizure usually is associated with organic lesions. Migraine and seizure can occur in the same patient; when they do, structural lesions, such as AVM, must be excluded, especially if the migraine is complicated and/or the seizure is focal.

Structural Causes

Although most structural lesions of the central nervous system cause chronic progressive headache, acute recurrent headache may ensue from disorders that cause increased intracranial pressure intermittently. For example, a pedunculated mass within a ventricle may cause recurrent hydrocephalus with headache and vomiting. Congenital lesions, such as an Arnold-Chiari malformation, may produce the same effect. Occipital headache and aggravation of the pain by Valsalva maneuvers are prominent features in such patients. Increased intracranial pressure also arises from lesions that cause intermittent subarachnoid hemorrhage, such as AVM, congenital berry aneurysms, or arachnoid cysts. Whereas the "thunderclap" (sudden, intense) headache of an acute subarachnoid hemorrhage is easily recognized, a less severe headache results when only a small amount of blood leaks into the subarachnoid space. A detailed neurologic examination is mandatory; a cursory examination misses subtle findings indicative of a structural lesion.

Hypertension

Hypertension is a very uncommon cause of recurrent headache. Intermittent or sustained hypertension in a patient with headache points toward a serious renal, cardiac, endocrine, or malignant disorder as the cause. Patients with vasculitis or pheochromocytoma frequently have headache that closely resembles migraine. Measurement of blood pressure is therefore an essential part of evaluating any patient with headache.

Carbon Monoxide Poisoning

Carbon monoxide poisoning may result in recurrent headache. This diagnosis should be suspected if a patient complains of headache only in cold weather or after sleeping in a particular room or if the headache disappears in a new environment.

Cluster Headache

Cluster headache, rarely seen in a general pediatric practice, presents with a dramatic and distinctive constellation of symptoms. Patients experience brief attacks of severe, unilateral eye pain with ipsilateral tearing, conjunctival injection, and nasal congestion; attacks occur daily over several days to weeks. The attacks frequently occur at night, prompting concern for a structural lesion. Unlike migraine, cluster headache has no familial component, boys are affected more often than girls, the pain does not improve with rest, and gastrointestinal complaints are mild. Some patients exhibit miosis and ptosis on the symptomatic side during an attack; otherwise the physical examination is normal.

Chronic Nonprogressive Headache

Headache that persists but does not progress is usually benign. Nonetheless it greatly disturbs parents and patients who fear brain tumors or other serious illnesses.

Tension-Type Headache

Tension-type headache is the most common cause of chronic nonprogressive headache. This type of headache has other names, such as muscle contraction headache or stress headache. The cause of tension-type headache is unknown. A popular theory points to sustained contraction of the head and neck muscles as the cause of the headache. However, electromyographic studies of scalp muscles in headache patients challenge this hypothesis.

Tension-type headache is common in teenagers and very infrequent in younger children. Patients complain of daily headache for weeks to months. The headache lasts for most or all of the day. The pain is felt in the forehead, temples, occiput, or muscles of the neck; it is mild to moderate in severity and is a dull, squeezing, or pressure-like sensation. Patients fall asleep despite the pain and do not wake from sleep because of headache (although it may be present upon awakening.) Unlike migraine, tension-type headache is not significantly improved by rest or sleep. Auras are absent, but prodromal symptoms of fatigue, pallor, anorexia, and irritability are common. Nausea and vomiting do not occur regularly in tension-type headache as they do in migraine. Patients are able to function despite the pain. The physical examination in patients with tension-type headache is normal, although tenderness or spasm of scalp and neck muscles is often present.

Psychosocial stress is an important factor in many patients with tension-type headache. In the past the term *psychogenic headache* was applied to patients with chronic nonprogressive headache who were depressed or experiencing other psychologic disturbances, such as anxiety, school phobia, and conversion or somatization disorder. Typically these patients have headache that is tension-type in character, offer multiple somatic complaints upon review of systems, and have missed a great deal of school. Although some patients with tension-type headache have no psychologic difficulties, physicians must explore all social and emotional aspects of a patient's history to detect a primary psychologic disorder in a patient with chronic headache. Private interviews with the patient and the parents are essential for this purpose.

Chronic Sinusitis

Parents and even physicians often blame frequent headache on "sinus trouble." One must ask, however, if chronic sinusitis is a *common* cause of chronic headache. In reviews of headaches in pediatric patients, chronic sinusitis receives only modest attention and is deemed an unlikely cause in the absence of respiratory symptoms. However, Faleck and others reported a series of 15 patients with daily nonprogressive headache, minimal respiratory symptoms, and radiographic evidence of sinusitis who had total resolution of their headache after treatment with antibiotics and decongestants. Patients with chronic headache and risk factors for sinus disease, such as allergies, cystic fibrosis, immotile-cilia syndromes, or immunodeficiencies, merit careful evaluation for sinusitis even in the absence of prominent respiratory symptoms.

Ocular Disorders

Recurrent headache is often ascribed to ocular problems. However, eye strain resulting from uncorrected refractive errors or astigmatism, for example, is associated with eye pain more often than headache. The pain is induced by reading, playing video or computer games, watching television, and doing schoolwork. This complaint resolves with use of proper corrective lenses. Glaucoma is an uncommon cause of headache and more often causes severe eye pain.

Disorders of the Teeth and Temporomandibular Joint

Caries, dental abscesses, and temporomandibular joint (TMJ) dysfunction cause headaches but do so infrequently. They cause facial pain that is well localized to the affected area.

Postlumbar Puncture Headache

Headache after lumbar puncture occurs when there is a tear in the dura that allows cerebrospinal fluid (CSF) to leak into the epidural space. Patients complain of generalized or occipital headache and nausea when they sit or stand. Their symptoms improve when they lie down. Sometimes the history shows that the lumbar puncture was difficult to perform. The neurologic examination of affected patients is normal.

Posttraumatic Headache

Headache after minor head trauma is common and usually resolves quickly. Because head trauma is frequent in children, a given incident of injury preceding the onset of headache may be immaterial. However, chronic nonprogressive headache may occur after mild to moderate head trauma, particularly if the patient lost consciousness or suffered posttraumatic amnesia. The headache occurs frequently and is dull or throbbing. It may be felt over the entire head or over the site of the injury. Companion problems include vertigo, impairment of concentration and memory, depression, and fatigue. Both migraine and tension-type headaches may begin after head injury.

Chronic Progressive Headache

Chronic progressive headache is the least common headache type. However, it is the most serious type; headache that occurs frequently and grows worse over time is usually due to a serious neurologic illness (Box 5-1). A patient with this pattern of headache warrants immediate evaluation. Selected causes of chronic progressive headache are detailed in the following sections.

Brain Tumor

Brain tumors cause increased intracranial pressure, which in turn generates traction on pain-sensitive structures (Fig. 5-1). Headache is the consequence of this process. Parents of children with headache are often worried about brain tumors, and headache is common in patients with brain tumors. However, children rarely have headache as the *sole* symptom of a brain tumor or other mass lesion.

Headache from brain tumors is usually chronic and progressive in character. The headache may evolve over weeks to months. Initially the pain may not occur daily, but over time it becomes more frequent. Tumors located in the posterior fossa tend to cause pain in the occiput and neck; the pain may also be felt over the tumor itself. The pain is usually dull and may be mild to moderate in severity. Key historic clues to increased intracranial pressure include headache that wakes the patient from sleep, is present when the patient wakes in the morning, worsens when the patient lies down, improves when the patient is standing, is associated with early morning vomiting, and starts or worsens because of Valsalva maneuvers (coughing, laughing, straining, or exer-

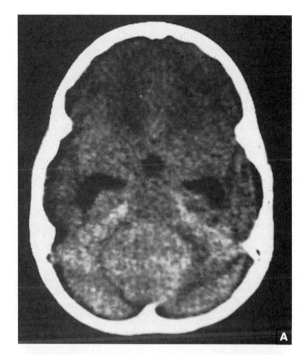

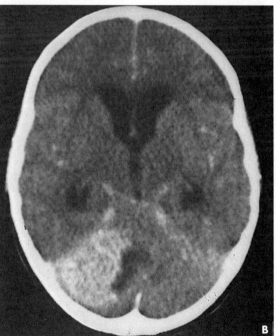

FIG. 5-1 Cerebellar neoplasms. *A,* Midline ependymoma filling the fourth ventricle and invading the cerebellar vermis. *B,* Glioblastoma of the right cerebellar hemisphere. (*A* Courtesy Dr. Michael Painter, Children's Hospital of Pittsburgh; *B* courtesy Department of Neuroradiology, University of Health Center of Pittsburgh.)

cising). These features and the inevitable appearance of other symptoms and signs, such as irritability, personality changes, seizures, weakness, papilledema (Fig. 5-2), sixth nerve palsy, or ataxia, are the hallmarks of brain tumors and other mass lesions.

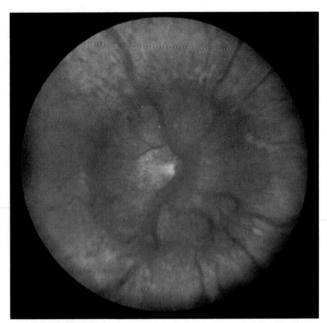

FIG. 5-2 Acute papilledema characterized by blurred disc edges, an absent physiologic cup, and intraretinal exudates.

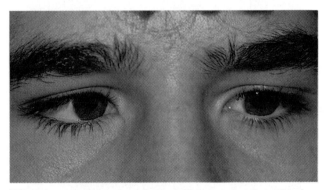

FIG. 5-3 Left abducens (sixth cranial nerve) palsy. This boy had headache and diplopia and was found to have papilledema and a left abducens palsy. Note that his left eye cannot move past the midline on left lateral gaze. (Courtesy Dr. Kenneth Cheng, Children's Hospital of Pittsburgh.)

Hydrocephalus

Hydrocephalus is a cause of chronic progressive headache. It may occur as a result of increased CSF production, obstruction of CSF flow within the ventricular system, or decreased CSF absorption in the arachnoid granulations. Papillomas and other tumors of the choroid plexus, for example, cause increased amounts of CSF. If ventricular obstruction occurs rapidly, the headache evolves rapidly also. Other symptoms of hydrocephalus include confusion, double vision, poor balance, nausea, and vomiting. The physical examination reveals papilledema, diplopia, and ataxia. Also, infants and toddlers may have macrocephaly, widened sutures, and a bulging anterior fontanelle.

BOX 5-3

Disorders Associated With Pseudotumor Cerebri

Infection
Mastoiditis
Sinusitis
Otitis media

Vitamins and Minerals
Hypervitaminosis A
Hypovitaminosis A
Nutritional rickets
Iron deficiency anemia

Drugs
Tetracycline
Steroid use or withdrawal
Oral contraceptives

Endocrine
Obesity
Pregnancy
Adrenal disorders
Congenital adrenal hyperplasia
Adenomas
Addison disease

Pseudotumor Cerebri

Pseudotumor cerebri, also known as *benign intracranial hypertension,* is a clinical syndrome of chronic progressive headache in patients with elevated intracranial pressure, normal CSF, and a structurally normal brain. It is associated with many different disorders, yet the exact pathophysiologic cause is unknown (Box 5-3). Associated symptoms include vomiting, diplopia, and blurred vision; papilledema and sixth nerve palsy (Fig. 5-3) are common findings on physical examination. This is not a benign condition. Permanent visual loss may occur if it is untreated.

Central Nervous System Infection

Subacute infection of the brain or meninges is associated with chronic progressive headache. Brain abscesses are more likely in patients with cyanotic heart disease, pulmonary arteriovenous fistulas, penetrating brain injury, frontal sinusitis, and mastoiditis. Fever is not always present. Other disturbing symptoms, nocturnal headache and morning vomiting, for example, are common in patients with brain abscesses. The neurologic examination reveals evidence of increased intracranial pressure, such as papilledema, sixth nerve palsy, hyperreflexia, and ataxia.

Chronic progressive headache is also the dominant symptom in patients with chronic meningitis. Again, fever is not always present in patients with chronic central nervous system (CNS) infection, especially if the patient has received oral antibiotics. Tuberculosis is the most common cause of chronic meningitis. In children and adolescents, CNS infection with *Mycobacterium tuberculosis* is preceded by pulmonary tuberculosis. Thus a history of chronic cough is significant. Immunodeficient patients are at risk for chronic CNS infection by unusual organisms, such as *Cryptococcus, Aspergillus,* and *Candida* species.

History

The interview of the patient with recurrent or chronic headache is the most important part of the diagnosis. The patient should be invited to describe his or her headache; even young children can describe important details. The examiner should look carefully for clues to serious causes of headache. As with all complaints, a systematic approach works well (Box 5-4).

An excellent beginning is identification of the temporal pattern of the headache. The examiner should ask how the headache began and how frequently it occurs. Did it begin after head trauma? Does it occur a few times each month, several times a month, more than once a week, or daily? Migraine occurs a few times or more each month. Tension-type headache occurs several times a week or daily for weeks to months and is monotonous. Headache from intracranial lesions occurs with increasing frequency. Are the headaches getting worse? Progression in severity implies an intracranial lesion. On the other hand, if a patient has had headache for more than 4 to 6 months without any progression in severity, he or she is unlikely to have a serious cause of headache. The physician should ask if the patient has more than one type of headache; migraine may coexist with tension-type headache, especially in teenagers.

The duration of the headache should be established. Most attacks of migraine last several hours, although on occasion they may last 1 to 3 days. Tension-type headache persists for many hours for days on end. Headache from intracranial lesions may last for brief periods to several hours.

The examiner should determine the *evolution* of the severity of the pain. Does it begin slowly, build to a peak, and slowly get better? This is typical of migraine. Does it become severe immediately at the beginning of the headache? This suggests a structural cause, such as a vascular malformation that is bleeding. The pain of tension-type headache is monotonous; it begins, progresses, and ends slowly.

How severe is the pain? This is an important question; it can be difficult to obtain clear and objective answers from patients and parents. In grading the severity of headache pain, the examiner should assess the severity of the pain, whether the pain interferes with routine activities, and how often the pain occurs. Numeric pain scales are not as useful in children as they are in adults. Does the headache interfere with normal activity or cause the child to stop playing? What can the child do during a headache? Mild to moderate pain is usually found with tension-type headache; severe or incapacitating pain is typical of migraine and acute vascular accidents. The physician should ask parents if the child appears normal between episodes of headache.

The location of the pain furnishes etiologic clues. The examiner should ask the patient to point to the area that hurts. Patients with tension-type headache often sweep a hand across the forehead. Patients with migraine commonly point to one side of the head or the other, both temples, or the forehead. The location of migraine pain changes. Unilateral pain

---

BOX 5-4

The Headache Interview: Twenty-Five Essential Questions

1. Tell me about your headache.
2. How and when did your headache start?
3. Do you have different types of headache?
4. How long have you had a headache?
5. How often to you get a headache? Daily or less often?
6. Where is the pain located? Show me where it is.
7. Does the location change?
8. What does the pain feel like, and is it always the same?
9. Does the pain come on all at once or build gradually?
10. What can you do when you have a headache? What can't you do?
11. Are your headaches getting worse?
12. Can you or your parents tell if a headache will begin? If so, what is your warning signal?
13. Do you hear, smell, or feel anything unusual before a headache?
14. Does anything give you a headache?
15. What makes your headache better or worse?
16. What do you do when you get a headache?
17. Is your headache worse with exercise, coughing, laughing, straining, or bowel movements?
18. Do you feel sick to your stomach, vomit, or have stomach pains with your headache?
19. What time of day or night does your headache occur?
20. Does your headache wake you from sleep?
21. How long does your headache last?
22. How do you feel after the headache is over, and how long does this feeling last?
23. Have you ever had motion sickness?
24. Who gets headache in your family?
25. How are things going at home and at school?

Modified from Rothner AD: The evaluation of headaches in children and adolescents, *Semin Pediatr Neurol* 2:109-118, 1995.

that never varies is suspicious for a structural lesion. Is the complaint actually of facial pain rather than headache? Patients with pain from eye strain point to the eye(s); patients with TMJ abnormality point to the ear, temple, or jaw. A patient with a brain tumor or an Arnold-Chiari malformation might complain of occipital pain.

The patient should be asked to describe the pain. If open-ended questions fail (i.e., What does your pain feel like? or Can you tell me about your pain?), questions should be directed to particular descriptions. Is the pain pounding or throbbing, as in migraine? Is it an aching, squeezing pain or bandlike feeling? Does it feel like pressure? These adjectives are typical of tension-type headache. The headache from a brain tumor may be throbbing or aching. Pain that is boring or burning occurs in cluster headache.

When and where does the headache occur? Headache that wakes patients from sleep or occurs in the early morning and improves as the day goes on is typical of structural lesions, such as brain tumors. Migraine may occur at any time but is infrequently nocturnal. Also, headache after a seizure is common; patients who convulse during sleep may wake up with a headache as the only remaining clue that a seizure occurred. If the headache occurs only at school, a psychologic disturbance may exist.

The examiner should ask parents and patients about signals that warn that a headache is imminent. Parents may note pallor, irritability, or anorexia shortly before the child has a migraine. The patient should be asked if anything strange or unusual happens before the headache. Is there anything, such as a food or activity, that causes the headache? Knowing the "triggers" of a headache is valuable for both diagnosis and management.

The physician should always ask the patient what makes the headache better or worse. Patients with migraine report improvement with rest or sleep and sometimes feel better after they have vomited. Light and sounds greatly disturb patients with migraine. If a headache is caused or aggravated by coughing, laughing, straining, exercising, or changing position, increased intracranial pressure should be considered as the source of the pain. Chewing and bruxism increase the pain of dental abscess, TMJ abnormalities, and maxillary sinusitis.

The examiner must *always* ask if the patient is having a new or different type of headache. Patients with migraine or tension-type headache are not immune to uncommon but serious disorders, such as meningitis, intracranial hemorrhage, and brain tumors. A major change in a previously established headache pattern demands an expedient and thorough evaluation.

A comprehensive review of systems is imperative in all patients with headache. The examiner should ask about neurologic function. Has the parent or patient observed changes in personality, memory, intellectual skills, vision, hearing, strength, gait, or balance? These functions are affected in patients with increased intracranial pressure. Adolescent patients with tension-type headache often complain of feeling "weak" and dizzy. The examiner must seek objective evidence to distinguish the patient who is tired and sensitive to postural changes from the patient with true weakness and vertigo.

A medication history is extremely important. The physician should obtain the name, dosage, frequency of use, and effect of all medications, prescription and nonprescription. When a patient with migraine or tension-type headache complains of worsening headaches, the examiner should ask if he or she has abruptly stopped taking analgesics after using them in large amounts; this pattern of drug use exacerbates headache and makes treatment very difficult. Teenagers should be asked about their use of birth control pills, cigarettes, alcohol, and illegal drugs.

A complete medical history includes information regarding pregnancy, labor and delivery, growth, cognitive and social development, allergies, and past illness or complaints. The examiner should ask about head injuries, even though minor head trauma is common in children and may be irrelevant. Has the child complained of motion sickness? This symptom can precede migraine by several years. Has there been school absence because of recurrent abdominal pain? Such a history is a flag for a stress-related headache.

A thorough family and social history is invaluable. When an established patient arrives with a new complaint of headache, the family's medical and social history should be reviewed for new information. The examiner should ask if either parent has headache, have the parents describe their headaches, and inquire about special concerns they may have. Has anyone in the family had a serious illness with headache as a major feature?

A private interview with adolescent patients is extremely important. Vital information about symptoms of anxiety or depression, drug use, sexual activity, peer relationships, and problems at home, in school, or with the community is more easily obtained when the parents are absent. Similarly a separate interview of the parents allows them to discuss their concerns and explore sensitive family matters.

Physical Examination

In most instances the physical examination of the child with recurrent or chronic headache is entirely normal. A complete examination, including a detailed neurologic assessment, is imperative and reassures patients and parents that the complaint is taken seriously. A patient complaining of headache for more than 4 to 6 months who has a benign history *and* normal general and neurologic examinations is highly unlikely to harbor a brain tumor or another serious disorder.

The patient's affect and interaction with his or her parents should be observed closely. Does the patient seem sad or withdrawn? If so, the possibility of depression or another psychologic disturbance should be considered. How does the patient interact with his or her parents? If both parents are present, important clues to marital stresses may be directly observed from their interactions.

The examiner should obtain measurements of height, weight, head circumference, and vital signs (including blood pressure) for all patients. Healthy children and adolescents sustain normal growth curves. Weight loss and lack of linear growth are clues to organic illness. The association of macrocephaly and headache raises concerns about hydrocephalus or mass lesions of the central nervous system. Fever suggests infection or inflammation. The finding of sustained or intermittent hypertension in patients with headache is important; serious renal, cardiac, or endocrinologic disorders present in childhood with hypertension. Absent femoral pulses and lower blood pressures in the legs are diagnostic of coarctation of the aorta.

The skin should be examined for pallor, petechiae, and bruises, which suggest malignancy. Alopecia, rashes, and painless oral ulcers are common in systemic lupus erythematosus (SLE); headache is common in SLE and other vasculitides. Multiple café au lait spots, especially if located in the axillae or inguinal areas, suggest neurofibromatosis, which is associated with an increased likelihood of brain neoplasms.

The head and neck deserve conscientious attention. The examiner should inspect the face for dilated scalp veins, frontal bossing, downward deviation of the eyes ("sunsetting"), and other signs of increased intracranial pressure. The skull should be auscultated for vascular bruits. The scalp and neck muscles should be palpated for the tenderness and spasm common in patients with tension-type headache. The sinuses and teeth should be percussed; tenderness is a clue to infection which can lead to facial pain and headache. Masseter muscle spasm and restricted jaw opening may be present in patients with TMJ dysfunction. Nuchal rigidity is a finding of great significance and should be looked for in every patient with recurrent or chronic headache.

In all patients with recurrent or chronic headache, the examination of the nervous system is of paramount importance. This includes assessment of mental status, cranial nerve function, motor strength, deep tendon reflexes, sensation, cerebellar function, and the optic fundi. Lethargy, confusion, disorientation, memory impairment, extraocular muscle dysfunction, weakness, spasticity, hyperreflexia, clonus, positive Babinski reflex, ataxia, and papilledema are evidence of organic causes of headache. An abnormal neurologic examination mandates urgent evaluation of the patient.

Approach to the Patient

Does the patient have a serious intracranial or systemic cause of his or her headache? This is the first question the physician must answer. Fortunately, most recurrent and chronic headaches are benign. A correct diagnosis of a particular headache type often evolves from a careful history and physical examination alone. Accurate headache identification, in the office of the primary care practitioner, need not be an exercise in "diagnosis by exclusion." For most patients, skull radiographs, electroencephalograms, and imaging studies of the brain and skull are unnecessary. Only a small number of patients require testing and referral to subspecialists.

What are the key historic features of recurrent and chronic headaches caused by serious disorders (Box 5-5)? Recognizing the temporal pattern of chronic progressive headache is critical. Frequent headache that is getting worse is highly associated with serious problems. Brain tumors often cause mild headache, but the headache's severity increases with time. Headache that wakes patients from sleep or is present in the morning is worrisome. The child who repeatedly wakes in the morning, vomits, and feels better after standing is a classic example of a child with a brain tumor. Headache

---

BOX 5-5

Key Clues to Serious Headache

History

Headache worsening in severity and frequency
Nocturnal headache
Morning headache with vomiting
Severe pain at headache onset
Fixed location, occipital pain
Pain worse with Valsalva maneuvers, recumbent position, or change in position
Change in headache pattern
Headache in patients with ventriculoperitoneal shunts
Neurologic symptoms or signs
   Lethargy, confusion, irritability
   Vomiting
   Visual/sensory changes, weakness, ataxia
   Headache *before* seizure
   "Migraine" headache with seizure

Physical Examination

Impaired mental status
Papilledema, retinal hemorrhage
Cranial bruit, nuchal rigidity
Cranial nerve palsy
Strabismus, diplopia, decreased visual acuity
Weakness, hyperreflexia, Babinski reflex
Ataxia, wide-based gait, positive Romberg sign
Neurocutaneous lesions
Macrocephaly

Modified from Barlow CF: *Headaches and migraine in childhood*, London, Spastics International Medical Publications, Philadelphia, 1984, JB Lippincott; and Prensky AL, Sommer D: Diagnosis and treatment of migraine in children, *Neurology* 29:506-510, 1979.

---

pain that is severe within seconds of onset suggests bleeding from an arteriovenous malformation. Pain that is fixed in location, even though all other features suggest migraine, points to a vascular or other structural lesion. Occipital headache may be caused by tumors of the posterior fossa or an Arnold-Chiari malformation. If the headache is precipitated or aggravated by Valsalva maneuvers and positional changes, increased intracranial pressure is likely. Has there been a change in a previously established pattern of headache? Although not always associated with serious disorders, such a change justifies aggressive pursuit of an organic diagnosis. Does the patient have risk factors for structural causes of headache, such as a ventriculoperitoneal shunt?

In addition a careful review of neurologic symptoms is very helpful in determining the likelihood of increased intracranial pressure. Have there been any changes in consciousness or personality? Is the child or adolescent lethargic in the morning and more alert after several hours out of bed? This history may be obtained from a patient with increased intracranial

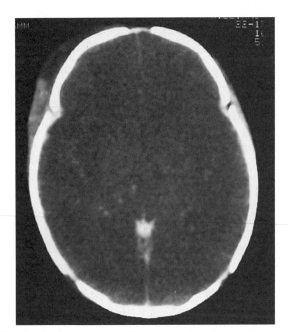

FIG. 5-4 Cerebral edema. CT performed 24 hours after severe hypoxic-ischemic injury. Note obliteration of the cerebral ventricles, loss of gray-white differentiation, and homogeneous "ground-glass" appearance. (Courtesy Department of Neuroradiology, University Health Center of Pittsburgh.)

pressure or posterior fossa tumor, for example. Is the headache accompanied by vomiting, weakness, poor balance, blurred or double vision, numbness, or gait changes? Several important causes of headache are associated with such features, including brain tumors, vascular malformations, and migraine with neurologic deficits, among others. Has the headache been associated with unusual movements that could be seizures? The presence of any or all of these features usually mandates consultation with pediatric subspecialists and imaging studies of the brain.

Similarly the neurologic examination is of paramount importance in the evaluation of the child or adolescent with headache (Box 5-5). Abnormal neurologic findings always require investigation beyond a meticulous history and general physical examination. Impaired mental or visual function, papilledema, sixth nerve palsy, weakness, and ataxia are the most common findings in the pediatric patient with headache caused by a brain tumor.

If there is concern for a serious intracranial cause of headache, what is the next step? If the patient is unstable in any way, emergency evaluation with a brain imaging study and consultation with a pediatric neurologist and/or neurosurgeon must proceed without delay. A computerized axial tomography (CAT) scan of the brain and skull is a reliable study often available more rapidly than other imaging modalities. In the unstable patient with suspected increased intracranial pressure, a CAT scan can identify cerebral edema (Fig. 5-4), acute hemorrhage, hydrocephalus, subdural fluid, brain abscess, and hemispheric tumors. Magnetic resonance

imaging (MRI) may not be available as rapidly as CAT scanning to evaluate the unstable patient. It is, however, a superior study for detection of Arnold-Chiari malformations, posterior fossa tumors, or low-grade hemispheric neoplasms. Detection of arteriovenous malformations and aneurysms is often difficult and may require magnetic resonance angiography (MRA).

A normal CAT scan or MRI in a patient with clinical evidence of increased intracranial pressure points to pseudotumor cerebri. Measurement of CSF pressure is necessary for diagnosis. After a mass lesion has been excluded, the pressure is measured with the patient in the lateral recumbent position. An opening pressure greater than 200 mm H_2O is abnormal. Routine studies (glucose and protein levels, differential cell count, Gram stain, and bacterial culture) are normal in patients with pseudotumor cerebri.

A lumbar puncture is also indicated in a patient with suspected chronic meningitis. In addition to routine CSF studies, special stains and cultures for unusual organisms may be required. Finally, a venous lead level should be obtained in patients with a history of pica or other risk factors for lead poisoning.

If a serious cause of headache is found and is systemic rather than intracranial, the physician must evaluate the underlying illness. For example, discovery of hypertension in a child with headache dictates an investigation focused on the source of the hypertension. Treatment of the primary illness generally alleviates headache symptoms as well.

If there is no serious intracranial or systemic problem causing the headache, the next step is categorization of the headache by temporal pattern. The initial history is sometimes inadequate for this purpose. In this case, if the physical examination is normal and the patient attends school regularly, the examiner should ask the patient to keep a diary of headache symptoms for 3 to 6 weeks and review the information during a return visit. The patient and family should be instructed to record the following features of each headache: the location, duration, severity, and character; associated symptoms before, during, and after the headache; dosage and frequency of medications used for the headache; school attendance; and whether any social activities were missed because of headache. If the patient has frequent headache, a normal physical examination, and poor school attendance, the examiner should ask the patient to return with the diary after a shorter period of time. Once the temporal pattern is known, the appropriate differential diagnosis is formed. Some patients have features of both migraine and tension-type headaches.

The temporal pattern of headache in most pediatric patients is acute recurrent. The most common cause of this pattern is migraine without aura. If the patient has headache with typical features of migraine with or without aura, a family member with migraine, a normal physical examination, and no evidence of a systemic disorder that is associated with migraine (such as SLE), no further evaluation is required for diagnosis. Other causes of acute recurrent headache are uncommon. A careful history and physical examination usually suggest the diagnosis and other appropriate diagnostic measures. For example, a child with recurrent bouts of headache associated with fever and upper respiratory tract symptoms in all likelihood has recurrent sinusitis. Sinus radiographs or CAT scanning of the sinuses may be helpful in this case. On the other hand, in a patient with recurrent occipital headache and neck pain, the physician must exclude a structural lesion of the posterior fossa or craniocervical junction; consultation with appropriate subspecialists regarding diagnosis and management is warranted. If clinical evidence suggests the patient is having seizures with resultant headache, an electroencephalogram and consultation with a pediatric neurologist are indicated.

Chronic nonprogressive headache is usually a tension-type headache. The history and physical examination are often so typical that the diagnosis is readily apparent to the physician. No other diagnostic efforts are necessary unless the physician suspects a primary psychologic disturbance, such as major depression. In such cases additional evaluation by a pediatric psychologist or psychiatrist is indicated. However, convincing families that no serious physical cause of the headache exists and that brain imaging studies are unnecessary is challenging because the chronicity of the complaint greatly alarms patients and parents. Physicians invite frustration by ordering unnecessary tests and imaging studies in response to a family's anxiety. Additional time spent discussing the diagnosis and its benign nature is more beneficial than a fruitless search for structural disorders. Most other causes of chronic nonprogressive headache are uncommon and readily apparent from a good history and physical examination.

SUMMARY

In conclusion, recurrent and chronic headaches are common in the pediatric population. Migraine without aura and tension-type headache are the most common disorders. Grave intracranial and systemic causes of headache are uncommon, but detection of these serious disorders is vital. Despite advances in imaging studies of the brain, the most powerful diagnostic tools still available to clinicians are a comprehensive history and a meticulous physical examination.

ILLUSTRATIVE CASES

Case 1. D.S. is a 9-year-old boy referred for evaluation of headache. He complains of daily, nonprogressive, throbbing headache localized to the right forehead, since 6 weeks before presentation. Analgesics and sleep do not relieve the pain. He denies an aura, nausea, vomiting, abdominal pain, or visual complaints; his parents describe him as "unusually irritable." He is on no medications and has no other medical problems. His father has ophthalmoplegic migraine, and his mother has tension-type headache. The family denies any stressors. D.S. has been out of school for 4 weeks at this time. His physical examination is normal. A complete blood count, sinus radiographs, and a CAT scan of the head obtained by the referring physician are normal.

The initial differential diagnosis is tension-type headache versus migraine. In favor of the former is the daily occurrence of the headache; lack of migraine-associated symptoms, such as nausea and vomiting; and failure of the pain to abate with rest or sleep. In favor of migraine is the location of the headache, the throbbing quality of the pain, and the family history of migraine.

The family is reassured that the physical examination is normal and agrees to a trial of propranolol. After several weeks, D.S. reports no improvement in his symptoms. A second visit is used to explore family issues in more depth. The family confides having extreme worries about their oldest daughter who has recently been arrested for shoplifting. There are multiple areas of conflict between family members, and the father is under tremendous stress at work. D.S. is the youngest child, an honor student, and "a model child" who "absorbs all the family stress." At this point, medications are discontinued, the family is referred for psychologic counseling, and D.S. is evaluated at a local pain clinic where he is trained in the use of a transcutaneous nerve stimulation unit (TENS). He returns to school and becomes asymptomatic after several weeks.

As this case illustrates, important information about family relationships is vital to diagnosis and is not always apparent at the first visit. Also, patients may have features of both migraine and tension-type headache, and this poses difficulty in both diagnosis and treatment.

Case 2. C.M. is a previously healthy 8-year-old girl who came to an emergency room with acute and rapid onset of a severe headache. She describes a severe, pounding headache located above her left eye. She is nauseated but denies abdominal pain or visual complaints. There is no history of head trauma or prior headache, and her review of systems is unremarkable. The headache began after she ate chocolate cake at a birthday party, and she recalls "feeling funny" just before the headache began. Her mother has a history of migraine since adolescence. Her own headache occurs 3 to 4 times per year, is usually localized to her right forehead, is triggered by "too much sleep," and is preceded by scotomata. The patient's physical examination shows her to be in severe pain but is otherwise normal. Because of the severity of C.M.'s pain, a CAT scan of the head is obtained and is normal.

A diagnosis of migraine is considered based on the headache character, associated symptoms, and positive family history. Her headache resolves with the use of ibuprofen and sleep. The patient is advised to avoid chocolate. Multiple episodes of similar headache occur over the next several weeks; repeat physical examinations are normal. Headache prophylaxis with propanolol is begun, and the headaches resolve. The medication is discontinued after 1 year, and the patient remains asymptomatic.

This case illustrates two challenges in migraine diagnosis. First, recurrence is a mandatory feature for migraine diagnosis; thus migraine cannot be diagnosed with certainty at the first attack. Secondly, the severity of the initial migraine compels some patients and parents to seek medical attention emergently because they fear a serious problem exists. In any setting, but particularly in an emergency room, a physician faced with a patient with a new onset of a severe headache must consider structural causes.

Case 3. A 16-year-old obese girl was well until 4 weeks before presentation, when she developed a mild headache in the frontal and occipital areas. The headache occurred daily and gradually worsened in severity. After 2 weeks, she complained of double vision and refused to drive a car. She denies all other symptoms, including fever, weight loss, morning nausea or vomiting, cough, weakness, ataxia, and neck pain. She has taken no medications, denies recent head trauma, and her only surgery was removal of a benign thyroid cyst just before her headache began.

Physical examination reveals an obese, healthy girl with normal vital signs, including blood pressure. Her general physical examination is normal. Her neurologic examination is normal with the exception of diplopia, which resolves when she covers one eye, and bilateral papilledema.

A CAT scan of the head performed with and without contrast is normal. A lumbar puncture is performed and reveals a markedly elevated opening pressure. Her diplopia resolves and her headache improves by the end of the first lumbar puncture. She is treated for several months with repeat lumbar punctures until her headache resolves entirely.

This case is an example of a chronic progressive headache. The indications for investigation included worsening headache, a worrisome neurologic symptom (diplopia), and an abnormal finding on physical examination (papilledema). Although pseudotumor cerebri was suspected, a CAT scan of the head was performed to exclude a mass lesion before proceeding with a lumbar puncture. In this case lumbar puncture was both diagnostic and therapeutic for pseudotumor cerebri or benign intracranial hypertension.

ANNOTATED BIBLIOGRAPHY

Bille B: Migraine in school children, *Acta Paediatr Suppl* 51(136):1-151, 1962.
  Thirty-five years after publication this remains the most comprehensive study of headache in childhood.

Elser JM: Easing the pain of childhood headaches, *Contemp Pediatr* 8:108-123, 1991.
  An excellent article focusing on the clinical evaluation and treatment of common headache types in children.

Prensky AL: Differentiating and treating pediatric headaches, *Contemp Pediatr* 1:12-45, 1984.
  This is an essential review of headaches for students, pediatricians, and family practitioners.

BIBLIOGRAPHY

Barlow CF: Headaches and migraine in childhood, London, Spastics International Medical Publications, Philadelphia, 1984, JB Lippincott.

Blau JN: Migraine: theories of pathogenesis, *Lancet* 339:1202-1209, 1992.

The Childhood Brain Tumor Consortium: The epidemiology of headache among children with brain tumor, *J Neurooncol* 10:31-46, 1991.

Chu ML, Shinnar S: Headaches in children younger than 7 years of age, *Headache* 23:15-19, 1983.

Cohen BH: Headaches as a symptom of neurological disease, *Semin Pediatr Neurol* 2:144-150, 1995.

Faleck H, Rothner AD, Erenberg G, et al: Headache and subacute sinusitis in children and adolescents, *Headache* 28:96-98, 1988.

Frischberg BM: The utility of neuroimaging in the evaluation of headache in patients with normal neurologic examinations, *Neurology* 44:1191-1197, 1994.

Honig PJ, Charney EB: Children with brain tumor headaches, *Am J Dis Child* 136:121-124, 1982.

Linet MS, Stewart WF, Celentaro DD, et al: An epidemiologic study of headache among adolescents and young adults, *JAMA* 261:2211-2216, 1989.

Maytal J, Bienkowski RS, Patel M, et al: The value of brain imaging in children with headaches, *Pediatrics* 96:413-416, 1995.

Oleson J: Clinical and pathophysiologic observations of migraine and tension-type headache explained by integration of vascular supraspinal and myofascial inputs, *Pain* 46:125-132, 1991.

Oleson J, Friberg L, Olsen TS, et al: Timing and topography of cerebral blood flow, aura and headache during migraine attacks, *Ann Neurol* 28:791-798, 1990.

Prensky AL, Sommer D: Diagnosis and treatment of migraine in children, *Neurology* 29:506-510, 1979.

Rothner AD: Headaches in children: a review, *Headache* 18(3):169-175, 1978.

Rothner AD: Pathophysiology of recurrent headaches in children and adolescents, *Pediatr Ann* 24:458-466, 1995.

Rothner AD: The evaluation of headaches in children and adolescents, *Semin Pediatr Neurol* 2:109-118, 1995.

Sheth RD, Riggs JE, Bodensteiner JB: Acute confusional migraine: variant of transient global amnesia, *Pediatr Neurol* 12:129-131, 1995.

Silberstein SD: Advances in understanding the pathophysiology of headache, *Neurology* 42(suppl 2):6-10, 1992.

Singer HS, Rowe S: Chronic recurrent headaches in children, *Pediatr Ann* 21:369-373, 1992.

6

The Limping Child

S A R A   C .   McI N T I R E   &   J O H N   D .   F A R R E L L

 Key Points

- Limp is never normal and is usually organic in origin.

- Gait analysis is a key step in the diagnosis of the cause of a limp.

- The differential diagnosis of the cause of limping is best divided into two categories—painful and nonpainful limping.

The child with a limp often has a history and physical examination that are diagnostic for a common and benign problem. When the initial history and examination do not reveal the diagnosis, however, attention must be given to less common and potentially more serious disorders. Limp is never normal and is usually organic in origin; on rare occasions it signifies mimicry or a conversion disorder. This chapter describes the evaluation of the pediatric patient with the symptom of limping. For the purposes of this chapter, a limp is any change in gait that is new and deviates from expected patterns for the age of the patient. The emphasis is on the patient with persistent limping.

Gait Analysis

At some point in evolutionary history a descendant of modern humans rose up on two legs and created the bipedal gait. Not long after, the first bipedal limp appeared and the opportunity for gait analysis was created. The science of gait analysis has come a long way since that time with the technologic capabilities of video recording and computers to analyze both normal and pathologic gaits. Primary care physicians are called on to analyze gaits frequently; aside from education, our tools are similar to those of the early cave dwellers—observation and examination.

A firm understanding of gait analysis begins with a systematic categorization of the normal gait. This is a complex process requiring integration of both the nervous and musculoskeletal systems.

Normal gait has two major phases—the stance phase and the swing phase. The stance phase begins with the heel striking the floor and ends with the toe leaving the ground. It is the weight-bearing phase of gait and makes up 60% of the gait cycle. Tachdjian subdivides the stance phase into four major stages: (1) heel strike, (2) flat foot, (3) push off with knee bend, and (4) toe off. The swing phase is divided into three stages: (1) the initial swing, continuation of the toe-off part of the stance phase, (2) midswing, beginning as the swing limb passes the contralateral limb, and (3) deceleration, where gravity and muscular exertion slow the forward limb in preparation for the heel strike.

Gait analysis is complicated by the changes in gait that accompany normal childhood development. Helpful milestones include the following: the ability to walk begins between 12 and 14 months of age, alternate step climbing begins by 17 to 21 months of age, and the ability to balance on one foot for 1 second develops by 30 to 36 months of age. Also, in contrast to a more mature gait, the toddler has a wide-based gait, no reciprocal arm movement, and no heel strike initiating the stance phase. This produces a staccato gait and contributes to the origin of the word *toddler* for children between 1 and 3 years of age.

Gait assessment is critical to the diagnosis of the cause of limping. In every patient with this complaint, the clinician must observe the patient walk, run, climb stairs, and balance on each foot separately whenever possible. Also, performance of the heel walk, toe walk, and tandem walk gives valuable information about the patient's neurologic and musculoskeletal states.

There are a number of different gait types that are clues to the specific underlying pathology (Table 6-1). The most common gait disturbance is the antalgic gait. This gait consists of a shortened stance phase of the affected limb, and it indicates a painful cause of limping. Clinical observation of this gait may pinpoint the location of the painful process. For example, the heel strike may be absent in a patient with a foreign body in the heel.

The Trendelenburg symptom, or gluteus medius lurch, is correlated with weakness or paralysis of the gluteus medius muscles. This pattern is seen in patients with developmental dysplasia of the hip and in Legg-Calvé-Perthes disease. In some patients this gait is not evident until they have walked for some time, but as the muscle fatigues, a dropped pelvis on the side of the swing phase limb becomes evident. The Trendelenburg test is performed with the patient standing on one leg. The gluteus medius muscle of the nonweight-bearing side normally elevates the suspended hip. A positive test reveals a lower pelvis on the nonweight-bearing side.

Back or vertebral pathology is suggested when the patient's gait is stiff. Pelvic rotation is decreased, and the trunk is held rigidly while the patient walks slowly and deliberately. This is typical of patients with symptomatic spondylolysis, diskitis, or osteomyelitis of the spine.

The most common neurologic causes of gait abnormalities are spasticity and ataxia. A spastic gait may be secondary to hypertonicity, incoordination of muscle groups, and/or contraction deformities. Lower limb hypertonicity often produces toe walking with no heel strike at any point in the gait cycle. Increased tone of the adductor muscles causes the knees to cross one another during walking and produces a scissor gait. Cerebellar disorders produce a broad-based, unsteady, and irregular or ataxic gait. Tandem walking is impossible for these patients who also have a positive Romberg test. Paralysis of ankle dorsiflexion produces a drop-foot gait. This gait is characterized by an abnormality at the end of the stance phase and the initial swing phase. To clear the toes the patient elevates the entire leg, flexes the knee, and externally rotates the hip.

Muscular dystrophy also causes gait disturbances. The patient waddles with bilateral Trendelenburg signs and an exaggerated lumbar lordosis. A positive Gowers sign is typical and points to weakness of hip and knee extensor muscles (Fig. 6-1).

In a short-leg limp the entire body dips down toward the side of the lower limb. This occurs when one leg is pathologically short or long.

Finally, the gait of a patient with a conversion disorder deserves mention. A conversion gait often appears peculiar to the clinician. It is typically narrow-based yet very unsteady. The patient may shuffle and demonstrate very exaggerated upper body movements as if to maintain balance. No anatomic explanation is consistent with the gait, and when carefully tested the patient has no true abnormalities of strength, tone, reflexes, or sensation.

Differential Diagnosis

Tunnessen divides the differential diagnosis into painful and nonpainful limping. Both groups may be categorized by the

TABLE 6-1
Pathologic Gaits

Gait	Problem
Antalgic	Trauma, infection
Trendelenburg	Hip dysplasia, Legg-Calvé-Perthes disease
Stiff	Spondylolysis, diskitis, osteomyelitis
Spastic	Cerebral palsy
Ataxic	Cerebellar lesions, drugs
Drop-foot gait	Paralysis of ankle dorsiflexion
Waddling	Muscular dystrophy, bilateral hip dysplasia
Short-leg limp	Leg length discrepancy
Conversion gait	Psychiatric disorder

BOX 6-1
The Limping Child: Differential Diagnosis

Painful Limping	Nonpainful Limping
Traumatic	Muscle
Mechanical	Joint
Infectious	Bone
Inflammatory	Neurologic
Neoplastic	Psychologic
Hematologic	
Intraabdominal disorders	

pathophysiologic cause of the limping (Box 6-1). Renshaw categorizes limp by one of three mechanisms—pain, weakness, and mechanical or structural disturbances. The most common cause of painful limping is trauma. Nonpainful limping is usually caused by musculoskeletal disorders.

Painful Limping

Traumatic Causes

Traumatic causes of limping—lacerations, bruises, pain from immunizations, sprains, fractures, and injuries to cartilage and ligaments—are usually apparent from the history and physical examination. The gait is painful (antalgic), and the affected bone, joint, muscle, or other soft tissue is identified by gait observation, inspection, palpation, and assessment of stability, strength, and range of motion. This is challenging in the nonverbal toddler who may cry or resist with examination of all areas, but the art of distraction serves the clinician well in this situation.

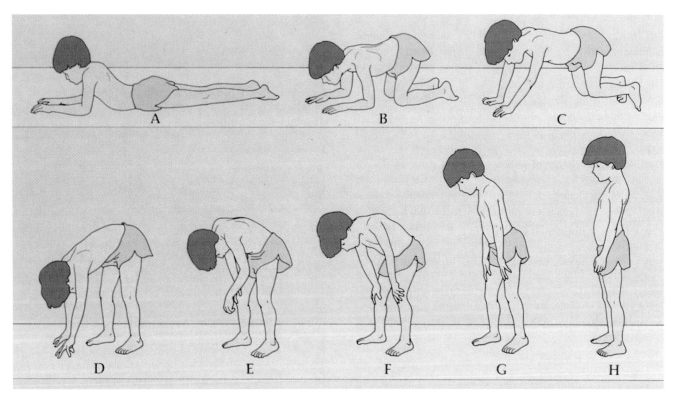

FIG. 6-1   Gowers maneuver. This series of diagrams illustrates the sequence of postures used in attaining the upright position. *A to C,* First, the legs are pulled up under the body, and then the weight is shifted to rest on the hands and feet. *D,* The hips are then thrust in the air as the knees are straightened and the hands are brought close to the legs. *E to G,* Finally, the trunk is slowly extended by the hands walking up the thigh. *H,* The erect position is attained.

An important point to remember when evaluating young children with painful limping after an injury is that children are more likely to sustain growth plate fractures (Salter-Harris type I) than ligament or muscle strains because of the relative weakness of the epiphyses compared with the surrounding bones, ligaments, and tendons. A toddler's fracture is a spiral fracture of the tibia that may occur after seemingly minor trauma; plain radiographs may be normal if taken soon after the fracture occurs. Also, a high index of suspicion is required to detect intentional trauma; a history that is inconsistent with the injury and/or evidence of other old injuries must be regarded as potential signs of abuse.

Knee injuries are extremely common in pediatric patients, especially those involved in sports. Although acute knee injuries do occur, inflammation and repetitive microtrauma ("overuse syndromes") account for a large number of patients with chronic knee pain with or without painful limping. Acute knee injuries, such as tears to the cruciate ligaments, are not addressed in this chapter.

A number of minor problems of the feet are associated with painful limping. Such problems include shoes that are too tight or stiff, paronychia, ingrown toenails, lacerations, plantar warts, and calluses. These conditions are easily diagnosed through careful inspection of the shoes and the feet. Also, a foreign body embedded in the foot or shoe leads to an antalgic gait. A careful search of the foot for such an object or its entry site is warranted. Only those foreign bodies that are radiopaque will appear on plain radiographs; on rare occasions, surgical exploration is necessary to locate a radiolucent object.

Repetitive Microtrauma

A number of injuries can be grouped under the category of repetitive microtrauma and result in avascular necrosis or sclerosis of the affected bones and ligamentous attachments. Repetitive exercise is a key feature of patients with this type of injury. In the following sections these injuries are discussed by anatomic location.

Spine

Disorders of the spinal column and its contents may cause painful gait disturbances and back pain (see Chapter 2). Spondylolysis is a stress fracture of the pars interarticularis of the vertebra, typically involving the fifth lumbar vertebra. Boys and girls are affected equally, with the age of presentation beginning around 10 years and extending into early adulthood. The injury often occurs during participation in sports, such as gymnastics or rowing, with repetitive hyperextension of the back. In addition to back pain this lesion causes pain in the gluteal muscles, producing a stiff gait that is slow and shortened. Patients also have paraspinous muscle spasm, decreased flexion of the lumbar spine, and hamstring tightness, leading to an inability to touch the toes on forward bending. Plain radiographs of the spine, including anteroposterior, lateral, and oblique views, confirm the diagnosis. A small number of patients with spondylolysis progress to spondylolisthesis, which is forward slippage of a vertebral body, usually L5 upon S1. This latter condition is also evident on plain radiographs and may require surgical correction if severe.

Hip

Legg-Calvé-Perthes disease (LCP) is avascular necrosis of the femoral head. It may arise from repetitive microtrauma, but the cause is not completely understood. LCP may be unilateral or bilateral and may present with a painful or nonpainful limp. The pain may be felt in the lateral aspect of the hip, groin, thigh, or knee. Affected children are usually 3 to 10 years old, and it affects boys more often than girls. The history may include a prior episode of toxic synovitis of the hip or family members with LCP. Clues on physical examination include an antalgic gait, mild leg length discrepancy, and decreased internal rotation and abduction of the hip(s). There may be a positive Trendelenburg test, indicating the child is unable to stand on the affected side. Anteroposterior and frog-leg radiographs of the hips reveal increased density and flattening of the femoral head (Fig. 6-2). Very early avascular necrosis can be diagnosed by bone scan or magnetic resonance imaging (MRI) before changes are visible on plain radiographs. A complete blood count and an erythrocyte sedimentation rate are normal.

Slipped Capital Femoral Epiphysis. Slipped capital femoral epiphysis (SCFE) may be a painless or painful disorder. SCFE is discussed in the section on nonpainful limping.

Knee

Chronic knee pain from repetitive exercise is a very common complaint among runners and other athletes. In the pediatric literature a variety of terms are used to describe this phenomenon, including *chondromalacia patellae, runner's knee,* and *patellofemoral arthralgia or stress syndrome,* for example. Regardless of the term used, what is described is an injury to the posterior surface of the patella that results in limping and knee pain. The pain is located under the patella and is aggravated by running, climbing stairs, and performing deep knee bends. The knee also frequently buckles. This disorder is most often seen in active adolescents. Plain radiographs of the knee, including anteroposterior, lateral, and tunnel views, are usually normal, yet they are necessary to exclude another lesion, such as a tumor. Patellar tendonitis is another source of chronic anterior knee pain, but patients with this disorder often do not limp.

Osteochondritis Dissecans of the Knee. Osteochondritis dissecans (OD) describes the process in which cartilage with a segment of bone attached to it separates from the surrounding bone and ligaments. The separation may be partial or complete. The cause is unknown, but it is likely that repetitive microtrauma plays a significant role. Avascular necrosis of the bony segment occurs with variable revascularization and repair. Boys are twice as likely to be affected as are girls. OD affects both children and adolescents. The knee is the most common site of involvement. Patients experience intermittent pain in the joint after strenuous activity, occasionally with stiffness, knee "clicking," "locking" of the knee in flexion or extension, and buckling or "giving way" of the knee. The physical examination reveals an antalgic gait and tenderness localized to the lateral surface of the medial femoral condyle on palpation. Wilson

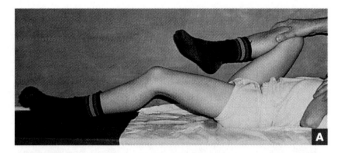
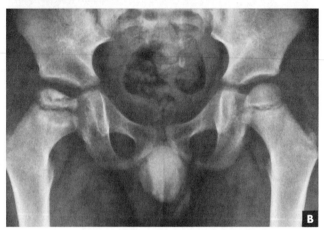

FIG. 6-2 Legg-Calvé-Perthes disease. *A,* Full flexion of the opposite hip eliminates lumbar lordosis and accentuates the contracture. This is an indication of irritation of the hip joint caused by the disease and associated synovitis. *B,* In this anteroposterior radiograph the right femoral epiphysis is flattened and fragmented. The proximal femur is also displaced inferiorly and laterally.

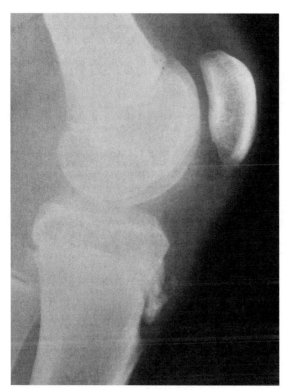

FIG. 6-3 Osgood-Schlatter disease. Irregularity and fragmentation of the tibial tubercle are seen in this radiograph. In less severe cases of shorter duration, soft tissue swelling or irregularity of ossification may be the only finding.

sign is elicited by flexing the knee to 90 degrees and rotating the leg medially; a positive sign consists of pain produced in the anterior aspect of the medial femoral condyle and relieved with extension of the knee. Plain anteroposterior and lateral radiographs usually reveal well-circumscribed fragments of bone, although special views (tunnel and oblique) may be necessary to detect the fragment. This is an important cause of knee pain, and referral to an orthopedic surgeon is indicated.

Tibia: Osgood-Schlatter Disease

Osgood-Schlatter disease is characterized by tenderness and swelling of the patellar tendon and excessive enlargement of the proximal tibial tubercle. It is seen in preadolescents, and boys are affected more often than are girls. It is caused by traction stress from the quadriceps muscle and patellar tendon on the tibial tubercle. Kneeling, marching, jumping, or running produces a pulling force on the tubercle with subsequent detachment of cartilage fragments. Patients complain of intermittent unilateral or bilateral knee pain that worsens with activity and improves with rest. The gait is usually minimally antalgic and may be normal. Palpation reveals a thickened patellar tendon and enlargement of the tibial

tuberosity. The pain is worse with squatting or deep knee bends. The knee joint itself is otherwise normal with full range of motion. Plain radiographs reveal soft tissue swelling and occasionally osseous fragments anterior to the tibial tuberosity (Fig. 6-3).

Shin Splints and Stress Fractures. Shin splints cause lower leg pain with or without limping. They are the result of repetitive trauma incurred in sports, such as long-distance running or basketball. They are most likely to occur when athletes overtrain after a period of relative inactivity. A typical complaint is an aching pain that increases with exercise and greatly improves with rest. On examination there is diffuse tenderness on palpation over the distal posteromedial tibia and excessive pronation of the feet when the patient walks. The athletes at risk for shin splints may also incur stress fractures of the tibia or fibula. The complaints are nearly identical, but the patient with a fracture has more localized tenderness on physical examination. If plain radiographs in the anteroposterior, lateral, and oblique views are normal, technetium 99 bone scintigraphy is likely to demonstrate the fracture.

Ankle: Sever Disease

Sever disease (or Sever apophysitis) results from repetitive microtrauma and is believed to represent subsequent avascular necrosis of the calcaneus at the insertion of the Achilles tendon. However, some authors believe it represents a stress fracture through the calcaneus. It is more common in boys than in girls. The gait is antalgic, and there is tenderness localized to the heel on palpation.

Achilles Tendonitis. Patients with Achilles tendonitis complain of chronic aching pain over the Achilles tendon. Runners are particularly vulnerable to this injury that results from microscopic tears in the tendon. On examination there is tenderness to palpation over the tendon; mild swelling and crepitus may exist also. The rest of the examination is normal, and radiographs are unnecessary.

Foot

Osteochondritis Dissecans. Children with OD of the foot have a history of a chronically "sprained ankle" with painful limping and buckling of the ankle. Plain radiographs with mortise views of the ankle are required for diagnosis. Computed tomography (CT) and magnetic resonance imaging (MRI) fully delineate the extent of the lesion.

Stress Fractures. Stress fractures of the second and third metatarsal bones may occur after repetitive trauma, such as that experienced by ballet dancers. These fractures may not be visible on plain radiographs; technetium 99 bone scintigraphy detects early lesions.

Freiberg Disease. Freiberg disease (also known as *Freiberg infraction*) is a disorder of adolescence in which the second metatarsal head is painful and appears "crushed in" on plain radiographs. It is far more common in girls than in boys. Ballet dancers frequently suffer this injury. The exact cause is unknown, but it may be due to chronic vascular insufficiency leading to avascular necrosis. Stress and repeated trauma are postulated causes of the vascular insufficiency. The diagnosis is evident from the history and physical examination and is confirmed by plain radiographs.

Kohler Bone Disease. Kohler disease is avascular necrosis of the tarsal navicular bone. It usually occurs in young boys around 3 to 6 years of age who have an antalgic gait and tenderness localized to the medial aspect of the midfoot. Plain radiographs are diagnostic and show flattening and sclerosis of the tarsal navicular bone.

Mechanical Causes

Deformities of the foot also cause painful limping. Coalition of two or more tarsal bones is a congenital lesion that may cause painful limping. Walking on uneven ground is especially difficult for patients with this deformity. On examination the affected foot is painful, stiff, and flat. The peroneal muscle is in spasm as well. The most common lesions are between the calcaneus and the tarsal navicular bones and between the talus and calcaneus bones. Plain radiographs in the anteroposterior, lateral weight-bearing, and oblique views should be ordered first. CT scan is also useful for detecting this condition. Congenital vertical talus is an uncommon foot deformity that is usually diagnosed in the newborn because the foot looks abnormal; if it is missed early on, it becomes apparent when the child walks because the foot is rigid. The diagnosis is confirmed by a plain radiograph in the anteroposterior and lateral weight-bearing view and in a lateral view of the foot as it is maximally plantar-flexed. Congenital vertical talus is associated with myelodysplasia and other anomalies, so a comprehensive examination is required when this deformity is recognized.

Other mechanical causes of painful limping include accessory navicular bones, hypermobile flatfeet, adolescent bunions, "growing pains," and popliteal (Baker) cysts.

Infectious Causes

When faced with a suspected infectious cause of limping, it is important to differentiate bone and joint infections from localized soft tissue infections. Pyogenic osteomyelitis and arthritis are conditions with high morbidity if the diagnosis is delayed. Consultation with orthopedic surgeons experienced in the care of patients with bone or joint infections is usually necessary for the diagnosis and management of these disorders.

Osteomyelitis

The presentation of the pediatric patient with osteomyelitis ranges from the obvious to the subtle. Involvement of the vertebral column, disk space, sacroiliac joints, pelvic bones, and any bone of the lower extremity can cause painful limping. Moreover the bony infection extends into the joint space and soft tissues when treatment is delayed.

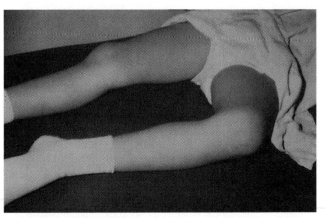

FIG. 6-4 Acute osteomyelitis. Fever, hip and thigh pain, and refusal to walk were the chief complaints of this 5-year-old girl with osteomyelitis of the proximal femur. On inspection she lay still, holding the left leg externally rotated and flexed at the hip and knee. This same position also is adopted by children with acute arthritis of the hip.

The predominant infecting organism in osteomyelitis is *Staphylococcus aureus.* This organism accounts for 80% of all cases in which a cause is confirmed. Other infectious agents must be considered in specific settings. For example, penetrating injury to the foot is associated with *Pseudomonas aeruginosa* osteomyelitis just as sickle cell anemia is associated with osteomyelitis caused by *Salmonella* species. The most commonly involved long bones are the femur and the tibia. Other bones for the clinician to consider when faced with a limping child include the fibula, the bones of the feet, and the bones of the pelvis and spine.

After infancy, boys are affected twice as often as girls. A history of blunt trauma is often obtained, but the significance of such an injury is unclear. Localized complaints, such as limping and pain over the affected bone, predominate early on in the disease. Pain at rest and increased pain with motion are common complaints. Nighttime pain occurs also. Fever and other constitutional symptoms, such as fatigue and anorexia, may be present. The absence of fever does not exclude osteomyelitis. Occasionally, patients are very ill at initial presentation and their toxic appearance suggests another diagnosis, such as meningitis or septicemia.

On physical examination, the physician may find warmth, redness, and swelling over the affected bone. The bone is exquisitely painful on palpation, and muscles adjacent to it may be in protective spasm. Infection of the spine or sacroiliac joint may be accompanied by scoliosis. Infection of the proximal femur causes the patient to hold the leg in flexion, abduction, and external rotation (Fig. 6-4). The patient either refuses to bear weight or has an antalgic gait.

Once osteomyelitis is suspected, laboratory and radiographic evaluations are mandatory. A complete blood count (CBC) with differential and platelets is a customary test for evaluating children with suspected infections; however, al-

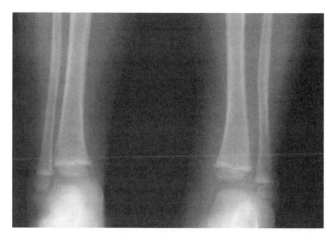

FIG. 6-5 Acute osteomyelitis. Radiographic changes lag behind the clinical in osteomyelitis. The first noticeable change, occurring about 3 days after onset, is deep soft tissue swelling, seen here adjacent to the metaphysis of the distal tibia on the left. (Courtesy Dr. Jocelyn Ledesma-Medina, Children's Hospital of Pittsburgh.)

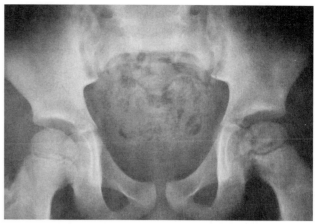

FIG. 6-6 Acute osteomyelitis. Radiographic changes lag behind the clinical in osteomyelitis. The epiphysis and proximal metaphysis of the left femur have a moth-eaten appearance in this older child. (Courtesy Dr. Roderigo Dominguez, University of Texas.)

though leukocytosis is typical of patients with osteomyelitis, a normal white blood cell differential count may be present. A Westergren method erythrocyte sedimentation rate (ESR) is greater than 30 mm/hr in more than 95% of cases and is very useful in following the resolution of the infection. The examiner should always obtain a blood culture because it is likely to reveal the infecting organism in approximately half of all patients. The tests of choice for isolation of the organism are Gram staining and culture of bone aspirate. Antimicrobial sensitivity testing of the organism is necessary as well.

Even though early plain radiographs may be normal, these films should always be obtained first. Although not specific for osteomyelitis, soft tissue changes may be noted as early as the third or fourth day of the illness (Fig. 6-5). Changes in the bone, such as periosteal new bone formation and resorption at the metaphysis, are often evident by the seventh day (Fig. 6-6). Of note, early antibiotic therapy may mask or eliminate the typical radiographic findings.

The triphasic technetium 99 methylene diphosphonate bone scan is the radiographic test of choice for the diagnosis of early acute osteomyelitis. Abnormal findings are present early in the course of the disease (see Fig. 2-8), and this test can usually differentiate soft tissue from bone infections. If better discrimination between inflammation of the bone versus the joint space is required, MRI is suitable.

Pyogenic Arthritis

Pyogenic arthritis is yet another consideration when evaluating a patient with fever and painful limping or refusal to bear weight. The joint most frequently involved in pediatric patients is the hip. Hematogenous spread of bacteria, usually *S. aureus* or *Streptococcus pyogenes,* accounts for most joint infections. When multiple joints are involved, consideration of other organisms, such as *Neisseria gonorrhoeae,* is

appropriate. Arthritis after an animal bite is likely the result of infection with *Pasteurella multocida.* Chondrolytic enzymes released from the leukocytes are destructive to articular cartilage. The inflammatory response also creates an effusion that raises intracapsular pressure; if the joint is not emergently drained, avascular necrosis may result.

The clinical presentation of the child with pyogenic arthritis is often one of rapid onset of pain, equally rapid progression to painful limping, and more often absolute refusal to bear weight on the affected side. The child may appear toxic with high fever and listlessness. Rash may be present if the infecting organism is a toxin producer. In a child with an infected hip, the leg is held flexed, abducted, and externally rotated; this position is most comfortable because it decreases intracapsular pressure. An infected knee is usually held in flexion (Fig. 6-7). Swelling, warmth, erythema, and decreased range of motion of a joint are clues to infection but may be observed in noninfectious inflammatory joint diseases also.

As with osteomyelitis, a CBC, ESR, and blood culture should be obtained. Plain radiographs of the joint may demonstrate a widened joint space (Fig. 6-8), or they may be normal. If the hip joint is involved, ultrasound examination is very useful in detecting an effusion. Aspiration of the joint may confirm the presence of an effusion, but open surgical drainage is required for optimal management. It is imperative that material obtained by aspiration and open drainage be sent for Gram staining, bacterial culture, and sensitivity testing.

Lyme Disease

Intermittent chronic monoarthritis, particularly of the knee, is a feature of untreated stage 3 Lyme disease. In general, Lyme disease is an overly diagnosed condition. However, children who live in an area endemic with *Borrelia*

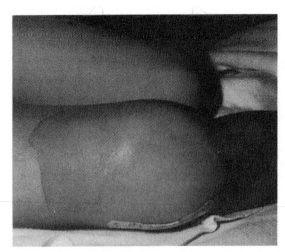

FIG. 6-7 Septic arthritis. This 8-year-old boy awoke suddenly at 3 AM with severe knee pain. By 8 AM he was febrile and had marked swelling and extreme limitation of movement. There was no overlying erythema. Examination of joint fluid revealed gram-positive cocci in chains, with a white blood cell count of 24,000/mm³. Cultures were positive for group A streptococci.

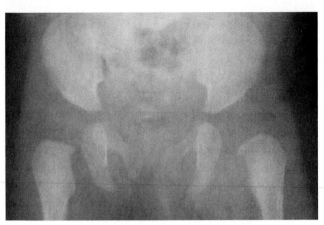

FIG. 6-8 Radiographic findings characteristic of septic arthritis. Although radiographs may be normal early on, joint-space widening can be detected in most cases. In this infant who showed fever, toxicity, and refusal to move the left leg, capsular swelling and lateral displacement of the proximal left femur are readily apparent. (Courtesy Dr. Roderigo Dominguez, University of Texas.)

burgdorferi and who present in the summer or fall with sudden onset of knee pain and swelling are quite likely to be infected with *B. burgdorferi*. A history of a tick bite followed by the characteristic erythema chronicum migrans rash is pathognomonic for Lyme disease (Fig. 6-9).

Soft Tissue Infection
Bacterial infections of the skin or muscles may also cause painful limping. Cellulitis of the foot, for example, after varicella infection, may be due to either *S. pyogenes* or *S. aureus*.

Diskitis
Although there has been debate about the cause of diskitis, many authors now believe that diskitis is a bacterial infection of the intervertebral disk space and is self-limiting in many cases (see Chapter 2). In general, patients have low-grade fever, back pain, and either a stiff gait or refusal to walk. An antecedent upper respiratory tract infection or gastroenteritis is a frequent historic finding. The physical examination reveals only mild to moderate back tenderness and decreased range of motion of the spine. If the patient will walk, the gait is stiff. Walking and climbing stairs makes the pain worse, and rest only partially relieves it.

The diagnosis of diskitis is confirmed by appropriate laboratory and radiographic studies. A CBC, ESR, and differential count are helpful but are not diagnostic by themselves. A normal or slightly elevated white blood cell count and an ESR less than 50 mm/hr are expected. Blood cultures are usually sterile in patients with diskitis.

Plain radiographs of the spine are usually normal early in the illness but after several weeks reveal narrowing of the disk space and irregularity of the vertebral body endplates. Early in the illness, technetium 99 bone scintigraphy is a sensitive method for localization to the disk space. MRI is yet another method for radiologic diagnosis.

The most controversial aspect of the diagnosis of diskitis is the decision about whether or not to aspirate the disk space. This procedure has been reserved for those patients who do not improve with conservation management. However, each case ought to be considered individually in consultation with colleagues in orthopedic surgery.

Other Infectious Causes
Systemic viral infections are associated with arthritis and occasionally with painful limping. Hepatitis B and Epstein-Barr virus both cause a mild arthritis of the large joints. Rubella infection and immunization are both associated with arthritis of the knee. Other viral infections, such as influenza, induce calf tenderness sufficient to cause limping.

Inflammatory Causes

Transient Synovitis of the Hip
Transient synovitis of the hip, also known as *toxic synovitis*, is another important cause of limping in the young child. It is more common in boys, and the peak age of affection is between 3 and 10 years. It is believed to represent a postinfectious, reactive arthritis of the hip. Common antecedent events include viral upper respiratory tract infections, acute gastroenteritis, and immunization with live-virus vaccines.

The progression and severity of transient synovitis is different from that of osteomyelitis. Patients endure the gradual onset of a mildly painful limp, usually bear weight on the affected side, and appear only mildly ill. Again, like other patients with hip disorders, knee pain may be the chief com-

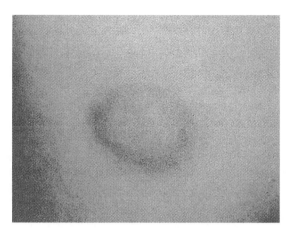

FIG. 6-9 Erythema chronicum migrans in a patient with Lyme disease. The lesion may be a large erythematous macule with central clearing, occurring singly or multiply.

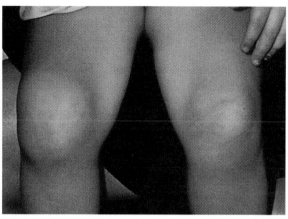

FIG. 6-10 This toddler with pauciarticular JRA has unilateral knee swelling with slight erythema. The right knee demonstrates loss of the normal anatomic landmarks.

plaint. The physical examination is notable for normal temperature or low-grade fever and a resting posture in which the hip is held in flexion, abduction, and external rotation. Internal rotation of the hip is diminished, the child's gait is antalgic, and there may be mild tenderness of the hip joint on palpation and compression.

The primary challenge in the evaluation of a child with fever, limp, and an abnormal hip examination is to differentiate transient synovitis from pyogenic arthritis, osteomyelitis, and Legg-Calvé-Perthes disease (among others). Clinical and laboratory features suggestive of toxic synovitis include a relatively well-appearing patient, low-grade fever, the willingness to bear weight (albeit with an antalgic gait), a normal or mildly elevated white blood cell count, and an ESR less than 30 mm/hr. In patients with transient synovitis, plain radiographs of the hips are either normal or show mild widening of the joint space because of increased fluid. Ultrasound examination of the hip joint is a highly effective method for detecting an effusion. Aspiration of the hip must be seriously considered in all febrile children with a hip effusion. Consultation with an orthopedic surgeon, regarding the need for aspiration in a patient with possible transient synovitis, is strongly recommended.

Rheumatologic Disorders

Rheumatologic disease is an important category of the inflammatory causes of limping (Box 6-2). A comprehensive treatment of this subject is beyond the scope of this chapter, but the salient features of the more common disorders are offered instead.

Of the three subtypes of juvenile rheumatoid arthritis (JRA), pauciarticular JRA is the most likely to have limping as the predominant manifestation of the illness. By definition

---

BOX 6-2

Rheumatologic Causes of Limping

Juvenile rheumatoid arthritis
    Pauciarticular JRA
    Polyarticular JRA
    Systemic-onset JRA
Acute rheumatic fever
Seronegative spondyloarthropathies
    Juvenile ankylosing spondylitis
    Reiter syndrome
    Psoriatic arthritis
Systemic lupus erythematosus
Inflammatory bowel disease
Henoch-Schönlein purpura

---

there are fewer than four joints involved; the arthritis is asymmetric and most often involves the knees, ankles, and elbows (Fig. 6-10). Type I pauciarticular JRA is more common in young girls (ages 2 to 5 years), and they frequently have a positive antinuclear antibody (ANA) test. These girls are at risk for chronic iridocyclitis. Hip involvement is rare. Type II pauciarticular JRA is more common in older boys, and their tests for ANA are negative. These patients are not at the same risk for chronic iridocyclitis as the patients with type I pauciarticular JRA. Hip and sacroiliac arthritis is more likely in type II pauciarticular JRA, and more than half of patients test positive for HLA-B27.

Systemic-onset JRA rarely presents with limping as the only sign of the illness. This subtype is characterized by polyarthritis and systemic features of fever and rash. Generalized stiffness and gel phenomenon (joint stiffness after rest) may be seen. Other organ involvement (liver, heart, bone marrow, etc.) is common in systemic-onset JRA. Boys and girls are affected equally. Tests for rheumatoid factors and ANA are negative.

Rheumatoid factor–negative polyarticular JRA is usually seen in girls without prominent systemic manifestations. Any joint may be affected, but arthritis of the small joints of the hand is typical. A small number of patients have a positive ANA test. Rheumatoid factor–positive polyarticular JRA, on the other hand, is a more severe polyarthritis with conspicuous systemic features, such as weight loss. All of these patients have a positive rheumatoid factor test, and a very high number also have a positive ANA test.

Acute rheumatic fever occurs after untreated streptococcal pharyngitis, and joint complaints are a prevailing feature. Large joints are predominantly affected, and migration is a key feature of the arthropathy of acute rheumatic fever. Often the arthritis is symmetric. Pain is moderate to severe and often out of proportion to the degree of objective joint involvement. A careful evaluation for carditis, subcutaneous nodules, erythema marginatum, and minor criteria is warranted. The revised Jones criteria should be carefully reviewed.

The seronegative spondyloarthropathies include juvenile ankylosing spondylitis (JAS), Reiter syndrome, and psoriatic arthritis. Back and sacroiliac joint pain and enthesitis (inflammation and pain at the insertion sites of ligaments and tendons) are clues to JAS, whereas conjunctivitis and urethritis are features of Reiter syndrome. A scaly rash and nail pitting are very suggestive of psoriatic arthritis. A thorough examination of every patient with limping is always superior to a cursory inspection of the area where there is pain or swelling.

Several systemic diseases are accompanied by an inflammatory arthritis. Inflammatory bowel disease, systemic lupus erythematosus, and sarcoidosis, for example, are well known for their association with joint complaints. Usually the systemic features are prominent in these conditions (fever, weight loss, diarrhea, rash, anemia, erythema nodosum, etc.), but occasionally arthritis and/or limp may be a presenting complaint, similar to that of pauciarticular JRA.

Henoch-Schönlein purpura (HSP) is another inflammatory process with pronounced joint involvement. Patients may complain of severe pain in the elbows, wrists, knees, and ankles and yet have only mild swelling. Abdominal pain, hematochezia, purpuric rash on the buttocks and extensor surfaces of the arms and legs, and hematuria complete the classic picture of HSP (see Fig. 23-17).

Two uncommon causes of painful limping worth mentioning are plantar fasciitis and thrombophlebitis. Inflammation of the plantar fascia is occasionally seen in adolescents, especially runners. A characteristic complaint is heel pain that is at its very worst in the morning when the patient wakes and takes his or her first steps; the pain then improves with motion. On examination the physician finds tenderness over the calcaneus at the insertion of the plantar fascia. This is a clinical diagnosis, and radiographs, which will be normal, are unnecessary. In thrombophlebitis, affected veins are usually superficial in location and are visibly tender, swollen, and erythematous.

Neoplastic Causes

Painful limping may be the chief complaint of patients with malignant and benign tumors of bone. In addition, nighttime pain is a frequent and significant complaint in many children with bone tumors. Acute lymphocytic leukemia and acute myelogenous leukemia sometimes cause bone pain and joint swelling even before the development of overt hematologic abnormalities.

Osteosarcoma, the most common malignant tumor of bone, is correlated with bone growth. Thus the onset typically occurs in adolescence during a growth spurt. Boys are affected more often than girls. The tumor arises at the metaphyseal ends of long bones; the femur is the most commonly involved bone. Patients often have vaguely described yet localized pain at the site of the tumor. Frequently the pain is ascribed to minor antecedent trauma. Involvement of the femur and pelvis produces a disturbance of gait well before a palpable mass is present. There are usually no systemic signs or symptoms associated with osteosarcoma. For this reason, all children (especially adolescents) with unexplained painful limping that persists deserve plain radiographic studies of the involved extremity. The radiographic appearance is highly characteristic, particularly if the tumor has eroded through the periosteum, the so-called sunburst sign (Fig. 6-11). Open biopsy of the tumor secures definitive diagnosis, and other studies are performed to assess the extent of the tumor spread, if any.

Ewing sarcoma is a small round cell tumor of bone that occurs in young children and adolescents. The incidence is higher in boys, and it is almost nonexistent in African-American patients. It arises in flat bones and long bones, usually in the diaphysis. In addition to an antalgic gait, patients with Ewing sarcoma experience pain and swelling at the site of the lesion. Many children also have systemic symptoms, including weight loss and fever, especially if metastatic disease exists. An "onion skin" appearance of the lesion on plain radiographs strongly suggests the diagnosis, but definitive diagnosis is obtained by tissue biopsy.

The cause of aneurysmal bone cysts is controversial; whether they arise *de novo* or as secondary phenomena stemming from underlying malignancies is unsettled. Nonetheless these are aggressive lesions that cause painful limping and pathologic fractures visible on plain radiographs.

Eosinophilic granuloma of bone, Langerhans cell histiocytosis, is a benign neoplasm of bone. The femur, vertebrae, and pelvis are common sites for this tumor; patients have painful limping, and swelling may be evident on inspection. A CBC is usually normal, but the ESR is often elevated. Plain radiographs may expose a lucent lesion, and technetium 99 bone scanning localizes some but not all lesions that are not

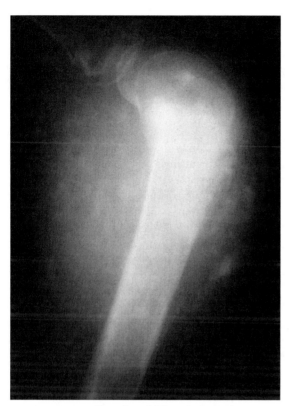

FIG. 6-11 An x-ray film of a child with osteosarcoma shows soft tissue swelling, calcification, cortical bone destruction with increased osteodensity, and new bone formation (Codman's triangle). (Courtesy Dr. Jocelyn Ledesma-Medina, Children's Hospital of Pittsburgh.)

evident on standard radiographs. The diagnosis is confirmed by tissue pathology, and consultation with colleagues from orthopedics and oncology is necessary.

Osteoid osteoma is a benign tumor of bone that may present in a way that suggests malignancy. It occurs most commonly in preadolescent children. Boys are affected more often than are girls. The child with osteoid osteoma gives a history of severe, constant pain that is typically worse at night. The pain is almost always completely relieved by aspirin; if aspirin fails to relieve the pain, an alternative diagnosis is likely. Most osteoid osteomas occur in the femur and tibia. Patients complain of groin, thigh, knee, or tibial pain and have an antalgic gait. On physical examination the joints are normal, and there may be pain on palpation of the bone over the tumor site. Patients with vertebral osteoid osteomas complain of back pain and may have a stiff gait. Plain radiographs of the long bones reveal a radiolucent area (or "nidus") encompassed by sclerotic bone. Vertebral lesions can be difficult to see on plain radiographs; consultation with colleagues in orthopedic surgery and radiology is helpful in selecting other imaging methods and in planning therapy.

Benign osteoblastoma is a very uncommon tumor seen in older children and adolescents that causes painful limping. It typically occurs in the femur and tibia but may occur in the foot. Plain radiographs reveal the lesion.

Nonossifiying fibroma is another benign tumor of bone that causes localized pain and limping without constitutional symptoms or signs. The diagnosis is evident from plain radiographs.

Hematologic Causes

Two inherited hematologic disorders are uncommon but important causes of painful limping. Patients with hemophilia endure recurrent bleeding into joints and may have painful limping and a swollen and tender joint, usually the knee joint. Children and adolescents with sickle cell anemia, are vulnerable to microinfarcts of long bones often causing intense pain and limping. Infants and toddlers with sickle cell anemia chiefly suffer from hand and foot involvement ("dactylitis").

Deep venous thromboses are very uncommon in children and adolescents; their presence may be related to risk factors, such as pregnancy or the use of birth control pills, nephrotic syndrome, inflammatory bowel disease, or inherited disorders of coagulation. Painful limping accompanied by a swollen and tender extremity ought to prompt consideration of a thrombus. Rare causes of painful limping include lead intoxication and hypervitaminosis A; both of these disorders cause bone pain with a paucity of findings on physical examination of the legs.

Intraabdominal Causes

Pediatricians and family practitioners must also consider the possibility that a child with painful limping may have an intraabdominal disorder rather than a disorder of the lower extremity. Painful limping is one of the many symptoms of both appendicitis and psoas muscle abscesses, for example. An antalgic gait or refusal to bear weight, hip pain, and findings consistent with hip inflammation (such as the frog-leg position and decreased internal rotation of the hip) may be seen with appendicitis or a psoas muscle abscess. Pelvic abscess is an uncommon cause of painful limping but deserves consideration in sexually active girls. Careful attention to the history and the abdominal and rectal examinations helps to distinguish these problems from disorders of the hip. Similarly, patients with inguinal hernias, lymphadenitis, and testicular torsion occasionally have painful limping. These problems are easily diagnosed by a complete physical examination and are just as easily missed by a brief look at only the legs and feet.

Nonpainful Limping

Muscle Disorders

Children with inherited disorders of muscle, such as Duchenne muscular dystrophy, often have a gait disturbance. The muscular dystrophies tend to appear in a subtle fashion during early to late childhood. There may be a history of delayed motor milestones, and the gait is waddling. Pseudohy-

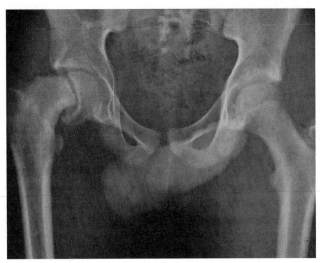

FIG. 6-12 Slipped capital femoral epiphysis. In this anteroposterior radiograph the right femoral head is displaced medially in relation to the femoral neck as a result of epiphyseal separation.

pertrophy of the calves is a striking feature of Duchenne muscular dystrophy as is the presence of a Gowers sign (Fig. 6-1). An elevated serum creatinine phosphokinase level is present in most but not all of the muscular dystrophies. Electromyography and muscle biopsy are other important tests for the diagnosis of the muscular dystrophies.

Bone Disorders

Leg Length Discrepancy

Differences in the lengths of the legs are associated with nonpainful limping. Such discrepancies caused by an abnormally short leg can be an isolated, idiopathic condition or arise from pathology, such as avascular necrosis of the femoral head, coxa vara, neoplasia, growth plate injury from previous trauma or infection, or metabolic bone disease. When a discrepancy occurs because one leg is abnormally long the cause may be a vascular malformation, hemangioma, or neurofibroma. Measurement of the lower legs from the anterior iliac spine to the tip of the medial malleolus takes little time and is essential to detect important differences in length. Two or more centimeters difference is significant, and referral to a pediatric orthopedic surgeon is warranted in this situation.

Coxa Vara

Coxa vara is defined as an angle of less than 120 degrees between the shaft and neck of the femur. Normally this angle is 150 degrees. It may be unilateral or bilateral. Clinical clues to unilateral coxa vara include a nonpainful Trendelenburg limp, a positive Trendelenburg sign, and limited external rotation and decreased abduction of the involved hip. A waddling gait and a positive Trendelenburg test bilaterally are observed when there is bilateral coxa vara.

Slipped Capital Femoral Epiphysis

Slipped capital femoral epiphysis (SCFE) is an uncommon but certainly not rare orthopedic disorder that usually affects obese and/or very tall boys and girls between the ages of 10 and 16 years. It is a fracture of the growth plate in which the capital femoral epiphysis slips off of the femoral neck in the posteromedial direction. SCFE is bilateral in a large number of cases. Classically these patients have limping and an externally rotated hip; many are perceived as "clumsy." Some but not all also complain of pain in the thigh, knee, or groin. Clues on physical examination include painful hip abduction and limitation of internal rotation. Plain radiographs of the hip, including anteroposterior and frog-leg views, demonstrate widening of the growth plate and medial slip of the capital epiphysis (Fig. 6-12). CT scanning also confirms the diagnosis of SCFE. This condition is an emergency, and patients must not be allowed to bear weight (even en route to the radiology department) until surgical fixation is accomplished.

Children with Blount disease, which refers to bowing of the tibia(s) resulting from a growth disturbance of the medial portion of the proximal tibial physis, may have an awkward gait that is not painful. Plain radiographs document the "beaking" of the tibia and the degree of deformity.

Scoliosis

The pelvis is normally level, but with moderate to severe degrees of scoliosis of the spine it is not level and nonpainful limping may occur. While standing, patients demonstrate an uneven pelvis, and scoliosis is evident when the patient bends over.

Joint Disorders

Developmental Dysplasia of the Hip

Formerly called *congenital dislocation of the hip*, developmental dislocation or dysplasia of the hip causes nonpainful limp in toddlers who have just begun to walk. The term *developmental dysplasia of the hip* represents a range of pathology, including acetabular dysplasia, hip dislocation, and hip subluxation. Ideally this condition is diagnosed in the first few weeks to months of life because early recognition and treatment are associated with the best prognosis. However, in a small number of children the development of acetabular dysplasia can occur in such a gradual and elusive fashion that routine hip examinations in the first year of life appear normal and only when the toddler begins to walk is a problem suspected. This disorder is more common in girls and in infants born in the breech position.

On physical examination, affected toddlers limp without pain and have limited hip abduction, tight adductor muscles, and asymmetric thigh folds. Unilateral developmental dysplasia of the hip results in a Trendelenburg gait. Children with bilateral hip dislocation display a wide perineum, waddling gait, and hyperlordosis. At this stage, plain radiographs in the anteroposterior and frog-leg views are diagnostic. Referral to an orthopedic surgeon is mandatory.

Contractures

Joint contractures of the hip, knee, or ankle cause non-painful limping. When multiple joints are involved, the physician should consider rare conditions associated with contractures, such as arthrogryposis and the mucopolysaccharidoses.

Joint Hypermobility

Joint hypermobility in children and adolescents who are normal in all other regards is occasionally associated with limping, which generally is not painful. Excessive joint hypermobility is a feature of connective tissue disorders, such as the Marfan and Ehlers-Danlos syndromes; a complete physical examination reveals evidence of these disorders.

Neurologic Conditions

Involvement of the central or peripheral nervous system at any level can disturb a patient's gait. The most common neurologic cause of an abnormal gait is static encephalopathy. Such patients demonstrate increased muscle tone, hyper-reflexia, and a spastic or "jerky" gait. Children with very mild spasticity appear to have a normal gait when walking, but running brings out abnormalities, such as flexion posturing of the upper extremities. Congenital spinal cord lesions, such as diastematomyelia, and acquired lesions, such as intraspinal masses, may present with limping secondary to weakness as a chief complaint. Focal CNS lesions such as a brain tumor, stroke, or spinal cord mass may cause limp because of weakness. Similarly a global process, such as a de-myelinating disorder, may also lead to limping because of weakness. Drug ingestion, cerebellar tumors, and CNS infections may cause ataxia in which the gait is wide-based and unsteady. Finally, although rare, flaccid paralysis of the lower extremity caused by poliomyelitis must be considered. Careful attention to the history and meticulous neurologic and musculoskeletal examinations differentiate these disorders from other causes of nonpainful limping.

Psychologic Disorders

Gait disturbance may be a presentation of a conversion reaction. Briefly, conversion reactions epitomize the unconscious expression of psychologic conflict through somatic symptoms. Office pediatricians and family practitioners observe these reactions most often in teenage patients and only occasionally in younger children. They are more common in girls than boys. Abdominal pain, chest pain, headache, and dizziness are common complaints of patients with conversion reactions, but gait disturbances are even more common. Key clinical features include a gait disturbance that is inconsistent with any identifiable anatomic or physiologic dysfunction, prolonged school absence, and either an indifferent or an overly dramatic attitude of the patient toward the symptom. Careful social and family histories reveal sources of conflict and often a model for the patient's symptom. For example, a close relative who has suffered a stroke and has an altered gait might serve as a model for a teenager who suddenly develops paralysis of a limb. Gold and Friedman recently reviewed this subject in-depth.

Reflex sympathetic dystrophy (RSD) is an unusual disorder of unknown cause. Many cases occur after minor trauma. RSD is characterized by limb pain associated with hyperesthesia, edema, color changes (erythema or cyanosis), and either very dry or moist skin. The pain is generally continuous and periodically worsens. Atrophy of skin, subcutaneous tissues, and muscle occurs if RSD persists for several weeks. It is more common in girls than in boys, and psychologic dysfunction is the rule. Laboratory studies (CBC, ESR, and serologies) and plain radiographs are normal. Bone scanning is abnormal. It is important to distinguish RSD from other organic diseases and conversion reaction.

History

The history is a key element in defining the cause of limping. First the examiner should ask if the limping is painful. All knee pain does not come from the knee; pain referred to the knee is common in hip disorders and has misled many fine physicians! Similarly, buttocks and thigh pain may be referred from the lower spine or sacroiliac joints. Is the pain constant or intermittent? Constant pain raises concerns for malignant tumors of bone and leukemia. Pain that is worse with motion and better with rest is more typical of traumatic and infectious causes of limping. Some inflammatory disorders, such as plantar fasciitis, improve with motion. Severe pain is more typical of osteomyelitis, pyogenic arthritis, malignancies, and fractures, whereas the pain of transient synovitis, JRA, and repetitive microtrauma is generally only mild to moderate. Pain may be entirely absent in patients with slipped capital femoral epiphysis.

Another critical element of the early history is a history of trauma and whether or not that history accounts for all the findings. A hallmark of child abuse is a history that is inconsistent with the injury. Details about the mechanism of injury, such as hyperextension or flexion of the knee, should be obtained. Even a history of minor trauma may be important; fractures occur more easily from "trivial" trauma when there is an underlying abnormality of bone, such as a bone cyst or tumor. Alternatively, major disability after minor injury is an indication of reflex sympathetic dystrophy. Does running or jumping produce the pain and limping? This suggests a stress fracture.

The examiner must determine if there are any other constitutional signs of infection or inflammation, such as fatigue, weight loss, night sweats, pallor, rashes, or diarrhea. The physician should ask about symptoms of rheumatologic disease, including joint swelling, morning stiffness, hair loss, alopecia, conjunctivitis, dryness of the eyes or mouth, oral ulcers, or urethritis. If the review of systems reveals nighttime pain, pallor, and easy bruising, a malignancy should be sus-

Abnormal Gait: Age of Onset

Preschool (Toddler to 5 Years)
Trauma
Toxic synovitis
Diskitis
Osteomyelitis
Developmental dysplasia of the hip

School Age (>5 Years to <12 Years)
Trauma
Legg-Calvé-Perthes disease
Ewing sarcoma
Osteogenic sarcoma

Teenage (>12 Years)
Trauma
Slipped capital femoral epiphysis
Osgood-Schlatter disease
Chondromalacia patellae
Osteogenic sarcoma
Conversion disorder
Reflex sympathetic dystrophy

pected. Similarly a history of back or abdominal pain indicates the possibility of an intraabdominal cause of limping.

The age, gender, and sports participation of the patient are very helpful in estimating the likely cause of limping (Box 6-3). Younger boys with painful limping are more vulnerable to Legg-Calvé-Perthes disease, whereas teenage boys are prone to slipped femoral capital epiphysis, for example. Teenage girls with knee pain frequently have Osgood-Schlatter disease. Gymnasts and tennis players of either gender are subject to spondylolysis and spondylolisthesis. Runners are vulnerable to plantar calluses, chronic knee pain, shin splints, and tibial stress fractures. If the patient participates regularly in a particular sport, the examiner should determine if the patient has recently increased the intensity of the activity; in the fall, new complaints of knee or leg pain may be the result of overtraining after a summer of relative inactivity.

Has the patient had a recent illness, such as an upper respiratory tract infection or gastroenteritis? These minor illnesses frequently occur before the onset of transient synovitis. Is there a history of a preceding pharyngitis that was untreated, and could the patient's complaints stem from acute rheumatic fever?

The past medical history must be complete because a number of problems predispose children to conditions that develop later in life and cause limping. Both rickets and transient synovitis, for example, may lead to limb length inequality. Transient synovitis of the hip is a precursor of Legg-Calvé-Perthes disease in some patients. Femoral artery

catheters placed in infants have been associated with interrupted vascular supply to and subsequent avascular necrosis of the femoral head.

A careful social history is especially important if there is any concern about abuse or neglect. Inquiry regarding school attendance and function is essential when a functional disorder is suspected. The examiner should also determine if there is a family history of rheumatic fever, systemic lupus erythematosus, juvenile rheumatoid arthritis, ankylosing spondylitis, Reiter syndrome, inflammatory bowel disease, sickle cell anemia, or hemophilia.

Physical Examination

The physical examination of the child with a limp is the proverbial road to riches, with a very high yield for clinicians. Although it is tempting to examine the lower extremities first, a host of systemic disorders may present with limping as a chief complaint. Therefore a thorough general examination is the recommended first step.

Growth parameters must not be overlooked. Weight loss and height deceleration are associated with subacute or chronic systemic diseases. The presence or absence of fever is equally important; the febrile patient is likely to have an infectious cause of limping, although the absence of fever does not exclude infection. Examination of the eyes, skin, hair, and nails may yield clues to rheumatic fever, systemic lupus erythematosus, Henoch-Schönlein purpura, and psoriatic arthritis, for example. Are there bruises in various stages of healing in unusual places? The examiner must always consider the possibility of abuse in patients with traumatic causes of limping.

Two other areas of the body merit meticulous attention—the abdomen and the back. In a child with fever and a right-sided antalgic limp, tenderness in the right lower abdominal quadrant may point to appendiceal inflammation as the source. Similarly, midline back tenderness and paravertebral muscle spasm raise concern for infection or inflammation of some element of the spinal column.

A complete neurologic examination is essential in patients with gait disturbances. Signs of nystagmus, truncal ataxia, incoordination of rapid alternating movements, weakness, absent reflexes, or tone abnormalities direct the examiner toward a neurologic cause.

Of course the examination of the lower extremities is paramount. This begins with observation of the child when entering the examination room. What is the activity level and general appearance of the child? What is the resting position of the lower extremities? Hip pathology, such as pyogenic arthritis or transient synovitis, produces inflammation within the joint capsule; to minimize pressure within the joint and decrease pain the child holds the limb in the FABERE (*f*lexed, *ab*ducted, *e*xternally *r*otated, and *e*xtended) position. All patients should be asked to climb onto the examination table so the examiner can observe which leg bears the weight of climbing. Does the patient need assistance in climbing? This can be a clue to weakness. When the patient rises to a standing position from a prone position, is there a Gowers sign, signifying gluteal muscle weakness or pain in the spine? Also, the examiner should ask the patient to sit up from the supine position; this is difficult for the child or adolescent with spine or hip inflammation. The legs should be inspected for evidence of trauma, foreign bodies, infection, arthritis, muscle atrophy, and pseudohypertrophy. The examiner should always have patients remove their shoes and socks. Common areas for subtle foreign bodies include the soles of the feet and the spaces between the toes. Are there foot deformities? Leg length should be measured from the anterior superior iliac spine to the medial malleolus. A discrepancy of 2 or more cm is clinically significant.

Active evaluation of the lower extremities is best started on the normal limb. The physician should examine each bone and joint for tenderness, erythema, and swelling. Stabilizing the knee while rotating the ankle in the opposite direction may elicit tenderness in a toddler's fracture where palpation was unrevealing. Both active and passive range of motion of the joints should be assessed. The examiner should always include the spine as a part of the joint examination. The sacroiliac joints should be palpated, especially in patients with back or hip pain. Muscle groups should be tested for tenderness, strength, and tone. Careful palpation of the insertion sites of tendons and ligaments identifies enthesitis, an important feature of seronegative spondyloarthropathies.

A key element of the examination is gait assessment. Whenever possible, the patient should be asked to walk, hop, run, and climb stairs. Is the gait antalgic, suggesting one of the more common causes of gait disturbance, such as trauma? Is the gait Trendelenburg, suggesting a disorder in the hip? Also, the examiner should ask the patient to balance independently on each leg and look for a Trendelenburg sign. Is the gait broad-based and unsteady, which is typical of a cerebellar disorder? If the patient refuses to bear weight at all, the physician should look closely for a very painful lesion, such as pyogenic arthritis. If the gait is completely normal in bare feet and only alters when the child wears shoes, the examiner should take a closer look at the shoes! Finally, if the patient has a normal physical examination and a normal gait in the office, reexamination when the symptom recurs is prudent.

Approach to the Patient

The approach to the patient with the symptom of limping is based on a careful history and complete physical examination. Once the mechanism of the disorder is ascertained (e.g., mechanical, infectious, neurologic, etc.), the physician may then decide if other diagnostic measures are appropriate.

In the afebrile child or adolescent with painful limping, particular attention should be given to the possibility of trauma. Overuse injuries are especially suspect if the patient

is an athlete. In some cases, when the cause is minor trauma, the diagnosis is evident on clinical grounds alone and no further investigation is necessary. In other cases, however, plain radiographs may be required to confirm a particular diagnosis. For example, both Osgood-Schlatter disease and osteochondritis dissecans cause chronic knee pain, and differentiation between the two may be difficult on clinical grounds alone. The physician should always order plain radiographs if a fracture or foreign body is suspected. However, not all foreign bodies are radiolucent! If child abuse is suspected, a skeletal survey or technetium 99 bone scan to detect occult fractures is recommended. Finally, plain radiographs are essential in the diagnosis of many other disorders, such as Kohler bone disease and tarsal bone coalitions. Limping secondary to a disorder of the spinal column always requires a comprehensive radiologic evaluation (see Chapter 2).

Plain radiographs should be the first step in imaging of the patient with painful limping, fever, or other evidence of an infectious, inflammatory, or neoplastic process and no history of trauma. Early in the course of osteomyelitis and diskitis, plain radiographs are normal or show only very subtle signs of soft tissue changes. However, technetium 99 bone scintigraphy permits diagnosis of osteomyelitis and diskitis if the patient presents early in the illness before overt signs of bone infection are evident on plain radiographs. An MRI study is useful if the bone scan is equivocal and osteomyelitis is strongly suspected. Plain radiographs may also reveal changes in the bones that point toward neoplastic causes of limping. For example, the child with acute lymphoblastic leukemia who limps because of bone pain may have "leukemic lines" visible on plain radiographs. Plain radiographs are also the first step toward the diagnosis of primary bone tumors.

The clinical diagnosis of a joint effusion may be confirmed by plain radiographs or by ultrasound examination. The presence of a joint effusion mandates consideration of aspiration of the fluid. If the physician suspects pyogenic arthritis, joint aspiration is required and there should be no delay in consultation with a pediatric orthopedic surgeon. Hip aspiration is also useful in children with transient synovitis of the hip to exclude the possibility of pyogenic arthritis.

Laboratory studies play an important role in the evaluation of the limping patient. In patients with fever and/or other constitutional symptoms, the examiner should always obtain a CBC with differential and platelet counts and an ESR. A blood culture is always appropriate in patients who are suspected to have an infectious illness, even if the patient has only low-grade temperature elevation. Liver enzyme assays, total protein and albumin levels, and uric acid and rheumatologic tests may be necessary as well. For example, ANA and rheumatoid factor tests are appropriate studies for a 4-year-old girl with limping and swollen knees because her presentation suggests the possibility of pauciarticular JRA. A throat culture and streptococcal antibody titers are mandatory tests in patients with suspected acute rheumatic fever. There are no tests diagnostic for Henoch-Schönlein purpura, but a CBC with differential and platelet count is indicated in any child with purpura to look for thrombocytopenia and other features suggestive of malignancy.

Plain radiographs also have a major role in the evaluation of patients with nonpainful limping. All children with a leg length discrepancy should have plain radiographs of the lower extremities, including the hip. Similarly, coxa vara, slipped capital femoral epiphysis, Blount disease, and developmental dysplasia of the hip are confirmed by plain radiography.

Children with muscular dystrophy and other neurologic disorders always require specialized tests referred to earlier. The examiner must be especially careful to exclude spinal column pathology in patients with limping, back pain, and/or an abnormal neurologic examination. The diagnosis of gait disturbances caused by psychologic dysfunction is particularly challenging. However, time invested in a careful social history may prevent a frustrating and unnecessary search for nonexistent physical ailments.

SUMMARY

Definitive evaluation of the limping child is always based on a careful history and a meticulous physical examination, which includes gait analysis. The experienced clinician knows that, although the cause may be relatively benign, limping is never normal and may be the first sign of a serious disorder. Trauma and infection are the leading causes of painful limping; disorders of muscles, bones, and joints are the chief culprits in patients with nonpainful limping. Judicious use of radiographic and laboratory testing allows prompt diagnosis and treatment of many disorders by the primary care physician and also confirms which patients require subspecialty consultation.

ILLUSTRATIVE CASES

Case 1. K.K. is a 2-year-old white boy who had a chief complaint of fever and limping. He was well until 6 days before presentation when he developed fever, nasal congestion, and rhinorrhea. The nasal symptoms resolved after 1 day, but he began to have daily temperatures as high as 105° F. Three days before presentation, he began to complain of left hip pain and his parents observed him limping. His pain worsened; he refused to walk and preferred to crawl.

On physical examination he appears nontoxic, is afebrile, and has normal vital signs. He initially refuses to stand but later walks with encouragement. His gait is antalgic with a decreased stance phase on the left leg. His general physical examination is normal. His abdomen and spine are without any tenderness to palpation. He is most comfortable in the supine position with his left hip held in flexion and abduction. He resists extension of the left hip, but all other joints are normal.

His initial evaluation included a CBC, which revealed an elevated white blood cell count with a predominance of polymorphonuclear cells, and an ESR of 61 mm/hr. Plain radiographs of the hips were normal. A technetium 99 bone scan revealed increased uptake in the left femoral head consistent with osteomyelitis. A blood culture obtained on the day of admission grew Streptococcus pneumoniae.

The differential diagnosis in this case includes pyogenic arthritis, toxic synovitis, and osteomyelitis. The indolent onset of the limp argues against pyogenic arthritis. However, the resting position of the patient (with the hip in flexion and abduction) could be consistent with pyogenic arthritis or osteomyelitis of the hip. High fever and the presence of a high ESR are not typical of toxic synovitis and suggest a bacterial cause. The plain radiographs were normal, which is expected in patients with early bone infection. Osteomyelitis was confirmed by bone scan, and the bacterial cause was identified by blood culture.

Case 2. B.W. is a 2-year-old boy with a chief complaint of limping accompanied by fever. He was well until 6 weeks before presentation, when he developed temperatures up to 102° F daily. The fevers continued for 2 weeks, and he was treated with an oral antibiotic for otitis media. After 2 days of treatment, his fever resolved for 3 days but then returned. At the same time, he began to limp. His parents remarked that he "favored" his right leg. Two days before admission, a blood culture was obtained and was sterile. On the day of admission to the hospital, he complained of foot pain bilaterally. There are no other symptoms and no history of trauma, pallor, fatigue, or swollen joints.

On physical examination, he is irritable but consolable. He is febrile to 101.5° F. His gait is antalgic. He has enlargement of his posterior cervical lymph nodes and a palpable spleen tip. His spleen and joints are normal, but he is tender to palpation over his left distal femoral epiphysis. A second blood culture is obtained and is sterile. A CBC reveals a white blood cell count of 9100/mm³ with 27% polymorphonuclear cells, 47% lymphocytes, 14% monocytes, and 12% band forms. The hemoglobin is 9.8 g/dl, and the platelet count is 174,000/mm³. The ESR is 60 mm/hr. Plain radiographs of the lower extremities and feet are normal. A bone scan reveals increased uptake in the left distal femur, L3 vertebral body, and several ribs. While considering aspiration of bone for culture, a repeat CBC reveals 12% lymphoblasts. A bone marrow biopsy is diagnostic for acute lymphoblastic leukemia.

This case underscores the protean manifestations of cancer in young children. Fever and bone pain from leukemia can occur before lymphoblasts appear in the peripheral blood. Also, a complete examination revealed lymphadenopathy and splenomegaly, whereas a cursory inspection of the extremities would have missed valuable clues to the diagnosis.

Case 3.   M.M. is a 14-month-old girl brought to a pediatrician with a chief complaint of limping. She had moved to the United States 1 month earlier after being adopted. The adoptive parents were told that she was in good health but were given no other medical information. They denied any history of trauma, fever, rash, joint swelling, or pain. One month after she arrived, she began taking steps independently at which point her parents noticed the limp.

On physical examination, she is an afebrile toddler in no distress. There are no signs of trauma, and her general physical examination is normal. The bones and joints of her feet and legs are not tender to palpation. The legs are of equal size and length. Her strength and deep tendon reflexes are normal. There is no Gowers sign when she stands up from a prone position. However, she has asymmetry of the creases in her thigh folds, limited abduction of her right hip, and a right-sided Trendelenburg gait. Plain radiographs of the hips in the anteroposterior and frog-leg views reveal dysplasia of the right hip.

This case illustrates the need for routine examination of the hips in infants and toddlers. The prognosis is directly related to the time of diagnosis; the child described here required surgery and will, in all likelihood, never have a completely normal right hip.

ANNOTATED BIBLIOGRAPHY

Gold MA, Friedman SB: Conversion reactions in adolescents, *Pediatr Ann* 24:296-306, 1995.

> *This article is a key reference for the practitioner who sees children and adolescents with perplexing chronic pain complaints and no apparent physical illness.*

Renshaw TS: The child who has a limp, *Pediatr Rev* 16:458-465, 1995.

> *This is an excellent general review of the most common causes of limping in children and adolescents.*

Sills EM: What's causing the back pain? *Contemp Pediatr* 5:85-96, 1988.

> *An excellent treatment of back pain in general and diskitis in particular is given in this article.*

BIBLIOGRAPHY

Aronson J, Garvin K, Seibert J, et al: Efficiency of the bone scan for occult limping toddlers, *J Pediatr Orthop* 12:38-44, 1992.

Chande VE: Decision rules for roentgenography of children with acute ankle injuries, *Arch Pediatr Adolesc Med* 49:255-258, 1995.

Christy C, Siegal DM: Lyme disease: what it is, what it isn't, *Contemp Pediatr* 12:64-86, 1995.

Correa AG, Morven SE, Baker CJ: Vertebral osteomyelitis in children, *Pediatr Infect Dis J* 12:228-233, 1993.

Crawford AH, Kucharzyk DW, Ruda R, et al: Diskitis in children, *Clin Orthop* 266:70-79, 1991.

Delbeccaro MA, Champoux AN, Beckers T, et al: Septic arthritis versus transient synovitis of the hip: the value of screening laboratory tests, *Ann Emerg Med* 21:1418-1422, 1992.

Erlich MG, Hulstyn M, d'Amato C: Sports injuries in children and the clumsy child, *Pediatr Clin North Am* 39:433-449, 1992.

Freiberg AA, Randall TL, Heidelberger KP, et al: Aneurysmal bone cysts in young children, *J Pediatr Orthop* 14:86-91, 1994.

Green NE, Edwards K: Bone and joint infections in children, *Orthop Clin North Am* 18:555-576, 1987.

Jackson DW, Wiltse LL, Cirincione RJ: Spondylolysis in female gymnasts, *Clin Orthop* 118:68-73, 1976.

Jonsson OG, Sartain P, Ducore JM, et al: Bone pain as an initial symptom of childhood acute lymphoblastic leukemia: association with nearly normal hematologic indices, *J Pediatr* 17:233-237, 1990.

Mooney JF, Emans JB: Developmental dislocation of the hip: a clinical overview, *Pediatr Rev* 16:299-304, 1995.

Orlowski JP, Mercer RD: Osteoid osteoma in children and young adults, *Pediatrics* 59:526-532, 1977.

Sherry DD, McGuire T, Mellins E, et al: Psychosomatic musculoskeletal pain in childhood: clinical and psychological analyses of 100 children, *Pediatrics* 6:1093-1099, 1991.

Special Writing Group of the American Heart Association: Guidelines for the diagnosis of rheumatic fever: Jones criteria 1992 update, *JAMA* 268:2069-2073, 1992.

Syriopoulou VPH, Smith AL: Osteomyelitis and septic arthritis. In Feigen RD, Cherry JA, editors: *Textbook of pediatric infectious diseases,* vol 1, ed 2, Philadelphia, 1987, WB Saunders.

Tachdjian MO: *Pediatric orthopedics,* vol 1, ed 2, Philadelphia, 1990, WB Saunders.

Tunnessen Jr WW: *Signs and symptoms in pediatrics,* Philadelphia, 1983, JB Lippincott.

Temperature

7

Prolonged Fever

J. CARLTON GARTNER, Jr.

Key Points

- The examiner must know the normal values for temperature and document fever before embarking on a detailed investigation.

- History, physical examination, cultures, and screening laboratory data are the most important tests in evaluating prolonged fever.

- Newer imaging techniques should not be used randomly but selectively to confirm suspicions developed from the history and physical examination.

Prolonged fever is a complaint frequently encountered by the physician and is one of the more common reasons for a visit to the pediatrician. Most commonly, children with fever lasting several days have an infectious, usually viral, cause of their symptoms. Several general definitions are important. Fever lasting less than 1 week without an obvious source on examination is termed *fever without localizing signs* (FWL). During the past two decades, FWL has been the subject of numerous articles dealing with the possibility of bacteremia, criteria that predict serious infection, role of expectant antibiotic therapy, outcome, and so on. There are now published "guidelines" for management of this problem. True fever of unknown (or unexplained) origin (FUO) is a less common disorder. Definitions vary; for adults the standard definition is that given in Petersdorf's original paper: fever lasting for at least 3 weeks with no cause found after 1 week in the hospital. A useful definition in pediatrics, although not used in any of the major clinical series, is fever lasting for more than 1 week in a patient whose initial history, examination, and laboratory evaluation fail to reveal a cause. In this chapter an approach to the patient with FUO is described. The key role of history, examination, and screening laboratory tests is emphasized.

Pathophysiology

Fever represents a resetting of the body's "thermostat." It is a response to numerous triggering mechanisms, including infectious agents, immune complexes, antigens, lymphokines, and others. Stimulated monocytes, fixed-tissue macrophages (such as Kupffer cells in the liver), and certain other tissue cells release an interleukin (probably but not definitively interleukin-1 [IL-1]), which was formerly known from pioneering experiments as *endogenous pyrogen*. IL-1 activates numerous acute-phase responses of the body's immune system, including the synthesis of prostaglandins in the anterior hypothalamus. Body temperature is then raised, with peripheral vasoconstriction, shivering, and the typical clinical picture of fever. Thus fever is a normal response that occurs throughout the animal kingdom. Several investigators, especially Kluger, have demonstrated the role of fever as a factor in resisting infection. Bacterial and viral replication slow, and body defenses are activated. In a poikilothermic animal, whose body temperature is dependent on the environment, failure to elevate body temperature in response to an infection significantly increases mortality. Data in mammals are less clear because extremes of fever (such as those in malignant hyperthermia, heat stroke, hemorrhagic shock/encephalopathy syndrome) may be hazardous. However, there is little to suggest that "normal" degrees of body temperature elevation are harmful, rather there are probably major benefits.

Literature Survey

Before initiating a review of FUO series, it is important to clarify what represents true fever. Two key longitudinal series are noteworthy. Bayley and Stolz evaluated healthy children up to 36 months of age in a daycare situation. Highest rectal temperatures tended to occur in the late afternoon at 18 months of age, with a mean temperature of 99.83° F in boys and a standard deviation of 0.89° F. Thus healthy children often had a rectal temperature close to 101° F. Similarly, Iliff and Lee studied children from birth to 18 years of age and found that the highest readings were in the youngest children. These normative data are important in approaching the child with apparent elevation of body temperature.

A detailed review of temperature measurement is beyond the scope of this chapter, but rectal thermometry remains the gold standard. Oral temperature is lower and influenced by several factors, including respiratory rate. Axillary temperature (often used clinically) is not accurate, and temperature strips are quite useless. The newest method uses infrared rays emanating from the middle ear, a site close to the hypothalamus and core temperature. Unfortunately, studies of this method (using several different instruments) have had somewhat conflicting results, and rectal temperature should be taken in important clinical situations. The digital thermometer units now standard in hospitals and offices should be checked and recalibrated on a regular basis to maintain accuracy.

A number of clinical series and several review articles deal with FUO. In adults the initial series of Petersdorf is quoted often and considered a "classic." As stated previously, these patients were hospitalized for at least 1 week and no diagnosis was established. Infectious disease, collagen vascular disease, and malignancy predominated, and the overall mortality was approximately 33%. Many of the patients with infection had tuberculosis. Biopsy was often necessary to establish a diagnosis. In a follow-up series published in 1982, diagnostic categories were similar except that collagen disorders were less frequent because newer serologies were available for rapid outpatient diagnosis. Indirect imaging methods were not as helpful as predicted, making the diagnosis in only about 10% of the cases. Mortality was even higher at 40%.

Pediatric series have been reviewed recently. Unfortunately, variable criteria for entry and different definitions of prolonged fever (ranging from 1 week as an outpatient to 1 full week in the hospital without a diagnosis) are used. In general the more stringent the entry criteria are, the more likely it is that the patient will have a "serious" cause for the fever. Younger children, such as those in Pizzo's series, generally have more self-limited illnesses, which often resolve without a diagnosis. This series is also useful because screening tests helped predict serious illness; elevated erythrocyte sedimentation rate (ESR) and/or reversal of the albumin/globulin ratio were present in the majority of patients with serious illness. (These findings are sensitive but not specific because these tests were also positive in many patients who had spontaneous resolution of illness.)

Differential Diagnosis

General diagnostic categories can be compiled using these different pediatric series. Infectious disease comprises about 50% of diagnoses, with one half of these confined to the respiratory tract. Other common locations for infection are the

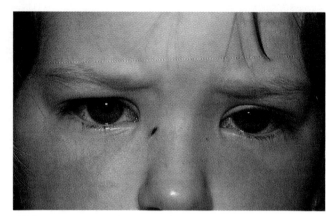

FIG. 7-1 Nonexudative, nonulcerative, bulbar conjunctivitis.

urinary tract, central nervous system, and bone. A careful search for localized infection, such as an abscess, is often important and rewarding. Unusual infections ("zebras" rather than "horses") are rare. Knowledge of **uncommon** presentations of **common** disorders is most helpful. A number of disorders with systemic presentations are important to recognize and may be bacterial, viral, fungal, or parasitic (rarely found in the United States). Some common examples include the following:

1. Bacterial—tuberculosis, syphilis (especially congenital), cat-scratch disease, enteric infection (*Salmonella* or *Yersinia* organisms), brucellosis, Q fever, leptospirosis and tularemia
2. Viral—Epstein-Barr virus and cytomegalovirus
3. Fungal—histoplasmosis and coccidioidomycosis
4. Parasitic—babesiosis and toxoplasmosis

Many systemic infections have multiple manifestations, such as rash, adenopathy, and pulmonary infiltrates, so that fever alone is not a common manifestation.

Collagen vascular disease is the second most common diagnostic category. The most likely disorders in children are juvenile rheumatoid arthritis (JRA), Kawasaki syndrome, systemic lupus erythematosus (SLE), and rheumatic fever. Other vasculitides, such as Wegener granulomatosis, Behçet disease, and others, are uncommon. Systemic JRA usually includes adenopathy, fever, anemia, and later arthritis. Some patients may have fever for many months before other disease manifestations occur. Kawasaki syndrome usually has multiple manifestations, but in young infants these symptoms may be recognized only partially or be present for only a brief period of time (Figs. 7-1 to 7-6). Coronary aneurysms have been reported in patients with minimal signs and symptoms. SLE occasionally presents with fever alone, but other manifestations become evident early in the course of disease. Rheumatic fever without arthritis may be a difficult diagnosis to recognize until major cardiac signs develop.

Malignancy is an obvious concern in patients with prolonged fever. The lymphoreticular neoplasms (leukemia or lymphoma) most frequently cause fever, but neuroblastoma may do so as well. Changes in the blood count, adenopathy,

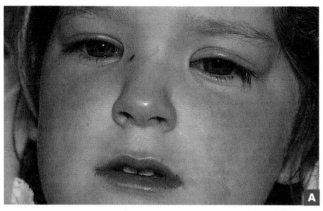 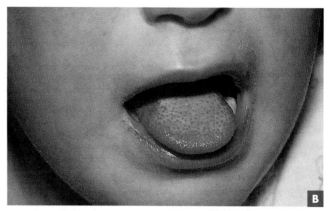

FIG. 7-2 *A*, Erythematous, cracked lips. *B*, "Strawberry tongue." *A* and *B* are oral findings of Kawasaki syndrome.

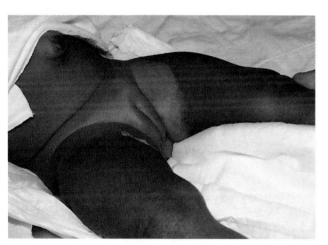 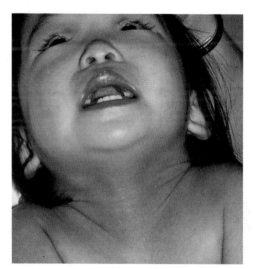

FIG. 7-3 Perineal rash with peeling.

FIG. 7-4 Neck rash with peeling. Note that peeling of intertriginous rash occurs before extremity peeling.

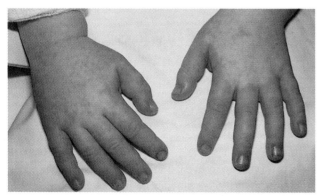 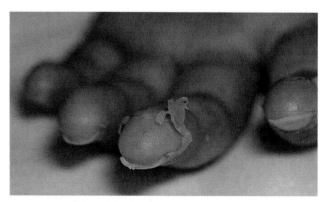

FIG. 7-5 Swollen, erythematous hands. Note fusiform appearance.

FIG. 7-6 Fingertip peeling in subacute phase of Kawasaki syndrome. (Modified from Centers for Disease Control: Kawasaki disease, *MMWR* 29:61-63, 1980.)

BOX 7-1

Differential Diagnosis of Fever of Unknown Origin

Infectious Disease (About 50% of Diagnoses in Most Series)

Localized

Respiratory tract

Upper—nasal passages, throat, sinuses

Lower—pneumonia, bronchitis, bronchiectasis, foreign body, etc.

Urinary tract—culture; without leukocytes, may be simply "bacteriuria" and not a cause of fever

Bone—bone scan may be helpful

Central nervous system—lumbar puncture

Abscess—especially abdominal; consider appendicitis, CT scan **if** suggested by history or examination

Generalized

Common—Epstein-Barr virus, enteric infection (*Salmonella* and *Yersinia* species, etc.), cat-scratch disease, tuberculosis, hepatitis, cytomegalovirus

Unusual—tularemia, brucellosis, leptospirosis, Q fever, Lyme disease, syphilis, toxoplasmosis, etc.

Collagen/Connective Tissue Disorders

Juvenile rheumatoid arthritis

Prolonged fever without joint complaints, anemia and leukocytosis, lymphadenopathy, elevated ESR

Kawasaki syndrome

Rash, conjunctival injection, mucosal changes, extremity changes, peeling diaper area; infants less than 1 year old may have few features

Systemic lupus

Adenopathy, mouth sores, hair loss, rash, joint complaints, chorea; serology (10% ANA negative, but anticytoplasmic antigens may be present)

Rheumatic fever

Revised Jones criteria

Collagen/Connective Tissue Disorders—cont'd

Other

Vasculitis syndromes, Behçet's disease, mixed connective tissue disease

Neoplasia

Lymphoreticular

Most commonly causes fever, may mimic rheumatoid arthritis with joint pain, perform bone marrow examination if two cell lines are decreased (e.g., anemia and thrombocytopenia)

Sarcomas

Neuroblastoma

Inflammatory Bowel Disease

Crohn disease

Poor growth, diarrhea, perianal changes, arthritis, rashes, digital clubbing, nocturnal bowel movements

Miscellaneous

Ectodermal dysplasia, thermoregulatory disorders, diabetes insipidus

Periodic Fever (Not Truly FUO, by Definition)

Common

Recurrent viral infections

Uncommon

Cyclic neutropenia, familial Mediterranean fever (serositis, arthritis), "pharyngitis with aphthous stomatitis" (Marshall syndrome), *Borellia* infection, familial dysautonomia

Pseudo FUO

Probably more common than true disease, prolonged low-grade fevers without findings on examination, multiple vague complaints, excessive school absence, normal screening laboratory tests

ANA, Antinuclear antibody test.

hepatosplenomegaly, and joint complaints may be clues to the diagnosis. Bone marrow examination should be considered if several cell lines in the peripheral blood are decreased.

Inflammatory bowel disease is not a frequent cause of FUO, but occasionally fever is the predominant manifestation. Usually the disorder is Crohn disease rather than ulcerative colitis, which universally has rectal (and symptomatic) involvement. Other prominent features of Crohn disease are growth deceleration, diarrhea (especially nocturnal), perianal disease, digital clubbing, joint involvement, and rashes.

There are other isolated causes of prolonged fever that are quite rare, including ectodermal dysplasia with inability to

sweat, diabetes insipidus with periodic dehydration in infancy, and central nervous system fever in children with severe brain injury. Occasionally, patients with disorders such as these experience periodic temperature elevation with normal intervening periods. Most children with periodic fever have recurrent "ordinary" infections, but a few disorders are truly associated with "periodic fever," including familial Mediterranean fever (serositis); relapsing fever (*Borrelia* species); cyclic neutropenia; and periodic fever, pharyngitis, aphthous stomatitis syndrome (as discussed by Marshall). This last disorder is probably more common than previously recognized.

TABLE 7-1

Summary of Six Pediatric Fever of Unknown Origin Series

Diagnosis	Number	Percent
Infection		
Respiratory	102	22.9
Other	97	21.7
Collagen disease	57	12.8
Resolved	56	12.6
Miscellaneous	54	12.1
No diagnosis	48	10.7
Neoplasm	25	5.6
Inflammatory bowel disease	7	1.6

Modified from Gartner JC, Jr: Fever of unknown origin, *Adv Pediatr Infect Dis* 7:1-24, 1992.

Any discussion of FUO would be incomplete without mention of the common "pseudo FUO" first described by Kleiman. Children with this disorder have multiple complaints, miss school frequently, and are "vulnerable children" similar to those described by Green and Solnit. Careful documentation of fever is critical to the investigation of these children. In a similar category is the patient who has very elevated body temperature at home but never in the office or hospital. Factitious fever is a significant possibility, and this may be one of the symptoms of Munchausen syndrome by proxy.

Box 7-1 summarizes the differential diagnosis of FUO. The percentages from the six major pediatric series are combined in Table 7-1.

History

The most important clues to the diagnosis of FUO are found in the history. First and foremost the physician must be certain that fever is truly present. As a general rule, if there is a question about a truly elevated body temperature just slightly above normal, there probably is no major disease process present. Documentation of fever is mandatory, and at times a patient must be hospitalized to be certain, which is a difficult task in the era of managed care. A temperature diary is helpful. Patterns of fever are rarely diagnostic, but slight elevation late in the afternoon or after exertion is often insignificant. Major temperature spikes once or twice per day with drops to the subnormal range in between suggest JRA.

The course of the illness is important. Careful attention should be paid to features such as a prodrome and associated symptoms, such as rash, cough, adenopathy, diarrhea, localized pain, and night sweats. A careful review of systems should be done, looking for clues to suggest a diagnosis. Specific questions should be asked about breaks in the skin (including bites or stings), animal exposure (including pets), travel outside the local environment, and drug therapy or use. Any drug may be the cause of prolonged fever, and occasionally all medications must be stopped for a time. Weight loss is important to document, and in prolonged fever a review of the growth curve over the past few years may be important.

A history of exposure to others with an illness, such as infectious mononucleosis, should be sought, as well as a history of previous surgery or dental work. Family history is occasionally useful in difficult cases, and social history may be crucial if the physician suspects that the history is unreliable or fabricated.

A number of specific questions may provide critical information about diagnostic possibilities and must be asked if certain initial information is provided. Examples are specifics of joint swelling, erythema if joint pain is a symptom, and descriptions of stool (color, mucus, blood, etc.) if diarrhea is present. Key questions in making an effective differential diagnosis are presented in Box 7-2. At times the history is not helpful, and the examiner must turn to the physical examination for clues.

Physical Examination

The examination must be meticulous, confirming findings suspected from the history or yielding information that suggests other diagnoses. Vital signs should be recorded carefully. Temperature elevation can be confirmed. Respiratory rate may be a clue to respiratory or cardiac involvement. Blood pressure may be elevated, suggesting certain tumors (neuroblastoma, pheochromocytoma) or renal involvement by the disease process. Growth and weight should be plotted on a curve to compare with previous measurements. Skin examination is often neglected but may provide important information, including rashes, nodules, skin breaks, papules, petechiae, bruises, and pallor (Figs. 7-7 to 7-12). It is important to search for older lesions that may be almost completely healed, for example, those found in cat-scratch disease (see Fig. 25-9). Eye examination may reveal subtle icterus, resolving conjunctival erythema, and splinter hemorrhages. Retinal examination may provide clues to hemorrhages or signs of increased intracranial pressure resulting from occult infection. Ear, nose, and throat examination should be performed carefully because infection in the sinuses is often overlooked and may be suggested by posterior mucopurulent discharge or tenderness. Ear examination with a pneumatic otoscope is mandatory, although otitis media is often overdiagnosed as a cause of fever. Adenopathy should be documented, and the question of localized versus generalized enlargement should be answered. Lung examination may reveal findings that suggest infection, and heart examination may reveal findings that suggest

Key Questions in Approaching Fever of Unknown Origin

1. Is fever truly present? A knowledge of normal temperature variation is important, and documentation of fever is mandatory.
2. Exposures? This includes travel to places or countries where unusual illness might be acquired.
3. Pets? Kitten exposure (with fleas) and exposure to other animals could be major clues.
4. Drugs? Any medication is suspect in a patient with prolonged fever.
5. Skin breaks? A puncture or laceration can be the source of numerous infections (i.e., bacteremia leading to osteomyelitis).
6. Insect bites? Tick exposure is the most common risk in recent times, but flies or mosquitoes also may carry disease.
7. Unusual or poorly prepared foods? Raw fish and unpasteurized milk are examples.
8. General history? Onset, periodicity, temperature curve, weight loss, and school absence should be noted.
9. Localized pain? If present, this may lead to a detailed investigation of a particular site.
10. Review of systems? Detailed questions about rashes, joint complaints, cough, and bowel movements may offer important clues to the diagnosis.
11. Have detailed cultures been performed? This is a mandatory starting point; blood, urine, stool, and perhaps throat cultures are important.
12. Complete blood count? This may be nonspecific, but inflammatory disorders usually lead to a rise in leukocyte count and eventually a rise in platelet count with a fall in hemoglobin level. Falling counts suggest a marrow process or peripheral destruction and warrant further hematologic investigation. In periodic fever, counts should be done during illness to evaluate neutropenia.
13. Screening laboratory procedures? More serious causes of FUO commonly cause a rise in sedimentation rate and a fall in albumin level with reversal of albumin/globulin ratio.
14. Tuberculin skin test with controls to evaluate anergy? The skin test may be normal early in the disease but remains one of the most useful tests for evaluating a disease.
15. Family history? Familial Mediterranean fever is rare, but streptococcal disease tends to cluster in families, and connective tissue disease may have genetic predisposition.
16. Is the physical examination normal? Investigation should focus on abnormalities detected by meticulous examination.

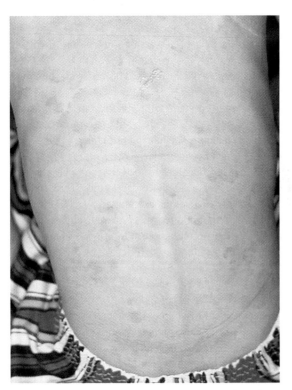

FIG. 7-7 Erythema marginatum rash in a child with acute rheumatic fever. Note the wavy margins in the distribution on the trunk.

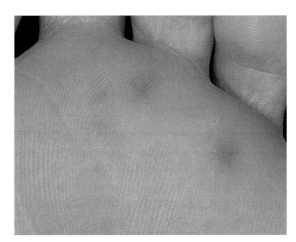

FIG. 7-8 Janeway lesions. A patient with bacterial endocarditis has small painless nodules on the sole.

rheumatic fever, endocarditis, or myocarditis. Important findings on abdominal palpation are organomegaly (see Chapter 24), tenderness, palpable bowel loops, and masses. The perianal area should be inspected closely. Skin tags, fissures, and drainage may suggest Crohn disease or an intraabdominal infectious process (see Fig. 1-2). In some cases a rectal examination is necessary to test for occult blood or to confirm ab-

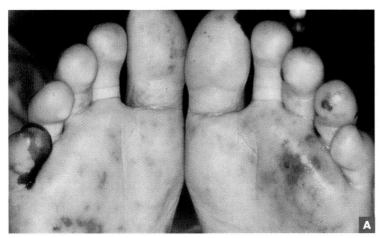
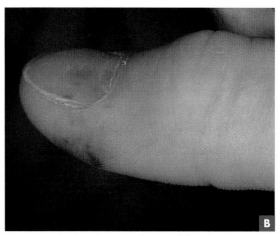

FIG. 7-9 *A,* Hemorrhagic lesions in a patient with acute bacterial endocarditis. *B,* Subungual splinter hemorrhages. (*A* Courtesy Dr. W.H. Neches, Pittsburgh.)

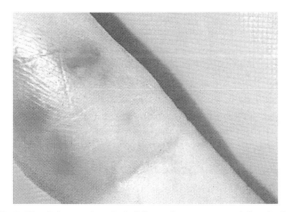

FIG. 7-10 Osler nodes. Painful erythematous nodular lesions resulting from infective endocarditis. (Courtesy Dr. J.F. John, Jr.)

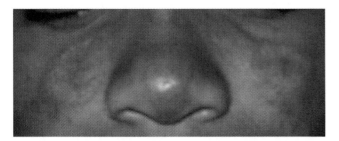

FIG. 7-12 Typical malar rash of SLE. Erythema, erosion, and atrophy are present. Note sparing of nasolabial folds.

FIG. 7-11 Rash of systemic-onset JRA is erythematous, macular, and often evanescent. It can be more prominent during periods of fever. The rash was pruritic in this patient.

normal findings suggested by the history. Extremities should be evaluated for clubbing, joint limitation, and tenderness. Observing the patient rise from a supine position and then observing gait may provide important data pointing to muscle, bone, or joint involvement. In selected cases individual palpation of vertebrae and other bones may be diagnostic (see Fig. 2-8).

Approach to the Patient

Completion of the history and physical examination usually produces a selected differential diagnosis. If no specific illness is suggested, cultures should be done and several screening tests performed. It is reasonable to culture urine, blood, and stool if infection is a possibility. Occasionally a throat culture is necessary. Initial screening tests should help; a major elevation of the ESR (greater than 30 mm/hr by either Westergren or Wintrobe method) or reduction of the albumin level suggests a non–self-limited illness. Although not specific, a standard complete blood count is reasonable and may distinguish an inflammatory process (increased white blood cells and platelets, low hemoglobin) from a bone marrow or destructive process (reduction in cell lines). If suggested by the history, several serologic studies also may be done initially, such as those for Epstein-Barr viral infection or the agent of cat-scratch disease.

The question that usually arises at this point is which of the newer imaging techniques should be routinely employed? *If suggested by the history and physical examination,* specific tests are very useful. A bone scan may confirm or support primary bone infection, and a computed tomography (CT) scan may definitively document an abscess collection. Magnetic resonance imaging (MRI) may supplant bone scans and CT in the future because the pictures are so complete and precise. However, caution should be used in the indiscriminate use of these techniques. In one study, abdominal CT scan was *not* helpful when no clues pointed to the abdomen as the source of possible infection. In a review studying the role of newer procedures (including ultrasound, CT, indium-tagged leukocyte scan, gallium scan, and bone scan) in the diagnosis of FUO, Steele and colleagues found that these techniques confirmed diagnoses already suspected clinically. Others have used procedures, such as gallium scans, to confirm a localized process. As a general rule, directed examination (i.e., the test is used to confirm a suspicion raised by the history or physical examination) seems to have the best results. Children who have generalized, nonfocal symptoms rarely have a diagnosis that is uncovered by a physician using newer imaging modalities.

In a stable patient whose initial evaluation has failed to yield a reasonable diagnosis, a period of observation is mandatory. Repeated examination and a search for new clues from the history may be rewarded with new diagnostic possibilities, or better still the patient may recover without a diagnosis as is well documented in all of the pediatric series. On some occasions, repeated cultures may be rewarded by a positive result. The course of certain illnesses, such as JRA, may require months of close follow-up before a diagnosis is made. Under these circumstances patience is critical. Being patient may be difficult for both the family and the physician.

If the patient has progression of hematologic abnormalities, especially falling hemoglobin level and platelet count without evidence of regeneration (low reticulocyte count, small platelets on smear), bone marrow examination may be important. In adults with prolonged fever, liver biopsy may prove useful in the diagnosis of granulomatous disease, especially histoplasmosis or tuberculosis. However, this theory has not been studied in children. In this chapter we have confined the discussion to the immune-competent host, but if the patient is not immunologically normal (e.g., immunodeficiency, chemotherapy, and neutropenia), unusual superven-

ing infection is the first priority, and repeated cultures (even of bone marrow) may be necessary.

SUMMARY

True fever of unknown origin is unusual in pediatric patients if a strict, adult definition is used. However, less stringent criteria, such as more than 1 week of fever without an evident diagnosis, significantly increases the number of patients categorized as having FUO. The majority of these children, especially infants and toddlers, have self-limited illness. Serious illness, however, does present as prolonged fever. In order of frequency, infectious disease, collagen vascular disease, malignancy, and inflammatory bowel disease should be considered. Many illnesses resolve spontaneously, despite a prolonged course. Factitious fever and pseudo FUO are possible as well. By taking a careful history, completing a meticulous physical examination, and using selected screening tests, the clinician may arrive at major diagnostic possibilities. An elevated ESR and low albumin level with elevated globulin fraction suggest more serious disease. Cultures, serologies, and selective use of imaging procedures in children who have focal findings on history or examination should ensure that diagnoses are not overlooked. A patient approach, using additional history and examination information to find clues, is the most likely course to a correct diagnosis.

ILLUSTRATIVE CASES

Case 1. K.H., a 9-year-old girl, was admitted for further evaluation of fever that had lasted for 5 weeks. Fever had been documented on numerous occasions in her pediatrician's office. She had night sweats and anorexia, with a weight loss of 12 pounds. Physical examination was normal except that weight was in the 25th percentile for age and height was in the 50th percentile. Outpatient evaluation included normal radiographs of the chest and sinuses, negative PPD, normal CBC and differential count, and normal blood, urine, and throat cultures. ESR was 100 mm/hr. A brief course of amoxicillin was given without a response.

Family, social, and past histories were normal. There were no pets. She had traveled to a rural area for vacation but was well for the 6 months afterward. Review of systems was not helpful.

During a 5-day hospitalization, temperature was above 39° C once or twice per day. Repeated cultures were negative. Laboratory tests disclosed the following values: CBC revealed mild anemia, 10.8 g/dl; ESR, 58 mm/hr; albumin, 3.3 g/dl; total protein, 7.1 g/dl; antistreptolysin O (ASO) titer was elevated at 680, but a cardiology evaluation revealed only a flow murmur and normal echocardiogram.

Over the next 4 months fever continued daily. She then developed a mild limp with pain in her right ankle and very minimal swelling. Laboratory tests disclosed the following values: hemoglobin, 8.1 g/dl; WBC, 12,000/mm³;

platelets, 633,000/mm³; ESR, 61 mm/hr; ASO titer, normal; and x-ray films of the ankle were normal. She was started on a nonsteroidal antiinflammatory agent with some response.

This patient was quite vexing to her physicians. She later developed a faint macular, evanescent rash and was presumed to have systemic-onset JRA. Eighteen months after the onset of her fever she suddenly developed acute swelling of multiple joints, including the knees, ankles, wrists, and elbows. She has required aggressive therapy with intraarticular and systemic steroids, methotrexate, and intravenous gamma-globulin. Despite this therapy, she has had major joint destruction.

Clues to the seriousness of this prolonged FUO were the elevated ESR and reversal of the albumin/globulin ratio. Bone marrow examination was considered, but elevation of the platelet and leukocyte counts suggested inflammation rather than replacement. Time and the eventual appearance of mild articular and skin involvement were helpful.

Case 2. A.B. is a 10-year-old girl transferred from her community hospital after 2 weeks of fever. Initial temperature was low-grade but then increased to 40° C, usually in the late afternoon. She had chills and night sweats. Initial physical examination was normal after the first week of fever. Tests in the community hospital disclosed the following values: hemoglobin 13 g/dl; WBC, 3100; platelets, 115,000/ mm³; differential cell count, 37 neutrophils, 60 lymphocytes, 2 monocytes, and 1 eosinophil; ESR, 10 mm/hr; blood, urine, and cerebrospinal fluid cultures were negative; as were x-ray studies of the chest and sinuses. Rapid test for infectious mononucleosis and antinuclear antibodies were negative. Liver enzymes were mildly increased as follows: AST, 174 IU; LDH, 666 IU; and GGTP, 174 IU. She was treated with parenteral cefotaxime without a response.

Further history on arrival at Children's Hospital revealed no travel or animal exposure. Parents remarked on a mild sore throat and puffiness around the eyes at the onset of the patient's fever.

Physical examination revealed a mildly ill girl with a temperature of 38.8° C. The liver was palpable 4 cm below the right costal margin with a span of 10 cm. The spleen tip was palpable. Laboratory evaluation disclosed the following values: hemoglobin, 11.4 g/dl; WBC, 8900; platelets, 191,000/mm³; differential cell count, 7 neutrophils, 3 stabs, 63 lymphocytes, 4 monocytes, 1 eosinophil, 1 basophil, and 21 atypical lymphocytes; ESR, 28 mm/hr; albumin, 3.2 g/dl; total protein, 6.2 g/dl; ALT, 174 IU; AST, 80 IU; GGTP, 77 IU; and LDH, 378 IU.

This girl did not appear seriously ill, and her thrombocytopenia was transient. Review of her blood smear confirmed atypical lymphocytes and no malignant cells. The history of periorbital puffiness (Hoagland sign) and sore throat at onset suggested infectious mononucleosis.

Epstein-Barr viral titers confirmed acute infection. The rapid tests for mononucleosis antibodies are excellent, but false negatives do occur and there is a window of time when this test will be positive. It tests only for heterophile antibody; it is not specific for the virus.

Case 3. B.P. is a 26-month-old boy who complained of fevers intermittently for 7 weeks. His initial symptoms included mild diarrhea without mucus or blood, temperature to 40° C, and cervical adenopathy. After 2 days, fever was low-grade. He was initially referred to a pediatric hematologist who found no major problem but was concerned about the diarrhea. The child's diarrhea improved when fruit juices were eliminated from the diet. Two courses of antibiotics were given, but the temperature continued to be elevated in the late afternoon. The child became irritable and a picky eater. Weight loss of 2 pounds occurred. There were no other complaints, and review of systems was not helpful. Family, social, and past histories were unremarkable. Examination revealed a healthy, "clingy" toddler with a normal examination.

Laboratory data disclosed the following values: albumin, 4.3 g/dl; total protein, 7.1 g/dl; ESR, 4 mm/hr; tuberculin test, negative; and CBC, normal.

This child appeared well. Stool smear and culture were unremarkable; no leukocytes were seen. The mother was asked to keep a daily temperature curve. Peaks occurred in the late afternoon, and the highest temperature was 38.4° C rectally. The mother had been taking the temperature regularly every 4 hours. With reassurance the child improved, and appetite and behavior returned to normal.

This patient had a brief illness, and the parental concern was increased by several courses of antibiotics. It was evident that the temperature was probably in the normal range for a child this age. Screening tests, in addition to a normal examination, were helpful in preventing overinvestigation.

ANNOTATED BIBLIOGRAPHY

Bayley N, Stolz HR: Maturational changes in rectal temperatures of 61 infants from 1 to 36 months, *Child Dev* 8:195-205, 1937.

This classic study of normal values for healthy children must be reviewed by those who evaluate prolonged fever. Highest mean temperatures were at about 18 months, and the mean temperature was almost 100° F.

Gartner JC, Jr: Fever of unknown origin, *Adv Pediatr Infect Dis* 7:1-24, 1992.

This article contains references to all the pediatric series on fever of unknown origin, as well as data on frequency of various major conditions.

Kleiman MB: The complaint of persistent fever: recognition and management of pseudo fever of unknown origin, *Pediatr Clin North Am* 29:201-209, 1982.

Much more frequent than true FUO is pseudo FUO. The practicing physician should recognize this condition so that detailed investigation is done only on patients with a major risk of organic disease.

BIBLIOGRAPHY

Atkins E, Wood WB, Jr: Studies on the pathogenesis of fever. II. Identification of an endogenous pyrogen in the bloodstream following the injection of typhoid vaccine, *J Exp Med* 102:499-516, 1955.

Baraff LJ, Bass JW, Fleisher GR, et al: Practice guidelines for the management of infants and children 0 to 36 months of age with fever without source, *Pediatrics* 92:1-12, 1993.

Buonomo C, Treves ST: Gallium scanning in children with fever of unknown origin, *Pediatr Radiol* 23:307-310, 1993.

Dinarello CA, Wolff SM: Molecular basis of fever in humans, *Am J Med* 72:799-819, 1982.

Hayani A, Mahoney DH, Fernbach DJ: Role of bone marrow examination in the child with prolonged fever, *J Pediatr* 116:919-920, 1990.

Iliff A, Lee VA: Pulse rate, respiratory rate, and body temperature of children between 2 months and 18 years of age, *Child Dev* 23:237-245, 1952.

Kluger MJ: Fever, *Pediatrics* 66:720-724, 1980.

Larson EB, Featherstone HJ, Petersdorf RG: Fever of undetermined origin: diagnosis and follow-up of 105 cases, 1970-1980, *Medicine* 61:269-292, 1982.

Lorin MI, Feigin RD: Fever without localizing signs and fever of unknown origin. In Feigin RD, Cherry JD, editors: *Textbook of pediatric infectious diseases*, Philadelphia, 1987, WB Saunders.

Marshall GS, Edwards KM, Butler J, et al: Syndrome of periodic fever, pharyngitis, and aphthous stomatitis, *J Pediatr* 110:43-46, 1987.

Norris J: Taking temperatures: the changing state of the art, *Contemp Pediatr* 2:22-39, 1985.

Petersdorf RO, Beeson PB: Fever of unexplained origin: report on 100 cases, *Medicine* 40:1-30, 1961.

Picus D, Siegel MJ, Balfe DM: Abdominal computed tomography in children with unexplained prolonged fever, *J Comput Assist Tomogr* 8:851-856, 1984.

Pizzo PH, Lovejoy FH, Smith DH: Prolonged fever in children: review of 100 cases, *Pediatrics* 55:468-473, 1975.

Rowley AH, Gonzalez-Crussi F, Gidding SS, et al: Incomplete Kawasaki disease with coronary artery involvement, *J Pediatr* 110:409-413, 1987.

Steele RW, Jones SM, Lowe BA, et al: The usefulness of scanning procedures for diagnosis of fever of unknown origin in children, *J Pediatr* 119:526-530, 1991.

Wood PR, Fowlkes J, Holden P, et al: Fever of unknown origin for six years: Munchausen syndrome by proxy, *J Fam Pract* 28:391-395, 1989.

Yetman RJ, Coody DK, West MS, et al: Comparison of temperature measurements by an aural infrared thermometer with measurements by traditional rectal and axillary techniques, *J Pediatr* 122:769-773, 1993.

Nervous System

8

Abnormal Head Size and Shape

JAMES A. NARD

Key Points

- Awareness of the pathophysiology of macrocephaly allows for a cost-effective evaluation and appropriate treatment.

- Recognition and accurate diagnosis of the familial influences on head size can be accomplished by using Weaver's curves, avoiding unnecessary evaluation.

- Infants with craniosynostosis should be recognized early in life and evaluated appropriately. Referral should be made in a timely manner.

Growth and development are the cornerstones of pediatric care. Measurements of growth, including height, weight, and head circumference, are routinely plotted on standard curves to assess the well-being of the pediatric patient. Deviations from the normal growth pattern may be the first sign of disease. This is especially true when evaluating a child's head size and/or shape; head circumference usually reflects brain growth. Brain growth is rapid during the first few years of life, and early identification of abnormal head size or shape allows rapid management of potentially treatable causes. In addition, in many syndromes, deviations in head growth are a major manifestation. Recognition of these conditions allows the clinician to counsel the family and patient regarding specific diagnosis, prognosis, and treatment. The multiple causes of variations in head size and shape require thoughtful investigation to arrive at a diagnosis in a timely and cost-effective manner.

Pathophysiology of Head Growth

Normal cranial contents include the brain substance, blood, and cerebrospinal fluid (CSF). A change in any of the major components is usually at the expense of the others and may result in abnormal head growth. With rare exception the actual cranial thickness plays a minor role in head growth.

Expansion of the CSF space is one of the most common causes of abnormal head enlargement. Under normal conditions, an equilibrium between CSF production and absorption is maintained. The absorption of CSF is variable, however, and may increase up to 3 times baseline in the presence of increased pressure. The arachnoid villi are responsible for most of the absorption, and other venous sinuses account for a small percentage. Approximately 70% of the CSF is produced by the choroid plexus. Transependymal movement of fluid from the brain into the ventricles accounts for the remainder. CSF production is variable; adults secrete approximately 750 ml per day, children secrete less, and newborns make as little as 25 ml per day. CSF turns over 3 to 4 times per day. There is almost always an impairment in absorption, rather than an overproduction, that leads to expansion of the CSF compartment (i.e., hydrocephalus).

Hydrocephalus is divided pathophysiologically into communicating and noncommunicating types, depending on whether CSF can flow from the ventricular system into the subarachnoid space (communicating) or the flow from one or more ventricles is blocked (noncommunicating).

Communicating hydrocephalus is usually secondary to impaired absorption. The impairment is commonly caused by inflammatory CNS processes (e.g., increased subarachnoid protein or blood from a subarachnoid hemorrhage) or malignant infiltrates (e.g., leukemia), which slow CSF absorption. Overproduction of CSF is occasionally the cause of communicating hydrocephalus. Central nervous system (CNS) tumors (e.g., choroid plexus tumor) increase CSF production enough to overwhelm the reabsorptive capacity of the system.

Noncommunicating hydrocephalus is due to obstruction of CSF flow out of the ventricles. Production of CSF is actually decreased because the rate of formation is sensitive to the increased pressure within the system. Obstruction may occur internally or externally as a result of forces anywhere along the flow of the CSF. However, the most common cause is aqueductal stenosis, accounting for 20% of noncommunicating hydrocephalus.

Alterations in brain substance may lead to alterations in head growth. Enlargement (megalencephaly) can lead to macrocephaly, or a paucity of brain tissue may cause microcephaly. When megalencephaly is the result of an increase in the number or size of cells, the condition is termed *anatomic megalencephaly*. Diseases that increase brain substance by depositing metabolic products over time are termed *metabolic megalencephaly*. Occasionally, changes in the blood space (arteriovenous malformations [AVM] or intracranial hemorrhage) may lead to macrocephaly. An even rarer cause of head enlargement is thickening of the skull, which may be seen with bone marrow expansion secondary to severe chronic anemias (thalassemia major) or primary bone disorders.

Microcephaly always signifies a small brain. The loss of normal brain substance is either primary, in which there is lack of brain development, or secondary, in which a normal brain is injured by any number of disease processes.

Differential Diagnosis of Head Growth

The differential diagnosis of abnormal head size is best discussed by looking separately at macrocephaly (head circumference more than 2 standard deviations *above* the mean) and microcephaly (head circumference more than 2 standard deviations *below* the mean). Standard head circumference curves include age and gender; prenatal curves include gestational age.

Macrocephaly

The main causes of macrocephaly are increases in the CSF space, hydrocephalus, and megalencephaly (an increase in brain substance) (Table 8-1).

Communicating hydrocephalus caused by decreased absorption of CSF is a secondary phenomenon resulting from a number of inflammatory CNS diseases. Any condition that leads to blood collecting in a subarachnoid space, such as subarachnoid hemorrhage or an intraventricular hemorrhage in premature infants, can slow the absorption of CSF enough to allow the development of hydrocephalus and macrocephaly (if the cranial sutures are open). A similar cause is seen with meningitis, resulting in a high CSF protein. An-

TABLE 8-1

Common Causes of Macrocephaly and Age at Clinical Presentation

Age	Cause
Birth-6 months	Hydrocephalus, subdural effusions, familial (normal variant)
6 months-2 years	Hydrocephalus, Dandy-Walker syndrome, subdural effusion, increased intracranial pressure, primary skeletal and cranial dysplasias (thickened or enlarged skull), megalencephaly
After 2 years	Hydrocephalus, megalencephaly, pseudotumor cerebri, familial (normal variant)

other cause is malignant infiltration, such as that seen in leukemia. Communicating hydrocephalus occasionally results from CNS tumors, such as a choroid plexus tumor that increases CSF production above the absorption capacity of the arachnoid villi.

Achondroplasia is an autosomal dominant form of dwarfism that is clinically apparent at birth. Characteristic features include macrocephaly, rhizomelic shortening of the limbs (proximal limbs are shorter than distal), and lack of endochondral bone formation at the base of the skull and face, giving the appearance of recessed facies. These children may be born with macrocephaly secondary to anatomic megalencephaly. Later in infancy, communicating hydrocephalus develops, further accelerating the macrocephaly. Small venous sinuses in a structurally small posterior fossa become obstructed, which causes increased venous pressure. The venous flow impairs CSF absorption, leading to communicating hydrocephalus and increased intracranial pressure (ICP).

Although achondroplastic dwarfs develop hydrocephalus as described previously, they may also have an Arnold-Chiari malformation (detailed under noncommunicating hydrocephalus). This commonly associated defect leads to respiratory control abnormalities. The apnea and upper airway difficulties are secondary to cervicomedullary compression.

Noncommunicating hydrocephalus is caused by obstruction of CSF flow out of the ventricles (Fig. 8-1). Obstruction may occur anywhere along the flow of CSF; however, the most common cause is aqueductal stenosis, accounting for 20% of noncommunicating hydrocephalus. The aqueduct that allows CSF flow between the third and fourth ventricles is a long, narrow tract (12.8 mm × 0.5 mm), making it vulnerable to internal obstruction and external compression. Isolated aqueductal stenosis accounts for 2% of congenital cases. This form may be inherited as an X-linked condition.

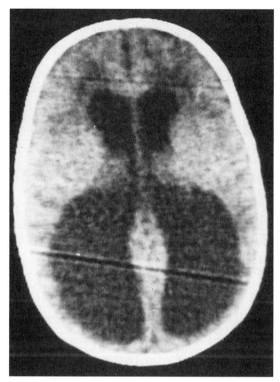

FIG. 8-1 CT scan of the head demonstrates a dilated ventricular system in an infant with hydrocephalus.

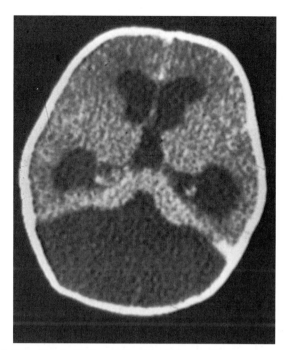

FIG. 8-2 Dandy-Walker deformity. CT scan shows a posterior fossa cyst, small cerebellar remnant, and hydrocephalus.

In the congenital form, hydrocephalus is present at birth along with signs of increased ICP, such as sunsetting of the eyes, split sutures, and cranial nerve palsies. This form can be diagnosed prenatally with sonography. Chromosome abnormalities and spinal dysraphism are associated problems that require further investigation. Spina bifida is concurrent in up to 70% of congenital cases. Acquired aqueductal stenosis is the result of postinflammatory lesions or is secondary to tumor compression.

Another cause of noncommunicating hydrocephalus is a group of anomalies that fall under the heading of Arnold-Chiari malformations. The following four types have been described:

Type I is a milder form of type II.

Type II causes caudal shifting of the cerebellum and medulla with kinking and compression of the upper spinal cord. This form is frequently seen and associated with myelomeningocele and aqueductal stenosis. The stenosis leads to hydrocephalus. This form of Arnold-Chiari malformation usually causes respiratory control abnormalities.

Type III is an occipital encephalocele with cerebellar protrusion through a posterior skull opening.

Type IV causes hypoplasia of the cerebellum. This may be a Dandy-Walker deformity (see next section).

A Dandy-Walker deformity is characterized by progressive cystic enlargement of the fourth ventricle, which is accompanied by enlargement of the posterior fossa, agenesis

or hypoplasia of the cerebellar vermis, and almost always development of hydrocephalus. Other associated anomalies are common, especially agenesis of the corpus callosum (Fig. 8-2). Clinically the onset of symptoms depends on the severity and speed with which the hydrocephalus develops. Although not always present at birth, noncommunicating hydrocephalus develops in 60% of cases by 2 years of age. In infancy, features of this malformation include a prominent occiput, rapidly increasing head circumference, a full fontanelle, and signs and symptoms of increased ICP. As the posterior fossa contents compress, apnea, truncal ataxia, nystagmus, cranial nerve palsies, and increased deep tendon reflexes appear. In children less than 1 year of age, transillumination of cysts may be demonstrated.

Vascular abnormalities, such as a malformation of the vein of Galen, may cause noncommunicating hydrocephalus. Enlargement of this vascular structure compresses the aqueduct, leading to hydrocephalus. Of affected infants, 80% are boys. Other mass lesions include abscess, hematoma, and tumor.

The most common findings are hydrocephalus and intracranial bruit, congestive heart failure secondary to high output, and unexplained hypoglycemia.

Benign enlargement of the subarachnoid space (also called *external hydrocephalus, extraventricular hydrocephalus,* or *benign subdural effusions*) is a relatively common condition, affecting up to 16% of infants, with boys having a higher incidence than girls. Macrocephaly may be the only feature present at birth. In early infancy the head size rapidly increases to greater than the 90th percentile but then runs parallel to the growth curves. The anterior fontanelle is full but pulsatile. There are no signs of increased ICP, and neurologic and developmental examinations are normal. The diagnosis is confirmed by enlargement of the subarachnoid space with normal ventricles on CT scan. The latter is important to rule out brain atrophy and *ex vacuo* changes as the cause of the expanded subarachnoid space. Close observation with serial head circumference measurements is required to ensure that head growth slows to a normal rate. Head growth velocity slows to a normal rate by approximately 6 months of age (Box 8-1).

Megalencephaly refers to enlargement of the brain substance. When this is due to an increased number of cells or their size, the condition is termed *anatomic megalencephaly*. Diseases that increase brain substance by deposition of metabolic products over time are termed *metabolic megalencephaly*.

Children with anatomic megalencephaly usually have a large head at birth that continues to enlarge. If this occurs in a familial form and is accompanied by normal development and neurologic function, the term *genetic megalencephaly* is applied. At birth the head may be normal or large, but the body size is normal. In infancy, head growth accelerates to greater than the 90th percentile, by as much as 2 to 4 cm, then parallels the normal growth curves. A CT scan of the head shows no abnormalities. Measurement of family members' head circumferences confirms that this is a familial trait. In the method described by Weaver, the examiner measures both parents' head circumferences and the standard deviations from the mean are then averaged. The average standard deviation is then plotted against the standard deviation of the child's head circumference using Weaver's curves. With this tool, it can be determined whether genetic influences alone explain the child's macrocephaly. Other than macrocephaly, the individuals are normal.

Megalencephaly with neurologic disorders is a heterogeneous group of entities with megalencephaly and cerebral dysfunction. Neurocutaneous syndromes are excluded from the grouping. At birth, the head is normal in size or macrocephalic, but the size increases in infancy. Learning disabilities, seizures, and mental retardation develop; these are static processes. Appropriate diagnosis involves ruling out any neurocutaneous syndrome. Imaging of the brain is normal or shows only a mild increase in the ventricular size. Agenesis of the corpus callosum is seen occasionally.

Cerebral gigantism (Sotos syndrome) is characterized by gigantism in early childhood and dysmorphic features. Mental retardation is common (affecting approximately 80% of patients). Children are born with a head size in the 75th to 90th percentile. In contrast to genetic megalencephaly, somatic growth is rapid in newborns, and it steadily increases until 3 to 4 years of age. Adults with Sotos syndrome are not giants. The typical dysmorphology consists of a prominent forehead, high arched palate, hypertelorism, dolichocephaly,

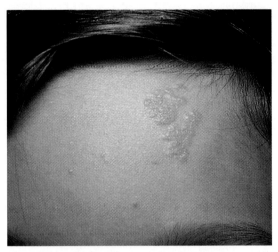

FIG. 8-3 Linear nevus sebaceous on the scalp of a child with seizures and mental retardation (linear sebaceous nevus syndrome).

BOX 8-1

Hydrocephalus

Communicating	Noncommunicating
Achondroplasia	Aqueductal stenosis
Postinflammatory	Arnold-Chiari malformation
Posthemorrhage	Dandy-Walker deformity
Vascular	Vein of Galen
AVM	Mass lesions
Venous obstruction	
Choroid plexus tumor	
Brain malformations	
Encephalocele	
Holoprosencephaly	
Porencephaly	
Benign subdural collection	

AVM, Arteriovenous malformation.

---

pointed chin, and large hands and feet. The syndrome is inherited in an autosomal dominant or recessive fashion but is more often sporadic. Sotos syndrome probably represents more than one specific entity. Diagnosis is based on the aforementioned pattern of growth and accompanying dysmorphic features. The CT scan typically shows a normal brain with slightly dilated ventricles. Endocrine abnormalities that cause the rapid growth cannot be found. On occasion, patients may have glucose intolerance. Somatomedin levels can be elevated during the first year of life. The bone age is advanced. Chromosomal studies should be obtained because fragile X syndrome has similar features.

Although neurocutaneous disorders usually cause typical skin findings, seizures, or developmental delay, macrocephaly is a prominent feature of these syndromes.

Hypomelanosis of Ito, first described in 1951, is a rare autosomal dominant disorder; however, girls are affected

Nonneurologic Manifestations of Neurofibromatosis and Tuberous Sclerosis

Neurofibromatosis

Skeletal
Sphenoid wing dysplasia, pseudoarthrosis, scoliosis

Arterial stenosis
Renal (hypertension), aorta, celiac, cartoid, cerebral

GI
Visceral neurofibromas

Lung
Neurofibromas

GU
Obstructive uropathy secondary to neurofibromas

Endocrine
Precocious puberty, pheochromocytoma, multiple endocrine neoplasia

Neoplastic
Acoustic neuroma (type II), optic glioma, sarcomas, Wilms tumor, leukemia

Tuberous Sclerosis

Kidney
Cysts, angiofibromas

Eye
Astrocytic hamartomas

Heart
Rhabdomyomas

Lung
Cysts

Megalencephaly

Anatomic
Genetic
Neurocutaneous syndromes
Megalencephaly and neurologic abnormalities
Achondroplasia
Sotos syndrome

Metabolic
Aminoaciduria
    Maple syrup urine disease
Leukodystrophies
    Canavan disease
    Alexander disease
Lysosomal storage disorders
    Tay-Sachs disease
    General gangliosidosis
    Mucopolysaccharidosis
    Metachromatic leukodystrophy

Neurofibromatosis and tuberous sclerosis are well-defined neurocutaneous entities, and macrocephaly may be part of the clinical picture. Details of these conditions can be found in standard texts (Box 8-2).

Children with metabolic megalencephaly have a normal head size at birth, and macrocephaly and increased ICP develop with time. Many inborn errors of metabolism have acquired macrocephaly as a feature. The head enlargement from accumulating metabolic products directly correlates with neurologic deterioration. Patients usually have degenerative neurologic disease (Box 8-3).

Microcephaly

Microcephaly is defined as a head circumference more than 2 standard deviations below the mean for age, gender, and gestation. A small head always signifies a small brain.

Genetic microcephaly (microcephaly vera) results in decreased growth of the brain. It is inherited as an autosomal dominant or autosomal recessive condition. Clinically the autosomal dominant form is milder. The facies are normal or only slightly dysmorphic, with receding forehead, upslanting palpebral fissures, and large ears. The intellect is normal to mildly retarded; however, learning disabilities are common. Other than microcephaly, somatic growth is normal.

The autosomal recessive form of this condition is severe. It is associated with moderate to severe mental retardation. Dysmorphology is a prominent feature along with short stature, a small skull-to-face ratio, small chin, large ears and nose, and redundance in the occipital area. Spasticity and seizures are seen. CT scan demonstrates only a small brain.

2.5 times more often than boys. Characteristic skin changes are bilateral asymmetric hypopigmented whorls found over different areas of the body. The hypopigmentation is usually present at birth and appears as a reverse image of incontinentia pigmenti. Associated anomalies of the CNS, eyes, integument, and skeletal system are found in about 75% of the cases. Megalencephaly occurs in the minority of patients. Spasticity, seizures, and mental retardation dominate the clinical picture.

Linear sebaceous nevus syndrome is recognized by the typical skin lesion of a unilateral sebaceous nevus on the scalp or face. Associated CNS and eye anomalies, developmental delay, and infantile spasms are common. Ipsilateral (to the nevus) hemihypertrophy may occur along with macrocephaly. The macrocephaly is either generalized or unilateral. CT scan shows asymmetry of the brain with enlargement of one hemisphere (Fig. 8-3).

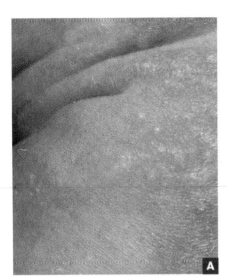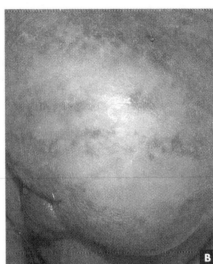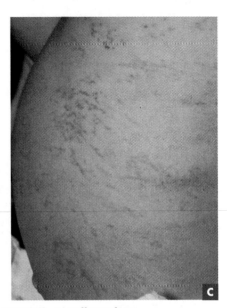

FIG. 8-4 The evolution of the skin lesions associated with incontinentia pigmenti. *A,* Bullous phase. *B,* Papular phase. *C,* Hyperpigmented phase.

Various chromosomal disorders cause microcephaly at birth. This is especially true when they are associated with major brain malformations. The combination of dysmorphic features and chromosomal analysis leads to a specific diagnosis.

Incontinentia pigmenti is an X-linked dominant disorder, and 95% of the cases affect girls. It was first described by Garrod in 1906. The typical skin lesions go through three stages. The first stage is a vesiculo-bullous eruption appearing during the first several weeks of life. This lesion develops a verrucous appearance after 6 weeks and finally changes to a hyperpigmented macular lesion during the first few years. The hyperpigmentation may fade throughout life and even eventually disappear. Neurologic abnormalities, such as mental retardation, seizures, and spasticity dominate the clinical picture. About one third of patients have associated microcephaly (Fig. 8-4).

A number of neural tube defects may lead to major brain malformations and resulting microcephaly. Anencephaly results in failure of the anterior neuropore to close and subsequent failure of the cerebrum to form. The skull and scalp are absent. The majority of anencephalic infants are stillborn or die shortly after birth. Diagnosis is obvious at birth. Prenatal diagnosis can be made by ultrasound. The recurrence rate ranges from 2% to 5%.

An encephalocele is a protrusion of a portion of the cerebral hemisphere or meninges through a skull defect. Encephaloceles occur in the occipital area 75% of the time, and the remainder are frontal. The size of encephaloceles varies greatly, and large defects are associated with microcephaly. As a general rule the more sessile forms usually have brain within them. Encephaloceles usually occur as one of multiple

brain malformations. Evaluation of the sac contents requires imaging with CT scan or MRI.

Another large group of conditions are categorized as cleavage and migration defects. Holoprosencephaly is caused by the forebrain failing to cleave and form two separate cerebral hemispheres. This failure leads to a small brain and microcephaly. Chromosomal abnormalities should be sought, especially trisomies, deletions, and rings of chromosomes 13 and 18. Associated defects include agenesis of the corpus callosum; midline defects of the eyes, nose, and palate; and malformations of the genitourinary and cardiac systems. Most children are severely affected and are stillborn or die shortly after birth. Microcephaly, hypotonia, seizures, and severe developmental delay are present. The diagnosis should be suspected in any child with a midline facial defect. Brain imaging confirms the diagnosis. Most lesions are incompatible with long-term survival.

Agenesis of the corpus callosum is an anomaly that often occurs in conjunction with other brain malformations. A specific syndrome described by Aicardi in 1965 showed an X-linked dominant pattern of inheritance. The features are agenesis of the corpus callosum, infantile spasms, chorioretinal lacunae, mental retardation, and vertebral anomalies. The syndrome is lethal to the male fetus and therefore affects only girls.

When agenesis of the corpus callosum is an isolated defect, patients appear normal unless specific psychometric testing is performed and demonstrates problems with the interhemisphere communications.

Other severe cellular migrational defects leading to microcephaly, severe psychomotor retardation, and seizures include schizencephaly, symmetric clefts within the cerebral

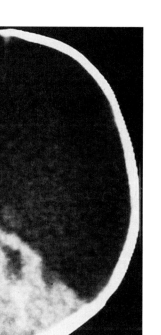

FIG. 8-5 Hydranencephaly. CT scan demonstrates massive replacement of brain substance with CSF.

BOX 8-4

Microcephaly

Primary
Genetic
Autosomal dominant
Autosomal recessive

Chromosomal

Neurocutaneous
Incontinentia pigmenti

Brain malformation
Encephalocele
Holoprosencephaly
Agenesis of corpus
  callosum

Porencephaly
Hydranencephaly

Migrational defects
Schizencephaly
Lissencephaly
Pachygyria

Secondary
Prenatal
Infections
Toxin exposure
Maternal disease
Vascular accidents

Perinatal
Hypoxic-ischemic insult
Vascular accidents
CNS infections

Postnatal
Severe chronic disease
Severe malnutrition
Same as perinatal

hemispheres, and hypoplasia of adjacent brain substance. Lissencephaly is incomplete gyral formation with resultant smooth brain and microcephaly. The term *pachygyria* applies to simplified gyral patterns with widening of the gyri and microcephaly.

Porencephaly refers to replacement of malformed or destroyed areas of the brain in the cerebral hemispheres by fluid-filled cysts. The cysts may or may not connect with the interventricular system. A congenital form of midline porencephaly exists and is characterized by congenital hydrocephalus, alopecia, and an encephalocele. The children have seizures and severe psychomotor retardation.

Either brain development failure or destruction may lead to absence of brain substance and replacement with CSF. This is termed *hydranencephaly*. Children with hydranencephaly may appear normal at birth except for microcephaly. Appropriate primitive reflexes are present because they are based at the subcortical level. Within a few weeks, developmental delay, hypertonia, and hyperreflexia become apparent. Transillumination of the skull demonstrates replacement of brain substance with CSF. This finding can be confirmed by CT scan or MRI (Fig. 8-5).

Secondary microcephaly occurs when an insult to normal brain results in destruction of the brain substance.

Prenatal causes of microcephaly may be broken down into four large categories. A multitude of intrauterine infections damage the fetal brain and cause microcephaly. Classically the well-described TORCH infections fall into this category. Intracranial calcifications seen on CT scanning may help to make this diagnosis, along with TORCH titers.

Although a host of toxins have been investigated, ethanol has been proved with certainty to impair brain growth. The result is fetal alcohol syndrome. When full blown, the syndrome is readily diagnosed by intrauterine growth retardation, short palpebral fissures, smooth philtrum, thin upper lip, microcephaly, and hypoplasia of the nails and distal digits. Milder forms exist, and a high index of suspicion is necessary to make the diagnosis (see Fig. 9-5).

Any maternal disease that results in placental insufficiency, such as chronic renal failure, severe insulin-dependent diabetes, or malnutrition, can cause microcephaly. However, head size is relatively spared and the weight is affected most, leading to the asymmetric small for gestational age (SGA) infant.

Intrauterine vascular insults lead to ischemic destruction of the developing fetal brain. Lesions, such as aplasia or thrombosis of major intracranial vessels, may result in infarction of brain with cyst formation. Occasionally, calcifications are in the cysts. If a significant portion of brain is destroyed, the infant may be born with microcephaly.

Insults at the time of delivery, or perinatal disorders, may result in brain injury severe enough to cause secondary microcephaly. Patients are born with normal head size; retarded brain growth becomes evident during infancy. Examples of such disorders include hypoxic ischemic encephalopathy, intracranial hemorrhage, CNS infections, and strokes.

Any of the perinatal problems that occur during the first few years of life may result in secondary microcephaly. In addition, early severe malnutrition, severe systemic disease (e.g., congenital heart disease, chronic renal failure), and infections that invade the CNS (e.g., HIV, meningitis) should be included in this category (Box 8-4).

Pathophysiology of Abnormal Head Shape

Internal Forces

Whereas head size is determined primarily by the intracranial contents, shape is mainly a function of forces exerted on the skull. The forces may be functionally divided into internal, external, and intrinsic. Internal forces are generated by intracranial contents in the skull with open sutures. Excessive enlargement or diminution of the brain substance, CSF space, or blood space can lead to alterations in the head shape. Examples are as follows:

1. Hydrocephalus—bowing of the forehead,
2. Dandy-Walker deformity—bulging of the occiput,
3. Subdural hematoma—bitemporal widening, and
4. Cerebellar agenesis—small posterior fossa.

External Forces

External forces are exerted on the skull by outward physical constraints. They can be intrauterine (e.g., abnormally shaped uterus), intravaginal (e.g., molding from prolonged delivery), or postnatal (e.g., poor head movement secondary to neuromuscular disease).

Intrinsic Forces

Intrinsic forces are usually the result of craniosynostosis, which is premature closure of one or more of the cranial sutures. Primary craniosynostosis results from premature fusion of single or multiple cranial sutures, causing deformation of the skull and face.

The pathologic bony defects begin in utero, restricting normal skull growth perpendicular to the affected suture. This may result in limited brain growth, increased intracranial pressure, and neurologic deficits. The cause of primary craniosynostosis includes a defect in the mesenchymal layer of the ossification sites within the skull. When part of a more global deficit, craniosynostosis syndromes are seen in conjunction with facial and skeletal anomalies.

Another factor that may cause craniosynostosis is intrauterine mechanical forces restraining adequate head growth (as described under external forces). A more controversial cause of craniosynostosis is deformity of the skullbase that alters tensile forces, which results in premature closure of the sutures.

Miscellaneous diseases with craniosynostosis include chromosomal disorders, blood dyscrasias with bone marrow hyperplasia, hypothyroidism, rickets, hypercalcemia, and hypophosphatasia (Box 8-5).

Secondary craniosynostosis is premature closure of the cranial sutures caused by a primary defect in brain growth, such as that seen in severe microcephaly or after ventricular shunting of massive hydrocephalus. Secondary craniosynostosis does not further impair the already defective brain growth in these children.

BOX 8-5

Disorders Associated with Craniosynostosis

Ataxia-telangiectasia
Familial hypophosphatemia
Hyperthyroidism
Idiopathic hypercalcemia
Mucopolysaccharidoses
Polycythemia vera
Rickets
Sickle-cell disease
Thalassemia major

Differential Diagnosis of Abnormal Head Shape

Most cases of craniosynostosis are isolated and sporadic. The prevalence is approximately 0.04% to 0.1%. Of isolated cases, 2% to 8% are familial, inherited as an autosomal dominant or autosomal recessive trait. A number of chromosomal and nonchromosomal syndromes have craniosynostosis as a prominent feature. These syndromes frequently occur with limb abnormalities, such as polydactyly and syndactyly.

Abnormal head shape may be the first sign of prematurely closed sutures because bone growth is disrupted in the plane perpendicular to the fused suture. Craniosynostosis is categorized by the suture that is involved and the resultant abnormal head shape (Table 8-2).

Sagittal synostosis results in elongation of the anteroposterior (AP) diameter, termed *scaphocephaly* (also called *dolichocephaly*). Premature sagittal fusion is the most common form of craniosynostosis (50% to 60%). Most patients are boys. The abnormal head shape is present at birth with ridging of the sagittal suture. Similar head shapes are seen in premature infants secondary to positional molding without synostosis.

Coronal synostosis, more common in girls, accounts for 20% of the cases of craniosynostosis. The head shape is termed *brachycephaly*. The skull is shorter in the AP diameter but is wide and high. There is flattening of the forehead and occiput. If untreated, coronal synostosis results in significant compromise of the orbits, globes, and vision.

Closure of a single suture, usually lambdoid or coronal, results in an asymmetric skull, called *plagiocephaly*. In lambdoid synostosis the ipsilateral ear is displaced anteriorly with one frontal bone larger than the other. The head takes on the shape of a parallelogram. This shape is also seen with congenital torticollis without craniosynostosis. During early infancy, torticollis restricts head movement, resulting in asym-

TABLE 8-2

Head Shape Terminology and Affected Suture

Term	Head shape	Suture
Scaphocephaly (or dolichocephaly)	Long and narrow	Sagittal
Brachycephaly	Broad with recessed forehead	Coronal
Plagiocephaly	Flattened on one side	Lambdoid
Trigonocephaly	Triangular with midforehead vertical ridge	Metopic
Oxycephaly	Pointed	All

BOX 8-6

Syndromes with Craniosynostosis (Sutures Frequently Affected)

Antley-Bixler (multiple)
Apert (coronal)
Baller-Gerold (metopic)
Carpenter (coronal, sagittal, lambdoid)
Crouzon (coronal, lambdoid, sagittal)
Fetal trimethadione
Pfeiffer (coronal, sagittal)
Saethre-Chotzen (coronal)
9p − (metopic)

From Jones KL: *Smith's recognizable patterns of human malformation*, Philadelphia, 1988, WB Saunders.

metry of the occiput and face secondary to the constant pressure. Clinically, torticollis is easily distinguished from lambdoid craniosynostosis by the classic head tilt toward the involved sternocleidomastoid muscle and the chin turned in the opposite direction.

Metopic synostosis results in a triangulated forehead with a midline ridge, called *trigonocephaly*. Hypotelorism accompanies the narrowed forehead. Some patients have significant abnormalities, including mental retardation, urinary tract anomalies, cleft palate, coloboma, and holoprosencephaly.

When coronal and sagittal sutures prematurely close, the skull shape is excessively high and narrow, termed *oxycephaly*. More importantly, increased ICP and severe neurologic sequelae develop. Optic atrophy, papilledema, exophthalmos, and choanal atresia may occur. In addition a narrowed external auditory canal results in hearing and vestibular dysfunction.

Common Syndromes With Craniosynostosis

Crouzon disease (craniofacial dysostosis) is an autosomal dominant disorder with a variable expression (Box 8-6). Approximately one fourth of the cases have negative family histories, and they are presumed to be new mutations. The most consistent clinical feature is shallow orbits with ocular proptosis. Strabismus and hypertelorism are other frequent findings. The maxilla is hypoplastic, and the nose is parrotlike. Craniosynostosis is present and usually involves the coronal, lambdoid, and sagittal sutures. The diagnosis is based on recognizing the typical facies in conjunction with a positive family history (25% have a negative family history).

Acrocephalosyndactyly is a group of syndromes with common features, consisting of craniosynostosis, fusion of the phalanges, and varying degrees of mental retardation.

Apert syndrome consists of brachycephaly, syndactyly, high forehead, and small mandible. Absence of the corpus callosum and abnormalities of the limbic system are associated CNS defects. Inheritance may be autosomal dominant, but the majority of cases represent new mutation. Advanced paternal age is a risk factor in sporadic cases.

Main features of Carpenter syndrome are brachycephaly and lateral displacement of the inner canthi with or without inner canthal folds. Brachydactyly, polydactyly, and syndactyly are accompanying limb abnormalities. Obesity and hypogonadism are prominent findings. This syndrome is presumed to be an autosomal recessive disorder.

Saethre-Chotzen syndrome, originally described in the early 1930s, may be the most common inheritable disorder in which coronal craniosynostosis is an associated feature. Craniofacial anomalies include brachycephaly, presumably caused by synostosis of the coronal suture; maxillary hypoplasia; facial asymmetry; shallow orbits; hypertelorism; and ptosis of the eyelids. Small ears with prominent ear crura are common. The large fontanelles close late. Usually, partial syndactyly of the second and third fingers and/or third and fourth toes occurs. There is a mild degree of brachydactyly of the small distal phalanges. The great toes and thumbs are broad. Rarely the craniosynostosis is severe enough to cause increased ICP. Patients also may have some mental deficiency, although normal intelligence is more common. It is believed that Saethre-Chotzen syndrome is an autosomal dominant disorder with a wide variance in expression. Saethre-Chotzen syndrome has been mapped to chromosome 7p.

Pfeiffer syndrome consists of brachycephaly with craniosynostosis of the coronal and occasionally sagittal sutures and accompanying high forehead. There is hypertelorism, antimongoloid upslanting palpebral fissures, and a small, low nasal bridge. The thumbs and big toes are typically broad. There may be partial syndactyly of the second and third fingers and the second, third, and fourth toes. Usually, intelligence is within normal ranges. Occasionally, hydrocephalus and Arnold-Chiari malformations are noted. It is believed that this is an autosomal dominant disorder, and many new mutations are being seen. There are three forms of Pfeiffer syndrome: type 1 (classic) is described here; type 2 is associated with cloverleaf skull. Type 3 may be overlooked because it causes extreme ocular proptosis in the absence of a cloverleaf skull. Visceral anomalies are common. Types 2 and 3 generally result in severe neurologic compromise and early death.

History and Physical Examination

As with any diagnostic problem, a thorough history is the key to directing the physical examination and reaching a final diagnosis. Children with abnormally sized or shaped heads may or may not have head size or shape as the chief complaint. The physician must be able to recognize the associated history and physical findings that accompany disorders of cranial size and shape. Because the differential diagnoses of macrocephaly, microcephaly, and abnormal head shape are quite different, each is covered separately in this section.

Macrocephaly

Macrocephaly is noted when the child's head size exceeds the 95th percentile. Even more important is the rate of rise and associated symptomatology (signs and symptoms of increased ICP, neurodevelopmental assessment, and dysmorphic features), which can be the key to the diagnosis.

If macrocephaly is secondary to the enlargement of the CSF space (hydrocephalus), the signs and symptoms of increased ICP are seen. In infancy the history includes complaints of a rapidly growing head size, bulging fontanelle, irritability, and sunsetting of the eyes. The older child typically complains of progressive headache that worsens with lying down or Valsalva maneuvers. The headaches are accompanied by vomiting and progressive lethargy.

Typically, children with benign subdural effusions initially have rapid head growth that eventually parallels the 97th percentile. Importantly, neurodevelopmental assessment is normal and there are no signs of increased ICP (Fig. 8-6).

Children with megalencephaly fall into two major categories—anatomic (enlarged and/or increased number of cells) and metabolic (secondary to accumulation of metabolic byproducts in the brain substance). Timing of the onset is important in distinguishing the differences in the two categories early in the course. Patients with anatomic megalencephaly usually have large heads at birth that increase in size postnatally. If this occurs on an inherited basis (genetic megalencephaly), one or both parents have macrocephaly. Through the use of Weaver's curves the parental influences on the child's head circumference can be estimated. Other forms of anatomic megalencephaly include the important group of

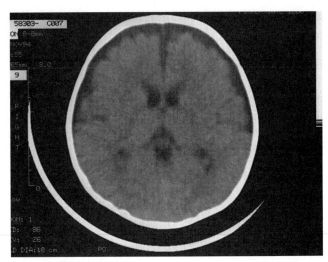

FIG. 8-6 Benign subdural effusion on CT scan with enlargement of the subarachnoid space (especially frontal) and normal ventricles. (Courtesy Dr. Marsha Stein, Youngstown, Ohio.)

conditions termed *neurocutaneous disorders*. Each syndrome in this group has characteristic skin and extradermal manifestations. The infant may have a history of multiple hypopigmented or hyperpigmented macules at birth, increasing in number with age, which points to a neurocutaneous disorder.

Children with metabolic megalencephaly have head circumferences in the normal range at birth, but they increase over time. The increase in head size coincides with the degenerative neurologic disease seen in these patients.

A few disorders may cause skull thickening of enough magnitude to result in macrocephaly. Typically, conditions in which anemia is severe enough to cause bone marrow proliferation in the skull have severe anemia as a chief complaint. Another causative disorder to consider is primary bone disease (Box 8-7).

Family history is important because a number of conditions are inherited. This includes X-linked aqueductal stenosis, genetic megalencephaly, neurocutaneous disorders, and metabolic megalencephalies. Other important aspects of the family history that may aid in the diagnosis include unexplained or early deaths in the family, mental retardation, and seizure disorders.

On past medical history, previous illnesses predisposing to hydrocephalus should be sought. Such conditions include bacterial meningitis and posthemorrhagic hydrocephalus secondary to intracranial hemorrhage. This is particularly true in the preterm infant with an intraventricular hemorrhage leading to noncommunicating hydrocephalus.

A detailed developmental history may elucidate a degenerative neurologic process, such as those seen in the metabolic megalencephalies. Static encephalopathy accompanies a number of megalencephalic conditions, such as megalen-

Conditions with Macrocephaly Secondary to Thickened Skull

Severe hemolytic anemia
Dysostosis
    Cleidocranial
    Orodigitofacial
    Pyknodysostosis
Osteopetrosis
Rickets
Hyperphosphatasemia
Russell dwarf
Osteogenesis imperfecta
Epiphyseal dysplasia

Modified from DeMeyer W: Megalencephaly: types, clinical syndromes, and management, *Pediatr Neurol* 2:321-328, 1986.

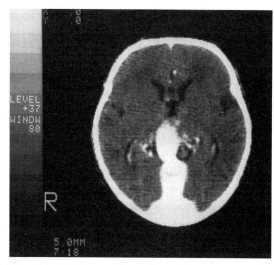

FIG. 8-7   Vein of Galen malformation. A large aneurysmal sac is visible on contrasted CT scan. (Courtesy Dr. Marsha Stein, Youngstown, Ohio.)

cephaly with neurologic abnormalities, neurocutaneous syndromes, and cerebral gigantism.

Physical examination begins with documentation of the macrocephaly by careful measurement of the occipitofrontal circumference (OFC). Although a thorough physical examination includes evaluation of all organ systems, particular detail should focus on the general appearance of the child, any abnormal skin manifestations, and the neurologic examination.

The general appearance of the child should be inspected for dysmorphic features. In particular, abnormal facies is seen in conditions such as Sotos syndrome. Patients with this condition have a prominent forehead, dolichocephaly, hypertelorism, and a pointed chin. Other dysmorphic features include hemihypertrophy, which may be seen in linear sebaceous nevus syndrome or neurofibromatosis. Rhizomelic limbs signify achondroplasia as a possible diagnosis.

The skin is examined for characteristic markings of neurocutaneous syndromes. After inspection, Wood's lamp examination of the skin is necessary to reveal subtle abnormal pigmentation. In particular the lesions of neurofibromatosis (café au lait spots), tuberous sclerosis (hypopigmented macules), and nevus sebaceous (seen in linear sebaceous nevus syndrome) should be sought.

Signs of congestive heart failure (gallop rhythm, hepatomegaly, and tachypnea) coupled with a cranial bruit raise concerns about vein of Galen malformation as a diagnosis. Hepatosplenomegaly is also seen in a number of storage diseases (Fig. 8-7).

A careful neurologic examination is required, looking for signs of increased ICP, such as bulging anterior fontanelle, split sutures, sunset eyes, papilledema, and increased tone. Any of these findings points to an increase in the CSF or blood space within the cranial vault. Spasticity with neurologic regression typifies the metabolic megalencephalies.

Microcephaly

Microcephaly is the physical manifestation of a small brain. A history should first focus on the onset of impaired brain growth (i.e., prenatal versus postnatal). Causes of microcephaly vary, depending on the timing of the brain insult that resulted in the final common manifestation.

Evaluation of the prenatal history includes inquiry about inappropriate intrauterine growth and movement. This history and a history of any significant maternal illnesses, such as infection or toxin exposure, point to a prenatal cause of the microcephaly. These children are born with small head circumferences. If the disorder is caused by placental insufficiency (severe diabetes, toxemia, etc.), the infant is asymmetric and SGA (weight is affected more than length, and length is affected more than head circumference). When a symmetric, SGA infant is born, the cause is typically genetic, chromosomal, early intrauterine infection (TORCH), or toxin exposure. Therefore obtaining growth parameters from birth is invaluable in evaluating the microcephalic infant.

Children with secondary microcephaly usually have an obvious inciting event or severe chronic disease as the cause. Hypoxic-ischemic encephalopathy any time within the first few years of life is a common cause of impaired brain growth. Other causes include CNS infection early in life (bacterial meningitis or HIV), stroke, and chronic diseases, such as cardiac disorders (cyanosis or chronic congestive heart failure), renal failure, or any condition leading to severe malnutrition.

Family history may reveal a genetic pattern of the microcephaly, in which the parents or other family members also have microcephaly. Patterns of autosomal dominant (with mild mental retardation) and autosomal recessive (with severe mental retardation) microcephaly are seen. Developmental history can be quite varied; a normal pattern is seen occasionally, but more often delays and learning disabilities are documented.

Physical examination must first confirm the microcephaly through accurate measurement of the OFC. Other growth parameters and any previous measurements should be obtained and plotted on standard curves in an attempt to differentiate a prenatal from a postnatal insult.

The search for dysmorphic features revolves around the presence of midline anomalies, such as those seen in association with holoprosencephaly. Anencephaly or an encephalocele is seen readily on inspection. As a general rule the more sessile the encephalocele, the more likely it is to contain brain tissue. Chromosomal anomalies, especially trisomies 13 and 18, cause microcephaly present at birth and other features, including major brain malformations, abnormalities of the extremities, and severe cardiac defects. An example of a nonchromosomal disorder is fetal alcohol syndrome, which causes short palpebral fissures, smooth philtrum, hypoplasia of the nails, and thin upper lip.

Abdominal examination may reveal hepatosplenomegaly, which can occur with the TORCH infections and resolves with time. During the acute infection, "blueberry spots" appear on the skin secondary to extramedullary hematopoiesis. Depending on the child's age, incontinentia pigmenti may present with any of the three stages of skin lesions.

Because most children with microcephaly are developmentally delayed, neurologic findings are common. Focal motor deficits, such as stroke, accompany focal CNS lesions. However, more often, findings are global in nature. Abnormalities of the fundi, such as chorioretinal lacunae, are important in the diagnosis of Aicardi syndrome.

Specific chronic diseases have typical findings compatible with the underlying disorders. Cardiac lesions include cyanosis and/or symptoms of congestive heart failure. The only findings in malnutrition may be loss of subcutaneous fat and overriding cranial sutures.

Abnormal Head Shape

Because head shape is determined by the play of forces exerted on a cranium with open sutures, history is aimed at revealing which forces are the major determinants of the abnormal head shape.

Internal forces are exerted by the intracranial contents (CSF, brain substance, and blood space). Questions pertaining to changes in intracranial contents are used to evaluate these forces. A history compatible with increased ICP and hydrocephalus may alter head shape significantly. External forces, such as abnormalities in uterine shape, can cause constraint severe enough to alter head shape. Other external forces, such as prolonged labor with severe molding or caput formation, should be sought routinely. Also, poor extrauter-

ine or intrauterine movement allows for compression and flattening of the malleable neonatal skull. This may represent significant neuromuscular disease or hypotonia caused by severe prematurity.

Craniosynostosis, an example of abnormal intrinsic forces, presents with an abnormal head shape that grows perpendicular to the closed suture. Signs of increased pressure are seen only when multiple sutures are closed. If synostosis is suspected, a history of polydactyly and syndactyly is frequently present. These findings may represent a number of recognizable syndromes. Family history may identify other members of the family with craniosynostosis syndromes, such as Crouzon, Apert, Carpenter, Saethre-Chotzen, or Pfeiffer syndromes. Developmental history demonstrates normal to varying degrees of mental retardation, depending on the primary syndrome.

Physical examination readily identifies a head shape that corresponds to synostosis of a specific suture (Table 8-2). A ridge palpated over the involved suture is a late finding and may never be seen.

Dysmorphic facies may point to any one of the known syndromes associated with craniosynostosis. Typically, abnormalities in the orbits with proptosis are seen. Other accompanying features may be coloboma, abnormalities in the nose, and abnormally shaped and placed ears. Torticollis should be noted because it may lead to plagiocephaly if untreated for a prolonged time.

The extremities should be inspected carefully for polydactyly and syndactyly. Bowing of the legs, short stature, and craniosynostosis can be seen with rickets.

Neurologic examination reveals signs of increased ICP if there is craniosynostosis of multiple sutures. Multiple focal and general CNS findings are seen, depending on the extent of brain involvement. In simple craniosynostosis, neurologic examination is usually normal.

Approach to the Patient

Diagnostic Approach

After a thorough history and physical examination, the cause of macrocephaly usually can be placed into one of three large categories—increased CSF or blood space, megalencephaly, or thickened skull.

Imaging of the head (CT or MRI) defines the cause as communicating or noncommunicating hydrocephalus. There may be associated defects, such as Arnold-Chiari malformations, Dandy-Walker deformity, and absence of the corpus callosum. Vascular lesions require contrasted MRI studies or angiography. Benign subdural effusions show only enlargement of the frontal subarachnoid space.

Imaging in patients with anatomic megalencephaly is usually normal or demonstrates minor abnormalities, such as agenesis of the corpus callosum or mild ventricular dilation. However, if neurocutaneous syndromes are suspected, imaging may reveal the tubers of tuberous sclerosis or asymmetry

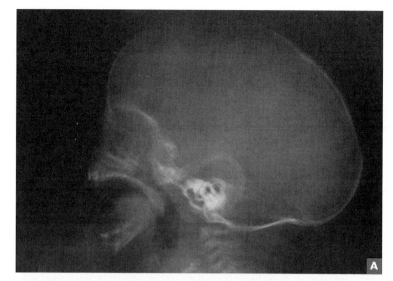

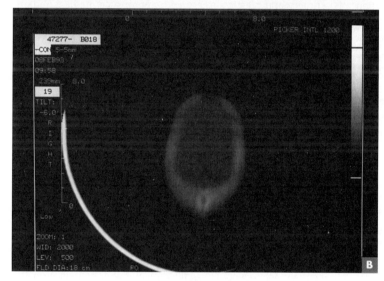

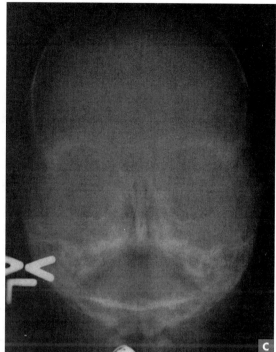

FIG. 8-8 *A,* Bony bridging of the sagittal suture seen in plain films in a child with isolated sagittal craniosynostosis. *B,* CT scan bone windows demonstrating increased bone density along the sagittal suture. (Courtesy Dr. Marsha Stein, Youngstown, Ohio.)

of the cerebral hemispheres as seen in patients with linear sebaceous nevus syndrome. If neurocutaneous disease is suspected, careful examination of the patient's skin is mandatory. In addition, the parents and siblings should be given thorough physical examinations.

Genetic megalencephaly has a positive family history of macrocephaly, and imaging of the head is normal. Developmental assessment is important because mental retardation can be seen in association with megalencephaly and the neurocutaneous disorders. When degenerative neurologic disease is apparent in association with macrocephaly, an evaluation for the metabolic megalencephalies is required. Appropriate evaluation of metabolic megalencephalies includes collection of blood, urine, and biopsy specimens to identify the metabolic defect. Additional evaluation may include chromosomal analysis and EEG because seizures may be present in a number of conditions.

Imaging of the microcephalic head is most useful when development is abnormal. Scans may be normal (microcephaly vera) or may show major anomalies, such as holoprosencephaly, cerebral infarction, or defects in cellular migration. Other findings include periventricular calcifications, such as those seen in intrauterine cytomegalovirus infections. If TORCH infections are suspected at birth, serology and cultures are helpful. Significant dysmorphology requires chromosomal analysis because microcephaly is a major finding in a number of conditions.

The diagnosis of chronic disease severe enough to result in microcephaly is usually straightforward. Abnormal head shape should always raise suspicions of craniosynostosis. Palpation of the sutures may reveal ridging of the involved suture, and x-ray films demonstrate a band of increased density along the suture line. However, CT scan with bone windows is the best diagnostic test. CT scans of the head should be performed when multiple sutures are involved or increased ICP is suspected (Fig. 8-8).

When significant dysmorphic features, especially abnormalities of the extremities, are present in association with craniosynostosis, a specific syndrome may be present. These syndromes include Crouzon and acrocephalosyndactyly.

Chromosomal analysis and genetic and craniofacial consultation are helpful. Imaging of the head and facial structures is important to identify synostosis and accompanying severe facial and orbital derangements.

Therapy

Therapies for abnormal head size are largely supportive. Patients with hydrocephalus usually require mechanical shunting (ventriculoperitoneal [VP] shunt). Conditions such as Dandy-Walker syndrome require special consideration. The cyst should be shunted and a VP shunt placed. Failure to shunt both the cyst and ventricles usually results in recurrence of symptoms.

Children with Arnold-Chiari malformations and cardiorespiratory symptoms secondary to brainstem compression require careful monitoring. They should undergo suboccipital craniotomy to decompress the brainstem. A VP shunt is then required to relieve hydrocephalus.

If congenital aqueductal stenosis is detected early, intrauterine ventriculoamniotic shunting is performed to relieve the severe progressive hydrocephalus. After birth, a more permanent shunt may be placed. When compression of the ventricular system is secondary to an external mass, such as tumor, resection and mechanical shunting are necessary. If compression is secondary to a vascular structure, such as the vein of Galen, both the surgical repair and intravascular occlusion may be attempted. Both these interventions carry a high morbidity and mortality. Infants with benign subdural effusions, on the other hand, require no therapy for this self-limiting condition. However, reevaluation is mandatory if developmental delays, signs of increased ICP, or the head circumference continue to increase at a rapid rate.

Macrocephaly caused by megalencephaly has no specific treatment. Patients with the genetic form are normal and require no therapy. Other forms, such as megalencephaly with neurologic symptoms or the neurocutaneous syndromes (hypomelanosis of Ito or linear sebaceous nevus syndrome), often have seizures that respond to antiepileptic medication. These children also require special education for their learning disabilities or mental retardation. In addition to seizures, neurofibromatosis and tuberous sclerosis cause extraneuronal manifestations that require ongoing monitoring and possible treatment (Box 8-2). Control of the seizures is also important in degenerative metabolic megalencephalies. There is no specific therapy for this group of disorders, and patients eventually succumb to their disease. Genetic counseling is important for patients with this group of inherited conditions.

Primary microcephalies are often accompanied by a significant seizure disorder that may require neurologic consultation and antiepileptic medications. Physical therapy may be beneficial because spasticity usually ensues in these conditions.

Neurosurgical evaluation is required when an encephalocele is suspected. Children should be delivered by cesarean section so as not to traumatize the involved area. Closure of the sac and its contents is performed. Prognosis depends on the amount of brain substance present within the defect. Often, ventricular shunting is required for the accompanying hydrocephalus. Other severe brain malformations, such as anencephaly or hydrencephaly, are incompatible with prolonged life. Other than comfort measures, no treatment should be instituted.

Therapy for the secondary microcephalies is limited to treatment of seizures, special education, and physical therapy. Treatment of extranervous system manifestations may be required for some syndromes, especially those in which significant heart anomalies are seen (e.g., rubella).

In general, no therapeutic intervention is required for simple craniosynostosis. As a rule, surgery is indicated for significant cosmetic problems or when signs and symptoms of increased ICP are seen. When craniosynostosis syndromes are the cause of abnormal head shape, a team (craniofacial) approach to therapy is best. Usually this includes neurosurgery and plastic surgery with appropriate medical and ancillary personnel. Multiple craniofacial surgeries are required for cosmetic and functional correction. Families should also receive genetic counseling regarding their recurrence risk.

SUMMARY

Evaluation of head growth on each visit is part of routine pediatric care. Abnormalities of growth can be divided into macrocephaly, microcephaly, and abnormal head shape. In the case of macrocephaly it is most important to recognize increased intracranial pressure or hydrocephalus early; megalencephaly may be familial or genetic or secondary to metabolic or neurocutaneous disorders. Close attention to skin and general physical and developmental examinations aids in the diagnosis. Neuroimaging is frequently critical in decision making, unless history and normal development point to genetic megalencephaly. Microcephaly usually indicates poor brain growth and is commonly associated with anatomic, genetic, or infectious causes. Developmental delay is common. The most important first consideration in abnormal head shape is craniosynostosis, often indicated by ridging of the sutures on physical examination. A number of known syndromes should be considered if other dysmorphic features are present.

Close attention to the history and physical examination often suggests the correct diagnosis and the appropriate evaluation of patients with abnormal head size or shape.

ILLUSTRATIVE CASES

Case 1. An 8-week-old boy was found to have a head circumference greater than the 95th percentile at his well child care visit. On review of the previous head circumference measurements, it is obvious that head growth velocity has been increasing rapidly since shortly after birth (head circumference = 36 cm). On examination, length and weight velocities are normal as is the child's development. The general examination is normal other than a full pulsatile fontanelle; there is no sign of increased ICP. Both par-

ents have a head circumference in the 50th percentile. A CT scan of the head demonstrates enlargement of the subarachnoid space with normal ventricles.

This case demonstrates the typical history, physical examination, and CT scan findings of a child with benign enlargement of the subarachnoid space. Serial head circumference measurements showed slowing of the head growth velocity at 4 months of age, at which time the curve began to parallel the 95th percentile.

Case 2. A 4-month-old infant being followed by her pediatrician was noted to have a head circumference less than the 2nd percentile at her well child care visit. The head circumference had been small since birth (31 cm), although the length and weight have been tracking at the 75th percentile. Physical examination and development are normal, and the child is otherwise well. The mother's head circumference is 3 standard deviations below the mean, and the father's is 1 standard deviation below the mean. Of note, the mother had learning problems in school and was in learning disability classes. The pediatrician suspected that the child had genetic microcephaly by using the technique described by Weaver.

In this child with normal development and somatic growth with microcephaly, using Weaver's formula, the average of the standard deviations of the parents' head circumferences are plotted against the child's (-3 SD $+$ -1 SD/2 $=$ -2 SD). Clearly the child's microcephaly is explained solely by parental influences. No further evaluation is needed.

Case 3. A 6-month-old infant is brought to the pediatrician's office by the parents who are worried because they can no longer feel the child's anterior fontanelle. They were told by friends that this was not normal. The child is otherwise healthy and thriving. On examination the fontanelle is closed, and it is obvious that the head shape is abnormal, with frontal bossing and a narrow bitemporal diameter. A ridge is felt along the sagittal suture. The other sutures are normal as is the head circumference. Neurologic and developmental examination are normal. The pediatrician believes this is simple sagittal suture synostosis (scaphocephaly). A CT scan with bone windows confirms the diagnosis.

This child has the most common form of simple craniosynostosis. The main problem facing the parents and child is the cosmetic deformity if left untreated. The child was therefore referred to the craniofacial team for surgical correction.

ANNOTATED BIBLIOGRAPHY

Cohen MM: Craniosynostosis update 1987, *Am Med Genetics Suppl* 4:99-148, 1988.

The epidemiology, etiology, and pathophysiology of craniosysnosto-

sis syndromes and prenatal diagnosis of craniosynostosis are covered in this very detailed review.

Lorber J, Priestly BL: Children with large heads: a practical approach to diagnosis in 577 children, with special reference to 109 children with megalencephaly, *Dev Med Child Neurol* 23:494-504, 1981.

The authors review the natural course of megalencephaly as a significant subset of macrocephaly. Particular attention is placed on head growth velocity and developmental outcomes.

Weaver DD, Christian JC: Familial variation of head size and adjustment for parental head circumference, *J Pediatr* 96:990-994, 1980.

A very useful article looking at the influence of parental head size on their children's head growth. A method is presented that allows the physician to determine these influences.

BIBLIOGRAPHY

Aicardi J, Lefebvre J, Lerique-Koechlin A: A new syndrome: spasm in flexion, callosal agenesis, ocular abnormalities, *Electroencephalogr Clin Neurophysiol* 19:609-610, 1965.

Albright AL, Byrd RP: Suture pathology in craniosynostosis, *J Neurosurg* 54:384-387, 1981.

Chervnak FA, Berkowitz RL, Tortora M, et al: The management of fetal hydrocephalus, *Am J Obstet Gynecol* 151:933-941, 1985.

Clancy RR, Kurtz MB, Baker D, et al: Neurologic manifestation of the organoid nevus syndrome, *Arch Neurol* 42:236-240, 1985.

Cohen MM: Pfeiffer syndrome update: clinical subtypes and guidelines for differential diagnosis, *Am J Med Genet* 45:300-307, 1993.

DeMeyer W: Megalencephaly: types, clinical syndromes, and management, *Pediatr Neurol* 2:321-328, 1986.

Fenichel GM: *Clinical pediatric neurology: a signs and symptoms approach*, Philadelphia, 1988, WB Saunders.

Garrod AE: Peculiar pigmentation of the skin in an infant, *Trans Clin Society* 39:216, 1906.

Haslam RHA, Smith DW: Autosomal dominant microcephaly, *J Pediatr* 95:701-705, 1979.

Ito M: A singular case of naevus depigmentosus systematicus bilateralis, *Tohoku J Exp Med* 55:57-59, 1952.

Jones KL: *Smith's recognizable patterns of human malformation*, Philadelphia, 1988, WB Saunders.

Kuznieky RI, Watters GV, Watters L, et al: X-linked hydrocephalus, *Can J Neurol Sci* 13:344-346, 1986.

Mueller SM, Reinertson JE: Reversal of emissary vein blood flow in achondroplastic dwarfs, *Neurology* 30:769-772, 1989.

Nickel RE, Gallenstein JS: Developmental prognosis for infants with enlargement of the subarachnoid spaces, *Dev Med Child Neurol* 29:181-186, 1987.

Swaiman KF: *Pediatric neurology*, St Louis, 1989, Mosby–Year Book.

Wit JM, Breemer FA, Barth PG, et al: Cerebral gigantism (Sotos syndrome): compiled data of 22 cases—analysis of clinical features, growth, and plasma somatomedin, *Eur J Pediatr* 144:131-140, 1985.

Yokota A, Matsukado Y: Congenital midline porencephaly: a new malformation associated with scalp anomaly, *Child Brain* 5:380-397, 1979.

9

Developmental Delay

DENA HOFKOSH ❦ LISA M. NALVEN

 Key Points

- Developmental disorders (e.g., mental retardation, cerebral palsy, sensory impairment, autism, learning disabilities, attention-deficit hyperactivity disorder, and language disorders) are the most common chronic problems of childhood.

- Developmental surveillance is the recommended process for evaluating development in children and is based on careful interview of parents; observations of the child's behavior, play, communication, and motor skills over time; and use of standardized developmental screening tests.

- The pediatrician must be able to elicit parents' concerns about development, recognize the significance of developmental delay, make appropriate use of community resources for developmental assessment and early intervention, and serve as an advocate for families as they cope with their child's chronic condition.

Role of the Pediatrician

Developmental disorders, which typically present as the delayed acquisition of developmental skills, are the most prevalent chronic problems encountered by the general pediatrician. Pediatricians must be able to recognize developmental delay to detect developmental disorders as early as possible. The detection of developmental disorders requires an elicitation of parents' concerns, an ongoing evaluation of the child's developmental progress, an understanding of the patterns of normal child development, and an appreciation for the distinction between variation within the normal range and truly abnormal development. Pediatricians are in an ideal position to identify early signs of developmental disorders because of the longitudinal nature of their relationship with the child

and family and their understanding of how individual characteristics and the child's environment influence the emergence of developmental skills. The pediatrician should recognize the significance of developmental delay, initiate a diagnostic evaluation when appropriate, and make judicious referrals for more specific assessment and intervention.

The pediatrician should be aware of the professional resources in the medical and educational community, including developmental pediatricians, child psychologists, educators, and speech, physical, and occupational therapists who provide further assessment of child development and behavior. The pediatrician may initiate a diagnostic evaluation to establish a specific cause of developmental delay or refer to a developmental pediatrician, geneticist, or child neurologist for consultation regarding the selection and interpretation of medical testing. If specialty consultation is sought in the evaluation of the child with developmental delay, the pediatrician serves the family best if he or she retains responsibility for discussing the purpose of such consultation with the family and preparing the family for what they may expect from the consultant. The primary pediatrician plays an important role as the coordinator of subspecialty, therapeutic, and educational services and as an advocate for the family as they cope with their child's chronic disabling condition.

In the sections that follow the prevalence of developmental disorders is reviewed, and the critical components of early detection which include using a standardized method of evaluating developmental progress and eliciting parents' concerns, are discussed. The chapter presents the basic pathophysiology of abnormal development and suggests an approach to formulating a differential diagnosis of developmental delay. The elements of the history and physical examination that are particularly useful in determining the contributors to developmental delay are discussed, and an approach to the selection of medical tests is presented. Whether the primary pediatrician initiates the diagnostic evaluation of developmental delay or refers for specialty evaluation, the differential diagnosis and the rational selection of tests should be well understood by the pediatrician so that he or she can serve as a resource for the family. Finally, some of the issues involved in working collaboratively with the families of children with developmental disabilities are discussed.

Pathophysiology

Development reflects the maturation of the child's central nervous system (CNS) under the continual influence of the child's environment. The ongoing interactions between the child and his or her environment have been called *transactions,* implying that the child and the environment continually influence each other so that the nature of the interactions changes with time. Qualities with which the child is born, including genetic endowment, temperament, and experiences during fetal development, contribute to the pattern of acquisition of developmental skills. Likewise, qualities of the environment, including the parents' experiences and expectations of parenting, their temperamental style, their responses to the child's behavior, and the nature and amount of stimulation available in the home, influence the pattern and quality of development. Environmental factors are operative whether the underlying biologic structure and function of the CNS is normal or abnormal and must be considered in the evaluation of developmental delay.

In view of the transactional nature of development, it is important to consider both biologic and environmental contributions rather than assess environmental factors only after "ruling out" numerous medical problems. Skills that are the least dependent on environmental influences, such as gross motor skills, are the most predictable in terms of sequence and timing of emergence. Therefore delay in the acquisition of gross motor skills is probably primarily related to CNS dysfunction, although environmental factors must be considered. Language and social skills in contrast are highly dependent on reciprocal interactions with the environment and therefore are much more variable in their pattern and rate of acquisition. Environmental factors must be assessed carefully in the evaluation of delayed language or social development.

Severe abnormality in CNS function results in severe developmental disability, regardless of the influence of the environment. Severe dysfunction in the environment, such as physical or emotional abuse, neglect, chronic illness, or long-term hospitalization, may also result in severe developmental disability, even though the child's CNS may have been normal in structure and function at birth. The nature and severity of developmental problems that result from milder dysfunction in the CNS or the environment are much more difficult to predict. The impact of biologic risk factors, such as prematurity, perinatal asphyxia, or prenatal drug exposure, on the pattern and rate of skill acquisition may be minimized by an environment that supports learning and promotes emotional growth. Developmental disability is much more likely to be severe when the child experiences a biologic insult and lives in an environment unable to provide the consistency, stimulation, and nurturance necessary for optimal develop-

ment. Children who have experienced both biologic and environmental risk factors are said to be at "double hazard" and require particularly careful developmental surveillance. Although risk factors by definition increase the risk of developmental disability, they do not necessarily predict future developmental problems.

Scope of the Problem

Developmental disorders or disabilities are chronic conditions related to impairment in cognitive, language, motor, or self-care domains manifested during childhood. Delayed development in infancy or early childhood may occur because of underlying chronic illness or environmental deprivation or may be the presenting sign of a primary developmental disorder affecting CNS development. The developmental disabilities, including cerebral palsy, mental retardation, sensory impairment, and learning disabilities, occur in 10% to 17% of American children. Low-prevalence and high-severity disabilities, including cerebral palsy (1 to 2 per 1000), severe or profound mental retardation (3 per 1000), visual impairment or blindness (12 per 1000), hearing impairment or deafness (15 per 1000), and autistic disorder (1 per 1000), can be identified in infancy or early childhood. High-prevalence and low-severity disabilities, including attention-deficit hyperactivity disorder (5 per 100), learning disabilities (7 to 10 per 100), and mild or moderate mental retardation (2 to 3 per 100), may present in early life with only mildly delayed development or subtle differences in behavior. They are therefore more difficult to recognize early and may not become apparent until the child enters school and struggles or fails.

Detection: Developmental Surveillance or Screening

The early detection of developmental disorders requires that pediatricians make accurate judgments about the rate and pattern of development, based on a comparison of the individual child's skills and behaviors with age-appropriate expectations. Developmental screening tests have been developed to identify children who require more extensive developmental evaluation, adding objectivity to the physicians' assessment of development. The most widely used screening instrument, the Denver Developmental Screening Test II, has been extensively revised and expanded and is more sensitive in identifying delays than the previous version. Despite the availability of several standardized screening instruments, only 30% of pediatricians actually use a developmental screening test for the routine evaluation of children. Instead, pediatricians often base their assessment of development on informal observations of the child's behavior in the office. Unfortunately, physicians' informal, subjective impressions of development are fairly unreliable. Physicians who rely solely on their impressions may overlook up to 50% of children with developmental disabilities. Therefore the use of a standardized screening instrument is recommended as an integral component of pediatric practice.

In contrast to physicians, parents are both sensitive and specific in identifying developmental disorders, including mental retardation, in their children. Parents in a pediatric primary care clinic were asked to list developmental concerns they had about their children before a developmental screening test was administered. The parents of 80% of children who failed the developmental screen had identified developmental concerns, whereas the parents of 94% of those who passed the screen had no concerns. Parental worries about development are very common, and the importance of respecting parents' concerns about their child's development cannot be overemphasized. The most valuable developmental history begins by exploring any concerns the parents have about the child's progress. Parents in pediatricians' waiting rooms are often more concerned about their child's development, behavior, or personality than medical issues. Glascoe suggests "that when parents are concerned about their child's development, healthcare professionals should pay attention."

Developmental surveillance, the continuous process of evaluating child development, is based on a partnership with parents and includes careful questioning to elicit and explore parents' concerns, identification of risk factors, and observations of the child's behavior, play, communication, and motor skills in the pediatrician's office. Although surveillance does not require the use of a particular screening instrument, the use of such an instrument can enhance the pediatrician's ability to detect developmental problems that otherwise might not have come to attention. Developmental surveillance allows for an appreciation of the child's individual "developmental curve," similar to a growth curve, in which the important concept is the rate of development over time, rather than skills at a single point in time. Development is typically assessed according to the following specific domains: motor skills (gross and fine), language skills (receptive and expressive), social skills, adaptive skills (feeding, dressing, toileting), and cognitive skills. Recognition of the particular pattern of developmental delay, involving only certain domains or all domains of development, is important in forming a differential diagnosis and may suggest a particular diagnostic approach.

Differential Diagnosis

The approach to establishing a diagnosis for children with developmental disorders requires two separate diagnostic processes. The *developmental diagnosis* is based on a characteristic pattern of delay or deviance in the affected developmental domains. Developmental disorders may be global, affecting all developmental domains, or may involve only specific domains while development in other domains may be normal. Mental retardation, language disorders, autism, and cerebral palsy are examples of developmental diagnoses.

The *medical diagnosis* refers to the cause of the developmental disorder and includes chromosomal abnormality, metabolic disease, hypoxic-ischemic encephalopathy, and infection of the CNS. The developmental diagnosis may be describable, but in many cases a medical diagnosis cannot be established (Table 9-1).

Developmental disorders can also be classified according to the static or progressive nature of the disorder. Static disorders reflect an alteration in structure or function of the CNS of prenatal, perinatal, or postnatal origin and are characterized by the steady but slower-than-normal acquisition of developmental milestones. The severity of the delay, expressed as the ratio of the child's developmental age/chronological age, or developmental quotient (DQ), remains constant over time. In contrast, progressive disorders are characterized by developmental regression (the loss of previously attained skills), resulting in a decreasing DQ. These disorders may be congenital or acquired and are much less common than disorders of a static nature.

The following discussion of the differential diagnosis of developmental delay is organized according to developmental diagnoses, followed by a brief discussion of the associated medical diagnoses. There is considerable overlap among the categories and great variability in the mode of presentation. Within each category of developmental diagnosis both static and progressive processes are considered. Disorders presenting as global delay are considered first, followed by a discussion of disorders involving only specific domains of development.

Static Global Developmental Delay: Mental Retardation

Mental retardation is defined as significantly subaverage intellectual functioning that is accompanied by significant limitations in adaptive functioning. Intellectual functioning is measured by performance on standard tests of intelligence, such as the intelligence quotient (IQ), although the limitations in adaptive function typically bring the child to attention. According to the definition of significantly subaverage intelligence, 3% of the general population is mentally retarded, with scores on standardized IQ tests of less than 70. Before the age of $2\frac{1}{2}$ to 3 years, when a formal IQ test can be administered, children with significantly subaverage intellectual and adaptive functioning are described as developmentally delayed. If the delay is significant and persists over time, the developmentally delayed child should be considered by the physician to be at risk for a later diagnosis of mental retardation.

Most people who are mentally retarded have mild to moderate retardation with IQ in the range of 55 to 70 for a classification of mild and 40 to 55 for moderate retardation. Individuals with mild retardation typically are able to achieve academic skills, including reading and arithmetic, at a grade-school level. With great individual variation, they may have adequate social and adaptive skills to live and work indepen-

TABLE 9-1

Differential Diagnosis of Developmental Delay

Presentation	Conditions	Associated features
Static global delay/ mental retardation	Chromosomal abnormalities or genetic syndromes	Dysmorphic features, +/− hypotonia, +/− short stature
	Prenatal exposure to toxins or teratogens	Dysmorphic features (FAS, fetal hydantoin syndrome)
	Congenital infection	Microcephaly, intrauterine growth restriction, hearing impairment (CMV), chorioretinitis (toxoplasmosis)
	Hypoxic-ischemic encephalopathy	Focal neurologic signs, motor delay
	Structural brain malformation	Dysmorphic features, microcephaly, other major malformations
	Idiopathic mental retardation	—
Progressive global delay	Inborn errors of metabolism	Developmental regression, visceromegaly, failure to thrive
	Neurodegenerative disorders	Developmental regression, loss of motor skills, dementia, seizures, hypotonia followed by spasticity, blindness
	Rett syndrome	Girls with loss of functional hand use, progressive dementia, spasticity, hand wringing, mouthing, acquired microcephaly
	AIDS encephalopathy	AIDS risk factors, failure to thrive, recurrent illness
	Congenital hypothyroidism	Constipation, lethargy, poor growth, delayed closure of posterior fontanelle, coarse facial features
Language disorders	Hearing impairment	Associated with several genetic syndromes, congenital CMV
	Language processing, expressive language disorders	Normal nonverbal (problem-solving) skills, gestural communication
	Pervasive developmental disorder or autistic disorder	Poor social interaction, unusual behaviors
	Landau-Kleffner syndrome	Seizures, loss of language
Gross motor delay	Cerebral palsy	Focal neurologic signs, +/− cognitive impairment, normal strength
	Peripheral neuromuscular disorders	Weakness, +/− decreased or absent deep tendon reflexes

AIDS, Acquired immunodeficiency syndrome; *CMV*, cytomegalovirus; *FAS*, fetal alcohol syndrome; +/−, with or without.

dently or with minimal supervision. Individuals with moderate retardation generally are able to perform activities of daily living but need support and supervision for living and work. Only 0.3% to 0.5% of the general population has severe to profound retardation with an IQ less than 40. The functional abilities of these individuals are more limited, although skills can be learned, and supervision is typically needed for activities of daily living.

The cause of mild to moderate mental retardation is idiopathic in 45% to 65% of cases. However, because mild to moderate mental retardation may have a medical basis, a thorough evaluation is warranted, even though the yield may be low. In contrast a specific, definable cause can be identified in 60% to 70% of cases of severe to profound mental retardation; 30% to 40% are idiopathic. The differential diagnosis of severe to profound mental retardation includes chromosomal abnormalities (30%); multiple congenital anomaly syndromes without identifiable chromosomal abnormality (4% to 6%); injury to the CNS, including prenatal exposure to toxic or teratogenic agents, prenatal and perinatal infections, and hypoxic-ischemic injury (15% to 20%); structural brain malformations (10% to 15%); and endocrine and metabolic disorders (3% to 5%).

Genetic Syndromes

The physical features of Down syndrome, the most common chromosomal abnormality (Table 9-2), are easily recognized, and in most infants the diagnosis is confirmed by karyotype shortly after birth. Down syndrome occurs in 1 in 800 live births. The majority of individuals with Down syndrome function in the mild to moderate range of mental retardation. Fragile X syndrome is another common identifiable cause of mental retardation with a prevalence of 1 in 1250 males and 1 in 2500 females in the general population. In ad-

Syndromes Associated With Development Delay

Syndrome	Dysmorphic features	Cognitive/behavioral features	Genetic defect
Down	Short stature, hypotonia, microcephaly, flat occiput, upslanting palpebral fissures, epicanthal folds, Brushfield's spots, single palmar crease, congenital heart disease	Moderate mental retardation	Trisomy 21
Fragile X	Prominent ears, long narrow face and jaw, hyperextensible joints, macroorchidism at puberty	Moderate mental retardation, hand flapping and other autistic-like behavior, hyperactivity, family history of mental retardation, autism, learning disabilities, hyperactivity	Mutation in FMR-1 gene on X chromosome
Prader-Willi	Short stature, hypogonadism, small hands and feet, hypotonia during infancy with failure to thrive, followed by obesity	Moderate mental retardation, behavior problems, unregulated appetite	15 deletion (paternal) in 50%
Turner	Short stature, webbed neck, low posterior hairline, broad chest with wide-spaced nipples	40% mild mental retardation, hearing impairment	XO, mosaic forms XX/XO
Williams	Short stature, epicanthal folds, blue eyes with stellate pattern, prominent thick lips with open mouth, congenital heart disease (supravalvular aortic stenosis)	Mild to moderate mental retardation, verbal skills much better than perceptual-motor skills, friendly loquacious personality	7 deletion
Noonan	Short stature, broad forehead, ptosis, low-set ears, low posterior hairline, cryptorchidism, shield chest, congenital heart disease (pulmonic stenosis)	Mild mental retardation, 75% in normal range of intelligence	—
Sotos	Tall stature of prenatal onset, large hands and feet, macrocephaly, prominent forehead, hypertelorism, downslanting palpebral fissures, prognathism	Mild to moderate mental retardation	—
Klinefelter	Tall slim stature, long limbs, hypogonadism	Late speech onset, mild mental retardation, behavior problems	XXY
Angelman	Ataxia and jerky movements, seizures, prognathism, large mouth with tongue protrusion	Severe mental retardation, paroxysms of laughter	15 deletion (maternal)
Cornelia de Lange	Short stature, failure to thrive, microcephaly, bushy eyebrows and synophrys, long curly lashes, micrognathia, hirsutism, failure to thrive, hypoplastic nipples	Severe mental retardation, hearing impairment	—
Beckwith-Wiedemann	Large size at birth, large tongue, microcephaly, prominent occiput, neonatal hypoglycemia, large fontanelle, visceromegaly, advanced bone age	Mild to moderate mental retardation, may have normal intelligence	—

dition to cognitive deficits, boys with fragile X syndrome may have behavior problems, such as hyperactivity, impulsivity, short attention span, and low frustration tolerance. They may also have features suggestive of autism, including hypersensitivity to sensory stimulation, hand flapping, language delay, and poor eye contact, although they may not meet formal diagnostic criteria for autistic disorder. Specific dysmorphic features, including prominent ears, hyperextensible joints, flatfeet, prominent forehead, long face, and macrocephaly, are associated with fragile X syndrome, but these features may be

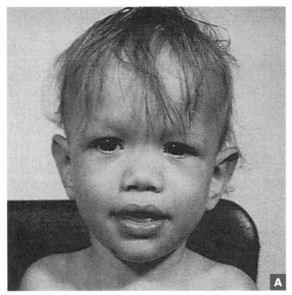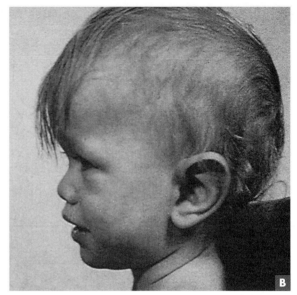

FIG. 9-1   Physical findings in fragile X syndrome. *A* and *B,* Note the long, wide, and protruding ears, elongated face, and flattened nasal bridge. (From Simko A, Hornstein L, Soukup S, et al: Fragile X syndrome: recognition in young children, *Pediatrics* 83(4):547-552, 1989.)

quite subtle in infants and young children. Hypotonia with associated mild delays in motor development, recurrent otitis media, and refractive errors are also common. After puberty, macro-orchidism and a prominent jaw are also noted. Girls who are carriers of the mutation may have normal IQs, although mild mental retardation is reported in about 50% of carrier females, and learning disabilities, language delays, depression, and other psychiatric symptoms are common, even among those with normal IQs (Fig. 9-1).

Numerous other genetic syndromes are characterized by mental retardation and specific dysmorphic features, but the pattern of dysmorphic features may be subtle, thus delaying diagnosis until the child has developmental problems. Among the more common of these conditions is Prader-Willi syndrome, which has clinical characteristics, such as hypotonia, feeding problems, and failure to thrive in infancy, that evolve to unregulated appetite, obesity, short stature, mild to moderate mental retardation, and behavior problems, beginning at 2 to 3 years of age (Fig. 9-2).

Williams, Noonan, and Turner syndromes, with specific patterns of dysmorphic features, may also be associated with mild to moderate mental retardation. However, cognitive function may be within the normal range in individuals with these syndromes.

Tall stature, motor incoordination, behavioral difficulties, and mild to moderate retardation are features associated with Sotos syndrome (cerebral gigantism) and Klinefelter (XXY) syndrome.

Angelman syndrome is characterized by severe mental retardation, movements that are described as jerky and ataxic or "puppetlike," a pleasant disposition, paroxysms of laughter, seizures with characteristic electroencephalogram (EEG) findings, and dysmorphic features, including microcephaly, a

prominent jaw, irregularly spaced teeth, and a large mouth. These children typically have severe developmental delay in infancy when the dysmorphic features may be difficult to recognize (Fig. 9-3).

Neurocutaneous syndromes are genetically determined conditions resulting from abnormal development of embryonic ectoderm, which develops into skin and neural tissue. The neurocutaneous disorders, including neurofibromatosis and tuberous sclerosis, are characterized by specific skin markings and neurologic abnormalities, such as mental retardation and seizures. The most common of these conditions is neurofibromatosis, which may be associated with mild mental retardation (Fig. 9-4). Attention-deficit hyperactivity disorder and learning disabilities, particularly visual-spatial deficits, are also common.

Injury to the Central Nervous System

Prenatal Exposure to Toxins or Teratogens. Fetal alcohol syndrome (FAS) is the most common preventable cause of mental retardation, occurring in 0.3 to 0.5 per 1000 live births. The diagnosis of FAS is based on specific criteria, including abnormalities in each of the following three categories: growth deficiency, which is often of prenatal onset, craniofacial dysmorphic features, and evidence of CNS dysfunction, in the context of a history of maternal alcohol use during the pregnancy. Because a safe threshold of alcohol consumption during pregnancy has not been established, it is not possible to state with certainty the amount of maternal alcohol use that poses a risk of FAS. Many children with FAS are born small for gestational age and continue to grow poorly after birth. The dysmorphic features, including microcephaly, short palpebral fissures, flattening of the midface, short nose, poorly developed philtrum, and smooth,

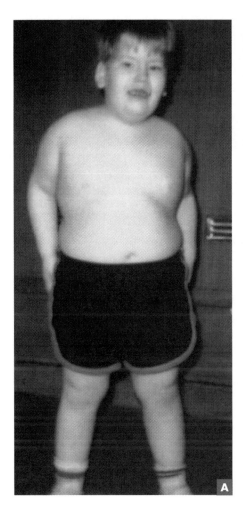
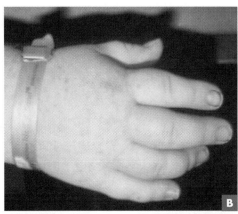
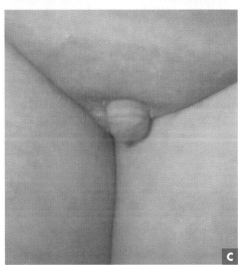

FIG. 9-2 Prader-Willi syndrome. *A,* This patient demonstrates the characteristic marked obesity. Excess fat is distributed over the trunk, buttocks, and proximal extremities. *B* and *C,* Small hands (and feet) and hypoplastic penis and scrotum are other typical features. (*A* Courtesy Dr. Jeanne M. Hanchett, The Rehabilitation Institute of Pittsburgh; *B* and *C* courtesy Dr. Holly W. Davis, Children's Hospital of Pittsburgh.)

thin upper lip, may be subtle at birth and during infancy (Fig. 9-5). The diagnosis may be difficult to make definitively until the dysmorphic features are apparent but should be considered in children with poor growth, developmental delay, and maternal history of alcohol or other substance use. The average IQ is 65 to 70, within the mild range of mental retardation, although IQ is within the normal range in 40% of children with FAS. Other manifestations of CNS dysfunction among children with FAS include hyperactivity, problems with information processing, and poor memory. *Fetal alcohol effects* (FAE) is a term used to describe children with abnormalities in one or two but not all three of the diagnostic categories for FAS and a questionable history of prenatal alcohol exposure. Recently, it has been suggested that the FAE designation be abandoned because it implies that alcohol has caused the symptoms, although the history of maternal alcohol use may be only suspected. *Alcohol-related birth defects* (ARBD) is the current preferred terminology for children with a history of alcohol exposure and some but not necessarily all of the features of FAS.

A teratogenic effect has been established for a number of drugs (other than alcohol) to which a fetus may be exposed.

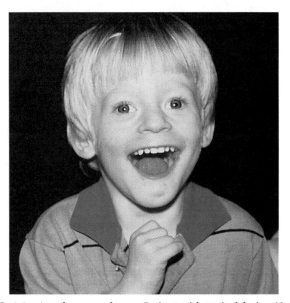

FIG. 9-3 Angelman syndrome. Patient with typical facies. Note the maxillary hypoplasia, large mouth (often with protruding tongue), and prognathism. (Courtesy Drs. C.A. Williams and J. Hendrickson, University of Florida, Gainesville.)

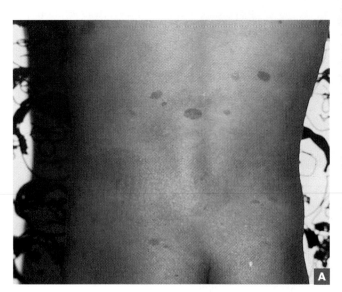
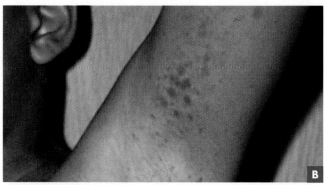
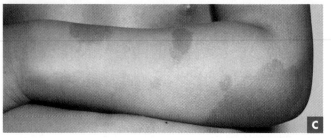

FIG. 9-4 Neurofibromatosis. Clinical manifestations of cutaneous pigmentary abnormalities. *A,* The most common abnormality is multiple café au lait spots over the trunk. *B* and *C,* Axillary freckling or extensive areas of hyperpigmentation are also seen. (Courtesy Dr. Michael Sherlock, Baltimore.)

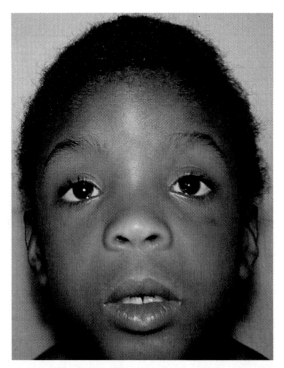

FIG. 9-5 Fetal alcohol syndrome. Note the poorly formed philtrum; slightly narrow, wide-spread eyes, with inner epicanthal folds and mild ptosis; hirsute forehead; short nose; and relatively thin upper lip.

Fetal hydantoin syndrome, for example, is characterized by mental retardation, nail hypoplasia, and facial features similar to those of ARBD.

Prenatal exposure to drugs other than alcohol may result in CNS dysfunction as a direct toxic effect of the drug on developing brain. Exposure to opiates, cocaine, and other typically abused drugs may be associated with cognitive deficits and behavior problems. Prenatal exposure to some drugs is associated with intrauterine growth restriction resulting from chronic hypoxia (nicotine) or poor placental blood flow (cocaine) that may be severe enough to affect brain growth. However, the specific effect of the drug may be difficult to determine because of the presence of confounding variables related to the social context in which drug abuse typically occurs. Women who use drugs prenatally are more likely to be poorly nourished, to have higher life stress, to have fewer social supports, and to have had more negative previous obstetrical histories than women who do not use drugs. Each of these variables is individually associated with poorer birth outcome and thereby with increased developmental morbidity independent of drug use. In addition, the rearing environment of children prenatally exposed to drugs is likely to be less than optimally supportive of growth and development. In assigning a specific cause to developmental delay, it may be impossible to separate the impact of prenatal drug exposure from the influence of other factors in the prenatal and postnatal environment of the child. Therefore a history of prenatal drug exposure should be considered a risk factor for developmental disorders but a cause-and-effect relationship has not been firmly established.

Congenital Infection. Children with congenital infection are typically ill at birth, with evidence of hepatic, hematopoietic, and other systemic disease. Congenital infections with rubella virus, herpesvirus, and *Treponema pallidum* are rarely subtle in their presentation during the neonatal period. However, the majority of infants with congenital cytomegalovirus (CMV) and *Toxoplasma gondii* infection are asymptomatic at birth. Infants affected by either of these agents may present in later infancy or childhood with cognitive impairment, hearing loss, visual problems, or seizures, reflecting earlier CNS injury. Clues to the early diagnosis of congenital CMV infection include microcephaly and intrauterine growth restriction. The diagnosis of congenital CMV should be considered in the evaluation of children with microcephaly, hearing impairment, and developmental delay, particularly in the context of a maternal history of infection during pregnancy or neonatal illness. Unfortunately, the diagnosis is difficult to make with certainty beyond the neonatal period because postnatal infection with CMV, which has no impact on development, is common and humoral evidence of infection or culture of the virus cannot determine whether the infection was acquired prenatally or postnatally. Calcifications of the basal ganglia and other brain structures visible on computed tomography (CT) are common in congenital CMV infection and should be considered indirect evidence of congenital infection. Although congenital toxoplasmosis is symptomatic in only 10% to 25% of affected neonates, the majority develop neurologic or visual impairment related to chorioretinitis in later childhood. Toxoplasmosis should be considered in the child with developmental delay and visual impairment.

Hypoxic-Ischemic Encephalopathy. Hypoxic-ischemic encephalopathy is discussed in the section on motor delay because children who have sustained hypoxic or ischemic injury to the CNS typically have delay in the acquisition of motor skills and focal findings on neurologic examination, although they may also have cognitive deficits.

Structural Brain Malformations

The presentation of structural malformation of the CNS can be nonspecific, but the diagnosis is most common in a child with mental retardation, microcephaly, and abnormal neurologic signs. As discussed earlier, abnormalities of CNS development resulting in structural malformations account for 10% to 15% of cases of severe to profound mental retardation. These cases include disorders of neural proliferation, migration, and/or organization identified on neuroimaging as structural defects of brain. The underlying cause of these structural brain defects may be vascular, genetic, or infectious, although it is usually impossible to determine precisely. The process that disrupts normal brain development may also disrupt organogenesis in other organ systems, resulting

in the dysmorphic features and malformations commonly associated with structural brain anomalies. Disruptions at specific stages of brain development result in specific brain malformations. The group of disorders that arises earliest in the first trimester is the failure of closure of the neural tube and ranges in severity from spina bifida occulta to meningomyelocele to anencephaly. Depending on the severity of the defect, the spinal cord level involved, and associated features, such as hydrocephalus, a child may be asymptomatic with normal intelligence, have isolated motor defects, or have significant global impairment.

Disorders of cleavage of the forebrain, arising in the early to mid first trimester, result in the spectrum of holoprosencephalies, which varies in severity depending on the extent of cleavage. The most severe of these disorders is associated with seizures, hypothalamic dysfunction, and severe developmental delay. Associated midline defects may be noted, including hypotelorism, midline cleft lip, cleft palate, flattened nose, and other organ malformations.

Defects of neuronal migration to the outer layers of cerebral cortex result in deficient formation of gyri and gray matter heterotopia, in which abnormal islands of gray matter that should have migrated outward accumulate in the deeper white matter. Lissencephaly (the absence of gyri resulting in smooth brain) and pachygyria (thick gyri that are reduced in number) are two of the more common migrational defects associated with mental retardation and seizures.

Idiopathic Mental Retardation

In cases in which a definitive cause for mental retardation is not evident, a diagnosis of "idiopathic" mental retardation is often made. In this context, the term *idiopathic* implies that, although there is an underlying difference in brain structure or function, the difference cannot be identified or measured by current technology. As discussed earlier, this occurs in a large proportion of cases of mild to moderate mental retardation. Moreover, mild mental retardation is often multifactorial in cause, with both biologic and environmental components, neither of which is always clearly defined.

The fact that mild mental retardation is more common among socioculturally disadvantaged individuals reflects the important role of environmental stimulation for the optimal expression of development. An environment that does not provide appropriate cognitive stimulation and verbal communication may not allow the optimal maturation of the CNS or attainment of developmental milestones. Studies have demonstrated that poverty is associated with delayed language skills and a related decline in DQ, beginning in the years when language acquisition is rapidly emerging. Although there is a clear environmental contribution to mild mental retardation, individuals with the genetic predisposition to mild mental retardation are more likely to live in poverty because they may lack the functional skills needed to achieve higher socioeconomic status. In addition, these individuals are likely to raise their families in poverty, making it very difficult to separate the influences of genetics and the environment on development.

Developmental delay may also be transient, occurring in the context of severe, acute illness; poor nutrition; and psychologic or emotional distress associated with abuse, loss of a parent, birth of a sibling, or a change in the living situation. The rate and pattern of skill acquisition may return to normal when the child recovers from illness, nutrition improves, or the psychosocial issues are resolved. The physician must evaluate the individual child's pattern of development, much as he or she would evaluate physical growth, to make an accurate statement about the likelihood of "catch-up."

Progressive Global Developmental Disorders

Progressive developmental disorders are characterized by a period of normal development followed by slowing in the rate of acquisition of skills, plateauing in the rate of progress, and ultimately loss of previously acquired skills. These conditions may be overlooked in the early stages before it becomes clear that the child is actually losing skills. The duration of the phases of developmental regression is highly variable and depends on the nature of the underlying condition and the age of the child. Most of the progressive disorders eventually affect all areas of development, although the initial presentation may be loss of cognitive, motor, or language skills. The progressive disorders of the CNS are far less common than the static encephalopathies discussed previously.

Only a few of the conditions characterized by developmental regression can be successfully treated, but early diagnosis is critical because there may be associated medical problems and implications for genetic counseling and prenatal diagnosis. The diagnosis of a progressive disorder also has important implications for prognosis in the affected child. Although they are rare, the conditions associated with developmental regression are discussed briefly because they should be considered in the differential diagnosis of a child with global developmental delay.

Inborn Errors of Metabolism

Metabolic disorders should be considered in the evaluation of a child who has developmental delay and poor feeding, poor growth, recurrent illness, developmental regression, or parental consanguinity. Metabolic disorders are caused by single gene abnormalities, usually autosomal recessive or X-linked in inheritance, that result in synthesis of an abnormal protein or deficient synthesis of a normal protein, usually an enzyme. Abnormal function or absence of the enzyme results in blockage of a critical metabolic pathway, with deficiency of metabolic products after the block and accumulation of metabolic products before the block. Unlike genetic syndromes associated with dysmorphic features, in which entire chromosomes or multigene segments of chromosomes are abnormal, single gene abnormalities are rarely associated with dysmorphic features, and affected children typically ap-

pear and act normal at birth. Although they should always be considered, inborn errors of metabolism rarely explain developmental delay in a child whose growth and health are normal and who is acquiring developmental skills at a steady, though slow rate.

Metabolic disorders may present in early infancy with poor feeding, vomiting, failure to thrive, or catastrophic illness when the abnormal metabolic process is associated with acidosis, hypoglycemia, and/or hyperammonemia. In contrast, when the metabolic abnormality results in the accumulation of abnormal metabolites that are toxic to the CNS, the presentation is typically a period of normal development followed by developmental regression. In addition, all of the conditions that usually cause early, catastrophic illness may have a more indolent course and present in later infancy or early childhood with developmental regression. A high index of suspicion regarding the possibility of metabolic disease is warranted in the evaluation of developmental delay in infancy and early childhood because many of these disorders have no major systemic symptoms, and slowing in the rate of developmental progress or actual loss of skills may be difficult to recognize early in the course of the disorder. Metabolic conditions that typically result in developmental regression in later childhood are not discussed here.

Neurodegenerative Disorders

Neurodegenerative disorders can be classified with the inborn errors of metabolism because they reflect abnormal metabolism and accumulation of toxic metabolites. However, it may be useful to classify them separately because they primarily involve degeneration of the CNS, and although some of these conditions are characterized by visceromegaly and other signs or symptoms, systemic signs are usually less prominent than neurologic findings. The age of presentation varies widely; some of the neurodegenerative conditions become evident after only a few months to a year of normal development (Tay-Sachs, Krabbe, and Canavan diseases), whereas others typically present in preschool to early school age (adrenoleukodystrophy).

The neurodegenerative disorders eventually evolve to affect all developmental domains, but the initial presentation can usually be classified as the loss of cognitive skills (dementia), personality change, and seizures, reflecting initial gray matter involvement, versus the development of spasticity, ataxia, and visual impairment, reflecting initial degeneration of white matter. There is typically diffuse cerebral involvement as the disease progresses, and the separation into gray versus white matter disease becomes irrelevant.

Rett Syndrome. Rett syndrome is a neurodegenerative disorder of unknown etiology that affects primarily girls. Girls with Rett syndrome develop normally for the first 6 to 12 months of life and then begin to show evidence of developmental regression. They lose functional use of their hands and develop stereotypic hand wringing and mouthing movements. They develop spasticity of the lower extremities and may lose or never gain independent ambulation. The rate of head growth slows, resulting in acquired microcephaly. Verbal communication rarely develops. The cause of Rett syndrome is not known, and there are currently no medical tests that are diagnostic. The diagnosis of Rett syndrome is relatively easy to make in the child 5 to 6 years of age, when the clinical picture is well developed. In infancy and early childhood, however, the presentation may be a subtle slowing in the rate of acquisition of new skills in a girl with no obvious dysmorphic features, no signs or symptoms of chronic or acute illness, and normal physical and neurologic examinations. The lack of verbal communication and stereotypic hand movements may erroneously lead to a diagnosis of autistic disorder. Because autism is much rarer among girls, the diagnosis of Rett syndrome should be considered in any girl with features of autistic disorder.

AIDS Encephalopathy. In children the encephalopathy associated with human immunodeficiency virus (HIV) infection is most often related to HIV infection of the brain rather than to secondary opportunistic infection. Acquired immunodeficiency syndrome (AIDS) encephalopathy has been reported to be delayed in onset for up to 5 years after infection with the virus, although the typical presentation is in the toddler years. The encephalopathy is characterized by developmental regression, poor head growth, and spasticity, but the course can be indolent, and the child may seem to have a static encephalopathy. Children with AIDS encephalopathy may have opportunistic infections and failure to thrive, but the CNS symptoms and signs may be the first presentation of the disease. For these reasons, AIDS encephalopathy should be considered in the evaluation of children with developmental delay and regression, in the context of risk factors for HIV infection.

Congenital Hypothyroidism. Congenital hypothyroidism is classified with the progressive disorders because it causes deterioration of CNS function. However, the typical presentation in infancy is slower-than-normal acquisition of skills consistent with a static encephalopathy. Thyroid hormone is required for normal brain development, particularly during the period of rapid brain growth during the first 2 years of life. Before the availability and widespread use of neonatal screening tests, congenital hypothyroidism was a leading cause of severe to profound mental retardation. Neonatal screening for congenital hypothyroidism is sensitive, but false-negative results do occur; therefore the physician should consider congenital hypothyroidism in the evaluation of developmental delay. Congenital hypothyroidism is associated with lethargy, constipation, and feeding and respiratory problems in the majority of affected infants, but a partial deficiency of thyroid hormone can be delayed in onset and cause much milder symptoms. Because early treatment with thyroid hormone is critical for optimal outcome, hypothyroidism should be considered in the evaluation of infants with delayed development and poor growth, even in the absence of specific signs or symptoms usually associated with the condition. Acquired hypothyroidism presenting after 2 years of age is less commonly associated with developmental problems.

Language Disorders

Children who are mildly to moderately mentally retarded may have little or no delay in the acquisition of motor skills, and therefore concerns may not be raised until the preschool years when language milestones are not met. Because language development reflects cognitive ability, delayed language development is often the sign of global developmental delay or mild to moderate mental retardation. The differential diagnosis of language delay also includes hearing loss, specific language processing problems or expressive language disorders, and autistic disorder. Children with delayed expressive language warrant an assessment of receptive language ability, cognitive skills, social skills, and behaviors to determine whether the delay in expressive language indicates global delay, a specific language problem in the context of normal cognition, or a disorder of impaired language and social interaction.

Hearing Impairment

Hearing loss should always be considered in the child with delayed language because early intervention with amplification and/or specific educational techniques is critical for future functioning. Children with normal receptive language (i.e., children who follow verbal directives) rarely have a significant hearing loss. However, the gestures that accompany verbal communication and the familiar context of communication in the home may allow a hearing-impaired child with normal cognitive skills to respond appropriately, even though he may not have heard what was said. Typically, children with isolated hearing loss and normal cognition develop a form of communication using gestures so they may communicate effectively, even though their speech is delayed.

Language Processing or Expressive Language Disorders

A child who seems to have normal cognitive ability and normal hearing but is delayed in receptive or expressive language skills may have a language processing disorder. Language processing disorders are disorders of CNS function that result in difficulty translating auditory signals into meaningful concepts. These disorders may affect language comprehension and/or language production. Children with language processing disorders typically take longer to respond to instructions or questions and therefore may be considered lazy, stubborn, or inattentive. Multiple-step or complex tasks are often difficult because the child may seem to forget what she is doing, when in fact, she may not have understood what was said. A delay in verbal responses to questions may be secondary to word retrieval or sequencing difficulties. Children often develop strategies to help them process information, including repeating instructions to themselves or using pauses and fillers ("um" or "uh") in their speech to provide extra time for processing.

A specific expressive language disorder should be considered a diagnostic possibility in a child with normal cognition, normal hearing, and normal receptive language. Typically these children demonstrate appropriate responses to verbal directives but have delayed verbal output and develop functional communication with gestures. Their ability to communicate may be greatly facilitated by learning to sign. Children with disorders of language processing or expressive language may develop behavior problems because of the frustration related to difficulty understanding verbal communication and/or difficulty communicating needs or emotions. The behavior problems associated with abnormal language development may be so severe that the diagnosis of autism may be considered.

Although the disorders of language processing and expressive language seem to reflect abnormal brain function in a very localized area, neuroimaging is usually normal and the specific medical diagnosis can rarely be established.

Pervasive Developmental Disorders

Autistic Disorder. Autistic disorder is the most common of the pervasive developmental disorders, which are characterized by delayed development of communication skills and reciprocal social interactions and unusual stereotypic behaviors. The diagnosis of autism should be considered in children with delayed or deviant development in the following three domains: (1) language, (2) social interaction, and (3) imagination and spontaneous play. These deviations may be manifest by unusual behaviors, including absent language or unusual speech patterns; avoidance of eye contact; difficulty making transitions from one activity to the next; perseveration on specific tasks or topics; and a limited repertoire of behaviors. The prevalence of autistic disorder, which is more common in boys than in girls, has been reported to be 0.4 per 1000, but with the recent increase in recognition and inclusion of milder cases the prevalence is closer to 1 to 1.5 per 1000. Some children with autism are reported by their parents to have been different since early infancy, with unusual behaviors including lack of social gaze or reciprocal vocalizations and an aversion to cuddling. In other cases parents report that the child seemed to be developing normally until 18 to 24 months of age and then appeared to lose language and social skills. It is important to note that autistic disorder is a condition with a wide range of severity. A child does not have to be totally withdrawn and rocking, for example, to warrant a diagnosis of autism. The diagnosis of pervasive developmental disorder, not otherwise specified, should be considered in children who have a severe and pervasive impairment in the development of social interaction or communication skills or unusual, repetitive or stereotypic behaviors but do not meet the criteria for autistic disorder.

The diagnosis of autism is usually made by a physician, but there is often a long interval between the time the parents expressed concerns and the time a physician made the final diagnosis. The diagnosis should be considered in children with delayed language, poor eye contact, unusual interactions with peers, and unusual speech patterns. The Checklist for Autism in Toddlers (CHAT) is a recently developed instrument to assess the likelihood of autistic spectrum disorder among young children. The instrument includes nine yes or no questions for parents to answer and five observations for the physician to make of the child's behavior in the office. It is intended for use by primary care physicians and takes only a few minutes to score. The questions focus the physician's attention on aspects of behavior and social development that typically may not be included in a routine developmental history.

Autistic disorder is rarely associated with specific medical conditions, although fragile X syndrome may be diagnosed in 1% to 2% of children with autism. As discussed earlier, the diagnosis of Rett syndrome should be considered in girls with symptoms of autistic disorder. The specific cause of autistic disorder has not been described, but the evidence suggests that it is a biologic condition of abnormal brain function involving several areas of the CNS. Older theories of cold, rejecting parents causing autism are not supported by current research.

Landau-Kleffner Syndrome. Landau-Kleffner syndrome, or acquired epileptiform aphasia, is a rare disorder characterized by a period of normal development until the age of 3 to 7 years, followed by loss of language and development of seizures. The EEG abnormalities are characteristic. Although rare, the diagnosis is important to distinguish from autistic disorder because it may respond to anticonvulsant or steroid therapy.

Gross Motor Delay: Central Versus Peripheral Neuromuscular Origin

In addition to considering the static or progressive nature of the condition, a useful approach to the evaluation of the child with gross motor delay is to determine whether the underlying abnormality is of CNS or peripheral nervous system (PNS) origin. Delayed motor development reflects abnormal function of the areas of CNS and/or PNS that are responsible for control of movement, including motor cortex, corticospinal tracts, cerebellum, basal ganglia, anterior horn of the spinal cord, peripheral nerves, myoneural junction, and muscle. Characteristics suggestive of a central origin include a history of prenatal or perinatal events associated with brain injury. In addition the delays reflecting a central origin may be isolated to the motor system or associated with delays in cognitive, social, and language development, depending on the severity, location, and extent of the abnormality. Finally, findings on neurologic examination consistent with central or upper motor neuron abnormality include spasticity, hyperreflexia, and abnormal posturing. These findings are characteristic of cerebral palsy, the prototype of a central static process resulting in motor delay. Disorders of the PNS are characterized by muscle weakness and delayed motor skills in the context of normal or near-normal cognitive, language, and social skills.

Cerebral Palsy

Cerebral palsy is defined as a nonprogressive disorder of the immature brain, affecting movement and posture. Cerebral palsy can be classified as spastic (70%), dyskinetic or choreoathetoid (20%), and ataxic (10%). The developmental diagnosis of cerebral palsy does not imply a specific cause but can occur after hypoxic or ischemic injury, trauma, or infection of the CNS. The origin of cerebral palsy is believed to be prenatal in most cases. Prematurity, low birth weight, and perinatal asphyxia are all associated with an increased risk of cerebral palsy, although the majority of children with these risk factors do not develop cerebral palsy. Low Apgar scores and other factors suggesting perinatal asphyxia are associated with an increased risk of developmental disability, but the majority of children with cerebral palsy have had uneventful deliveries with Apgar scores above 7. Therefore the diagnosis of cerebral palsy should be considered in children with delayed motor skills and abnormalities of muscle tone, even in the absence of specific historic risk factor.

Spastic cerebral palsy is the neurologic residual of injury to subcortical and periventricular white matter containing fibers of the corticospinal tract. The resulting neurologic findings are related to a loss of higher cortical inhibition of reflexes and motor patterns that originate in the spinal cord. The subcortical white matter in the full-term infant and the periventricular white matter in the preterm infant represent the "watershed" areas of the brain, which are particularly vulnerable to hypoxic-ischemic injury because of the vascular anatomy in the regions. Injury to other areas of the CNS involved in control of movement, including the basal ganglia, cerebellum, and associative fibers, may result in less common forms of cerebral palsy, including dyskinetic or choreoathetoid, ataxic, and mixed. Kernicterus, now extremely rare because of the aggressive preventive and therapeutic approach to Rh hemolytic disease and other conditions associated with hyperbilirubinemia, is associated with dyskinetic or choreoathetoid cerebral palsy because of the vulnerability of the basal ganglia to bilirubin toxicity. Hypotonia and athetosis are the most striking neurologic findings in kernicterus, in association with hearing impairment and gaze abnormalities. Cognitive deficits occur, but mental retardation is rare.

Peripheral Neuromuscular Disorders

Weakness is characteristic of disorders of the PNS, including disorders of the anterior horn cell of the spinal cord, peripheral neuropathies, disorders of the myoneural junction, the muscular dystrophies, and congenital myopathies. Cognitive development is typically normal in these disorders, although there may be associated cognitive deficits. For example, learning disabilities are more common among boys with Duchenne muscular dystrophy than in the general population. The presentation of these conditions varies from severe weakness and hypotonia noted at birth to normal appearance and activity in infancy followed by progressive weakness and the loss of previously attained motor skills. The extensive differential diagnosis of conditions associated with hypotonia and muscle weakness is discussed in detail elsewhere in this book (see Chapter 11).

History

Developmental History

The pediatrician must obtain an accurate and detailed developmental history to determine the domains of development affected, the rate and pattern of acquisition of skills, and the existence of any developmental regressions. The developmental history should begin with the parents' description of the child's current skills in all developmental domains, which is much more valuable than asking parents to recall the age at which particular milestones were achieved. The pediatrician should begin with open-ended questions (e.g., How does she move around? How does he use his hands? How does he let you know what he wants? What does she understand of what you say? What can you tell him to do that he will do? What does she like to play with? How does she play with that toy? How does he interact with other children?), which are of great value in eliciting descriptions of the child's abilities and do not convey any judgment to the parents about whether or not the child should have attained a particular skill. These can be followed by more specific questions (e.g., How long has she been doing that? Is there anything that he used to do that he no longer does well? What new skills has he learned recently?) to elicit detailed information about the pattern of attainment of developmental milestones. The pediatrician should ask the child's age when parents first became concerned about development to get a sense of the severity of the problem and the parents' level of anxiety. The developmental history should include information about the child's current behavior and aspects of the child's behavior in early infancy with particular reference to the quality of alertness and responsiveness. Parents may report normal development up to a particular time, raising concern about progressive disorders. With careful questioning, it may become apparent that the child was relatively inactive, less responsive, or extremely irritable in early infancy, suggesting a disorder present at birth that has become more obvious over time as expectations for development have increased.

Once the pediatrician has obtained an accurate developmental history, he or she can appreciate the significance of the developmental delay by estimating a developmental quotient (DQ). As mentioned earlier, the DQ represents the developmental age (the age at which the averge child accomplishes the skills) in months, divided by the index child's chronologic age, multiplied by 100. For example, a 12-month-old child who has just become able to sit independently, is reaching for and transferring objects from hand to hand, bangs in play, and has just started to babble is demonstrating skills appropriate for a 6-month-old. Her developmental age therefore is 6 months, and her developmental quotient is 50. At this time, she is functioning at 50% of expected levels. Although the continued slower than normal acquisition of developmental skills suggests a developmental disability, performance on developmental assessment instruments during infancy does not necessarily predict IQ scores or functional ability in later childhood. It is clear, however, that an infant whose development is extremely delayed (DQ less than 50) will probably continue to demonstrate a low level of functioning at school age. The child in the example is at risk for a later diagnosis of mental retardation, although her future functional ability cannot be accurately predicted.

Perinatal History

Information should be obtained regarding the possibility of in utero exposure to toxins or teratogens, maternal illness or trauma, or other complications of pregnancy. The quality of fetal movement should be described because the absence of fetal activity suggests a primary neuromuscular disorder or CNS malformation and a decline in the amount of fetal movement suggests an hypoxic or ischemic event. Complications at the time of labor and delivery should be described, although a history of perinatal complications does not necessarily imply the cause of developmental disorders. Parents often seek an explanation for their child's delays in events around the time of birth; therefore the difficulty in establishing a specific causative relationship between perinatal events and developmental disorders requires discussion with the family. Apgar scores were developed to describe the neonate's physiologic status in the immediate postnatal period and guide resuscitative measures; they were not intended to be predictive of developmental morbidity and are poorly correlated with developmental outcome. Of more importance than Apgar scores is a history of neurologic compromise after birth, manifested as seizures, poor feeding, or abnormalities of muscle tone. Growth parameters at birth, including head circumference, should be obtained. Poor head growth implies poor brain growth and may be the result of a genetic abnormality, brain malformation, or intrauterine infection. Poor fetal weight gain suggests placental dysfunction, which may also be associated with developmental delay.

Medical History

The medical history should include information regarding the nature and frequency of illness, as well as the quality of feeding and growth. Children who are frequently ill may develop slowly because they have limited energy and opportunities for learning. Frequent, recurrent illness is a common feature of metabolic disorders, as are poor feeding, vomiting, and failure to thrive. Infants with cerebral palsy may have a history of poor coordination of sucking and swallowing, resulting in a weak or inefficient suck or excessive drooling. Poor growth may reflect poor nutritional intake or, as in hypothyroidism and other metabolic disorders, the inability to use consumed calories for growth. Concerns about vision and hearing should be explored because children with sensory impairment do not develop optimally unless the impairment is recognized and remediated. In addition the presence of visual or hearing impairment may provide some insight into

the underlying cause of developmental delay. For example, hearing impairment is associated with congenital CMV infection, several of the mucopolysaccharidoses, and several genetic syndromes. Visual impairment may be associated with structural brain malformation, white matter degenerative disease, and congenital toxoplasmosis.

Family History

A thorough family history of illness, sensory impairment, and developmental disorders, including mental retardation, mental illness, language problems, and learning disabilities, should be sought. Specific patterns of inheritance may suggest particular genetic abnormalities. For example, a history of learning disabilities, autistic behavior, or mental retardation among male relatives on the maternal side should prompt an evaluation for fragile X syndrome. A family history of the need for special education services during childhood may be indirect evidence of familial mild mental retardation, even if the affected individuals did not have a specific diagnosis made. Parental consanguinity increases the risk of disorders characterized by autosomal recessive inheritance, such as most of the single gene abnormalities, including metabolic disorders.

Physical Examination

In addition to the routine pediatric examination to discover signs suggesting acute or chronic illness, the pediatrician evaluating a child with developmental delay should pay careful attention to growth patterns, search for dysmorphic features and skin stigmata of neurocutaneous disease, and perform a thorough neurologic examination to evaluate brain function (Table 9-3).

Growth Parameters

Poor weight gain suggests an underlying chronic illness, metabolic disease, or feeding difficulties related to neurologic impairment. Short stature and developmental delay occur in association with many dysmorphic syndromes, including Down syndrome, Prader-Willi syndrome, Williams syndrome, and Noonan syndrome, among many others. The association of developmental delay and tall stature occurs in several syndromes, including Sotos syndrome, Beckwith-Weidemann syndrome, and Klinefelter syndrome. Microcephaly is a nonspecific sign that can be consistent with normal development, but it may reflect abnormal brain growth secondary to brain injury (hypoxic-ischemic encephalopathy), congenital infection, genetic syndromes, or brain malformation. Macrocephaly is a common finding among children with neurofibromatosis and fragile X syndrome. A few very rare neurodegenerative disorders of the CNS are associated with macrocephaly, including Alexander and Canavan diseases.

TABLE 9-3

Findings on Physical Examination

Finding	Diagnostic considerations
Growth Parameters	
Poor weight gain	Chronic illness, metabolic disorders, feeding difficulties secondary to neurologic impairment
Short stature	Down syndrome, Prader-Willi syndrome, Williams syndrome, Noonan syndrome, Turner syndrome, Cornelia de Lange syndrome
Tall stature	Sotos syndrome, Beckwith-Wiedemann syndrome, Klinefelter syndrome (XXY)
Microcephaly	Many genetic syndromes, injury to the CNS (hypoxic-ischemic encephalopathy, prenatal exposure to toxins/teratogens, congenital infection), structural brain malformation
Macrocephaly	Hydrocephalus, neurofibromatosis, fragile X syndrome, Alexander disease, Canavan disease
Skin	
Café au lait spots	Neurofibromatosis, tuberous sclerosis, ataxia-telangiectasia
Hypopigmented macules	Neurofibromatosis, tuberous sclerosis
Hemangiomas	Sturge-Weber syndrome, Beckwith-Wiedemann syndrome
Telangiestasias	Ataxia-telangiectasia
Axillary freckling	Neurofibromatosis
Eye Findings	Homocystinuria (cataracts, dislocatable lens), mucopolysaccharidoses (corneal clouding), cerebral palsy (strabismus)
Cardiac Abnormalities	Down syndrome (atrioventricular septal defect), Williams syndrome (aortic stenosis), Noonan syndrome (pulmonic stenosis), fetal alcohol syndrome (ventricular septal defect), Hurler syndrome (valve defect)
Visceromegaly	Glycogen storage disease, mucopolysaccharidoses, Gaucher disease type II, Niemann-Pick disease type A, Sandhoff disease
Hypogonadism	Prader-Willi syndrome, Noonan syndrome, Klinefelter syndrome (XXY)

Dysmorphic Features

A careful search for dysmorphic features may reveal a pattern of subtle features consistent with a particular syndrome (see Chapter 29). Some syndromes, such as Down syndrome, are easily recognized because of the familiar pattern of unusual features. However, in many of the less common syndromes, the pattern of dysmorphic features may be difficult to recognize. Therefore it is important to look at each feature individually, describe it, measure it if applicable, and then compare the description or measurement with a standard reference. Particular attention should be paid to the size and placement of the pinnae (low-set, posteriorly rotated, cupped, small, or prominent); the size, shape, and distance between the eyes (small palpebral fissures, hypotelorism or hypertelorism, and upslanting or downslanting palpebral fissures); the size and shape of the nose (broad nasal bridge, short nose, and anteverted nares); the forehead (frontal bossing and low anterior hairline); the mouth (fullness or thinness of the lips and downturned corners); the chin (prominent or small); the hands and feet (clinodactyly, syndactyly, nails, or palmar and plantar crease pattern); and the genitalia

(hypogonadism). If the child has an unusual appearance, it may be useful to ask the parents which family member the child resembles and examine a family photograph. Even if the unusual feature is a family trait, the child who has an unusual appearance and developmental delay may have an identifiable syndrome that is worth pursuing by referral to a geneticist.

Skin

Examination of the skin for stigmata of neurocutaneous disease, including café au lait spots, hypopigmented macules, hemangiomas, telangiectasias, and axillary freckling is an important component of the physical examination. The use of a Wood's lamp may make hypopigmented macules appear more obvious and is recommended.

General Examination

The child should be examined for signs of chronic illness that may contribute to delayed development. The eyes

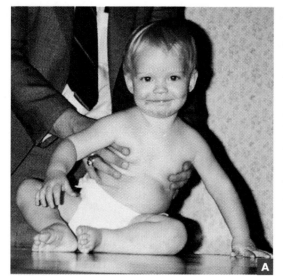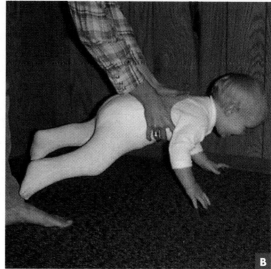

FIG. 9-6 *A,* Protective equilibrium response. As the child is pushed laterally by the examiner, he flexes his trunk toward the force to regain his center of gravity and extends one arm to protect against falling (lateral propping). *B,* Parachute response. As the examiner allows the child to free-fall in ventral suspension, the child's extremities extend symmetrically to distribute his weight over a broader and more stable base upon landing.

should be examined for the presence of retinopathy, cataract, or corneal clouding. If there are any concerns about vision or ophthalmologic findings on examination, a complete examination by an ophthalmologist is warranted. Cardiac abnormalities are common in several genetic syndromes, including Down, Noonan, and Williams syndromes, and may be asymptomatic when the developmental delay is first recognized; therefore careful auscultation of the heart is worthwhile in every child with developmental delay, particularly if he or she has dysmorphic features. The presence of organomegaly suggests an inborn error of metabolism in which enlargement of the liver and spleen is due to storage of metabolites in these structures (e.g., mucopolysaccharide or glycogen) or liver injury (e.g., congenital CMV or AIDS). The genitalia should be examined because several genetic syndromes, including Prader-Willi syndrome, are associated with hypogonadism.

Neurologic Examination

The neurologic examination is of particular importance in the evaluation of developmental delay. The standard pediatric neurologic examination, including the assessment of muscle tone and strength, deep tendon reflexes, sensation, cranial nerves, and gait, should be supplemented in infancy by the assessment of the presence of the primitive reflexes and the automatic equilibrium and protective reactions (Fig. 9-6). Equilibrium reactions can be elicited by slowly tilting the child's body to the side and observing for the compensatory movement of the head and trunk to keep the body in the midline. Protective reactions can be elicited by quickly displacing the child's trunk to the side and observing for the rapid

extension of the arm on that side to block the fall. These responses are typically well-developed enough by the age of 7 to 8 months to allow independent sitting. By 9 to 10 months, rapid forward displacement of the trunk should elicit the forward protective reaction in which both arms extend to break a fall. Delay in the emergence of these automatic reactions suggests neurologic abnormality.

Cerebral palsy is a clinical diagnosis based on the pattern of abnormalities on neurologic examination. The typical abnormalities leading to the diagnosis of cerebral palsy have been summarized as a mnemonic—POSTER (Table 9-4). Abnormalities of posture include fisting with adducted thumbs, hyperextension and adduction (scissoring) of the lower extremities, and hyperextension of the trunk (arching). Poor oral-motor coordination may be manifest in early infancy by poor suck-swallow coordination, poor lip closure on the nipple, difficulty handling textured foods, or excessive drooling. Older children may have problems with chewing, drooling, or articulation. Strabismus is commonly associated with cerebral palsy. The typical alterations in muscle tone associated with spastic cerebral palsy include increased resistance to passive movement of the extremities and decreased axial tone. However, some children have hypertonia of the axial and appendicular musculature. Children with dyskinetic or ataxic cerebral palsy may have fluctuating muscle tone. Delayed integration of the primitive reflexes, including palmar grasp, Moro, and asymmetric tonic neck reflexes, and delayed evolution of the protective and equilibrium reactions are also characteristic of children with cerebral palsy. Deep tendon reflexes are typically brisk, with clonus when spasticity is severe. Infants with findings in four or more of these categories are likely to receive a diagnosis of cerebral palsy in later childhood.

TABLE 9-4		

Features of Cerebral Palsy

	Abnormality	Characteristic
P	Abnormal posture	Fisting with adducted thumbs, hyperextension and adduction of lower extremities, hyperextension of trunk
O	Oral-motor incoordination	Poor suck, drooling, tongue thrust, choking with solids, poor articulation
S	Strabismus	—
T	Abnormal muscle tone	Hypertonia, hypotonia
E	Delayed integration of the primitive reflexes	Persistent palmar grasp, Moro, ATNR
	Delayed evolution of the automatic responses	Poor equilibrium, delayed protective responses
R	Deep tendon reflexes	Hyperreflexia, clonus

ATNR, Asymmetric tonic neck reflex.

In early infancy, children with spastic cerebral palsy may be diffusely hypotonic, with particularly poor head and trunk control. The spasticity that characterizes injury to the corticospinal tracts may evolve over the first year of life, as myelination of the injured CNS pathways develops. Therefore children with hypotonia and delayed development should be carefully observed over time so that an accurate diagnosis can be made. Children who will develop athetoid or akinetic cerebral palsy typically remain severely hypotonic for a longer period of time than those who will develop spastic cerebral palsy.

Muscle strength must be carefully evaluated in the child with delayed motor skills, particularly if the child has poor muscle tone, although the distinction between hypotonia and weakness can be difficult to appreciate in infancy. Peripheral neuromuscular disorders should be seriously considered in the context of muscle weakness or hypotonia so severe that the assessment of strength is equivocal.

Of note, hypotonia is common in children with abnormal CNS function, even in the absence of localizing neurologic signs. Hypotonia may be considered a nonspecific sign of CNS dysfunction when muscle strength and deep tendon reflexes are normal and other abnormal neurologic findings are absent. The descriptive diagnosis of benign congenital hypotonia may be considered in the hypotonic child with delayed gross motor skills, if there are no other abnormal neurologic findings and cognitive, language, and social skills are age appropriate. If this diagnosis is used, the child should be followed carefully to ensure that there is continued progress in all developmental domains, including motor skills, and that cognitive, language, and social skills remain age appropriate.

Approach to the Child and Family

Value of the Diagnosis

Once the developmental diagnosis is clearly established, the pediatrician must discuss the implications for future functioning with the family. However, because it is difficult to pre-

dict later abilities on the basis of early developmental assessment, it is important to allow the family of an infant or young child with delayed development to remain hopeful yet realistic about the child's future abilities. A pediatrician who is uncertain as to the significance of the developmental delay may decide to temporize and see if the child will "outgrow" the problem rather than worry the family unnecessarily. The physician may have the impression that the family will be alarmed by his or her concern that the child may be delayed in development and the implications of a future diagnosis of mental retardation. On the contrary, most studies suggest that parents are often already concerned and therefore grateful to the physician for the opportunity to discuss their worries about the child. Because parents are often very troubled by the uncertainty about future development inherent in the diagnosis of a developmental disorder, the pediatrician may be tempted to try to predict the child's developmental course. This prediction, if it cannot be made with certainty, may offer false reassurance or prematurely "label" a child and encourage parents, therapists, and teachers to have low expectations for the child's performance, creating a self-fulfilling prophecy for poor function. If the future implications are not known, it is best to be honest about the uncertainty and to be available to the family for support. Consultation with a developmental pediatrician or child neurologist should be considered if the pediatrician is unsure about the significance of the delay or its functional implications.

The fact that specific treatment is rarely available for developmental disorders has led to questions about the extent to which a specific medical diagnosis should be pursued in the evaluation of developmental delay. Although most conditions associated with developmental delay are not medically or surgically remediable, there are some notable exceptions, including hearing impairment, hypothyroidism, phenylketonuria, and several other disorders of amino acid metabolism. Even though no effective treatment may be available, a specific diagnosis may be valuable because it may enable identification of associated medical problems that may require intervention. Examples include the genetic syndromes associated with cardiac anomalies and the brain malformations associated with cardiac, renal, and skeletal anomalies. Seizure disorder is common in children with structural brain malformation, Rett syndrome, and other neurodegenerative disorders. In addition, many of the developmental disorders have a well-described inheritance pattern that may allow the physician to determine the recurrence risk and counsel the family accordingly.

Even when the diagnosis has no implications for treatment, identification of associated medical problems, or genetic counseling, a specific diagnosis may allow the family to plan for the future and resolve their uncertainty about responsibility. Families grieve when they acknowledge that their child's development is not and may never be "normal." This grieving process is often extended and difficult to resolve when there is uncertainty regarding the cause of the disability and the prognosis for future functioning. If a specific diagnosis is made, the family can learn much more about their child's condition, including how the same disorder has affected other children, and this may allow the grieving process to proceed in a healthy manner. Whether or not a specific diagnosis can be made, the physician can serve as a child and family advocate by coordinating medical, therapeutic, and educational services and supporting the family through the process of diagnosis and long-term management of the child.

As discussed earlier, the pediatrician may initiate a diagnostic evaluation and refer the child to a developmental pediatrician, geneticist, or child neurologist for further consultation, depending on the results of the initial studies. Alternatively the pediatrician may refer the child early in the diagnostic process for a comprehensive assessment of developmental skills, an interpretation of unusual developmental patterns or behaviors, and guidance regarding the appropriate selection and interpretation of medical tests. The diagnostic studies described in the next section represent a selected group of tests that may be useful in the initial assessment of the child with developmental delay. This is not intended to be a complete listing of available studies that can be ordered by a specialist. It is expected that beyond the initial diagnostic assessment, most general pediatricians will seek consultation from their colleagues in the appropriate specialties to guide further medical evaluation.

Diagnostic Studies

Because 60% to 70% of individuals with severe to profound mental retardation have a definable cause that may have implications for prognosis and genetic counseling, an extensive medical evaluation is warranted. The likelihood of identifying a specific cause for mild to moderate retardation is lower, but a diagnosis is so valuable to families that some testing should be considered. Recent advances in medical genetic testing and neuroimaging techniques have yielded a specific diagnosis in a higher proportion of chil-

dren than previously reported. A thoughtful approach minimizes unnecessary tests.

Genetic Studies

Chromosomal abnormalities, the most common identifiable cause of mental retardation, are usually associated with dysmorphic features. Although chromosome testing is normal in the many genetic syndromes associated with dysmorphic features that do not yet have identifiable genetic markers, among children referred to a developmental center for evaluation of developmental delay, 20% of those with dysmorphic features had an abnormality revealed on chromosome testing. Therefore a karyotype should be ordered for children with dysmorphic features, even if a specific pattern is not recognized. The use of genetic studies in children with developmental delay and no dysmorphic features is more controversial because the yield may be as low as 2%.

Specific testing for fragile X syndrome should be obtained in the evaluation of children with developmental delay and autistic qualities or a maternal family history of mental retardation, learning disabilities, or autism, even in the absence of dysmorphic features because the features associated with fragile X syndrome may be subtle in infancy and early childhood. The recommended assessment for fragile X syndrome is a deoxyribonucleic acid (DNA) probe for the area of mutation on the X chromosome. DNA probes have replaced cytogenetic testing because of the enhanced sensitivity.

A recent advance in medical genetics is the availability of *fluorescent in situ hybridization* (FISH) DNA probes, which are sensitive probes for the small genetic deletions and duplications that characterize certain syndromes. FISH probes are currently clinically available for Angelman syndrome, cri du chat syndrome, DiGeorge or velocardiofacial syndrome, Miller-Dieker syndrome (lissencephaly), Prader-Willi syndrome, Smith-Magenis syndrome, Williams syndrome, and Wolf-Hirschhorn syndrome. The clinician must inform the laboratory what syndrome to "FISH for" because specific probes are used for each syndrome. FISH probes and a DNA probe for fragile X must be specifically requested because they are not included in a routine karyotype.

Neuroimaging

Neuroimaging should be obtained in children with focal neurologic signs or severe global delay in the absence of an identifiable genetic syndrome or other obvious explanation. CT scan adds little diagnostic information to the evaluation of children with developmental delay in whom history and physical examination revealed no specific cause, although nonspecific CT findings of cortical atrophy are seen in up to 20% of children with developmental delay. CT scan is the most useful neuroimaging tool for the detection of intracranial calcification and therefore is the technique of choice when congenital infection is a major diagnostic consideration. Magnetic resonance imaging (MRI) is well designed to reveal abnormalities in gray-white matter differentiation, including defects of neuronal migration and abnormalities of myelination associated with hypoxic-ischemic injury and demyelinating diseases. It is therefore the technique of choice in the evaluation of children with focal neurologic signs, a history of prematurity, a history of prenatal or perinatal hypoxic-ischemic encephalopathy, or symptoms of white matter degenerative disease. Children who have normal findings on MRI scan, despite focal neurologic deficits consistent with localized CNS dysfunction, are presumed to have abnormalities in brain structure and function at a cellular or axonal level that cannot be detected with current neuroimaging techniques.

Information from the CT or MRI scan rarely leads to specific treatment for the affected child. However, the findings may provide the family with an explanation they will find valuable in understanding and coming to terms with their child's disability and planning for their child's future.

Metabolic Studies

As discussed previously, inborn errors of metabolism and neurodegenerative disorders should be considered in the evaluation of children with developmental delay. Most of these disorders are associated with a combination of systemic symptoms and signs, including poor feeding, poor growth, recurrent illness, visual impairment, localizing neurologic signs, or visceromegaly. These disorders are also typically associated with developmental regression, but this may be difficult to detect early in the course, and abnormal metabolism can underlie some cases of static encephalopathy. The general pediatrician should consider consulting a specialist in the evaluation of children with developmental delay in the context of any of the symptoms or signs noted previously.

For children with severe developmental delay in whom history and physical examination reveal no specific cause, the physician should consider the possibility of metabolic disease even in the absence of developmental regression or any other signs or symptoms suggestive of metabolic disorders. Tests that are often suggested as the initial step in the evaluation of suspected metabolic disease include an ammonia level, liver function tests, electrolytes, and total CO_2 or venous blood gas level to determine the presence of an anion gap acidosis. A supplemental newborn screen (available in some states) includes assays for more than 30 disorders, including many of the amino and organic acid disorders, and may be less expensive and more efficient as an initial step in screening for metabolic disorders. Although a panel of metabolic screening tests can be performed on a random urine sample in many laboratories, the sensitivity and specificity of these urine metabolic screens vary widely. If metabolic disease is suspected, definitive testing rather than the urine metabolic screen is recommended. Positive results on screening must be followed by definitive testing, including quantitative assays for organic acids, amino acids, mucopolysaccharides, or specific enzyme assays in leukocytes or skin fibroblasts. These studies are best selected and interpreted by a specialist in the evaluation of metabolic disease.

Other Studies

Formal audiologic evaluation should be considered for every child with global or specific language delays. Hearing impairment, with significant implications for language development, may go undetected with subjective, informal testing in the physician's office. Any concerns regarding vision require ophthalmologic evaluation.

Because early treatment is critical, evaluation for hypothyroidism should be considered in children with developmental delay and poor growth, even in the absence of other systemic signs and symptoms. A combination of thyroxine (T_4) and thyroid-stimulating hormone (TSH) levels detects infants with primary and secondary hypothyroidism (TSH deficiency). If abnormal levels are detected, the child should be referred to an endocrinologist for further evaluation.

Significantly elevated blood lead levels are associated with acute neurotoxicity that may cause dementia, hyperactivity, hearing loss, or behavior problems, and lower levels may be associated with more subtle cognitive impairment. Children with cognitive deficits may ingest inedible substances (pica), increasing the risk of lead exposure. If routine lead screening has not been performed, determination of a venous lead level should be considered in children with developmental delay and unusual behaviors.

The child with muscle weakness warrants referral to a child neurologist for the selection of tests, including electromyography, nerve conduction velocity, and muscle biopsy, to evaluate neuromuscular disorders (see Chapter 11).

Value of Early Intervention

While the diagnostic evaluation is proceeding the primary physician should seriously consider referring the family to community-based early intervention or special education services. Early intervention programs in most communities accept a referral on the basis of the physician's judgment that the child is developmentally delayed. A developmental assessment is then scheduled to determine whether the delay is severe enough to make the child eligible for early intervention services. In many communities the eligibility criteria for early intervention services is a delay of 25% below age expectations in at least one developmental domain.

Early intervention refers to any services initiated before 36 months of age for the purpose of enhancing the development of a handicapped, biologically at risk, or socioeconomically disadvantaged child. The clearest positive impact of early intervention is seen in programs that provide environmental enrichment for youngsters from impoverished backgrounds (e.g., Head Start). It has been argued that early intervention for children with developmental disabilities may be futile because of the inability of these services to cure the disability by influencing CNS structure. Although they acknowledge that developmental disabilities are not cured by these services, many investigators in this area take a broader view of the impact of early intervention. When the impact of early intervention is evaluated in terms of improved functional skills, easier handling, and enhanced parental competence and confidence in parenting a disabled child, most studies suggest a benefit, particularly when the parents are involved in the program. Low birth weight infants at risk for developmental disabilities have improved IQ scores at 36 months and fewer reported behavior problems when they are involved in early intervention services that include a parent component.

Since the passage of Public Law 99-457 in 1986 (revised as Individuals with Disabilities Education Act [IDEA] 102-119 in 1991), physicians have become more knowledgeable about the availability and usefulness of early intervention services. PL99-457 ensures children with developmental delay and their families access to publicly funded early intervention services to optimize the child's potential and thereby minimize the need for special education services at school age. The focus of PL99-457 is support of the family's ability to provide an appropriately nurturing and stimulating environment for the child through coordinated community-based services. The law provides many opportunities for involvement of healthcare providers in the identification of developmental disabilities, referral for early intervention services, and ongoing collaboration with the early intervention system. Optimal benefits of early intervention services are realized when the physician is an advocate for families and works collaboratively with the service agencies in all stages of the process, including identification, referral, and monitoring of developmental progress.

SUMMARY

The high prevalence and significant morbidity of developmental disorders require that physicians be vigilant in monitoring developmental progress during childhood. Standard developmental screening methods are recommended, although the most important aspect of developmental surveillance is the evaluation of development over time via a partnership between physicians and families. Once a child is identified as delayed, the physician should initiate or refer for an evaluation to determine the developmental diagnosis (based on the pattern and severity of delay in each developmental domain) and, if possible, the medical diagnosis (the underlying cause of the delay). Families and children with developmental problems are best served by physicians who are able to listen carefully to parents' concerns, understand the variations of normal development and appreciate the mutual contributions of the environment and the child to developmental progress, recognize delays in the expected rate or deviance in the expected pattern of development, formulate a useful differential diagnosis, initiate a diagnostic evaluation and/or refer for more specific evaluation, and provide support to the family during the period of uncertainty regarding the child's future functional abilities. Physicians can serve as strong advocates for families when they are aware of the available early intervention and educational services in their communities and when they develop working relationships with the other professionals who provide services to the child and family.

ILLUSTRATIVE CASES

Case 1. A.B. *is a 3-year-old boy who does not use words to communicate. He points and grunts or cries to indicate his wishes. He will take an adult's hand and lead the adult to what he wants.*

The developmental history reveals the age-appropriate acquisition of motor skills; A.B. walked at 11 months and is able to climb steps and run without difficulty. His fine motor skills are also normal. He is able to manipulate small objects with dexterity and takes apart radios and other pieces of machinery. He babbled at 6 months, but his expressive language has progressed very slowly since that time. He uses no words spontaneously, although he repeats some things that are said to him. He can sing several entire songs that he has heard on Barney *and sometimes repeats entire television commercials.*

At 2 years of age, he was not responding to any familiar commands, and his pediatrician ordered an audiologic evaluation, which was normal. He turns inconsistently when his name is called. A.B. prefers to play by himself and does not interact when he is around other children. His play is repetitive; he spins the wheels of toy cars and lines up his cars and trucks. He does not engage in pretend or imaginative play.

A.B. was born at 42 weeks gestation with a birth weight of 3800 g. There were no complications of the pregnancy, labor, or delivery. Fetal movement was reportedly normal. He has been a healthy child with no episodes of illness, a good appetite, and normal growth. There is a maternal uncle with a history of learning and speech problems.

A.B. lives with his parents and a 6-year-old sister who is developing normally. Both parents work outside the home, and he is cared for by his maternal aunt when both parents are at work. There are no obvious psychosocial stressors.

The physical examination reveals height and weight at the 50th percentiles for age and head circumference at the 90th percentile. The ears are somewhat prominent, but there are no distinctly dysmorphic features. There are no neurocutaneous markings. Genitalia are normal. There is no organomegaly. The neurologic examination is without focal findings. A.B. became quite upset during the examination and was extremely difficult to distract or console.

In summary, A.B. is a 3-year-old boy with significant delays in language skills, difficulties with social interaction, and a limited repertoire of behaviors. His development is deviant in several domains (characterized by behaviors that are not normal at any age). The differential diagnosis includes hearing impairment (ruled out by a normal audiologic evaluation), mental retardation, language processing disorder, and autistic spectrum disorder.

The unusual social behaviors, lack of social interaction with peers, and extreme and intense negative reactions suggest that autistic spectrum disorder is likely. The family history of developmental problems on the maternal side raises the possibility of fragile X syndrome.

This child requires evaluation by a specialist or team of specialists in the diagnosis and treatment of autistic spectrum disorder and should be referred to a developmental program for further evaluation. The pediatrician may make a referral for special educational services while the diagnostic evaluation is proceeding. Audiologic evaluation would be indicated, if it had not been done previously. DNA probe for fragile X should be considered. Other medical testing depends on the results of psychologic testing and more detailed neurologic and physical examination.

Case 2. R.A. is an 11-month-old girl whose mother is concerned because she does not yet sit without support. Her parents became concerned about her development when she was 6 months old and was unable to maintain a sitting posture even briefly. She is able to roll from front to back but not from back to front. She pulls herself along on her belly using her arms and dragging her legs behind her. She reaches for objects and transfers from hand to hand. She prefers to use the left hand and keeps the right hand loosely fisted. She uses a whole-hand grasp to feed herself and to manipulate objects. She drinks from a sippy cup and has no difficulty with sucking or swallowing, although she sometimes chokes on chunks of food. She babbles with intonation and has several words, including "mama," "dada," "baba," and "duck," which she uses spontaneously and specifically. She waves "bye-bye," claps hands, and plays peekaboo. She has always been and continues to be an alert and socially interactive girl who is interested in her surroundings and clearly distinguishes her parents from unfamiliar people.

R.A. was born at 34 weeks gestation with a birth weight of 2000 g. Before the onset of preterm labor, there were no complications of the pregnancy. She had some early temperature instability and was kept in a warm bed for 2 days, after which she was discharged home. She has had three ear infections but no other illnesses. She has been growing well. The family history is unrevealing.

The physical examination revealed all growth parameters at the 25th percentile for age adjusted for prematurity, the 5th percentile for chronological age. The general examination was entirely normal without dysmorphic features, neurocutaneous markings, or signs of acute or chronic illness. The neurologic examination was significant for decreased axial muscle tone characterized by excessive head lag on pull to sit, excessive slip through at the shoulders in vertical suspension, and a rounded back in sitting and ventral suspension. Resistance to passive movement of the extremities was increased (lower extremities greater than upper, right greater than left). The right hand was kept loosely fisted. Deep tendon reflexes were brisk throughout,

and there were several beats of clonus at the right ankle. When the head was turned to the side in supine or sitting position, the asymmetric tonic neck reflex could be elicited.

This case demonstrates the salient features of cerebral palsy. Although born prematurely and with mild temperature instability, there were no other indicators of neonatal compromise, thus the cause is most likely a prenatal event resulting in hypoxic-ischemic injury of cerebral white matter. The history and evaluation reveal significantly delayed gross and fine motor skills, but social, cognitive, and language skills seem age appropriate. The examination reveals the abnormalities of muscle tone and deep tendon reflexes and persistence of primitive reflexes that characterize spastic cerebral palsy.

A neuroimaging study may be very useful in this situation to document underlying CNS injury suggested by history and examination. In this case MRI of the brain revealed immature myelination of the periventricular white matter and thinning of the corpus callosum and lateral ventricles at the upper limits of normal, which is suggestive of atrophy. These findings are consistent with a prenatal or perinatal hypoxic-ischemic event leading to damage to the periventricular white matter and interruption of the corticospinal tracts.

R.A. should be referred to an early intervention program for physical and occupational therapy to optimize her functional skills and enhance her parents' caregiving. She may require additional services, such as speech and language therapy, in the future; these skills should be carefully monitored over time.

Case 3. J.R. is an 18-month-old boy seen by his pediatrician for a routine well child care visit. He was last seen at 9 months of age, having missed several interval appointments. His mother reports that he has been walking for the past few months, but that he does not say any words. He points and grunts to get what he wants. He throws things and bangs in play. He has recently begun to push a truck along on the floor but otherwise does not engage in pretend play. He will wave "bye-bye" and respond with arms up to "so big," but he does not know body parts or respond to other directives. He likes to play alongside other children and responds with affection to familiar caregivers. There has been no loss of skills. The perinatal history is unremarkable. There have been no significant medical problems, and J.R. has always grown well.

J.R.'s mother is 17 years old, and before she left high school she was in special education classes for learning disability or mild mental retardation. He lives with his mother and 4-month-old sister in a small apartment. The maternal grandmother is not consistently available.

The physical examination reveals growth parameters at the 50th percentiles, no dysmorphic features, no neurocutaneous markings, and no signs of acute or chronic illness. The neurologic examination is completely normal.

This boy has cognitive and language skills at about a 12-month level, with motor skills somewhat less delayed. There are no medical risk factors obvious from the history. The cause of this child's global developmental delay is likely multifactorial with both genetic and environmental contributors. A search for a specific medical cause may be worth pursuing, but the pediatrician should certainly refer this child for early intervention services and refer the family to a community agency that provides social support. Further medical evaluation can be pursued depending on the rate of progress over the next few months with these additional supports in place.

ANNOTATED BIBLIOGRAPHY

Crocker AC: The causes of mental retardation, *Pediatr Ann* 18(10):623-636, 1989.

This article describes a useful approach to the pathogenesis of mental retardation and formulation of a differential diagnosis. A valuable discussion of "uncertain" or idiopathic mental retardation is also provided.

Dworkin PH: British and American recommendations for developmental monitoring: the role of surveillance, *Pediatrics* 84(6):1000-1010, 1989.

This article provides a detailed and clear discussion of the various methods of tracking developmental progress in pediatric practice. The process of developmental surveillance is described.

First LR, Palfrey JS: The infant or young child with developmental delay, *N Engl J Med* 330(7):478-483, 1994.

This is an excellent review of the major issues of early identification of developmental delay. It contains a summary of developmental "red flags," a brief review of available screening tests, and a list of key elements of the history and physical examination that may provide clues to diagnosis.

BIBLIOGRAPHY

Baron-Cohen S, Allen J, Gillberg C: Can autism be detected at 18 months? The needle, the haystack, and the CHAT, *Br J Psychiatry* 161:839-843, 1992.

Blackman JA, Healy A, Ruppert ES: Participation by pediatricians in early intervention: impetus from public law 99-457, *Pediatrics* 89(1):98-102, 1992.

Braddock SR, Braddock BA, Graham JM, Jr: Rett syndrome: an update and review for the primary pediatrician, *Clin Pediatr* 32:613-626, 1993.

Brooks-Gunn J, Gross RT, Kraemer HC, et al: Enhancing the cognitive outcomes of low birth weight, premature infants: for whom is the intervention most effective? *Pediatrics* 89(6):1209-1215, 1992.

Chaves-Carballo E: Detection of inherited neurometabolic disorders: a practical approach, *Pediatr Neurol* 39(4):801-820, 1992.

Dworkin PH, Bernstein BA: Pediatricians' approaches to developmental problems: has the gap been narrowed? *J Dev Behav Pediatr* 15(1):34-38, 1994.

Frankenberg WK, Dodds J, Archer P, et al: The Denver II: a major revision and restandardization of the Denver Developmental Screening Test, *Pediatrics* 89(1):91-97, 1992.

Gilbride KE: Developmental testing, *Pediatr Rev* 16(9):338-346, 1995.

Glascoe FP, Altemeier WA, MacLean WE: The importance of parents' concerns about their child's development, *Am J Dis Child* 143:955-958, 1989.

Graham SM, Selikowitz M: Chromosome testing in children with developmental delay in whom the etiology is not evident clinically, *J Pediatr Child Health* 29:360-362, 1993.

Levine MS: Cerebral palsy diagnosis in children over age 1 year: standard criteria, *Arch Phys Med Rehabil* 61:385-389, 1980.

Levy SE, Hyman SL: Pediatric assessment of the child with developmental delay, *Pediatr Clin North Am* 40(3):465-477, 1993.

Majnemer A, Shevell MI: Diagnostic yield of the neurologic assessment of the developmentally delayed child, *J Pediatr* 127:193-199, 1995.

McInerny TK: Children who have difficulty in school: a primary pediatrician's approach, *Pediatr Rev* 16(9):325-335, 1995.

Parker S, Greer S, Zuckerman B: Double jeopardy: the impact of poverty on early child development, *Pediatr Clin North Am* 35(6):1227-1240, 1988.

Schaefer GB, Bodensteiner JB: Evaluation of the child with idiopathic mental retardation, *Pediatr Clin North Am* 39(4):929-943, 1992.

Simko A, Hornstein L, Soukup S, Bagamery N: Fragile X syndrome: recognition in young children, *Pediatrics* 83(4):547-552, 1989.

10

Spells and Unusual Movements

J. CARLTON GARTNER, Jr.

 Key Points

- The most important part of the initial approach to the child with spells is determining whether the events represent seizures.
- Movement disorders represent the largest group in the differential diagnosis of spells.
- Meticulous history (prodrome, timing, triggers, etc.), video electroencephalogram, and home videotape are the tools most likely to aid the diagnosis of difficult cases.

Parents frequently bring their child to the physician because they have observed recurring episodes that they cannot dismiss as normal variations of movement or behavior. Terms such as *funny movements, spells, passing out,* or *seizures* may be used to describe these events, and the family looks to the physician for assistance and guidance.

Most commonly the physician has a quick general diagnostic approach that approaches spells as follows: Is it epilepsy or some type of movement disorder (neurologic)? Is it syncope (cardiac)? Could it be a normal variant or behavior? In young infants the physician frequently asks what possible relation this episode(s) could have to sudden infant death syndrome. Is it an apparent life-threatening event?

To improve organization of the approach to paroxysmal events, discussion is arbitrarily separated into three chapters—Spells and Unusual Movements, Syncope (Chapter 12), and Recurrent Apnea (Chapter 13). In addition, further discussion of migraine, certainly one of the common paroxysmal disorders, is found in Chapter 5. It is important to review the problem of epilepsy in depth in these chapters because this diagnosis must be considered frequently in the clinical approach. When presented with a very complicated and difficult diagnostic problem, it is most helpful to review all of the aforementioned chapters.

In this chapter the term *spell* includes intermittent, paroxysmal episodes often accompanied by movements of one or more areas of the body. Many children with these disorders are mistakenly placed on anticonvulsant therapy, and epilepsy is often the main problem in differential diagnosis. Because there is no single pathophysiologic basis for these episodes, mechanisms are discussed under individual diagnoses.

Literature Survey

There are no retrospective, much less prospective, studies of children who have spells. The literature that is available generally is written by neurologists and emphasizes an approach that contrasts and compares various types of spells with true seizures. A seizure is of cerebral origin and includes a clustering of movements or behaviors caused by a sudden, excessive, rapid, and local discharge of gray matter. Epilepsy is categorized by type (generalized or partial) and cause (primary or secondary). There is also a category of "undetermined." In primary generalized epilepsies, both cerebral hemispheres are involved at the onset. In the partial epilepsies, clinical or electroencephalogram (EEG) onset is in one hemisphere. Consciousness is not impaired in simple partial seizures but is impaired in complex partial seizures. Features that suggest a true seizure are a prodrome (any sensation before the event), loss of consciousness (common, almost universal with seizure but rare with *most* spells), onset while lying down (favors seizure), and postictal phenomena (i.e., clouded consciousness, sleep, or drowsiness). Unfortunately, the interictal EEG is not specific for epilepsy and may be normal 50% of the time in the first recording. Also, EEG abnormalities may be seen in children who have no clinical seizures. Specific features of the history still provide the best approach to diagnosis. As discussed later, prolonged or video EEG along with home recording of spells may be of value in difficult cases. An additional tool may be the recently recognized rise in serum prolactin levels that occurs after a true seizure.

Differential Diagnosis

There are several ways to approach the differential diagnosis of paroxysmal episodes. Perhaps the most lucid approach is that provided by Barron in his recent review of spells. With certain additions and deletions this general schema is followed here. Table 10-1 provides an outline with key features.

Nonepileptic Neurologic Disorders

Movement Disorders

Disordered movement is the most extensive area for diagnostic possibilities and can include single or multiple muscle groups. The emphasis is on those disturbances that occur intermittently and not continuously so that they can truly be termed *spells.*

Tics. A tic is a brief, involuntary, repetitious, stereotyped, purposeless movement or vocalization. Simple tics are common in the pediatric population; about 24% of children have a tic at some time. Tics that persist for more than 1 year are chronic. When multiple tics are present for a year, the diagnosis is chronic motor tic disorder, and when vocal tics are present as well, Tourette syndrome must be considered. General diagnostic criteria for Tourette syndrome include onset before 21 years of age, chronicity (lasting longer than 1 year), multiple motor and one or more vocal tics, waxing and waning course, gradual replacement of old tics with new ones, and absence of other medical explanation. Attention-deficit hyperactivity disorder and obsessive-compulsive disorder are commonly associated.

Tics are not associated with loss of consciousness and can be suppressed by the patient at times. They tend to change over time; new tics develop and old ones may return. Simple motor tics (eye blinking, facial grimacing, shoulder shrugging, etc.) are most common, but complex movements (finger snapping, face wiping, etc.) may be present as well. Tics may improve during sleep but often do not disappear completely.

Myoclonic Syndromes. *Myoclonus* is defined as rapid, sudden muscle jerks that may be focal, multifocal, or generalized. It is the movement disorder most closely associated with epilepsy (Lennox-Gastaut syndrome, etc.) and appears to arise from cortical, subcortical, or spinal areas as opposed to most of the other movement disorders, which originate in the basal ganglia. Myoclonus is common, especially sleep myoclonus in infancy. Synchronous jerking movements of the

hands, or occasionally the feet, accompanied by flexion of elbows, wrists, and fingers occur in the early stages of sleep and disappear with awakening. Myoclonus is part of the normal development of the nervous system and generally disappears by 8 months of age.

Lombroso and others have described a form of benign myoclonus that occurs in infancy while the child is awake and resembles infantile spasms. These infants had normal EEG readings, and all had disappearance of the spells (which involved mostly the head and arms) by 2 years of age.

Another unusual and benign disorder is hyperekplexia, or exaggerated startle syndrome. This is a hereditary disorder characterized by generalized muscular hypertonicity in infancy, sleep myoclonus, and an exaggerated startle response. The last characteristic persists into adulthood so that individuals may fall suddenly after an unexpected stimulus.

Myoclonic encephalopathy of infancy, or myoclonus-opsoclonus syndrome, is familiar to pediatricians because of its association with neuroblastoma. In addition to myoclonic jerks, these patients have flurries of random, conjugate eye movements. The cause may be encephalitis, and spinal fluid examination often reveals mononuclear cells and an elevated protein level. The occult neural crest tumor may be located only by careful search (CT scan, urinary catecholamines), and prognosis for complete resolution is guarded even if the tumor is removed.

Myoclonus has a number of treatable causes that must be recognized. These are summarized in a recent review and include vitamin deficiencies, Wilson disease, metabolic disorders, drugs, infections of the nervous system, and rare tumors. A thoughtful and complete approach to this movement disturbance may be rewarded with an effective treatment.

Shuddering Spells. Shuddering spells consist of flexion of the head, elbows, trunk, and knees with adduction of the legs as if the child had suddenly become cold. Episodes may occur more than 100 times per day and usually present in the preschool toddler, although some parents notice stiffening in infancy. Excitement tends to encourage the episodes, which gradually decrease in frequency over time and occasionally disappear completely. There is a relationship to essential tremor, which may be present in the patient or family members.

Dystonia. Dystonia is characterized by involuntary, persistent muscle contraction that often causes abnormal posturing or twisting. In the early stages, abnormalities may be evident only with onset of movement, may be aggravated by anxiety or stress, and tend to disappear with sleep. Later the movements may be sustained and lead to hypertrophy of muscle. The initial description of torsion dystonia (originally known as *dystonia muscularum deformans*) was given by Oppenheim in 1911. The onset is usually late in the first or early in the second decade of life and often with intermittent posturing or gait abnormalities of one leg. At times this may be interpreted as a psychologic disorder because there are no neurologic abnormalities at rest. The condition is progressive and has a genetic basis. Management is difficult and best done under the guidance of a neurologist with experience

TABLE 10-1

Differential Diagnosis of Spells

Disorder	Characteristics
Epilepsy	Loss of consciousness, EEG
Nonepileptic Neurologic Disorders	
Movement disorders	
Tics	Brief, repetitious, purposeless; chronic, 1 year; vocal, Tourette syndrome
Myoclonic syndromes	Rapid jerks, focal or generalized
Sleep	Common in infancy
Benign	Resembles infantile spasms in infants, gone by 2 years
Hyperekplexia	Exaggerated startle response
Myoclonus-opsoclonus	Eye movements, neural crest tumor
Other	Metabolic disorders, vitamin deficiencies, drugs, infections, Wilson disease, rare tumor
Shuddering spells	Toddlers, "doused with cold water" appearance, essential tremor in family
Dystonia	Muscle contraction, posturing
Torsion (DMD)	Onset with leg posturing; genetic, progressive
Dopa responsive	Variant of torsion, good outlook
Transient	Onset during first months, certain positions, disappears
Torticollis	Paroxysmal, remember spasmus nutans
Sandifer syndrome	Reflux, head or neck dystonia
Drugs	Metoclopramide, neuroleptics
Dyskinesias	Paroxysmal, familial, occur with exercise or at rest
Metabolic/genetic	Multiple, see text and references
Reflex dystrophy	May precede pain, sympathetic symptoms
Nocturnal	Paroxysmal, rare, head turning
Physiologic	Posturing; fecal, urinary obstruction
Choreoathetosis	Random, rapid, purposeless
Benign	Common, improves second decade
Familial	Autosomal dominant
Paroxysmal	May respond to anticonvulsants
Sydenham	Major manifestations of ARF
Huntington	Parkinsonian features early
Drugs	Especially anticonvulsants
Severe BPD	Akathisia associated, hypoxia?
Other	Treatable, Wilson disease, SLE, hyperthyroidism
Benign paroxysmal vertigo	Brief episodes; loss of balance; emesis, nystagmus in 25%
Migraine	Confusion, ataxia, vertigo; positive family history
Parasomnias	Distributed nighttime or excessive daytime sleep
NonREM	*Pavor nocturnus, somnambulism/somniloquy,* enuresis
REM	Nightmares; narcolepsy—cataplexy, paralysis, hallucinations
Nonepileptic Nonneurologic Disorders	
Syncope	Chapter 12
Breathholding spells	Chapter 12
Behavioral/Psychiatric Disorders	
Pseudoseizures	Unusual triggers, absence of injury
Automatisms	Repetitive rocking, head banging; masturbation in infants/toddlers
Dyscontrol syndrome	Rare, rage toward individual or animal
ADHD	May stare, tantrums, behavior

ADHD, Attention-deficit hyperactivity disorder; *ARF*, acute rheumatic fever; *BPD*, bronchopulmonary dysplasia; *DMD*, dystonia musculorum deformans; *EEG*, electroencephalogram; *REM*, rapid eye movement; *SLE*, systemic lupus erythematosus.

using multiple pharmacologic agents. Several articles describe a variant of torsion dystonia that is levodopa responsive and generally has a much better long-term prognosis.

Transient idiopathic dystonia in infancy was originally described in eight otherwise normal children by Deonna and colleagues. These patients had onset of dystonic posturing in the first months of life that progressed for several months and later disappeared (by 3 months to 5 years of age). The head or limb posture was evident only in certain body positions or with change in position. Outlook for normal development was uniformly excellent.

Paroxysmal torticollis is seen in infancy with intermittent episodes lasting for minutes to days and probably represents a transient dystonia. It may be confused with spasmus nutans unless the characteristic nystagmus and head bobbing are recognized.

One relatively common condition associated with dystonia in infancy is Sandifer syndrome, which includes irritability, torticollis, and opisthotonic posturing associated with gastroesophageal reflux or esophagitis. If recognized and treated appropriately with medical or even surgical therapy, the movement disorder abates. Patients with underlying spasticity and developmental delay are especially likely to have this syndrome. Unfortunately, metoclopramide, which is used to treat reflux, may be one of the drugs that may cause dystonia. Additional inciting agents are neuroleptics, such as haloperidol and fluphenazine.

Paroxysmal dyskinesias occur in childhood and are often familial. These movements may be induced by exercise (kinesigenic) or occur at rest (nonkinesigenic) and usually resolve during sleep. Movements may have features of choreoathetosis and dystonia. Certain patients may respond to anticonvulsant therapy despite the generally normal EEG.

Dystonia may be found with other genetic and metabolic disorders that affect the nervous system, for example, Wilson disease, Hallervorden-Spatz disease, ceroid lipofuscinosis, aminoacidopathies, organic acidopathies (e.g., glutaric acidemia), and mitochondrial disorders. Rett syndrome, a progressive disorder of girls beyond infancy, is characterized by stereotyped hand movements, gait disturbance, dystonia, bruxism, and other extrapyramidal disturbances. In this and other conditions, additional findings on history or examination, especially neurodevelopmental delay or regression, should point away from primary dystonia.

The reflex sympathetic dystrophy syndrome is usually recognized by the presence of pain and vasomotor, sudomotor, and later dystrophic and atrophic changes in an extremity. There is often a history of minor trauma or injury. Recently Schwartzman and Kerrigan brought attention to the presence of dystonia and tremor, which may be the earliest manifestation of this disorder, occurring before the more typical findings. Their photographs demonstrate several dystonic hand and foot positions.

Nocturnal paroxysmal dystonia is a rare form of dystonia that occurs in nonREM sleep. Episodes usually last for minutes; the patients open their eyes, raise or turn the head, and then develop dystonic posture of the head, trunk, and extremities. They may have violent dyskinetic movements. EEG recordings are most frequently normal, but there is often an excellent response to carbamazepine.

In the category of dystonia there are several diagnoses not mentioned in the literature (which is usually written by child neurologists). Some children with apparent dystonia may have physiologic explanations for their symptoms, including constipation and obstructive uropathy, especially involving the urinary bladder. Stool retention may cause episodic gluteal and quadriceps muscle contractions while ambulating, and the gait may appear dystonic. Toddlers with intermittent squatting and grunting may actually have bladder contraction or difficulty voiding. A careful history may determine that these symptoms have a physical stimulus and that the child's apparent dystonia is a reaction to a visceral smooth muscle contraction. This variant of dystonic posturing should perhaps be called *physiologic dystonia.*

Chorea or Choreoathetosis. Choreic movements are random, brief, rapid, and purposeless jerking movements usually involving the extremities, face, tongue, and trunk. When slow writhing movements of one side of the body occur, the term *choreoathetosis* is used. The patient may be unable to sustain a grip and intermittently contract and relax (milkmaid phenomenon). Occasionally, children have choreiform movements on neurologic examination that improve during the second decade. These are benign, but there is a dominant familial choreoathetosis as well. Several authors have described paroxysmal choreoathetosis, which may respond to anticonvulsant therapy. The increase in rheumatic fever cases in the last decade has increased the awareness of Sydenham chorea (St. Vitus' dance), which is one of the major manifestations of this disorder and may occur late in the course after all signs of streptococcal infection have disappeared. Patients with this disorder may have a form of encephalopathy with behavior change, decreased school performance, and anxiety. Hypotonia is also a feature. Huntington chorea is a devastating hereditary disorder that begins as early as the first decade of life. Juvenile onset may be more associated with parkinsonian features, with chorea appearing later. Genetic and family studies are the key to diagnosis. Other disorders may have chorea as the major complaint, including Wilson disease, systemic lupus erythematosus, hyperthyroidism, and adverse effects of anticonvulsant drugs, to name just a few. Recently a report of a movement disorder occurring in premature infants with severe bronchopulmonary dysplasia was published by Perlman and Volpe. This disorder included choreiform movements and motor restlessness (akathisia). It usually started at about the third postnatal month. The outlook was variable with resolution or a static course. Hypoxia was postulated as a possible mechanism for the movement disturbance.

Benign Paroxysmal Vertigo

Benign paroxysmal vertigo is characterized by brief episodes of loss of balance that usually begin between 1 and

3 years of age. The child may become frightened and grasp for support of an object or parent; gait may be ataxic. Older children may complain of dizziness or a spinning sensation. Emesis and nystagmus occur in about 25% of the patients. There is no loss of consciousness and no postictal phase. Some children have a history of paroxysmal torticollis. The problem is self-limited but quite frightening to the patient and family.

Migraine

Migraine represents one of the most common paroxysmal conditions of childhood (see Chapter 5). Usually, in older children the typical headache helps make the diagnosis. Other important features are the family history and occurrence of associated phenomena, such as motion sickness. Several migraine variants deserve mention as the cause of unusual spells, including basilar artery migraine, acute confusional state, and the "Alice in Wonderland" syndrome. Basilar artery migraine may cause ataxia, vertigo, loss of postural tone, diplopia, and confusion. Acute confusional migraine may mimic drug intoxications, absence seizure, or postictal state. In the "Alice in Wonderland" syndrome there are disturbances of body image and space and time perception, as well as hallucinations. Fortunately, headache usually develops in these patients, and most often the family history is positive for migraine, or "sick headaches." Complicating the evaluation of migraine is the fact that nonspecific abnormalities of the EEG are common during and between attacks. The history and clinical findings remain the most important elements in the correct diagnosis.

Parasomnias

Parasomnias are characterized by disturbances during nighttime sleep or excessive daytime sleepiness, but unusual features (such as cataplexy) may make diagnosis difficult. It is easiest to divide the problems into those that affect rapid eye movement (REM) sleep and nonREM sleep.

NonREM Disorders. NonREM disorders are usually recognized by the physician who sees children regularly and include nocturnal enuresis (not further discussed here, see Chapter 21), night terrors *(pavor nocturnus),* and *sleepwalking or talking (somnambulism or somniloquy).* In night terrors, which usually begin at about 4 years of age, the child sits upright after 15 to 90 minutes of sleep and appears terrified, with associated sympathetic signs of mydriasis, tachycardia, and diaphoresis. The child usually returns to sleep in 5 to 10 minutes and does not remember the episode upon awakening the next day. There is no evidence for a primary emotional disorder, and long-term outlook is normal with reassurance the mainstay of management.

Sleepwalking affects about 15% of children between 5 and 15 years of age and is characterized by slow, trancelike ambulation. The patient may attempt to avoid others but generally goes back to bed quietly. Sleeptalking usually includes incomprehensible short syllables and not an intelligent dialogue.

REM Disorders. The REM disorders are nightmares and narcolepsy. Nightmares are common and distinguished from night terrors by the easy awakening of the patient and the vivid recollection of the event. Narcolepsy is characterized by excessive daytime sleepiness. Onset is usually in the second decade of life, although there are reports of earlier onset. Patients have frequent unrefreshing daytime naps, and approximately 50% have a family history of narcolepsy or disordered sleep. The classic tetrad includes sleep attacks, cataplexy (loss of postural tone, usually with laughter), sleep paralysis (inability to move when falling asleep), and hypnagogic hallucinations (vivid sensations when falling asleep or awakening). Cataplexy was present in all four preadolescent children described by Kotagal and others and serves as a useful symptom because only 20% of children have the complete tetrad. If the diagnosis is suspected, nighttime polysomnography and daytime sleep latency testing are diagnostic.

Nonepileptic Nonneurologic Disorders

There are two types of nonepileptic nonneurologic disorders—syncope (see Chapter 12) and breathholding spells. These disorders are certainly "spells," but the usual complaint from parents is that the child suddenly loses consciousness or "passes out." Often there is a question about asystole or bradycardia. These entities are discussed in Chapter 12.

Behavioral and Psychiatric Disorders

Children can have a number of simple and stereotyped patterns of behavior that mimic epilepsy and other neurologic syndromes. Awareness of these more common entities can often but not always avoid unnecessary and invasive diagnostic testing and allow a family- and office-based approach.

Pseudoseizures

Pseudoseizures can be difficult to diagnose because many of these patients have true epilepsy. Manifestations are multiple and may include staring, unresponsiveness, thrashing, and tonic-clonic movements. Several clues to the diagnosis are often present, including unusual aura, provocation and cessation by stimuli, failure of anticonvulsant therapy in excellent doses or breakthrough while on medication, absence of incontinence or injury from falls, absence of postictal state, and recent traumatic life events. Often these spells must be investigated using video EEG recording and various stimuli to provoke episodes. In a study of psychogenic seizures in normal children without prior epilepsy, Wylie and associates emphasized the positive outcome when the patient and family were told that the episodes were emotional in origin and referral was made to a child psychiatrist.

Automatisms

Repetitive body rocking, head rolling, and head banging are present in many normal children and tend to be present at certain times of day, often when the child is tired or going to sleep. Behavior ceases when the child is distracted. Masturbation in children is frequently misdiagnosed and not recognized by parents. Rhythmic rocking or rubbing with facial flushing is common, and at times a home video recording is diagnostic. This activity is commonly confused with either epilepsy or recurrent abdominal pain (see Chapter 1).

Episodic Dyscontrol Syndrome

Episodic dyscontrol syndrome consists of sudden rage directed at a person or animal and is often mistaken for a partial complex seizure. In one study the average age was approximately 27 years, but several pediatric patients were reported. The onset is abrupt, and the episode lasts minutes to hours. As opposed to epilepsy, the rage is directed at an individual and the patient may appear temporarily psychotic. There are no automatisms or other seizure manifestations and no postictal state. In adults this syndrome may have lethal consequences.

Attention-Deficit Hyperactivity Disorder

Although attention-deficit hyperactivity disorder is not a common cause of isolated spells, patients can have staring episodes, sudden change in behavior, tantrums, and sudden angry behavior directed at people or objects. Complete history should reveal the long-standing and complex nature of the child's problem.

Table 10-1 organizes the differential diagnoses with key features, which are further elucidated in the next sections of the text.

History

As in other chronic and recurrent disorders, the history is most likely to lead the examiner to the correct diagnosis. Time spent reviewing details of the episodes, both with the family and the patient, may prevent hastily ordered studies that may be of no real value. A number of questions may narrow the focus to one of several possibilities and allow definitive testing. Because epilepsy remains part of the differential diagnosis for many types of spells, the physician should inquire carefully about those characteristics that support or reject this diagnosis. A series of questions about the episodes should be thorough. Some of these are detailed in a review by Rothner.

When was the onset of the spells? Were there episodes earlier in life that could have been paroxysmal? Can the patient tell when an episode will start? Is there a warning sign? Is there a trigger for the spell (crying, anger, boredom, anxiety, fever, trauma, etc.)? Do the episodes occur at a particular time (sleeping, awakening, or after meals)? How often do they occur? What is the duration? Are all episodes the same, or are there several types? What is the position at onset (standing or reclining)? Is the patient at rest, exercising, or initiating movement? Does he or she always fall if standing?

Does the patient injure himself or herself? Do the episodes occur at different places (school or home)? Are there different observers? Could any of these observers be contacted? Are there other associated symptoms, such as emesis, pallor, diaphoresis, change in gait or balance, nystagmus, or headache? Can you tell whether the child has lost consciousness? Does he or she speak during the spell? Does he or she recognize you or reach out his or her arms to be helped? Does the patient remember the spells afterward? Can you interrupt a spell? If so, how? What is the child like after the episode (postictal, confused, or alert)? Does he or she sleep? How long? Can the child describe what happens? What sensations does he or she perceive? Does anything happen at the end of a spell, such as fecal soiling or urination? Can the entire spell be described from onset to resolution by the parent or another observer? Also, are the episodes becoming more or less frequent? How is school attendance affected? Is there any change in other developmental skills? Are there any symptoms of systemic disease?

Family history is important. Many of the episodes described earlier have a tendency to be genetic. Does anyone else have similar episodes, migraine, tics or tremors, Tourette syndrome, sleep disturbance, epilepsy, or chorea? Is there a family history of rheumatic fever, streptococcal infection, degenerative disease, liver disease, or any problem with metabolism?

Past medical history and previous functioning should be reviewed. The movement disturbance may have a perinatal cause, such as that seen in severe bronchopulmonary dysplasia. Myoclonus is often difficult to distinguish from epilepsy; long duration and absence of developmental delay or regression favors a more benign diagnosis. Obviously, if chorea is suspected, the physician must question the patient about symptoms of rheumatic fever. If the patient is already under treatment, what tests are available for review? What medications, especially anticonvulsants, is the child taking?

At this time the examiner should have a good sense of the type of spell, although the possibilities may still include epilepsy along with others and some further testing may be warranted. Key questions are summarized in Box 10-1.

Physical Examination

Again, a thorough examination may be reassuring (if completely normal) or may provide clues to support specific diagnoses. General nutrition, growth, and vital signs are important. Is best to review growth over time if possible. It is extremely helpful to see a spell, and during the evaluation an attempt should be made to elicit an episode with the assistance and cooperation of the parents. If this is possible, what initiates spells in the office setting? Tics may be suppressed, but eventually (perhaps later in the waiting room or after the examiner leaves the room) a flurry of them may occur. Do episodes occur only with the initiation of move-

Key Questions in Approach to Spells

Time of onset (what month or year)?
Previous episodes that were unexplained?
Can you tell when an episode will start?
Warning signs before onset (aura)?
Trigger (crying, anger, or trauma)?
Timing (sleep, awakening, exercise, or with meals)?
Frequency (increasing or decreasing)?
Different types of episodes?
Position at onset (standing, fall, or injury)?
Initial and later movements? Can you describe them?
Where do episodes occur (school or home)?
Observers? Full event?
Other symptoms (emesis, pallor, confusion, or gait change)?
Headache?
Loss of consciousness?
Does he or she speak during episode? Coherent?
Recognize you?
Recall spell? Describe what happened?
Can you interrupt the episode?
State of awareness afterward (confused or sleepy)?
Nystagmus (during or after)?
Length of episode?
Events at end (soiling)?
School attendance?
Change in performance or developmental skills?
Sleep problems (night, excessive daytime, or sudden episodes of sleep)?
Family history (similar episodes, epilepsy, migraine, chorea, sleep problems, rheumatic fever/streptococcal infections, tremor, degenerative disorder, cirrhosis)?
Systemic symptoms (fever, weight loss, jaundice, lymphadenopathy, joint symptoms, rash, etc.)?
Medications (anticonvulsants)?
What tests have been done previously (EEG)?
Can you record an episode on video?

ment or at rest? The physician should observe the patient performing tasks (tying shoes, dressing or undressing, walking, and running if possible). A complete general physical examination should be completed with emphasis on neurologic and neurodevelopmental status. The physician must look for findings of neurocutaneous syndromes, such as neurofibromatosis and tuberous sclerosis, which are associated with epilepsy. Abnormalities of neurologic examination, especially signs of increased intracranial pressure (rare), certainly accelerate the use of consultants and neuroimaging procedures. It is very informative to observe interactions among family members and the effect that the spells have on them. What do they do during an episode, and how does the child appear? Unfortunately, few spells are observed in the controlled office environment.

Approach to the Patient

At this point in the evaluation, it is critical that the examiner know exactly what type of event or episode is being evaluated. The plan of further management is almost totally dependent on this. Certain spells are so characteristic that the history and physical examination are sufficient for therapy. Examples are night terrors, head banging, and simple tics. Other disorders are much more difficult, such as certain dystonias, myoclonic syndromes, and pseudoseizures. A key first step is to distinguish the spell from epilepsy, if possible. Clues that strongly suggest a seizure are prodrome or aura, absence of a "trigger" for the event, loss of consciousness, onset while reclining quietly, tonic-clonic movements, nondirected activity (such as rage), inability to interrupt or modify the spell, postictal state, and paroxysmal EEG. In a recently published study of adults the most useful feature to distinguish syncope from seizure was disorientation after the event. Very helpful at this stage, before initiating other testing, is a home video recording of the spell or spells over several days. If equipment is not available to the family, often the hospital's audiovisual department can either lend the family a video camera or arrange a brief outpatient taping. This less costly approach should precede detailed video EEG recording, which may still be necessary at a later time.

If after close review of an episode epilepsy remains a consideration, an EEG is indicated. If there is general certainty of this diagnosis, routine outpatient recording is sufficient. There are both false positives and false negatives; abnormalities are found in patients with migraine and in some otherwise normal children. Interictal EEG is often normal in patients with epilepsy. In a study of adults with known seizures the first interictal EEG was abnormal 50% of the time, the third was abnormal 84% of the time, and the fourth was abnormal 92% of the time. Spells that remain confusing should be evaluated by prolonged EEG and videotaping. In some institutions, ambulatory EEG recording (using a cassette) is available and may confirm ictal episodes before inpatient video EEG recording. If cardiac events are a consideration (see Chapter 12), monitoring of vital signs and cardiac rhythm is warranted. Another possible diagnostic test that may become available soon is the use of serum prolactin levels drawn within 90 minutes of a spell. Zelnik and associates found that serum prolactin levels in patients with epilepsy were significantly higher than those in patients with syncope, breathholding spells, or even febrile seizures. There was little overlap in the values, but this remains an observation that warrants more detailed study.

If the patient has episodes confined to sleep or the period just before sleep or awakening or there is excessive daytime sleep or cataplexy, a detailed sleep study is indicated to define possible disorders, such as narcolepsy or sleep-induced epilepsy. Sleep is a recognized time for epilepsy, so careful description of sleep events remains critical. The trancelike state of the sleepwalker is quite distinct from the stereotyped or clonic movements of the epileptic patient who is often agitated or confused afterward. Once again a simple video recording may obviate the need for an EEG if sleep myoclonus, night terrors, or another self-limited disorder is evident.

At the initial evaluation, in addition to searching for a central origin for episodes, the clinician should ask what treatable disorders could be overlooked. This demands that disorders in younger children raise suspicions of congenital metabolic disease and that older children with a movement disturbance be evaluated for Wilson disease, systemic lupus erythematosus, rheumatic fever, and other illnesses that have well-defined therapies. Urine for metabolic screening (amino acids, organic acids) is generally available and may be sent to reference laboratories by community hospitals. In children who are progressing normally there is much to be said for a prolonged period of observation when the diagnosis remains unclear, as long as progressive and treatable disorders are excluded.

Imaging of the nervous system is late on the list of procedures. Obviously, brain tumors and neurodegenerative diseases may cause movement disturbances but *rarely* with spells followed by a completely normal examination. If symptoms are progressive and/or accompanied by headache, loss of skills, change in sensorium, or other signs of increased intracranial pressure, an imaging procedure is indicated. MRI is rapidly replacing CT scan for accurate and complete evaluation.

Consultation with specialists is often quite helpful when the diagnosis of a particular spell remains questionable after initial evaluation. If a videotape is available, a consultant may give valuable input about the nature of what is recorded. At times a formal opinion is the best route, allowing the consultant time to review all the information available and assess the need for therapy.

SUMMARY

Spells are relatively common in pediatric patients and most often are confused with epilepsy or, in the case of syncope, cardiac events (see Chapter 12). A complete approach that includes detailed history of the event(s) and careful review of the family history and past medical history often produces the correct diagnosis. Videotaping an episode is invaluable in developing a reasonable plan of management. Evaluation may be complete at this point, but selected patients require more testing and referral, usually to a pediatric neurologist. Using this approach, the clinician will become familiar with the common variants of normal development and behavior and refer only patients who need more invasive testing.

ILLUSTRATIVE CASES

Case 1. J.D. is a 15-month-old girl referred for evaluation of episodes of abdominal pain that could possibly be seizures. At 6 months of age the parents noted stiffening of the lower extremities when the infant was on her side or

back. Later these episodes occurred while she was in a high chair with her legs lifted and straightened. Episodes were most frequent at bedtime but gradually began to occur daily for periods up to an hour in daycare. The child appeared to stare and be in pain during the spells but could sometimes be interrupted during an episode. The child was normal after an event but would often fall asleep in the evenings. There was no defecation or "gas" afterward. Growth, development, and physical examination were normal, and the child was sociable and interactive.

This history may suggest epilepsy, except that the child can be interrupted and distracted. Videotape strongly suggested masturbation, and further questioning of the mother supported this. The child often placed a blanket between her legs or pushed her perineal area onto the restraining strap in her stroller during episodes. With distraction and reassurance the episodes have lessened in frequency.

Case 2. A 12-year-old girl was referred for further evaluation of ataxia. One week before admission she had a brief episode of difficulty walking during a prolonged upper respiratory tract infection. Amoxicillin was prescribed for sinusitis, and she improved. The day before admission she had blurry vision and went to bed early. She could not walk the next morning and was brought to her pediatrician who noted nystagmus and referred her after obtaining a normal CT scan of the brain. Past history was unremarkable except that the mother mentioned a short episode of "balance problems" lasting for 24 hours, 1 year earlier.

Physical examination was remarkable for a well-nourished appearing, cooperative, oriented girl with nystagmus in all gaze positions, truncal and appendicular ataxia, past-pointing, and mild hypotonia. Funduscopic examination was normal. Lumbar puncture was normal, and after overnight observation the child's signs and symptoms completely resolved.

This child was thought to have acute cerebellar ataxia, but the rapid resolution was unusual. Drug screens of urine and serum were normal, prompting further history. Mother and daughter remembered more prominent headache than on first questioning but had been so concerned by the gait disturbance that they neglected to comment on it. Family history was positive for migraine in both the mother and her sister, and a diagnosis of basilar artery migraine was tentatively made.

Other data supporting migraine in this case are the recurrent episodes, blurry vision (which actually was more diplopia), and short duration.

Case 3. G.P. is an 8-year-old boy with episodes of difficulty standing up after sleeping. Past medical history is remarkable for microcephaly and developmental delay with autistic features. Detailed metabolic and genetic testing was not helpful. He was nonverbal and attended a special school.

Play included many repetitive activities. Episodes began 6 months before the office visit and usually occurred in the morning. He could not rise from bed; each time he attempted to stand, he would sit back on the bed and look downward. Attempts were numerous and lasted for up to 20 minutes. He would then get ready for school. He began to have some episodes of falling in school, and similar standing difficulties occurred after naps.

Examination revealed a fairly pleasant, autistic boy with no new findings on neurologic examination. Previous CT scan of the brain was reviewed and was normal.

Differential diagnosis in this patient was difficult. The events reviewed on videotape resembled disequilibrium with inability to stand. Paroxysmal vertigo was considered. Because of his developmental problems and the unusual videotape, a video EEG was obtained. Striking spike and wave discharges were seen associated with the episodes, which had a more prominent head drop than seen on the home video, and atypical absence epilepsy was considered the likely diagnosis. Anticonvulsant therapy has not completely eradicated the episodes, but they are less severe.

ANNOTATED BIBLIOGRAPHY

Barron T: The child with spells, *Pediatr Clin North Am* 38:711-724, 1991.
This is an excellent review and classification of the entire group of disorders that may present as spells.

Fleisher DR, Morrison A: Masturbation mimicking abdominal pain or seizures in young girls, *J Pediatr* 116:810-814, 1991.
This brief article is a particular favorite because several difficult cases were solved after close attention to the episodes described here.

Pranzatelli MR: An approach to movement disorders of childhood, *Pediatr Ann* 22:13-17, 1993.
This is the first of a group of articles in this issue of Pediatric Annals *that cover the most common neurologic causes of spells, including movement disorders (tics), myoclonic disorders, chorea, dystonia, tremor, and others.*

BIBLIOGRAPHY

Anderman F, Keene DL, Anderman E, et al: Startle disease or hypereflexia, *Brain* 103:985-997, 1980.
Butler IJ: Movement disorders of children, *Pediatr Clin North Am* 39:727-742, 1992.

Caplan LR: Migraine and vertebrobasilar ischemia, *Neurology* 41:55-61, 1991.
Deonna TW, Ziegler A, Nielson J: Transient idiopathic dystonia in infancy, *Neuropediatrics* 22:220-224, 1991.
Duchowny MS, Resnick TJ, Deray MJ, et al: Video EEG diagnosis of repetitive behavior in early childhood and its relationship to seizures, *Pediatr Neurol* 4:162-164, 1988.
FitzGerald PM, Jankovic J, Percy AK: Rett syndrome and associated movement disorders, *Mov Disord* 5:195-202, 1990.
Golden GS: Nonepileptic paroxysmal events in childhood, *Pediatr Clin North Am* 39:715-725, 1992.
Hoefnagels WAJ, Padberg GW, Overweg J, et al: Transient loss of consciousness: the value of the history for distinguishing seizure from syncope, *J Neurol* 238:39-43, 1991.
Kotagal S, Hartse KM, Walsh JK: Characteristics of narcolepsy in preteenaged children, *Pediatrics* 85:205-209, 1990.
Livingston S: Disorders simulating epilepsy. In: *Comprehensive management of epilepsy in infancy, childhood and adolescence*, Springfield, Ill, 1972, Charles C. Thomas.
Lombroso CT, Fejerman N: Benign myoclonus of early infancy, *Ann Neurol* 1:138-143, 1977.
Nanayakkara CS, Paton JY: Sandifer syndrome: an overlooked diagnosis? *Dev Med Child Neurol* 27:816-819, 1985.
Pedley TA: Differential diagnosis of episodic symptoms, *Epilepsia* 24(suppl 1):S31-S44, 1983.
Perlman JM, Volpe JJ: Movement disorder of premature infants with severe bronchopulmonary dysplasia: a new syndrome, *Pediatrics* 84:215-218, 1989.
Roddy SM: Bad habit, simple tic, or Tourette syndrome? *Contemp Pediatr* 6:22-36, 1989.
Rothner AD: Not everything that shakes is epilepsy: the differential diagnosis of paroxysmal nonepileptiform disorders, *Cleve Clin J Med* 56(suppl 2):S206-S213, 1989.
Salinsky M, Kanter R, Dasheiff RM: Effectiveness of multiple EEGs in supporting the diagnosis of epilepsy: an operational curve, *Epilepsia* 28:331-334, 1987.
Schwartzman RJ, Kerrigan J: The movement disorder of reflex sympathetic dystrophy, *Neurology* 40:57-61, 1990.
Vanasse M, Bedard P, Anderman F: Shuddering attacks in children: an early clinical manifestation of essential tremor, *Neurology* 26:1027-1030, 1976.
Woody RC: Home videorecording of "spells" in children, *Pediatrics* 76:612-613, 1985.
Woody RC: Sleep disorders in children, *Semin Neurol* 8:71-77, 1988.
Wylie E, Friedman D, Rothner AD, et al: Psychogenic seizures in children and adolescents: outcome after diagnosis by ictal video and electroencephalographic recording, *Pediatrics* 85:480-484, 1990.
Zelnik N, Kahana L, Rafael A, et al: Prolactin and cortisol levels in various paroxysmal disorders in childhood, *Pediatrics* 88:486-489, 1991.

11

Chronic Weakness

EUGENE M. MOWAD

Key Points

- Weakness is a distinct clinical entity with an extensive array of etiologic possibilities. The approach to a patient with weakness must begin with a thorough history and detailed general and neurologic examination.

- Historic questions and neurologic examination techniques should be framed by the child's developmental level. Based on the physical examination the examiner can often localize a lesion to a particular level of the neuromuscular system.

- Multitudes of diagnostic studies exist for the patient with weakness, but a logical, stepwise approach directed by the history and physical examination is the most effective.

Muscular strength is properly defined as the extent to which a muscle is able to shorten against a load. Any decrement in strength from an arbitrarily defined norm may therefore be termed *weakness*. The medical evaluation of weakness must begin with its accurate definition. Patients informally use the word *weakness* to describe such disparate entities as fatigue, malaise, hypotonia, and ataxia. These last two are also discrete neurologic entities that merit clear definition.

Tone is defined as the resistance to passive movement of a muscle and is best measured in a resting state. Strength differs in that it is defined in terms of maximal active effort. Ataxia is an abnormality in the smooth coordination of muscular movements. A patient with a staggering gait may state, "My legs are weak." It becomes imperative that the examiner separate the coordination of muscle actions from the strength of individual muscles to properly evaluate this problem.

It is the goal of this chapter to present an organized approach to the patient with weakness that may arise from a variety of anatomic locations along the motor system. Localiza-

tion of the source of weakness along the neuroaxis is a major step toward accurate diagnosis.

Because disease entities tend to occur at discete points along the motor system, a brief review of its anatomy is presented.

Pathophysiology

Anatomy of the Motor System

Motor impulses are initially generated by the motor neurons, which are located for the most part in the precentral gyrus of the cerebral cortex. Axons course through the ipsilateral cerebral white matter and brainstem until they reach the lower medulla. In the lower medulla the majority of these axons cross to the contralateral side. This decussation occurs just rostral to the pyramids of the medulla. The axons continue through the spinal cord in the lateral corticospinal tracts until they synapse with the anterior horn cell in the ventral spinal cord. This synapse marks the transition between upper motor neuron (UMN) and lower motor neuron (LMN) processes.

The anterior horn cell axon exits the spinal cord via the ventral root and terminates in a motor endplate. Chemical transmission occurs across the neuromuscular junction (NMJ) to excite muscle fibers, resulting in contraction.

There are numerous modulatory steps along the way, but these and the contribution of the afferent system to tone and strength are beyond the scope of this chapter.

Knowledge of the anatomy of the motor system is the basis for localization of lesions along the neuroaxis.

Localization

A lesion affecting the motor system anywhere from the cerebral cortex to the anterior horn cell results in a clinical syndrome associated with UMN pathology. This weakness is associated with hypertonia, hyperreflexia (and perhaps clonus), and an extensor plantar response if the lower extremities are involved. Acute onset of a UMN process, such as a stroke or trauma-related event, often results in a condition known as *spinal shock*. In this situation there is flaccid tone and hyporeflexia, and differentiation from LMN lesions becomes difficult. History of an acute event, presence of Babinski reflexes, and recognition of a sensory level in spinal cord processes, however, establish the UMN as the site of injury.

Hemiplegia (ipsilateral upper and lower extremity weakness) in isolation is usually the result of a unilateral cortical insult on the opposite side. If hemiplegia is accompanied by a sensory level, the ipsilateral spinal cord is the site of injury (see Brown-Séquard syndrome mentioned later).

Recall that cortical motor fibers decussate in the caudal medulla, whereas motor efferents of the cranial nerves innervate the ipsilateral side. For this reason, weakness of one side of the face with weakness of the opposite side of the body indicates a lesion in the brainstem (ipsilateral to the facial weakness).

Bilaterally symmetric weakness with UMN signs is almost always due to a spinal cord lesion. A careful search for a sensory level further pinpoints the lesion. Brown-Séquard initially described the clinical constellation that resulted from spinal cord hemisection. Whether caused by a traumatic event or a pathologic lesion that disrupts axonal integrity, the syndrome of weakness associated with loss of position and vibratory sense ipsilateral to the lesion and loss of pain and temperature sense contralateral to the lesion indicates unilateral spinal cord pathology. Involvement of the sacral spinal cord results in unilateral or bilateral lower extremity weakness with symptoms of bowel and bladder dysfunction.

Weakness associated with LMN lesions is characterized by diminished tone, hyporeflexia, muscle atrophy, and fasciculations. The diseases of the anterior horn cell, such as spinal muscular atrophy and poliomyelitis, have prominent loss of reflexes as an early sign.

Weakness associated with a peripheral nerve injury corresponds to the anatomic distribution of the involved nerve or nerves. An anatomically similar sensory loss may accompany peripheral neuropathies.

Diseases of the neuromuscular junction are notable for prominent extraocular muscle weakness and other cranial neuropathies. Deep tendon reflexes are spared, and extremity weakness if present is always less notable than the bulbar weakness.

Myopathies usually involve proximal musculature to a greater extent than distal musculature. Inflammatory myopathies and myositis are often associated with muscle tenderness.

Once a disease process is tentatively localized, a limited battery of ancillary studies is usually helpful in arriving at a specific diagnosis. The laboratory studies and tables of differential diagnoses included in this chapter are organized with respect to the anatomic areas previously discussed.

Literature Survey

The literature dealing with chronic weakness in childhood is quite diffuse. Countless articles present weakness as a symptom of a particular disease entity, but works that review the differential diagnosis and approach to the patient with weakness as an undiagnosed symptom are few.

Although nearly 20 years old, Spiro's review from *Pediatric Annals* superbly emphasizes a stepped approach to the patient with weakness, using clinical data, family history, biochemical data, electrodiagnostics, and finally biopsy specimens.

A more recent work by Lewis and Berman is a very useful review for the clinician who deals with progressive weakness. Their approach, which consists of careful history taking, detailed physical examination, anatomic localization, and supportive laboratory and electrodiagnostic studies, is most useful when faced with a patient with undiagnosed weakness.

There is some overlap between the entities that cause weakness and those that cause hypotonia, and Dubowitz's review of hypotonia is the most definitive work on the topic. The metabolic and neurodegenerative disorders present one of the most complex aspects in the evaluation of weakness, and Percy's article on clinical assessment of the heritable neurodegenerative disorders of childhood is a comprehensive and well-referenced review of this vast topic.

Differential Diagnosis

Upper Motor Neuron Weakness

The newborn examination is helpful for diagnosing many of the congenital causes of weakness (Table 11-1). Increased head circumference, a myelomeningocele, a sacral hair tuft, or a hemangioma should always prompt further evaluation. Klippel-Feil syndrome often presents in the newborn period with torticollis or a short, stiff neck (brevicollis) caused by congenital synostosis of two or more cervical vertebrae. A low hairline, genitourinary anomalies, congenital heart disease, and congenitally high scapulae (Sprengel deformity) may be associated.

Arnold-Chiari malformation type II often presents in the newborn period with hydrocephalus, myelomeningocele, and a foreshortened occiput. The type I variant may go unnoticed until adolescence because it does not usually cause hydrocephalus. This variant may cause headache, ataxia, incontinence, and lower extremity spasticity.

Focal UMN weakness suggests a focal insult (neoplastic, traumatic, or infectious) that should be supported by history.

Lower Motor Neuron Weakness

Spinal muscular atrophy can present in a severe, fatal infantile form known as *Werdnig-Hoffmann disease* or in a more chronic juvenile form known as *Kugelberg-Welander disease*

TABLE 11-1

Differential Diagnosis of Upper Motor Neuron Weakness

Cause	History/physical examination	Studies
Hydrocephalus	Head circumference	Sonogram, MRI
Basilar impression with platybasia	—	Skull radiograph
Dysraphism	Sacral tuft, sinus tract, or hemangioma	Radiograph, MRI, sonogram
Klippel-Feil syndrome	Sprengel deformity, torticollis	Radiograph
Arnold-Chiari malformation	Head size or shape, associated dysraphism	Sonogram, MRI
Abscess, mass, hematoma	Focal findings, fever, trauma	CT or MRI
Transverse myelitis	Rapid progression, bowel or bladder symptoms	LP
Neurodegenerative disease	Associated symptoms, family history	LP, enzyme assay

CT, Computed tomography; *LP*, lumbar puncture; *MRI*, magnetic resonance imaging.

TABLE 11-2

Differential Diagnosis of Lower Motor Neuron Weakness

Cause	History/physical examination	Studies
Anterior Horn Cell		
Spinal muscular atrophy	Areflexia, fasiculations	NCV/EMG
Polio and other enteroviruses	Asymmetric, perhaps monoparesis	LP, culture
Metabolic defects	—	Enzyme assay
Peripheral Nerve		
Guillain-Barré syndrome	Viral illness, ascending pattern	Albuminocytologic dissociation
Diphtheria	Cranial neuropathy, pharyngitis	—
Heavy metal poisoning	Exposure, rash	Serum screening
Charcot-Marie-Tooth disease	Stork legs, family history	NCV/EMG
Neuromuscular Junction		
Botulism	Constipation, mydriasis	EMG/NCV
Myasthenia	Maternal history, pupils normal, EOM decreased	Edrophonium test
Tick paralysis	Rapid, exposure history	Gravid tick
Organophosphate toxicity	Other anticholinergic symptoms, exposure	Cholinesterase level

EMG, Electromyogram; *EOM*, extraocular movements; *LP*, lumbar puncture; *NCV*, nerve conduction velocity.

(Table 11-2). Both are marked by fasciculations and early, prominent loss of reflexes.

Although paralytic poliomyelitis is now rare, the other enteroviruses are implicated in milder forms of often asymmetric LMN weakness associated with fever and a viral prodrome. Nonparalytic polio is characterized by muscle soreness and stiffness, including nuchal rigidity, but there is no weakness. Paralytic polio involves true weakness and depending on the muscle groups involved can be classified as bulbar, spinal, or bulbospinal.

Some of the many metabolic defects that result in weakness are listed in Table 11-3. These entities present with a mixed UMN and LMN picture. Notably, ataxia, developmental regression, and tone abnormalities accompany weakness in most of these disorders.

Guillain-Barré syndrome is an acute demyelinating polyneuropathy that often occurs 1 to 2 weeks after a viral illness. Paralysis is usually in an ascending pattern and involves distal muscles more than proximal muscles. Deep tendon reflexes are often lost early in the course of the disease. The characteristic finding in the cerebrospinal fluid is elevation of the protein level without a pleocytosis (known as *albuminocytologic dissociation*). The Miller-Fisher variant of this syndrome includes ophthalmoplegia, ataxia, and areflexia.

TABLE 11-3

Degenerative Diseases Presenting With Predominantly Motor Symptoms

Disease	Enzyme Defect	Inheritance	Age of onset	Weakness	Ataxia	Peripheral nerves	Other neurologic signs	Associated findings
Metachromatic leukodystrophy	Arylsulfatase A	Autosomal recessive	1-2 yr	+++ Spastic	+	++, Deep tendon reflexes	Mental regression, behavior changes, intention tremor	—
Neuroaxonal dystrophy	Unknown	Autosomal recessive	1-2 yr	+++ Hypotonic or spastic	−	+, Deep tendon reflexes	Mental regression, optic atrophy	—
GM$_1$ gangliosidosis (late infantile)	Beta-galactosidase	Autosomal recessive	1-5 yr	+++ Spastic	+	−	Mental regression, seizures, dysphagia	—
GM$_2$ gangliosidosis (juvenile or adult forms)	Hexosaminidase A	Autosomal recessive	4 yr-adult	+++ Spastic	+	−	Mental regression, myoclonic seizures, occasional neurogenic atrophy	—
Krabbe disease (late infantile or juvenile)	Galactocerebroside beta-galactosidase	Autosomal recessive	2-6 yr	+++ Spastic	++	−/+	Mental regression, dysarthria, seizures, optic atrophy	—
Gaucher disease (type 2 or 3)	Glucococerebroside-beta-glucosidase	Autosomal recessive	2-8 yr	+++ Hypotonic or spastic	+	−	Mental regression, ophthalmoparesis, dysphagia, seizures	Hepatosplenomegaly
Pelizaeus-Merzbacher disease (sudanophilic leukodystrophy)	Unknown	X-linked recessive	1 mo	+++ Spastic	++	−	Mental regression (late), nystagmus, choreoathetosis, seizures, mental regression, behavior changes, cortical blindness	—
Adrenoleukodystrophy/adrenomyeloneuropathy	Long-chain fatty acid defect	X-linked recessive	5-15 yr	+++ Spastic	++	+	—	Adrenal insufficiency
Niemann-Pick disease (types C&D)	Unknown	Autosomal recessive	2-8 yr	+ Spastic	+++	−	Mental regression, vertical gaze paresis, seizures	Splenomegaly
Ataxia telangiectasia	Unknown	Autosomal recessive	12-18 mo	+/−	+++	+, Deep tendon reflexes	Oculomotor apraxia, choreoathetosis, dysarthria	Immune deficiency, telangiectasis, sinopulmonary infection
Friedreich ataxia	Unknown	Autosomal recessive (variable)	5-20 yr	+	+++	++, Deep tendon reflexes	Dysarthria, nystagmus, *pes cavus*	Cardiomyopathy

From Lewis DW, Berman PH: Progressive weakness in infancy and childhood, *Pediatr Rev* 8:206, 1987.
+, Present and to what degree; −, not present or not involved.

TABLE 11-4

Differential Diagnosis of Muscle Weakness

Cause	History/physical examination	Studies
Muscular dystrophy	Family history	CPK, dystrophin
Periodic paralysis	Family history	Potassium level
Congenital myopathy	—	EMG/NCV
Mitochondrial disease	Liver failure in some	Anion gap acidosis, biopsy
Collagen vascular disease	Arthritis, rash	ESR, antibodies
Infectious myositis	Tenderness	CPK
Endocrine myopathy	Growth, specific symptoms of endocrine disease	Thyroid function studies, electrolytes, calcium, phosphate

CPK, Creatine phosphokinase; *EMG,* electromyogram; *ESR,* erythrocyte sedimentation rate; *NCV,* nerve conduction velocity.

Although these syndromes are often acute, chronic relapsing courses occur in 5% to 7% of cases and have been grouped under the term *chronic inflammatory demyelinating polyneuropathy.*

Diphtheria causes either a necrotizing pharyngitis or rhinitis characterized by a gray, thick, mucopurulent pseudomembrane. The *Corynebacterium* species elaborates a toxin that causes flaccid paralysis. The organism can be cultured from the involved site, but if suspicion is high, penicillin therapy should not be delayed.

Heavy metal poisoning, most notably lead and mercury, causes hypotonia, weakness, and sensory neuropathy. Lead poisoning is accompanied by a microcytic anemia, and mercury poisoning often causes a characteristic, acrally distributed, pink, desquamating rash.

There is a group of hereditary motor and sensory neuropathies, the most common of which is peroneal muscle atrophy, or Charcot-Marie-Tooth disease. The neuropathy affects mostly the tibial and peroneal nerve distribution, causing weakness in late childhood or early adolescence. Loss of muscle bulk in that distribution causes a "stork-leg" appearance. A less severe form is peroneal muscle atrophy type II, and a severe, rapidly progressive infantile form is peroneal muscle atrophy type III, also known as *Déjerine-Sottas disease.*

Neuromuscular Junction

In infancy, botulism occurs because of ingestion of *Clostridium* spores (Table 11-2). Addition of honey to infant formula is an epidemiologically associated phenomenon. In addition, breast-feeding is a risk factor probably related to differences in gut flora between breast-fed and formula-fed infants. There is global weakness; bulbar symptoms, including pupillary mydriasis; and associated constipation. Wound-related botulism is much rarer.

Myasthenia can occur as an acquired phenomenon, usually during adolescence, but it can also occur in the newborn because of passage of antibody across the placenta. Maternal history is obviously important in this situation. The extraocular movements are often the first and most frequently involved process. There is usually sparing of the pupillary reflex, which is not seen in patients with botulism. Improvement after injection of edrophonium (a short-acting cholinesterase inhibitor) is diagnostic of the myasthenic syndromes.

Certain varieties of ticks secrete a paralytic neurotoxin that can cause rapidly progressive weakness. The history of a tick bite or the finding of a tick on the patient is necessary for the diagnosis.

Organophosphates (usually found in insecticides) irreversibly bind to the acetylcholine receptor and in addition to weakness cause the classic signs of anticholinergic toxicity, such as pupillary dilation and a patient who is "red as a beet, dry as a bone, and mad as a hatter." Serum cholinesterase levels are elevated in organophosphate poisonings.

Muscle

The most common of the primary myopathic causes of weakness are the muscular dystrophies (Table 11-4). The muscular dystrophies are a group of heritable, progressive myopathies that cause weakness by degeneration and death of muscle fibers. Some of the most common types are summarized in Table 11-5.

Congenital myopathies are associated with static or occasionally only very slowly progressive weakness. There is usually a failure to attain motor milestones. In addition to weakness there is often profound hypotonia. Electromyography and muscle biopsy are the diagnostic tests of choice.

Familial periodic paralysis associated with abnormal potassium values is a rare, autosomal dominant inherited condition. Weakness may occur on awakening from sleep, with gradual recovery over several hours. Potassium levels are often low but may be elevated in a minority of patients.

Metabolic myopathy accompanies glycogen storage diseases, which are often associated with hypoglycemia, hepatomegaly, splenomegaly, and cardiomyopathy. Lipidoses and carnitine deficiencies have a similar presentation. These

TABLE 11-5

Clinical Features of the Muscular Dystrophies

Characteristic	Duchenne	Becker	Fascioscapulo-humeral	Limb-girdle	Myotonic
Inheritance	X-linked recessive	X-linked recessive	Autosomal dominant	Autosomal recessive	Autosomal dominant
Age of onset	Early childhood, adolescence	Late childhood	Variable, childhood through early adult life	Childhood to early adult	Highly variable
Pattern of weakness	Pelvic girdle, shoulder girdle	Pelvic girdle, shoulder girdle	Face, shoulder girdle	Pelvic girdle, shoulder girdle	Face, distal limbs
Rate of progression	Rapid	Slow	Very slow	Variable	Variable
Associated features	Pseudohypertrophy of calves	Pseudohypertrophy of calves	None	Pseudohypertrophy rare	Myotonia
Systemic features	Mental retardation, abnormal ECG, cardiomyopathy	Occasional mental retardation	None	None	Frequent mental retardation, heart block, cataracts, premature balding, testicular tubular atrophy, diabetes

disorders of lipid metabolism result in fatty infiltration of muscle tissue caused by defects in mitochondrial transport mechanisms.

Systemic carnitine deficiency results in a Reye syndrome-like illness with weakness, acidosis, hepatic failure, and low serum carnitine levels. Muscle carnitine deficiency has a presentation more restricted to weakness and normal serum carnitine levels, but low levels of carnitine are present in muscle tissue on biopsy. Another disorder is carnitine palmityltransferase deficiency, a condition that does not result in fatty replacement but causes prominent weakness and myoglobinuria, especially with sustained activity. Primary carnitine deficiency has been linked to short-chain and medium-chain acyl-CoA dehydrogenase deficiency.

Mitochondrial myopathies are diagnosed by electron microscopy of the mitochondria themselves. There are several forms, but most tend to be associated with central nervous system abnormalities, such as seizures, strokes, or retinitis. Myoclonic epilepsy with ragged red fibers, metabolic encephalopathy with lactic acidosis and strokelike episodes, Zellweger syndrome (Fig. 11-1) (cerebrohepatorenal syndrome), and Kearns-Sayre syndrome (acidosis and ophthalmoplegia) are examples of mitochondrial myopathies.

The collagen vascular diseases rarely present with weakness alone, though early on it may be the predominant complaint, especially in dermatomyositis and mixed connective tissue disease (Figs. 11-2 and 11-3). Clues from the history and physical examination should prompt an investigation of the autoantibody profile to allow the diagnosis of a specific syndrome.

Any of the classes of microorganisms (bacteria, viruses, parasites, and even fungi) may cause an infectious myositis. Focal tenderness and a history of an infectious prodrome support the diagnosis. Biopsy for direct visualization and culture of organisms along with serologic evidence of viral infections pinpoint the causative agent.

Addison disease, thyroid disorders, and parathyroid disease can be associated with generalized weakness and atrophy. Findings specific to the endocrinologic cause help to make these diagnoses. Thyroid function testing and electrolyte, calcium, and phosphorus levels are helpful in screening for endocrine myopathy.

Secondary Causes of Weakness

Weakness is a protean manifestation of many disease processes, and any chronic illness, especially if complicated by prolonged bed rest, may be accompanied by fatigue and global weakness. Weakness is also a common chronic symptom of a functional nature connected to ailments, such as chronic fatigue syndrome and depression. The treatment for this weakness is treatment of the primary condition and gradual resumption of a daily routine.

Similarly, depression is characterized by many psychosomatic complaints, and weakness is certainly no exception. Weakness is often global and mild. Often the weakness is out

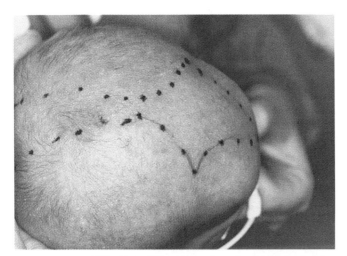
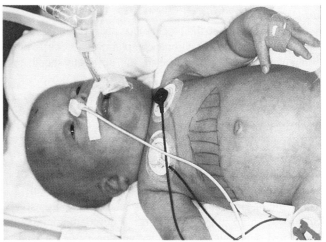

FIG. 11-1 This infant has the high forehead, enlarged fontanelles, and hepatomegaly seen with Zellweger syndrome. Affected infants also have hypotonia and weakness from a mitochondrial myopathy. (Courtesy Dr. J. Nard, Youngstown, Ohio.)

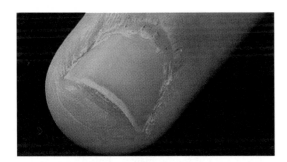

FIG. 11-2 Nailbed telangiectasia. Erythema can be seen around the nail edge. The pinpoint telangiectasia may require a magnifying lens to identify.

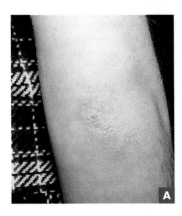
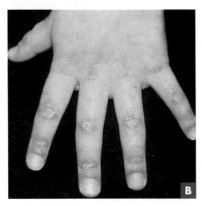
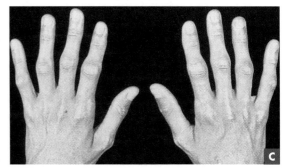

FIG. 11-3 Typical rash of dermatomyositis, as seen on the elbow (*A*) and the hands (*B* and *C*), showing erythema and pale, atrophic skin changes (Gottron papules).

of proportion to other neurologic signs and may be in an anatomically unusual distribution. Detailed investigation of the psychosocial background for triggers and stressors is of primary importance. In such circumstances, aggressive rehabilitation in association with psychologic counseling is indicated. However, organic illness, such as hypothyroidism, can cause weakness and depression and must be considered.

Although weakness may be a part of any of the somatoform disorders, the most common presentation is that of conversion reaction as a gait disturbance (see Chapter 6). Pathologic gait patterns that vary over time or those that recur with interspersed periods of normal gait should raise the suspicion of conversion reaction. Weakness and sensory findings may not correspond to any explainable anatomic distribution, and strength testing of the same muscle groups (with the patient lying down) may be completely normal. Spasticity of tone is absent, and patients may drag the involved leg rather than display the circumduction seen in a truly spastic gait.

Careful attention to the psychosocial history is indicated in the investigation of any chronic complaint. If an affective or somatoform disorder is suspected, the physician should involve psychiatric services early in the diagnostic process.

History

When evaluating a patient with weakness, Lewis and Berman state that the primary purpose of the history is to provide information concerning the pace of the disease process. In addition the history should completely characterize the nature of the weakness and through directed questioning pinpoint associated signs and symptoms that provide diagnostic clues. The contributions of family medical and social histories must not be overlooked.

The history should begin with a detailed and specific description of the weakness and how it began. The time of onset and rate of progression are very important. Certain diseases, such as transverse myelitis, are marked by rapid progression. Others, such as infantile botulism, are slowly progressive. In entities such as cerebral palsy the weakness is usually nonprogressive. When attempting to obtain a history of a slowly progressive or nonprogressive process in an infant, the physician should pose questions regarding the attainment of motor milestones. Knowledge of these milestones greatly facilitates history taking and the physical examination of the young infant. A standard approach is based on the Gesell developmental schedule.

The location of the weakness is important. Global weakness has a broad differential diagnosis, but weakness of a focal area lends itself much more easily to anatomic localization. As a somewhat oversimplified rule of thumb, proximal weakness is a hallmark of muscle disease and distal weakness is more often the result of neurologic disease.

If weakness is periodic, which it may be in metabolic diseases, cyclicity should be established. Any exacerbating and relieving factors should be documented because they often give important clues to the cause.

Several specific questions should be asked about associated factors. A history of major trauma merits consideration of a brain or spinal cord lesion, and weakness associated with chronic progressive headache should suggest a cause localized to the central nervous system. Inflammatory and infectious causes of weakness may be accompanied by fever. Tenderness of a muscle with no history of trauma suggests myositis or dermatomyositis. Neoplastic disease may present with a history of vague pains, weight loss, fatigue, and weakness. These factors and their implications are summarized in Table 11-6.

The past medical history is crucial when attempting to time the onset of a disease or to establish a congenital cause.

TABLE 11-6

Associated Symptoms and Their Implications

Historic finding	Implication
Fever	Inflammatory or infectious cause
Arthritis	Collagen vascular disease
Rash	SLE, dermatomyositis, viral cause
Tenderness	Infectious myositis, dermatomyositis
Tick exposure	Tick paralysis
Urine color change	Rhabdomyolysis
Weight loss	Neoplasia, eating disorder
Headache	CNS process
Trauma	CNS, cord injury, rhabdomyolysis

CNS, Central nervous system; *SLE,* Systemic lupus erythematosus.

Lack of movement in utero and breech presentation point toward a prenatal event. The circumstances of the birth and immediate neonatal period should be reviewed. Apgar scores, birth trauma or hypoxia, and history of "floppiness" in the neonatal period are important historic elements. After the birth history, a detailed developmental history should be obtained, with special attention paid to motor and cognitive milestones. Any significant illnesses or medication use should also be documented.

A careful family history should be obtained. For instance, the muscular dystrophies are a common example of heritable causes of weakness. Also, because many of the neurodegenerative diseases are inherited in an autosomal recessive fashion, the examiner should investigate the possibility of consanguinity and any fetal or neonatal deaths in the family.

The social history is useful for assessing the impact of the disease process on the family unit. Because many of the diseases are progressive, the social history is a starting point for investigating strengths in the therapeutic milieu for the patient's future. The physician should also be wary of red flags for potential child abuse and occult trauma or occult psychopathology in the patient.

Finally the coincidence of either onset of symptoms or exacerbation of symptoms with dramatic changes in the social environment points toward the diagnosis of a psychosomatic disorder.

Physical Examination

The physical examination is a powerful tool for localizing the anatomic source of weakness. It can also disclose important

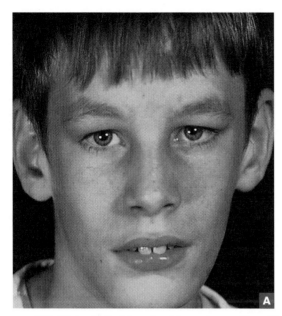 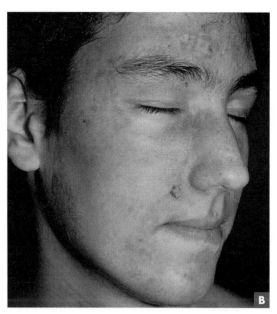

FIG. 11-4 *A,* Facial rash of dermatomyositis with a violaceous color around the eyes and malar region. *B,* More severe, erythematous, scaly rash involving almost the entire face. Note involvement of the nasolabial folds.

associated signs, such as the heliotrope rash of polymyositis (Fig. 11-4) or the "stork legs" of Charcot-Marie-Tooth disease (Fig. 11-5).

The general examination should be complete (Table 11-7). At first glance the examiner must establish the presence or absence of respiratory distress. If weakness has progressed to the point of respiratory insufficiency, the encounter assumes an emergency pace and the focus must shift from evaluation to immediate intervention. Assuming that respiratory distress is absent, the general examination should proceed as usual.

Growth velocity should be established to help determine the chronicity of the disease process, and dysmorphic features should be noted if present because they suggest a congenital cause of weakness. The presence of macrocephaly or microcephaly suggests a central nervous system cause. The skin should be meticulously examined for rashes, which may be hallmarks of the collagen vascular diseases, and ticks or tick bites. Pupillary reaction and extraocular movements should be noted because these are the first sites of involvement in the myasthenic syndromes. The thyroid should be palpated for the presence of a goiter. The importance of the pulmonary examination was noted earlier, but in addition to respiratory distress, the physician should note possible signs of chronic aspiration often present in the child with cerebral palsy or infantile botulism. Cardiovascular status should always be assessed, and the presence or absence of cardiomegaly, which occurs in some forms of muscular dystrophy, should be noted. Visceral organomegaly is a hallmark of many of the neurodegenerative storage diseases. The joint examination is obviously important if collagen vascular diseases are a possibility. The examiner should attempt to elicit muscle tenderness by squeezing the gastrocnemius

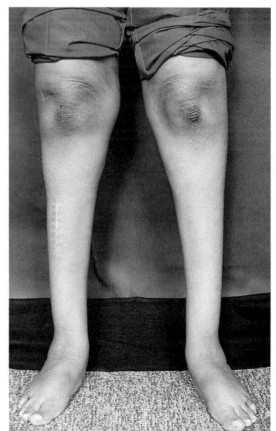

FIG. 11-5 Charcot-Marie-Tooth disease. Patient, age 15, with distal muscular atrophy of the lower extremities ("stork-leg" appearance).

TABLE 11-7

Physical Examination Findings and Their Implications

Finding	Implication
Growth pattern	Establishes chronicity, ability to feed
Dysmorphism	Genetic syndromes
Rash	Viral, SLE, dermatomyositis
Nailbed telangiectasia	Dermatomyositis
Pupil and EOM involvement	Myasthenia, botulism
Goiter	Hypothyroidism
Respiratory distress	Implies an emergency situation
Cardiomegaly	Muscular dystrophy
Organomegaly	Storage disease
Arthritis	Collagen vascular disease
Tenderness	Infectious myositis, dermatomyositis
Muscle wasting	Lower motor neuron etiology
Muscle absence	Congenital syndrome

EOM, Extraocular muscle; SLE, systemic lupus erythematosus.

and quadriceps muscles. Muscle tenderness is present in both polymyositis and infectious myositis. Finally, increased muscle bulk, such as the calf pseudohypertrophy of Duchenne muscular dystrophy (Fig. 11-6), muscle wasting, or frank absence of a muscle, should be noted. The significance of several features of the general physical examination are presented in Table 11-2.

It should come as no surprise that a complete neurologic examination is a must in the evaluation of weakness. The level of consciousness can easily be assessed even during the interview. A more formal mental status examination should be performed as soon as the child's age allows. Most preschoolers can participate in naming, following commands, memory tasks, and wordplay. The examiner must again develop development-specific standards through interactions with normal children.

A formal assessment of strength should document presence, specific location, and degree of weakness. In infancy, strength "testing" is often limited to observation for symmetric motor movements and resistance to the examiner. Strength in the toddler and early preschooler is best assessed by observation of normal play. By the age of 4 years, most children can cooperate with traditional motor testing. Strength can then be quantitatively graded on a 6-point scale (Table 11-8). In addition to testing functional muscle groups in each of the extremities, a special effort should be made to assess proximal muscle function. Climbing stairs and quickly rising from a sitting or lying position are effective ways to assess proximal motor strength. The Gowers sign, a classic indication of proximal muscle weakness, is shown in Fig. 6-1.

The differences between tone and strength were alluded to in the introduction to this chapter. The pull-to-sit maneuver and ventral suspension are simple, reliable tests for establishing truncal tone, and resistance to passive movement of the arms and legs is a reflection of extremity tone. Age-specific norms for tone must be established through practice. Standard developmental scales exist for comparison. Tone is one of the major discriminating factors in deciding whether a lesion involves the UMN or LMN (see section on localization); therefore it behooves the examiner to evaluate tone carefully.

The deep tendon reflexes are similarly useful in determining whether a lesion is in the UMN or LMN. They should be elicited in all four extremities and can be graded in a 4-point fashion (Table 11-9). Some pathologic processes cause early loss of deep tendon reflexes out of proportion to loss of strength. Guillain-Barré syndrome and spinal muscular atrophy are often suspected on this basis alone.

The cranial nerves should be examined in sequence. Cranial neuropathy indicates a brainstem component if it occurs in the company of UMN weakness. More often, however, it implies an LMN (as in Bell's palsy), neuromuscular junction (as in infantile botulism or myasthenia gravis), or myopathic (as in Fukuyama type congenital muscular dystrophy) process.

Cerebellar function should be noted because it may establish the diagnosis of ataxia rather than weakness. With the infant the physician is limited to observing reaching for toys with each hand in succession, truncal stability, and presence or absence of nystagmus. In the toddler, gait provides much additional information. In the older child, rapid repetitive movements can also be assessed.

Gait, in addition to providing information about coordination, can help characterize weakness. UMN lesions are accompanied by the stiff-legged, adducted, spastic gait. Toe walking that is persistent and inflexible or develops after a period of normal walking suggests increased tone in the lower extremities. LMN lesions affecting the ankle dorsiflexors result in a toe-to-heel "steppage" gait rather than the typical heel-to-toe gait. Proximal muscle weakness results in a shuffling, waddling gait with minimal elevation of the foot off of the floor.

The sensory examination is often neglected and can be quite difficult, especially in the young child. On the other hand, the detection of a sensory level in a patient with weakness is a diagnostic gold mine because it certainly localizes the pathology to the spinal cord. Light touch and pinprick tests should be attempted in all children. In older or cooperative children, position and temperature sense can be added. In the youngest or most uncooperative children, the examination may be limited to noting the withdrawal of an extremity in response to a mildly painful stimulus.

The examiner should attempt to elicit the Babinski reflex in every child because it implies UMN pathology. Similarly, fasciculations (uncontrolled rapid twitches of a motor unit) imply LMN pathology. Myoclonus (paroxysmally sus-

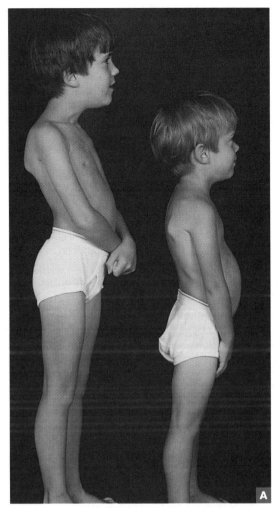
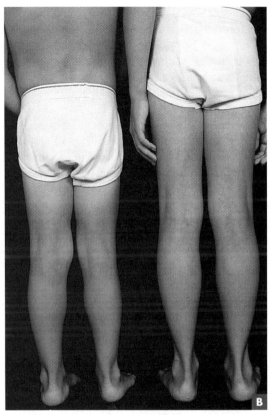

FIG. 11-6 Duchenne muscular dystrophy. *A,* These brothers, ages 5 and 8, show progressive compensatory postural adjustments, with broadening of stance, accentuated lumbar lordosis, and forward thrusting of the abdomen. *B,* Enlargement of calves.

TABLE 11-8

Strength Grading

Grade	Description
5	Maximal resistance to examiner
4	Suboptimal resistance to examiner
3	Resists gravity only
2	Movement after elimination of gravity
1	Only flickers of muscle activity
0	No muscle activity

TABLE 11-9

Reflex Grading

Grade	Description
4	Very brisk with clonus
3	Brisk with increased amplitude
2	Normal
1	Sluggish and low in amplitude
0	No reflexes

tained involuntary contraction of a muscle) should be sought because it is a hallmark of myotonic dystrophy. Myoclonus can be noted by the inability to release grip (e.g., in a handshake). It can also be elicited by percussion over the thenar eminence, which causes sustained abduction and flexion of the thumb in patients with myoclonus.

After a complete history and physical examination, the first step in narrowing the broad differential diagnosis is to anatomically localize the pathologic process. This step gives logical structure to further investigation.

Approach to the Patient

A detailed history and careful physical examination greatly narrow the differential diagnosis in patients with weakness. At this point in the evaluation, the nature and pace of progression of the weakness should be reasonably clear, as should its location of origin. Associated signs and symptoms should be reviewed for their diagnostic implications. Ancillary testing can then be used to investigate a particular anatomic area or to help establish a particular diagnosis. Laboratory and imaging studies should not be employed indiscriminately but in a limited fashion as suggested by the history and physical examination.

If a cerebral or spinal cord UMN process is suspected, MRI is the most effective and efficient diagnostic study. Cerebrospinal fluid (CSF) analysis is useful for culture or polymerase chain reaction to establish an infectious cause. Protein analysis of the CSF helps to diagnose demyelinating conditions, and cytologic examination may make a fairly noninvasive diagnosis in neoplastic processes.

Diagnostic studies in suspected LMN pathology are quite limited. Nerve conduction velocity testing documents a neuropathy if present, and occasionally the pattern of conduction impairment suggests a specific diagnosis. Specific enzymatic assays are available for the metabolic defects associated with LMN weakness (Table 11-3). Toxicologic and heavy metal screens can be performed when these specific diagnoses are suspected.

When a primary myopathic process is diagnosed, serum levels of creatine phosphokinase (CPK), aldolase, lactate dehydrogenase (LDH), and the transaminases can be used as nonspecific markers of cellular injury. CPK and LDH can be differentiated into isoenzymes that give some specificity with respect to cardiac versus skeletal muscle involvement. Urinalysis is indicated to look for myoglobin, a hallmark of rhabdomyolysis. A positive urine dipstick test for "blood" in the absence of red blood cells on a microscopic examination should raise the suspicion of myoglobinuria.

Electrolytes are useful to establish the diagnosis of the potassium-related periodic paralyses. Liver function testing, along with an electrocardiogram to investigate the possibility of a concomitant cardiomyopathy, are useful if a metabolic storage disease is suspected. Urinary total and free carnitine levels can be measured (and supplementation can be begun while awaiting the results).

The erythrocyte sedimentation rate (ESR) is elevated nonspecifically in inflammatory processes, but in the right clinical context an elevated ESR justifies more specific testing for the collagen vascular diseases or other inflammatory disorders.

Specific enzyme analyses are available for the metabolic myopathies, and detection of the dystrophin gene product that is absent in certain muscular dystrophies is now possible.

When combined with nerve conduction velocity testing, electromyography can help separate neuropathic and myopathic processes and can occasionally give a specific diagnosis.

Although certainly the most invasive diagnostic tests, open muscle biopsy and traditional and electron microscopy are often relied on to specifically diagnose a myopathic process. Before muscle biopsy, a neurologist and a muscle pathologist should be consulted to ensure proper specimen selection and handling.

SUMMARY

The differential diagnosis of chronic muscular weakness is vast and diverse but can be approached logically after a detailed history and physical examination. Localization of the pathologic process along the neuroaxis greatly narrows the differential diagnosis and suggests further testing. Careful attention to the pattern of the weakness, associated signs and symptoms, and limited diagnostic testing helps to establish a cause, upon which therapeutic decisions may be based.

Therapeutic interventions are as diverse as the differential diagnosis and are beyond the scope of this chapter. With chronic weakness, even when specific pharmacotherapy exists, it is seldom completely successful in isolation. Physical, occupational, and at times speech therapists should be employed early in the diagnostic process because their general contributions to rehabilitation are often as valuable as specific interventions once a diagnosis is established.

ILLUSTRATIVE CASES

Case 1. A 10-week-old African-American boy has increased fussiness and poor feeding. He did well until approximately 2 nights earlier, when he began feeding less vigorously. He is exclusively breast fed. He has had no vomiting or diarrhea. He normally stools 3 times per day, but he had only one stool 3 days ago and none since. His past medical history and birth history are unremarkable. He had no floppiness in the newborn period. His family history reveals no weakness. Developmentally, he had a social smile and lifted his head when lying on his belly; however, he has not done either of these for the last 2 or 3 days.

On physical examination, he is a whining, tired-appearing infant. He is afebrile with normal vital signs. He has a sunken fontanelle and sunken eyes. His ocular examination also reveals ptosis, sluggish pupillary responses, and slow extraocular movements. There is no nystagmus. On neurologic examination he is alert but drowsy. In addition to the ocular findings, his face is symmetric, but he will not smile. While attempting to drink an oral rehydration solution, he drools and then coughs and sputters. His tone is globally 1+, and his strength is 2+, even with maximal stimulation by the examiner. His tendon reflexes are 1+ and symmetric.

A blood count and electrolytes are within normal limits with the exception of a bicarbonate of 18 mEq/L and a BUN of 22 mg/dl. A urine toxicology screen is negative. His dehydration is corrected over a 24-hour period, and his eyes and fontanelle are no longer sunken. His examination is otherwise unchanged. On the second hospital day a stool is induced with a glycerine suppository. Assay of the stool is positive for Clostridium botulinum *toxin*. The infant is fed via nasogastric tube over the next 48 hours and monitored closely for signs of respiratory distress, which do not develop. His strength gradually improves, and he is restarted on oral feedings and discharged.

Here the discrete onset, history of breast-feeding and constipation, and loss of milestones point to an acquired phenomenon. The physical examination is consistent with disease of the neuromuscular junction because of prominent findings related to the extraocular and facial muscles. The laboratory values are due to mild dehydration from his poor oral intake. The loss of a functional swallow mandates the nasogastric feedings. Definitive diagnosis is based on the positive stool assay.

Case 2. A 6-month-old white boy was brought to the emergency room with labored respirations. He began breathing harder about 1 week prior, but this was attributed to a stuffy nose. His respirations have become slowly more labored over the week. He was born at term via caesarean section because of breech presentation. His birth weight was 3320 g, and his mother is 33 and primiparous. The pregnancy was uncomplicated. He has fed and grown well and has not seen his pediatrician other than for routine care and immunizations. Developmentally, he smiles socially, coos, and attempts to reach for objects but cannot hold onto them well after he grasps them. He has not yet rolled over or sat unsupported. Family history is unremarkable.

On physical examination he is an alert, cooing boy, lying in a frog-legged position. Vital signs are as follows: temperature, 37° C; pulse, 148; respirations, 48 and labored; blood pressure, 98/55. Length and weight are at the 50th percentile as is head circumference. General examination is remarkable only for tachypnea with mild retractions and nasal flaring. Lung fields are clear on auscultation. He does have a mucoid nasal discharge. On neurologic examination he has globally decreased tone manifested by head lag on the pull-to-sit maneuver, flexion at the waist on the ventral suspension maneuver, and minimal passive resistance in all extremities. During noxious parts of the examination, he attempts to push the examiner away. Strength is graded at 2+ . Despite persistent effort, tendon reflexes cannot be elicited. Cranial nerve examination is normal. There is no myotonia in the child or his parents.

Electrolytes and CPK level are within normal limits. Neurologic consultation is obtained, and EMG studies with nerve conduction velocity confirm the diagnosis of Werdnig-Hoffmann spinal muscular atrophy.

The child is observed and treated supportively for a presumed viral upper respiratory tract infection. His respiratory status gradually improved with the clearing of his rhinitis. He was discharged to home after in-depth discussion of his condition and the prognosis with the family. They elect not to have him intubated should an emergency occur.

Here the history of breech presentation suggests a prenatal onset. Examination is strongly suggestive of a neuropathic rather than a myopathic process with hypotonia and absent reflexes. A normal CPK supports this notion. The diagnosis is strongly suspected clinically, but in addition to the aforementioned studies, electron microscopy of muscle biopsy specimens and more recently genetic testing are also employed in the diagnosis of the spinal muscular atrophies.

Case 3. A 26-month-old white boy's parents bring him to the pediatrician for evaluation of clumsy walking. He was born at term after an uncomplicated antenatal course by vaginal delivery. His neonatal course was similarly uncomplicated, and he was never considered "floppy" by his family or the pediatrician.

He smiled socially at 2 months, cooed at about the same time, babbled at 9 months, spoke his first word (other than "mama" or "dada") at 11 months, and now has two binary word phrases. His pincer grasp (as evidenced by picking up a single Cheerio) first appeared at 9 months, and he is now able to zip and unzip but cannot button or unbutton. He sat unsupported at 8 months, pulled to stand at 13 months and did not take steps until nearly 18 months. He is unable to go up or down stairs and does not run more than a few steps.

His parents are concerned about his motor delay and also note that he trips over his own feet frequently. There is no known family history of clumsiness, weakness, or motor delay.

Physical examination reveals a happy, well-appearing 2-year-old with growth parameters at the 10th percentile consistently. His vital signs are all within normal limits. He is not dysmorphic, and a general physical examination is essentially unremarkable, though it is noted that his biceps, quadriceps, and gastrocnemius muscles are very well developed. He has no joint contractures. A neurologic examination is remarkable for weakness of the upper (grade 4) and lower (grade 3) extremities. He is unable to climb onto a two-step sliding board in the examination room. When arising from a prone position on the floor, he has great difficulty and does display Gowers maneuver. Muscle tone is normal, and bulk is increased as described above. Tendon reflexes and cranial nerve examination are normal. His sensation to light touch and pinprick is also normal. His walking gait is waddling, and he has an exaggerated lumbar lordosis when standing. When asked to run, he takes a few quick steps on his tiptoes then stops. He falls on a second attempt.

A CPK level returns at 7500 IU, and a preliminary diagnosis of Duchenne muscular dystrophy is made. The family is referred to a nearby regional muscular dystrophy center for coordination of services. Subsequently, genetic analysis returns and shows a deletion in the area of the dystrophin gene.

The history here points to a discrete onset in late infancy. The developmental history is appropriate for age in all areas except the gross motor domain. Physical examination highlights proximal muscular weakness, which as a rule is typical of myopathic processes. The marked elevation of the CPK essentially makes the diagnosis, which is later confirmed by the molecular genetic analysis.

ANNOTATED BIBLIOGRAPHY

Dubowitz V: *Muscle disorders in childhood*, St Louis, 1978, Mosby–Year Book.

Every chapter in Dr. Dubowitz's text is comprehensive and authoritative. The author gives excellent, in-depth reviews of muscular disorders, including the muscular dystrophies, congenital myopathies, poliomyelitis, and spinal muscular atrophies. This book is also the gold standard reference for the floppy infant syndrome.

Lewis B, Berman P: Progressive weakness in infancy and childhood, *Pediatr Rev* 8:200-208, 1987.

This is a crucial paper for the clinician. It is essentially the basis for the approach to diagnosis taken in this chapter. Well written and easily understood, it is a "must-read" article.

Swaiman: *Pediatric neurology*, ed 2, St Louis, 1994, Mosby–Year Book.

Although textual, this reference is quite pertinent for the clinician. The childhood neurologic examination is indeed an art form and Dr. Swaiman's text devotes substantial space to useful techniques in an age-based fashion. The text provides pearls from an experienced clinician.

BIBLIOGRAPHY

Asbury A: Diagnostic considerations in Guillain-Barré syndrome, *Ann Neurol* 9(suppl):1-5, 1981.

Cassidy, Petty: *Textbook of rheumatology,* Philadelphia, 1995 WB Saunders.

Dimauro S, Bonilla E, Zeviani M, et al: Mitochondrial myopathies, *Ann Neurol* 17:521-538, 1985.

Engel A: Myasthenia gravis and myasthenic syndromes, *Ann Neurol* 16:519-534, 1984.

Feigen RD, Stechenberg BW, Strandgard BH: Diphtheria. In *Pediatric infectious disease,* Philadelphia, 1992, WB Saunders.

Feigen RD, Stechenberg BW: Myositis. In *Pediatric infectious disease,* Philadelphia, 1987, WB Saunders.

Hobson A: Peripheral neuropathy in childhood: an update in diagnosis and management, *Pediatr Ann* 12:814-820, 1983.

Johnson R, Clay S, Arnon S: Diagnosis and management of infant botulism, *Am J Dis Child* 133:586-593, 1979.

Jones KL, editor: *Smith's recognizable patterns of human malformation,* Philadelphia, 1988, WB Saunders.

Knobloch H, Stevens F, Malone AF: *Manual of developmental diagnosis,* Hagerstown, NJ, 1980, Harper & Row.

Long S: Botulism in infancy, *Pediatr Infect Dis J* 3:266-271, 1984.

Menkes JH: *Textbook of child neurology,* Philadelphia, 1990, Lea & Febiger.

Percy AK: The inherited neurodegenerative disorders of childhood: clinical assessment, *J Child Neurol* 2:82-97, 1987.

Spika JS, et al: Risk factors for infant botulism in the United States, *Am J Dis Child* 143:828-832, 1989.

Spiro AJ: Approach to the diagnosis in the child with muscular weakness, *Pediatr Ann* 6:149-161, 1977.

Vanesse M, Dubowitz V: Dominantly inherited peroneal muscle atrophy in infancy and childhood, *Muscle Nerve* 4:26-30, 1981.

White RH, Robbins DL: Clinical significance and interpretation of antinuclear antibodies, *West J Med* 147:210-213, 1987.

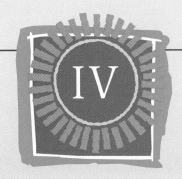

Circulatory

Syncope

J. CARLTON GARTNER, Jr.

 ## Key Points

- The most common cause of syncope in pediatric patients is vasovagal; a primary cardiac cause is quite rare.

- Clues, such as syncope with exercise or worrisome family history, should prompt further investigation.

- Tilt-table testing may be helpful in evaluating patients with unusual or confusing symptoms.

*S*yncope is defined as a transient, reversible loss of consciousness that is associated with the inability to maintain an upright posture. It is a relatively common problem in adults and the subject of fairly extensive study. In pediatric patients it is estimated that about 15% will experience a fainting episode by the end of adolescence. In one survey, 47% of college students reported syncopal episodes. Most of these episodes are benign, but all physicians are haunted by the issue of sudden death among children and worry that a serious underlying cause may be related to "passing out." About 25% of children who die suddenly have a prodromal syncopal event. Some children are described as feeling lightheaded or "almost fainting." Are they at the same risk as those who become completely unconscious? What about the adolescent who faints at the sight of blood? In this chapter an approach that should allow a well-reasoned plan of evaluation and management for patients with syncope is developed. Other chapters deal with closely associated paroxysmal events, such as spells (Chapter 10) and infantile apnea (Chapter 13), that may be relevant to the discussion.

Pathophysiology

The list of differential diagnoses for syncope would seem to make an approach to the physiologic mechanisms impossible (Table 12-1). However, the final common pathway for syncope is transient cerebral dysfunction usually from underperfusion. Most commonly this is caused by neurovascular mechanisms. The use of the tilt-table test (discussed later) is an attempt to reproduce this pathophysiology. Upright posture leads to pooling of blood in the lower body and decreased ventricular filling and decreased arterial pressure. Arterial and central baroreceptor reflexes then are activated, leading to increased heart rate and sympathetic tone. This state of decreased left ventricular volume and increased sympathetic tone may activate cardiac mechanoreceptors, triggering neural reflexes (vasodepressor or vasovagal) that lead to hypotension or bradycardia. The raised sympathetic tone has been confirmed by several studies that have documented increased urinary and plasma epinephrine and norepinephrine just before syncopal episodes. This finding led to the use of isoproterenol to enhance the rapidity and accuracy of the tilt-table test by further increasing sympathetic tone.

There are numerous recently published studies using various modifications of the tilt-table test (Fig. 12-1), and several include only children. Basically, patients undergo baseline measurements of heart rate, blood pressure, and continuous electrocardiogram (ECG). Most studies use noninvasive monitoring, but occasionally intraarterial catheters are inserted for blood pressure recording. The table is rotated, usually to an angle of 60 to 80 degrees (head up), and measurements are recorded for various periods of time. Symptoms are reproduced in some patients with syncope, and these patients are rapidly returned to a supine position (Fig. 12-2). The duration of the test may be prolonged (60 minutes), which is one factor that has led to the use of isoproterenol infusion followed by repeat measurements.

Of interest is a study demonstrating that during Valsalva maneuver patients with vasodepressor syncope demonstrate significantly greater drops in systolic and diastolic blood pressure and require more time to return to baseline values. Unfortunately, this study was done in a sophisticated laboratory with intraarterial pressure recording and does not provide a test that could become useful in more clinical settings.

TABLE 12-1

Differential Diagnoses of Syncope

Diagnosis	Characteristics
Neurovascular (Neurocardiogenic)	
Vasodepressor (vasovagal)	Prodrome, situational, "typical fainting spell"
Malignant	Prolonged asystole
Excessive vagal tone	Athletes, varying degrees of AV block
Reflex	Cough, stretch, defecate, etc.; pallid breathholding
Orthostatic hypotension	Hypovolemia, Addison disease, renal insufficiency
Cardiac	Sudden, no warning; exertion
Cardiomyopathies	IHSS, dilated cardiomyopathies
LV outflow obstruction	Aortic stenosis
Coronary artery	Aberrant right coronary
Marfan syndrome	Examination: tall, thin fingers, pectus, hyperextensible joints
Dysrhythmia	Palpitations
Prolonged QTc	Family history of sudden death, syncope, seizures
Wolff-Parkinson-White syndrome	Delta waves
Cyanosis	R to L shunt
Pulmonary	Primary pulmonary hypertension
Breathholding (cyanotic)	Typical spell, anger, frustration
Other Causes	
Epilepsy	Aura, movements, onset in prone position, postictal phase
Hyperventilation	Multiple symptoms, may be reproducible
Hysteria	Older children; other symptoms: gait disturbance, weakness, paralysis
Migraine	Headache, family history
Metabolic	Rare, hypoglycemia, fasting, time of day

AV, Atrioventricular; *IHSS,* idiopathic hypertrophic subaortic stenosis; *LV,* left ventricle; *QTc,* QT interval corrected for heart rate.

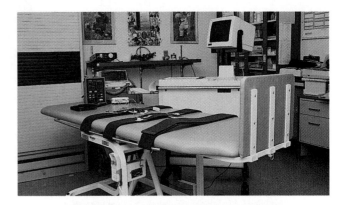

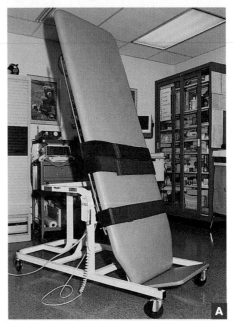

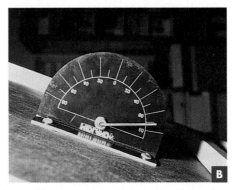

FIG. 12-1 *A,* The equipment in a testing laboratory demonstrates supine and upright positions of the table (*top* and *bottom*). *B,* The degree of tilt is measured accurately by the position device as illustrated.

All is not straightforward, however, in our understanding of vasodepressor syncope. A recent report demonstrated vasodepressor syncope in a heart transplant patient, a procedure in which the organ is always denervated. In addition, Kapoor demonstrated that normal adult controls were likely to have hypotension and bradycardia during tilt-table testing with isoproterenol. Perhaps it is most important to recognize the lack of key pieces of information regarding the neurally mediated cardiac reflexes. Once again, all studies that attempt to prove the cause of a disorder should be carefully

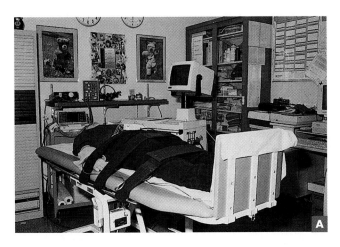

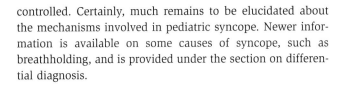

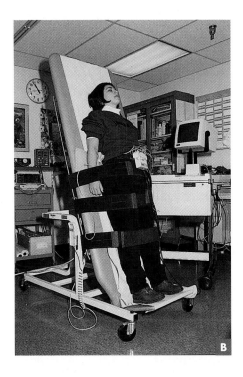

FIG. 12-2 The patient is undergoing tilt-table testing in the laboratory at Children's Hospital. Pulse, blood pressure, and oxygen saturation are monitored. An arterial catheter is often inserted for more precise monitoring, along with an intravenous catheter for administration of isoproterenol and other medications.

controlled. Certainly, much remains to be elucidated about the mechanisms involved in pediatric syncope. Newer information is available on some causes of syncope, such as breathholding, and is provided under the section on differential diagnosis.

Literature Survey

There are several review articles but no prospective studies of syncope in childhood. Some information is available from adult series that include some adolescent patients. The most comprehensive is that of Kapoor and colleagues, which included 204 patients. In simplified terms, after careful evaluation the groups were divided into cardiovascular (53), noncardiovascular (54), and unknown (97) causes. A key finding of this study is that the overall mortality at 12 months was strikingly higher for those patients with cardiovascular causes. Although the unknown group appears large, many of these patients may have had vasovagal syncope. A diagnosis of vasovagal (vasodepressor) syncope was made only if a definite precipitating cause, such as fear or pain, could be identified. Because most of the mortality in this study was from underlying heart disease, a general principle evolves—syncope in children is usually benign because underlying heart disease is much rarer in children than in adults.

One other large prospective study in adults deserves mention because of the large portion of patients who had psychiatric disorders. Koenig and colleagues prospectively studied 197 adults and included a structured psychiatric interview for many of the patients whose diagnosis remained questionable. Psychiatric diagnoses were made overall in 39% of the young (16- to 39-year-old) patients. Diagnoses included depression,

panic disorder, and conversion disorder. Hyperventilation (open mouth; slow, deep breaths [about 20 per minute]) often reproduced symptoms and was suggestive of a psychiatric diagnosis with a positive predictive value of 59%. Other studies have not used the detailed psychiatric interview, but the study also raises the question of "finding what you are looking for." Further study using detailed interviews may yield interesting results that may be applicable at least to adolescent patients.

Two studies in children are particularly useful. Gordon and others retrospectively looked at 73 children with syncope, 59 of whom had multiple episodes. Three patients were found to have underlying cardiac disorders, including primary myocardial disease, sick sinus syndrome, and nodal tachycardia. At an average follow-up of 2 years, there were no deaths. The authors looked at the total cost for procedures ($77,419) and hospital days ($141,568) and questioned the need for the extensive work-up in most of the patients. Pratt and Fleisher looked retrospectively at 77 children seen in their emergency room with syncope. Forty had true syncope, and 17 had "near syncope" in which there was a sensation of light-headedness but no complete loss of consciousness. Most patients had vasovagal episodes or postural hypotension that was easily treated. Of note is the fact that *no* abnormalities of laboratory or ancillary studies were found in the group with near syncope, thus making this a group that may not warrant further testing.

Differential Diagnosis

The differential diagnosis of syncope may be divided into three broad categories. We call the first major category "neurovascular" because that is where the essence of the problem lies, in the control and interactions between the autonomic nervous system and the cardiovascular system. "Cardiac" and "other" are the remaining large categories.

Neurovascular (Neurocardiogenic) Causes

Vasodepressor (Vasovagal)

Vasodepression is the leading cause of fainting in children (and the one most people refer to when they use the term *faint*). As mentioned previously the mechanism is thought to be related to hypovolemia, excessive sympathetic tone, and reflex arc involving the vagus nerve. The history is key in this diagnosis. There is usually a trigger or prodromal situation, such as hunger, fear, high room temperature, pain, anxiety, or fatigue. The patient has signs and symptoms, such as pallor, chills, sweating, dizziness, blurry vision, tunnel vision, nausea, and weakness. There is usually rapid recovery after a brief period in the supine position, and the patient is lucid with normal speech afterward, although pallor may remain. Observers often give good information about the events. Although such spells are often recurrent, there is no evidence that they are dangerous. Patients can often avoid situations associated with fainting in the past to help prevent episodes.

A strong positive family history of syncope may be valuable because the disorder tends to be familial. A Canadian study of children with vasodepressor or vasovagal syncope found that 27 of 30 had at least one first-degree relative with syncope, and in 11 of 30 cases both a sibling and parent had syncope (compared to 1 in 24 controls). Thus support for the diagnosis may come from the family history.

Recently, several investigators have described a condition termed *malignant vasovagal syndrome*. These patients have sudden "drop attacks" without the usual prodrome of vasodepressor syncope. When tested on the tilt table, they often have prolonged periods of asystole. Use of beta-blocking agents or even cardiac pacing may be necessary for this condition if recurrent and severe episodes occur.

Excess Vagal Tone

Bradycardia is common in highly conditioned athletes, who may occasionally have some degree of atrioventricular (AV) block. Some of these individuals have an increase in vagal tone with exertion and concomitant syncope. This group warrants very careful investigation because other, more dangerous causes of exercise-induced syncope may be present, such as occult dysrhythmia or obstructive cardiomyopathy.

Reflex Syncope

Bradycardia and rapid-onset syncope may occur with several triggers, including cough, stretching in adolescents, defecation, micturition, or swallowing. These presumably have a relationship to a reflex arc (carotid sinus) or to peripheral vasodilation. Key questions about the exact onset are obviously relevant. Also included in this group of reflex-induced syncope are pallid breathholding spells. As opposed to the more

typical cyanotic breathholding spells that occur after crying, pallid spells occur immediately after a sudden pain or injury, often to the head. The child rapidly becomes pale and faints. Onset of episodes is usually before 12 months of age, with a range of 6 to 24 months. These children have a much higher incidence of asystole as a response to ocular pressure, and several long-term follow-up studies have demonstrated an increased incidence of syncope in adulthood. Recent attempts to document abnormalities of the autonomic nervous system in pallid breathholding spells have demonstrated subtle differences from controls, such as significantly lower blood pressure when orthostatic testing is done. The rapid onset of symptoms without the prolonged crying period may make these episodes difficult to diagnose.

Orthostatic Hypotension

Several authors mention orthostatic hypotension as a cause of syncope. Although poorly documented, 20% of the patients in the Pratt series carried this diagnosis. It is critical to know the normal values and methods used to assess "postural changes." At least two studies have addressed this issue in pediatric patients. Castro and colleagues found that heart rate in normal children (2 to 12 years of age) often increased 30 to 40 beats per minute in a standardized supine-to-standing test. The largest increases occurred in the oldest children in the study. Fuchs and Jaffe repeated the study in an emergency room situation and found significant differences between dehydrated children (mean increase in heart rate was 29.1, ± 10.7) and controls (13.1, ± 8.5). Using a change of either 20 or 25 beats per minute yielded results with good sensitivity and specificity for hypovolemia. To further cloud the issue somewhat, a study in adults with syncope recently found that 31% had a significant fall in blood pressure (> 20 mmHg) with standing, and this was seen in all diagnostic categories, including vasovagal, cardiac, and reflex groups. It may be a general finding in individuals who faint.

It is still important to look for orthostatic changes in children who faint, using the following standardized method: at least 3 minutes supine, and then take measurements standing every minute for 5 minutes. A change in pulse of more than 20 to 25 beats per minute is probably significant. Chronic hypovolemia is unusual in pediatric patients, but again unusual but treatable disorders must be sought. Adolescents with eating disorders may purge or use diuretics and then develop fainting episodes. The child who becomes easily dehydrated with minor illness also may have subtle renal or adrenal dysfunction, leading to hypovolemia.

Cardiac Causes

Because of the risk of sudden death, much is written about the heart as the underlying cause of syncope. This is very uncommon in children but should be considered at least briefly in any patient with recurrent syncope or any patient who has a syncopal episode while exercising. Characteristically there is no warning for these spells, and the patient faints quickly without a prodrome. The group of children with recognized congenital heart disease, especially those who have had surgical repair, are at increased risk but are not discussed further here. This chapter concerns patients thought to be healthy who have syncope related to occult heart disorders. As mentioned previously, about 25% of patients with sudden death have a previous episode of syncope, usually during or shortly after exercise.

Cardiomyopathies

The most common disorder in this category is hypertrophic cardiomyopathy (previously known as *idiopathic hypertrophic subaortic stenosis,* or *IHSS*), which accounts for about 50% of the deaths in young athletes. These patients are usually believed to be completely well but may have a family history of the disorder, which is inherited as an autosomal dominant trait. In some patients a systolic murmur is audible and is accentuated by standing or with Valsalva maneuver. Certain variants of dilated cardiomyopathies may cause syncope, especially the type associated with right ventricular dysplasia.

Left Ventricular Outflow Obstruction

Although hypertrophic cardiomyopathy is the most common cause of obstruction, the examiner should also consider aortic stenosis, which may be at the level of the valve. Usually, such patients are referred because a murmur is heard along the right sternal border, along with an ejection click.

Coronary Artery Anomalies

Abnormal anatomic relationships, especially of the left coronary artery, may lead to poor myocardial perfusion during exercise. Occasionally this artery originates from the pulmonary artery or the right sinus of Valsalva, so that it may be compressed during exertion.

Marfan Syndrome

Marfan syndrome is associated with dilation of the aortic root, mitral valve prolapse, and aortic aneurysms. Sudden death and syncopal episodes are recognized associations. The stigmata of the disorder (tall stature, arachnodactyly, hyperextensibility, pectus excavatum, and dislocated lenses) may be subtle.

Dysrhythmias

Patients with the prolonged QT syndrome may have sudden syncope related to dysrhythmias, including ventricular tachycardia. (The corrected QT interval or QTc is calculated by dividing the QT interval by the square root of the RR interval; comparison is made with standard tables for age.) There may be a family history of syncope or sudden death because there are several familial forms of the disorder. The Romano-Ward syndrome is inherited as an autosomal dominant trait, and the Jervell and Lange-Nielsen syndrome is autosomal recessive and associated with sensorineural deafness. Recent genetic studies have associated markers on chromosome 11 with the long QT syndrome and demonstrated that a prolonged QT interval is not always a good screening test because there is overlap with unaffected family members. Of carriers of the gene, 63% had a history of syncope and 5% had aborted sudden death. In young children this disorder initially causes generalized seizures, presumably from unrecognized hypoxic events (Fig. 12-3).

Other Dysrhythmias

The Wolff-Parkinson-White (WPW) syndrome may be associated with sudden cardiac events, including ventricular fibrillation. Guidelines for the study and management of this disorder are available. When young patients are successfully resuscitated from cardiac arrest, later electrophysiologic studies may reveal occult tachyarrhythmias. This represents an extremely high-risk group that must be managed by a pediatric cardiologist (Fig. 12-4).

Cyanosis

Obvious congenital heart disease may be associated with spells, classically those associated with tetralogy of Fallot. A more subtle and ominous condition that may cause syncope or sudden cardiac arrest is primary pulmonary hypertension. Initial symptoms are fatigue and slowly progressive exercise intolerance. Patients with this disorder may have subtle findings on examination, such as a loud second heart sound, third and fourth heart sounds, and murmurs, especially tricuspid regurgitation.

Cyanotic Breathholding Spells

Cyanotic breathholding is the more typical type of spell recognized by families as a reaction to anger or frustration. Typically the child has an inciting event, begins to cry for a prolonged period, and then holds his or her breath in full expiration. The spell may resolve quickly after a brief period of cyanosis as the child takes a gasping breath, or the spell may progress to deep cyanosis, loss of postural tone, and opisthotonic posturing. Occasionally there is incontinence or seizure-like clonic movements. The episode resolves with a period of drowsiness. More than half of children with breathholding have the cyanotic form, and about 20% have the pallid type (see previous section); the rest have a mixed or uncertain form. Recent clinical and physiologic information on children with breathholding suggests they are different from a control or normal population. They have more nighttime sweating, different sleep patterns (arousals, non-REM sleep), and more and longer obstructive sleep apnea periods. More information over the next decade may further elucidate a set of physiologic differences in several types of childhood syncope.

Other Causes

Epilepsy

Epilepsy is part of the differential diagnosis of most paroxysmal disorders. There are some clues to an underlying seizure disorder. Episodes should occur while the

CHILDREN'S HOSPITAL OF PITTSBURGH
DEPARTMENT OF CARDIOLOGY

NAME

WARD-DOB

SERVICE

UNIT #

ELECTROCARDIOGRAPHY REPORT

RHYTHM: SINUS ☒ OTHER: AXIS **90** °

RATES: VENT. **80** /MIN.   ATRIAL **80** /MIN.

INTERVALS: PR **.12** SEC.   QRS. **06** SEC.   QTC **60** SEC.

INTERPRETATION:

ELECTROCARDIOGRAPHY REQUEST

ECG TAKEN IN LAB ☐ OPD ☐ WARD ☐

CLIN. DIAG.:   AGE

11-16-83

1.   **Prolonged Q-T segment.**
2.   **Abnormal S-T elevation and T wave.**

DATE: **6-18-96**
INTERPRETED BY:

_____ M.D.

MEDICATION. DIG. ☐ OTHER:
ORDERED BY

_____ M.D.

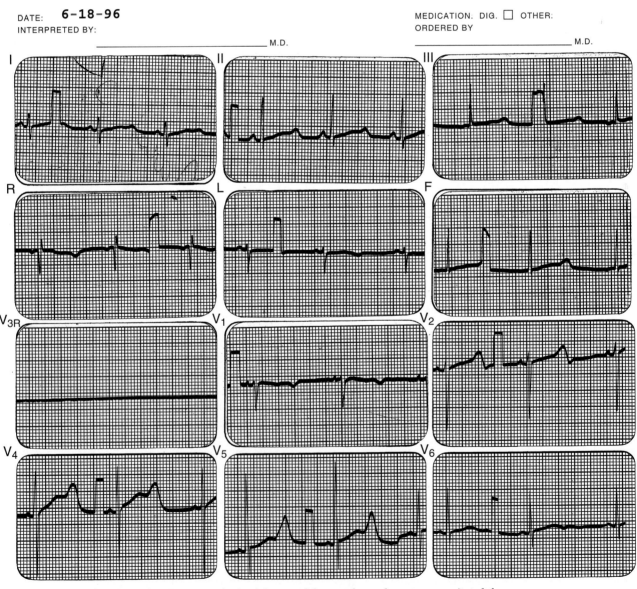

FIG. 12-3 This ECG was obtained in an adolescent boy who was resuscitated from a near drowning. He later died. Family studies confirmed numerous early sudden deaths, and subsequent family members have had documented prolongation of the QTc.

Patient:
Patient ID:
Time:
Date: 08-FEB-94
Comment: cont. strip

VENTRICULAR TACHYCARDIA
Run Length: 3 beats, Rate: 269 BPM
Heart Rate: 108 BPM

Strip 37

N   N   N   N   N   N   V   V   V   N   V   V   V   N   N   N   N

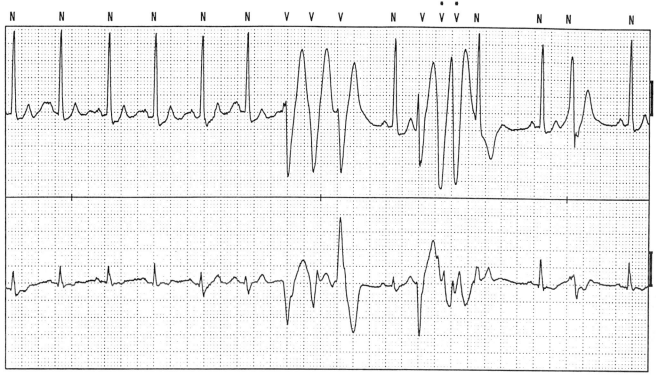

Patient:
Patient ID:
Time:
Date: 08-FEB-94
Comment: cont. strip

COUPLET

Heart Rate: 102 BPM

Strip 38

V N   N   N   N   N   N   N   V   V   N   V   2   N   V

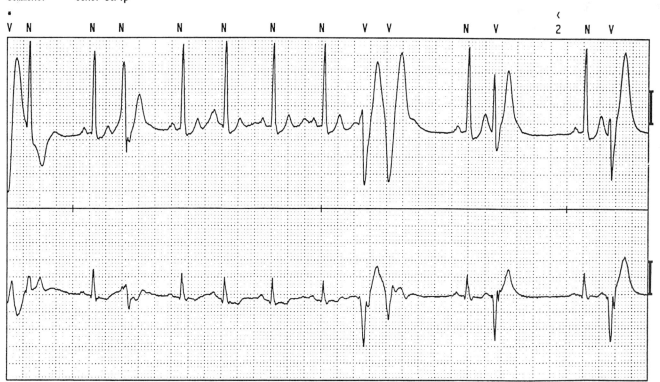

FIG. 12-4   This ECG is from an adolescent girl who was found unconscious in her bedroom by her mother. Bigeminy is illustrated, and she had clinical and ECG evidence of mitral valve prolapse.

patient is recumbent or upright. There may be a true aura, which is different from the usual weakness, nausea, or dizziness experienced by children with vasodepressor syncope. A postictal period may be present, and stereotyped or even tonic-clonic movements may occur. In difficult cases, prolonged electroencephalographic monitoring may be necessary, perhaps performed with video recording. Occasionally a seizure episode may occur after hypoxia from syncope, making diagnosis of the primary event more difficult. Tilt-table testing has been helpful in this situation; the seizure is found to be a secondary phenomenon.

Hyperventilation

Hyperventilation is probably underdiagnosed because it is not always evident at first evaluation and may be a chronic condition. As noted earlier, in the prospective study of Kocnig and colleagues, hyperventilation was associated with reproduction of syncopal symptoms in a large group of younger patients. This group was largely labeled "psychiatric" in cause. In addition to the typical breathing, tetany, and paresthesias, these patients may have a myriad of symptoms that may include weakness, chest pain, dizziness, stiffness, and muscle cramps. Complete loss of consciousness is rare, but the proper questions may lead to the diagnosis.

Hysteria

Hysteric reaction is unusual in younger children and generally becomes evident in preadolescence. The most common symptoms of conversion reaction are gait disturbance and weakness, but pseudoseizures and syncope may occur. Several observers have documented apparent loss of consciousness during tilt-table testing in patients who had no significant changes in pulse or blood pressure. In difficult cases this test may be helpful.

Migraine

Basilar artery migraine may rarely cause transient loss of consciousness. Usually, headache develops later in the episode, but in younger children there may be some difficulty in the diagnosis. Family history is almost always positive, and associated phenomena, such as motion sickness, may be present.

Metabolic Disorders

Several authors mention metabolic disorders as rare causes of syncope. One patient in the series of Pratt had a low blood sugar (40 mg/dl). More common in such patients is a significant prodromal period (hunger, sweating, etc.). In certain situations, such as diabetes mellitus, it may be reasonable to check laboratory findings, such as blood sugar levels.

Table 12-1 summarizes the differential diagnosis with key features of each possibility.

History

Despite the detailed discussion of life-threatening disorders, most children with fainting spells have a benign condition and an excellent long-term outlook. The initial questions should be directed to the issue of whether a *true* episode of unconsciousness occurred. Patients with light-headedness or dizziness do not seem to fall into a high-risk group and generally, unless the episode occurred during exercise, require minimal evaluation. Who witnessed the event(s)? Was the patient able to communicate throughout, or was he or she definitely unconscious? Did the patient suffer physical injury from the fall? (Patients with hysteria rarely do.)

The next important step is for the clinician to decide whether there is a potentially serious (cardiac) disorder. Once again exercise-related syncope is a "red flag" and warrants thorough investigation. Another feature of cardiac syncope is sudden onset without any warning or prodrome. Did the patient experience palpitations or chest pain? These symptoms may be related to myocardial ischemia or dysrhythmia. Is there a family history of sudden death or sensorineural deafness? The prolonged QTc syndrome may be lethal; estimates of about 70% mortality in undiagnosed cases have been made.

If cardiac-related syncope can be eliminated as a reasonable diagnosis, the more common causes can be considered. A careful search for a prodrome or trigger for the episode can be very valuable. What was the situation in which the spell began? Have there been other episodes that the patient could partially prevent? What was done to abort the episodes? Have any episodes occurred while in a recumbent position? (This would favor other conditions, such as epilepsy.) Did a color change occur? Most patients are slightly pale, but cyanosis is distinctly unusual and raises the issue of breathholding spells or cyanosis from heart or lung disease. Timing of the fainting episodes may be important. Do they occur only in the early morning, after prolonged fasting, during times of fatigue, or after stretching or micturition?

Questions about general health and emotional and psychologic status are indicated. Addison disease is characterized by lassitude, poor energy, gastrointestinal symptoms, and hyperpigmentation (the suntan that remains for a prolonged time). Syncope from psychologic causes may be accompanied by family stress, school or peer group difficulties, and, as usual, excessive school absence.

Although not mentioned previously, age of the patient may be a helpful screening test. Syncope is most common in the older population of children, preadolescents and adolescents. In the study by Pratt and Fleisher the mean age was 12.7 years. If breathholding is not a concern, the examiner must be somewhat more cautious before making the diagnosis of vasodepressor syncope in toddlers and early school-age children.

On most occasions the history is the driving force behind further investigation for more serious disorders. A summary of important questions is presented in Table 12-2.

Physical Examination

Although physical examination is most frequently normal, a careful evaluation may give clues to the correct diagnosis. Vital signs and growth parameters should be recorded, the latter as a sign of overall health. A number of additional office tests can be done; orthostatic pulse change and hyperventilation are generally safe. As noted earlier in the discussion of orthostasis, a change of more than 25 beats per minute is significant. Hyperventilation that reproduces symptoms may be a clue to psychiatric disorders and hyperventilation itself as a mechanism. The only caveat is that hyperventilation has produced asystole in several highly trained athletes who were undergoing preparticipation testing. Carotid massage and eyeball pressure have also produced asystole in certain types of syncope (reflex, pallid breath-holding); these maneuvers appear too dangerous for the office situation. Pulse rate and rhythm are important. Is there extreme bradycardia, tachycardia, or irregular beats? A thorough examination of the cardiovascular system is indicated, especially if this remains a prime diagnostic consideration. Standing and Valsalva maneuver may accentuate the murmur of IHSS.

The general examination should be thorough and include a search for features of Marfan syndrome and adrenal insufficiency, both of which have known associations with syncope. Neurologic status is important because abnormalities may suggest that a seizure disorder should be a diagnostic consideration.

Approach to the Patient

After completion of a history and physical examination, most patients are categorized as having vasodepressor syncope, several have recognized psychiatric causes, and the smallest group is at risk for underlying cardiac disorders. This is an important concept because many review articles discuss in great detail the invasive cardiac tests (described briefly here) and give the sense that all patients need such tests. In fact, patients who have definite, classic vasodepressor or vasovagal syncope need no further tests unless there is doubt about the diagnosis. Although an ECG is recommended by most authors, this should be routine only in situations that are questionable (i.e., patients who faint but have no trigger or prodrome).

Most attention in the past few years has focused on the tilt-table test. This is a useful tool for patients with syncope of unknown cause because vasovagal episodes may be reproduced and hysteria and hyperventilation may be recognized. Unfortunately, the use of isoproterenol is less clear, although it tends to shorten test time. The clinician should find a laboratory, generally under the direction of a pediatric or adult cardiologist, that will yield satisfactory results. It is very reassuring to reproduce a self-limited episode during the pro-

TABLE 12-2

Key Questions

Question	Value
Did the patient lose consciousness? Arouse instantly? Suffer injury?	If not, episode may not have been true syncope or was "near syncope"
What position at onset?	Syncope—upright; supine position suggests other disorder, such as seizure
Prodrome or warning?	Nausea, pallor, weakness common in vasovagal
Triggering event?	Fright, blood, micturition (vasovagal); also breathholding spells
Recurrent episodes during illness?	Orthostatic or hypovolemia (renal/adrenal disorders)
Exercise-related? Chest pain? Palpitations?	Red flags, cardiac causes possible
Family history of syncope? Sudden death? Hearing loss?	Prolonged QTc, vasovagal is also familial
Cyanosis?	Cardiopulmonary, breathholding spells
Confusion, somnolence afterward?	Epilepsy
Multiple symptoms, weakness, dizziness, cramps, paresthesias?	Hyperventilation
Family stress? School absence?	Hysteria, functional disorder
Headache or motion sickness?	Migraine (also family history)

cedure so that patient and family can be informed about the mechanism. Treatment of this group of patients is still under investigation, but adult patients (and a few children) have responded to measures to increase blood volume, such as fluorocortisone and salt supplementation. Beta-adrenergic blocking agents, such as propranolol or atenolol, have been used, as well as disopyramide, an anticholinergic and negative inotropic agent. Decisions about treatment of this group will become clearer over the next few years as studies are completed. It is important to recognize that many patients need no treatment except reassurance. Frequent, severe episodes associated with physical injury may warrant therapy.

Patients who have prolonged asystole during testing are a more difficult problem. If asystole is extreme, some investigators advocate permanent pacemaker insertion. Because the primary event is hypotension, however, pacemakers may not be effective. Decisions in this small and difficult group must be individualized.

Patients who have exercise-induced syncope or, in the most ominous group, patients who have required resuscitation need detailed and extensive investigation. Baseline ECG is indicated, looking for abnormal rhythm, evidence of ischemia, and also prolonged QTc. Prolonged rhythm monitoring using a Holter monitor may be helpful if rhythm disturbance is suspected. In adult patients, 24 hours of monitoring missed a significant number of patients who eventually were found to have paroxysmal events. More prolonged monitoring for 48 to 72 hours may be necessary. Also useful in this situation may be the newer transtelephonic ECG monitors that may be used by patient or parent during an episode.

If events are related to major exertion, a detailed exercise study under the direction of a consultant cardiologist may be useful to clarify the nature of the episode and the potential morbidity. If episodes are orthostatic without cardiac rhythm disturbance, more invasive study can be eliminated. Finally the most invasive study is direct intracardiac electrical monitoring and stimulation. In one study of young, apparently healthy patients who survived cardiac arrest and had completely normal evaluations afterward, intracardiac stimulation produced sustained tachyarrhythmias. In this group, antidysrhythmic drug therapy may be truly lifesaving.

SUMMARY

Fainting episodes are relatively common in the older pediatric population. Many may be "near syncope," recognized as such by the family, and never reported to the physician. When evaluating a patient with true syncope, the astute and careful clinician is able to categorize most patients into a very low-risk group after the history and physical examination. The high-risk group should have different features, such as a worrisome family history or exercise-induced episodes. Some patients who remain undiagnosed may benefit from newer methods of investigation. With rare exception, patients with syncope should have a benign long-term outlook.

ILLUSTRATIVE CASES

Case 1. A 14-year-old girl has been tired for several months and has lost 5 pounds. She has noted episodes of light-headedness, especially when standing quickly and quit her school basketball team because of loss of energy. She has had flulike symptoms for 2 days, with temperature to 101° F, rhinorrhea, loose cough, and mild diarrhea of two loose, watery stools per day. On the day of her emergency room visit she became unconscious at home for 1 minute after standing to walk to the bathroom.

*Examination reveals a thin, cooperative adolescent girl with dry mucous membranes and delayed capillary refill (3 seconds in a warm environment), associated with a pos-*tural change in heart rate of 25 beats per minute. She has mild hyperpigmentation of the skin and gums. She improves with intravenous infusion of normal saline over the next 4 hours.

This young woman may simply have adolescent fatigue and dehydration, but her clinical picture is out of proportion to her mild prodrome. Hormone testing confirmed a diagnosis of adrenal insufficiency, a potentially life-threatening disorder. The cause of her syncope falls into the category of orthostatic. (See Fig. 12-5 for examination findings in adrenal insufficiency.)

Case 2. A 10-year-old girl noted a swollen, pruritic eye and later in the day saw an ophthalmologist who diagnosed an allergic reaction. After the examination, the patient felt dizzy and had transient diplopia. As she walked out of the office she felt light-headed and "everything went black." She appeared pale, and her mother supported her as she lost consciousness. While resting supine, her heart rate was slow but regular and her respirations were normal. She was awake and oriented in less than 1 minute.

Previously the patient had two near syncopal episodes at the end of piano lessons. She was anxious during these lessons, which were taught by a family friend. ECG and examination were normal on the day of the syncopal episode.

This was an anxious girl who found the eye examination and her piano lessons very stressful. A presumptive diagnosis of neurovascular syncope was made and tilt-table testing was discussed with the family. It was decided to reassure and observe the patient for further episodes, which have not occurred over the past 6 months.

Case 3. A previously well 13-year-old boy fainted 30 minutes into his afternoon cross-country track team practice. He recovered over several minutes and remembered only a sudden "black-out." In the emergency room he appears somewhat anxious, but his examination and vital signs are normal, including postural changes in pulse and blood pressure. ECG is also normal. Past medical and family histories are unremarkable.

Although the initial evaluation in this boy is unrevealing, the association of the episode with exertion warrants further investigation. A cardiologist hears a soft systolic murmur while the patient is standing and also during Valsalva maneuver. Later ECG demonstrates findings consistent with hypertrophic cardiomyopathy.

ANNOTATED BIBLIOGRAPHY

Hardy CE: Syncope and chest pain: to worry, or not? *Contemp Pediatr* 11:19-42, 1994.

This is a useful review from a cardiologist's perspective with a number of illustrative cases.

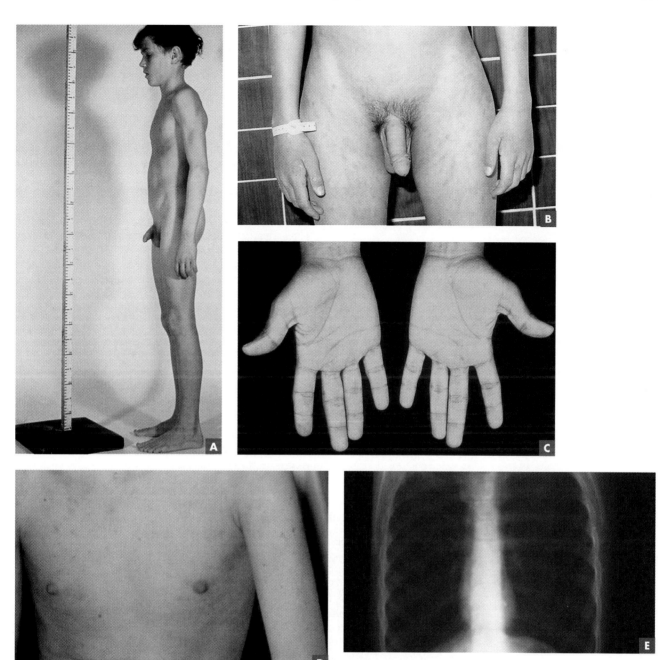

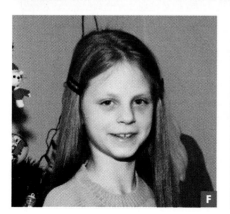

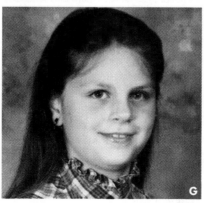

FIG. 12-5 *A*, This patient shows the thin habitus and ill appearance characteristic of Addison disease. *B* to *D*, Hyperpigmentation may be marked. *E*, Microcardia is characteristic on chest radiograph. *F*, Young girl with isolated ACTH deficiency shows wasting and pallor rather than excessive bronzing. G, The same girl after therapy. (*A* through *D* courtesy Dr. M. New, New York; *E* courtesy Dr. J. Medina, Pittsburgh.)

Koenig D, Linzer M, Pontinen M, Divine GW: Syncope in young adults: evidence for a combined medical and psychiatric approach, *J Intern Med* 232:169-176, 1992.

This is a nice contrast to Hardy's article. The authors describe a high frequency of psychiatric diagnoses in patients with syncope and discuss the usefulness of the "hyperventilation test" for diagnosis.

Pratt JL, Fleisher GR: Syncope in children and adolescents, *Pediatr Emerg Care* 5:80-89, 1989.

This is a review of pediatric emergency room experience with syncope. Vasovagal and orthostatic causes were most common, and patients with near-syncope had no abnormalities on further investigation.

BIBLIOGRAPHY

Atkins D, Hanusa B, Sefcik T: Syncope and orthostatic hypotension, *Am J Med* 91:179-185, 1991.

Camfield PR, Camfield CS: Syncope in childhood: a case control clinical study of the familial tendency to faint, *Can J Neurol Sci* 17:306-308, 1990.

Castro W, Skarin R, Roscelli JD: Orthostatic heart rate and arterial blood pressure changes in normovolemic children, *Pediatr Emerg Care* 1:123-127, 1985.

DiMario FJ: Breath-holding spells in childhood, *Am J Dis Child* 146:125-131, 1992.

DiMario FJ, Chee CM, Berman PH: Pallid breath-holding spells: evaluation of the autonomic nervous system, *Clin Pediatr* 29:17-24, 1990.

Fuchs SM, Jaffe DM: Evaluation of the "tilt test" in children, *Ann Emerg Med* 16:386-390, 1987.

Goldstein MA, Hesslein P, Dunnigan A: Efficacy of transtelephonic electrocardiographic monitoring in pediatric patients, *Am J Dis Child* 144:178-182, 1990.

Gordon TA, Moodie DS, Passalacqua M, et al: A retrospective analysis of the cost-effective workup of syncope in children, *Cleve Clin J Med* 54:391-394, 1987.

Kapoor WN, Brant N: Evaluation of syncope by upright tilt testing with isoproterenol, *Ann Intern Med* 116:358-363, 1992.

Kapoor WN, Karpf M, Wieland S, et al: A prospective evaluation and follow-up of patients with syncope, *N Engl J Med* 309:197-204, 1983.

Lagi A, Arnetoli G, Vannucchi PL, et al: The Valsalva maneuver in vasodepressor syncope, *Angiology* 40:958-963, 1989.

Lerman-Sagie T, Rechavia E, Strasberg B, et al: Head-up tilt for the evaluation of syncope of unknown origin in children, *J Pediatr* 118:676-679, 1991.

Missri J, Alexander J: Hyperventilation syndrome: a brief review, *JAMA* 240:2093-2096, 1978.

O'Marcaigh AS, MacLellan-Tobert SG, Porter CJ: Tilt-table testing and oral metoprolol therapy in young patients with unexplained syncope, *Pediatrics* 93:278-283, 1994.

Ruckman RN: Cardiac causes of syncope, *Pediatr Rev* 9:101-108, 1987.

Scherrer R, Vissing S, Morgan BJ, et al: Vasovagal syncope after infusion of a vasodilator in a heart-transplant recipient, *N Engl J Med* 322:602-604, 1990.

Scott WA: Evaluating the child with syncope, *Pediatr Ann* 20:350-359, 1991.

Thilenius OG, Quinones JA, Husayni TS, Novak J: Tilt test for diagnosis of unexplained syncope in pediatric patients, *Pediatrics* 87:334-338, 1991.

Vincent GM, Timothy KW, Leppert M, Keating M: The spectrum of symptoms and QT intervals in carriers of the gene for the long-QT syndrome, *N Engl J Med* 327:846-852, 1992.

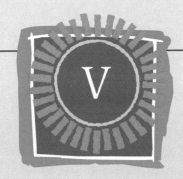

Respiratory

Recurrent Apnea

EUGENE M. MOWAD ❧ JAMES A. NARD

Key Points

- Neonatal apnea is a frightful event for parents and healthcare professionals. This fear is based on a popular, but as yet unproven connection between apnea and the sudden infant death syndrome. Because of this connection, apneic events require thorough investigation.

- Even after a careful history, physical examination, and directed ancillary studies, many cases of apnea remain idiopathic. Physicians should be aware of the pros and cons of home infant monitor use, especially in such cases.

- Obstructive apnea is based on a structural or functional lesion in or near the airway. Physical examination, imaging studies, and endoscopy, singly or in combination, often detect these lesions.

The infant who stops breathing creates a terrifying and emotionally charged situation for parents and physicians alike. This anxiety likely stems from the perceived connection between apneic episodes and the sudden infant death syndrome (SIDS). Although the true nature of SIDS remains a mystery to a certain extent, a long-standing popular hypothesis is that these apneic events are markers placing infants at high risk of subsequent death from SIDS. So ingrained is this perceived connection that the events we now term *apparent life-threatening events* (ALTE) (discussed later) were once known by the more emotional *near miss SIDS* terminology. Whether the apnea hypothesis of SIDS is eventually proven true or not is almost inconsequential in the minds of most parents. Because apnea and SIDS are inextricably linked, this chapter deals with the clinical approach to apnea largely in the context of the group of disorders that seem to have abnormal respiratory control as a common ground.

By way of definition, *apnea* as used here means a pause in respiration lasting 15 seconds or longer. Apnea occurring without any appreciable respiratory effort is termed *central apnea,* and apnea in the presence of ineffective respiratory effort, such as gasping or choking, is termed *obstructive apnea.* An ALTE as defined by the 1986 National Institutes of Health (NIH) conference panel is "an episode that is frightening to the observer and is characterized by apnea, . . . color change, . . . marked change in muscle tone, . . . choking, or gagging." In some cases the observer fears that the infant has died. A SIDS death is one that is sudden, occurs during the first year of life, and remains unexplained after a complete review of the case history; postmortem investigation, including autopsy; and examination of the death scene. *Periodic breathing* refers to a respiratory pattern characterized by periods of rapid ventilation separated by brief pauses (usually for less than 5 seconds). In periodic breathing the respiratory rate when calculated over a long period of time is normal, as is minute ventilation (Fig. 13-1). The NIH conference panel also defined the term *apnea of infancy* as an "unexplained episode of cessation of breathing for 20 seconds or longer, or a shorter respiratory pause associated with bradycardia, cyanosis, pallor, and/or marked hypotonia." To exclude those infants with apnea of prematurity, the term *apnea of infancy* should be restricted to infants greater than 37 weeks gestational age. In full-term infants, as much as 50% to 60% of apnea may fall into this idiopathic category.

This chapter does not deal with apnea of prematurity, but to establish a uniform understanding of this entity, it is defined as idiopathic apnea that occurs in infants less than 37 weeks gestational age. Apnea of prematurity usually disappears as an infant approaches term gestational age, but it may persist, in which case it is termed *persistent apnea of prematurity.* Because it is difficult to separate the causes of recurrent apnea from those of one-time events, both entities are discussed here.

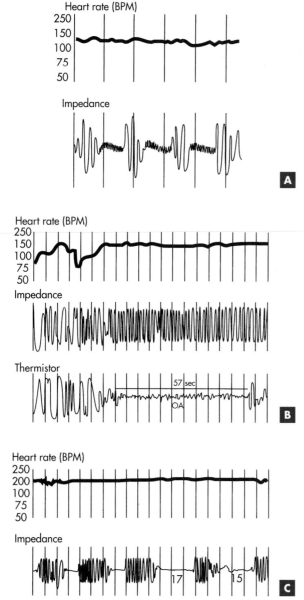

FIG. 13-1 *A,* Periodic breathing. Slow, deep breaths alternate with rapid, shallow breaths. *B,* A 57-second obstructive apnea. Note normal chest wall movement (impedance) and absent airflow (thermistor). *C,* Two central apneas lasting 17 and 15 seconds respectively. Note absent respiratory effort (impedance).

Pathophysiology

Physiologic control of respiration is accomplished through a complex feedback system. Much research is being conducted regarding the neural control of respiration, and what follows is a simplified approach to that system. Specialized receptor organs sense and relay information regarding blood pH, partial pressures of oxygen and carbon dioxide, amount of stretch in respiratory musculature, and presence of irritants in the airway. This information is processed in the central nervous system (CNS) and used to adjust rate and depth of respiration to meet the metabolic needs of the body. Hypoxia, hypercapnia, and acidosis all stimulate increased respiration.

The efferent pathway begins in an ill-defined population of neurons in the medulla oblongata termed the *central respiratory generator.* The central respiratory generator dictates firing patterns in two discrete groups of neurons also located in the medulla known as the *dorsal and ventral respiratory groups.* These neurons then project to spinal cord motor neurons that in turn drive the respiratory musculature.

The diaphragm is the major muscle of respiration, and the motor innervation is derived from the third through fifth cervical spinal cord segments. Thoracic and lumbar neurons innervate the intercostal and abdominal musculature that assists in respiration. Movements of the pharyngeal and laryngeal musculature must also be coordinated with respiratory movements to provide for unobstructed airflow. These structures are innervated by motor components of the vagus nerve (cranial nerve X).

During inspiration the diaphragm contracts and actively lowers intrathoracic pressure, resulting in airflow through the nasopharynx, trachea, main stem bronchi, and bronchial tree and finally into the alveoli where gas exchange occurs. Expiration is a more passive process accomplished as the respiratory musculature relaxes and intrathoracic pressure becomes positive. The direction of airflow is then reversed.

Apnea may result from a failure of neural mechanisms to initiate an inspiratory cycle at the appropriate time (central apnea) or from an impediment to airflow in the presence of a normal respiratory effort (obstructive apnea). These two mechanisms may occur in isolation, or they may overlap in what is termed *mixed apnea.*

Structural CNS defects involving the brainstem or cervical spinal cord can cause central apnea. These abnormalities may be grossly apparent and detectable on antemortem CNS imaging, but they also may be subtle microscopic changes detected only on autopsy. Central apnea also may occur in the absence of structural brainstem anomalies because of extrinsic compression of the brainstem in the Arnold-Chiari malformation or in association with osteogenesis imperfecta. Disordered control of respiration based on aberrant response to hypoxia can cause central apnea, as may the actions of toxic compounds, such as opiates, on the CNS. Abnormal responses to hypercarbia also may play some role in apnea, but the literature is divided on this issue.

Obstructive apnea results from static or dynamic lesions that obstruct the flow of air at any point from the nose to the alveoli. Obstruction may be due to a fixed structural lesion either intrinsic to the airway or extrinsic and causing compression. It may also be dynamic and functional, as in the case of infants with hypotonia and floppy airways that collapse during inspiration.

Reports on sleep positioning and its relationship to SIDS and obstructive apnea in the newborn have received much attention in pediatric and lay literature. The current state of understanding is that the prone sleep position is certainly an epidemiologic risk factor and perhaps a cause for SIDS. Before good head control is established, hyperflexion of the neck may occur when newborns ride in car seats, causing obstructive apnea and desaturation.

The pathophysiologic significance of periodic breathing as an isolated phenomenon remains unknown. In the absence of apnea or laboratory evidence of chronic hypoventilation (see section on approach to the patient), periodic breathing should simply be documented and followed closely.

Keeping these general concepts in mind, the physician can develop a broad differential diagnosis of causative factors leading to the final common pathway of apnea.

Literature Survey

The concept of apnea and its relationship to sudden infant death has existed for nearly 3000 years. Keens and Davidson Ward in their review of apnea and sudden infant death highlight the notion that these deaths were somehow due to suffocation, using a biblical quote, "And this woman's son died in the night because she laid on it."

The pediatric literature began to seriously assess the possible connection between apnea and infant death in the 1970s. The evolution from the entity of "near miss SIDS" to the concept of the ALTE was described previously. Brooks' review of ALTE and apnea of infancy catalogs the many efforts to delineate the epidemiology and clinical approach to ALTE. This paper is a well-written and crucial reference for the clinician who wishes to deal with the concept of the ALTE on more than an anecdotal basis. A number of papers produced in the 1980s and beyond intended to assign a cause to the infants in the so-called idiopathic ALTE group. Aberrant pulmonary mechanics, disordered respiratory control, gastroesophageal reflux, and occult metabolic diseases have all been implicated for subsets of infants. Another crucial document for the clinician is the 1986 NIH consensus report on infant apnea and home monitoring; it is the basis of several sets of guidelines and recommendations.

Like infant apnea, literary references to the obstructive sleep apnea syndrome occur throughout recorded history. The earliest scientific descriptions of the syndrome came from Gastaut in the 1960s for adults and Guilleminault in 1975 for children. Many of the contributions that addressed obstructive apnea in more general terms and expanded the differential diagnosis in infancy came from the surgical literature. Several excellent reviews of the topics of obstructive apnea and sleep apnea appear in the references at the end of this chapter.

Differential Diagnosis

Keeping in mind the pathophysiology of apnea, it is clear that this entity should be regarded merely as a symptom. The physician, through detailed history, physical examination, and selected tests, should be able to determine the cause of an apneic episode. The differential diagnosis of apnea is broad and can be divided in a number of ways. Two common approaches are the systems-oriented approach and separation of the causes of apnea into central versus obstructive causes. For the purposes of this chapter, a systems-oriented approach is used, and in the description of specific entities, apnea is characterized as central or obstructive wherever possible. This approach avoids confusion over entities, such as respiratory syncytial virus infection, that can cause either central or obstructive apnea.

CNS structural lesions cause central apnea beginning at birth that is nearly always irreversible. Other neurologic signs, such as hypotonia, cranial nerve dysfunction, or arthrogryposis, often accompany CNS structural lesions. Some of these lesions, such as Dandy-Walker malformation, are easily visible on computed tomography (CT) or magnetic resonance imaging (MRI) scans. Other lesions, such as congenital central hypoventilation syndrome (Ondine's curse), may result in brainstem gliosis or other subtle structural changes evident only on microscopic examination of brain tissue. Lesions that additionally cause elevation of intracranial pressure manifest with increased head circumference and hydrocephalus. Some specific examples of CNS structural lesions are listed in Table 13-1. These and many more examples are discussed in detail in Brazy's reference.

Other neurologic mechanisms that may result in apnea include seizures and severe neuromuscular disease. The presence of convulsive movements of the extremities or eyes is helpful in diagnosing an ictal phenomenon, but their absence does not rule out a seizure disorder as the cause of apnea, especially in the neonate. Hypertonia or tachycardia during an event should also raise suspicions of a seizure. The child with severe neuromuscular disease, such as spinal muscular atrophy (Werdnig-Hoffmann disease), may be too weak to initiate a respiratory effort, or the hypotonic airway may collapse during inspiration. The overall approach to such a child is addressed more completely in Chapter 11.

Metabolic lesions affecting the CNS may cause central apnea or hypoventilation that is reversible with correction of the metabolic defect. Examples are hypoglycemia and medication-related apnea from illicit or prescribed maternal opioids. Other metabolic defects that result in apnea are hypocalcemia, hypomagnesemia, and severe acidosis. The medium-chain acyl-CoA dehydrogenase (MCAD) deficiency is thought to be an explanation for some familial causes of SIDS. This disorder of lipid metabolism results in altered mental status, vomiting, acidosis, hyperammonemia, and nonketotic hypoglycemia.

Upper airway obstruction encompasses a diverse category of causes of obstructive apnea, ranging from congenital malformations to reversible infectious causes, such as viral croup. If obstructive apnea occurs in the neonatal period, congenital malformations, such as laryngomalacia or tracheobronchomalacia, and space-occupying lesions, such as cysts or tumors, should lead the differential diagnosis. Any of the various syndromes associated with craniofacial abnor-

TABLE 13-1

Differential Diagnosis of Apnea

Lesion	Comments	Diagnosis/management
Central Nervous System		
Dandy-Walker malformation	Congenital and central	CT or MRI
Arnold-Chiari malformation	Congenital and central, associated spina bifida	CT or MRI
Seizures	Convulsive movements, hypertonia, postictal	EEG, metabolic studies
Hypotonia, weakness	Stridor, labored breathing	EMG, CPK, (see Chapter 11)
Ondine's curse (congenital central hypoventilation syndrome)	Central, occurs during sleep, congenital	MRI (often normal), polysomnography
Metabolic/Toxic		
Hypoglycemia	Macrosomia, infant of diabetic mother	Blood glucose
Hypocalcemia	Athymic, DiGeorge syndrome	Blood calcium
Hyponatremia	Poor feeding, water supplements	Blood sodium
Acidosis	Lethargy, vomiting	Blood gas, HCO_3
Hypomagnesemia	—	Blood magnesium
Opioids	Iatrogenic or illicit use	Toxicology screen, naloxone
MCAD deficiency	Hyperammonemia, positive family history of SIDS	Ammonia, carnitine studies, consultation
Upper Airway		
Craniofacial syndromes	Congenital, dysmorphic	ENT referral
Laryngomalacia	Positional stridor	ENT referral
Rhinitis	URI symptoms/signs	Nasal suctioning
Choanal stenosis/atresia	Congenital, mouth-breathing, feeding difficulty	Pass feeding tube
Croup	Stridor, URI, barky cough	Steroids, mist
Adenotonsillar hypertrophy	Enlarged tonsils, OSAS	ENT referral
Epiglottitis	Stridor, fever, toxic appearance	Emergent evaluation
Postextubation	History of intubation	Steroids?
Vocal cord paralysis	Hoarse, stridor, aphonia	ENT referral
Anaphylaxis	Allergic history, urticaria	Epinephrine, steroids
Lower Airway		
Pneumonia	Fever, cough, rales	Chest X-ray films
Bronchiolitis	Fever, wheezing, URI	Nasal swab for RSV
Pertussis	Paroxysmal cough	Nasal swab
Cardiovascular		
Structural disease	Murmur, cyanosis	Echocardiography
Dysrhythmia	Abnormal heart rate, high index of suspicion	ECG, Holter monitor
Gastrointestinal		
Gastroesophageal reflux	Regurgitation, fussy after feeding	pH probe, upper GI
Miscellaneous		
Sepsis	Fever, toxic appearance	Emergent evaluation and therapy
Meningitis	Fever, lethargy, nuchal rigidity	Emergent LP and therapy
Munchausen syndrome by proxy	Vague history, no objective documentation of spells, medical training in mother	Exclude other causes, psychiatric referral

CPK, Creatine phosphokinase; *CT,* computed tomography; *ECG,* electrocardiography; *EEG,* electroencephalography; *EMG,* electromyography; *ENT,* ear, nose, and throat; *LP,* lumbar puncture; *MCAD,* medium-chain acyl-CoA dehydrogenase; *MRI,* magnetic resonance imaging; *OSAS,* obstructive sleep apnea syndrome; *RSV,* respiratory syncytial virus; *URI,* upper respiratory tract infection.

malities may also cause upper airway obstruction because of associated malformation of the nasopharynx, oropharynx, or tracheobronchial tree. The possible contribution of sleep position, discussed earlier, should be addressed.

In the older child the majority of obstructive apnea occurs mainly during sleep and is caused by adenoidotonsillar hyperplasia. Adenoidotonsillar disease may be manifest only in the face of acute infections, such as streptococcal tonsillopharyngitis or infectious mononucleosis.

Viral infections, such as nasopharyngitis and laryngotracheobronchitis (viral croup), also cause upper airway obstruction as a result of mucosal edema and increased secretions. Bacterial upper airway infections, such as bacterial tracheitis or epiglottitis, are infrequent and present with a toxic-appearing child with fever and signs of upper airway obstruction.

Many patients experience a brief episode of stridor after prolonged intubation. This is caused by mucosal edema in the upper airway. Persistent stridor in a postextubation patient suggests tracheal stenosis or an injury to the vocal cord. The recurrent laryngeal nerve may be injured during chest surgery, resulting in a vocal cord paresis and persistent upper airway obstruction.

Anaphylaxis results in acute, often severe, upper airway obstruction and must be immediately treated with epinephrine and corticosteroids. History of previous reactions and presence of urticaria should raise the suspicion of anaphylaxis. Exposure to an offending medication or an insect venom may be elicited, but in the case of food allergy, history of exposure is often complicated by "hidden allergens" in commercially prepared foods.

Infections of the lower respiratory tract, such as pneumonia, also cause apnea. Two specific agents, the respiratory syncytial virus (RSV) and *Bordetella pertussis*, should be mentioned with respect to apnea and respiratory infection.

RSV is the most common cause of bronchiolitis, an infection characterized by fever, coryza, tachypnea, and wheezing. As with any respiratory infection, copious secretions coupled with airway edema may cause obstructive apnea, but additionally, RSV may enhance neurally mediated apnea in infants by stimulation of laryngeal chemoreceptors. The experimental data come from studies conducted on infant lambs, but the results may be relevant to RSV-associated apnea in human infants. *Bordetella pertussis* is the causative agent of whooping cough. During infancy a paroxysm of coughing may not be followed by the classic inspiratory whoop but instead by apnea that can be prolonged and life threatening. Typically, hypoxia increases respiratory drive, but in these infants it leads to apnea. An immature central response to hypoxia is thought to be the pathophysiologic mechanism involved.

Cardiovascular disease can lead to apnea as a secondary phenomenon. Whereas cyanotic lesions and significant congestive heart failure are usually clinically apparent, cardiac dysrhythmias may be occult, episodic, and difficult to detect. A high index of suspicion and empiric testing are often nec-essary (see section dealing with the approach to the patient).

Reflux of gastric contents through the gastroesophageal junction is a common problem during the first year of life. Gastroesophageal reflux (GER) frequently but not always causes regurgitation of feedings into the oral cavity. Lesser degrees of reflux may result only in gastric contents reaching the lower third of the esophagus. Through a vagally mediated reflex arc, GER results in transient laryngospasm and obstructive apnea. Although GER resulting in regurgitation of feedings is easily diagnosed, radiographic means or esophageal pH monitoring may be necessary to diagnose lesser degrees of reflux.

Infections of the respiratory system may lead to apnea as described earlier, but severe systemic infections, such as sepsis and meningitis, may also lead to apnea. Because of the life-threatening nature of these infections, they should always be considered in the ill-appearing infant, and if any doubt as to their presence exists, empiric antibiotic therapy should be started promptly.

A history of recurrent infantile apnea in the presence of repeated unsuccessful attempts to document events in the hospital or with a home monitor should raise the suspicion of Munchausen syndrome by proxy. Usually the alleged event is seen only by a single caregiver, most often the mother. Often the medical history is long and complex yet vague. There is also frequently a history of "doctor shopping," and the perpetrator often has some medical training.

The differential diagnosis of apnea is summarized in Table 13-1.

History

To determine possible causes of an apneic event, the examiner must begin with a solid database. Caregivers are understandably emotional after an apneic event, so history taking should begin with an open-ended question aimed at clarifying exactly what happened to the infant. Pressing for specific details before the parents have had a chance to emotionally "unload" is seldom fruitful and more importantly may cause them to omit subtle details that may provide diagnostic information. After the caregivers have described the situation, the physician must ask specific questions to further document any circumstances of the event that will aid in the diagnostic approach. These questions should be guided by the differential diagnostic considerations outlined in the previous section.

The length of the pause in respiration is seemingly one of the most crucial pieces of information, yet it is often quite difficult to document because in such a stressful situation time is distorted, and seconds may seem like hours. Parents are also in fear for the child's life, and checking a watch is simply not a priority. Because the definition of an ALTE includes commentary on color and tone, these points must be addressed. Color changes often include cyanosis, but pallor also may occur. Similarly, hypotonia is a frequent finding at the time of the event, but hypertonia also may occur. If any resuscitative efforts, such as rescue breaths or chest compressions, were employed, these too should be documented because they are markers for more serious events.

It is diagnostically important to separate central from obstructive apnea, so careful history regarding any observed respiratory effort or unusual sounds, such as stridor or wheezing, associated with respiration must be noted as should the position of the child during the event, especially if it occurred during sleep. The child's state of consciousness before, during, and after the event aids in differential diagnosis.

The feeding history, including regurgitation after feedings, may raise suspicion of GER-mediated apnea. Vomitus in the oral cavity during or just after the event also makes aspiration a consideration.

A history of any previous respiratory problems or excessive snoring suggestive of chronic airway obstruction should be noted. A number of other symptoms are associated with the obstructive sleep apnea syndrome, including nocturnal enuresis, daytime sleepiness, and morning headache.

Any medications the child is taking and additionally any medications to which an older child might have access should be considered for their role in the event.

Any unusual movements and, in continent children, a loss of continence may point to the diagnosis of a seizure. The history of a subsequent postictal state is also supportive.

The past medical history should include a detailed birth history, including exposure to prenatal or perinatal infectious agents, maternal exposure to opioids (specifically for the neonate with apnea), and any difficulties during the birthing process, including traumatic deliveries. Any previous history of respiratory difficulties should be noted. Abnormal growth and development may be noted with congenital and chronic conditions. Immunization history may modify the degree of suspicion for infectious syndromes, such as pertussis.

The family history may help support the diagnosis of many genetic and metabolic disorders. A family history of such disorders or one that is notable for mental retardation, consanguinity, fetal loss, or neonatal death suggests this broad category of disease. History of SIDS in full siblings carries with it an increased risk of SIDS for the child in question, but no studies document an increased recurrence risk for more distant relatives.

The social history should include documentation of all people who provide significant amounts of care to the child because exposure to drugs, medications, and physical abuse may occur in social situations outside the confines of the nuclear household. Previous involvement of the family with child protective services is a red flag for factitious causes of ALTE, including suffocation in the most dramatic situations.

Physical Examination

The physical examination must first be geared to detect any immediate, life-threatening emergency. In the child with ongoing cardiopulmonary compromise, a septic appearance, or active convulsions, rapid intervention takes precedence over a detailed physical examination. In the majority of cases, however, the apneic event has ended and the child is conscious at the time of presentation. In these cases the physical examination can take on a more typical pace and should be complete with specific focus on the cardiopulmonary and neurologic systems.

Length, weight, head circumference, and any dysmorphic features may support a congenital cause for an apneic event. Poor skin perfusion; cool, mottled extremities; and delayed capillary refill are signs of compensated shock. Bruising should raise suspicion of physical abuse.

The nasal cavity should be examined for any secretions indicative of an upper respiratory tract infection or for any causes of possible obstruction, such as septal deviation or polyps. If any obstruction is suspected at the nasal level, the examiner should attempt to pass a nasogastric tube through each nostril. The structure of the lips, palate, and tongue should be noted, and the tonsils should be closely examined for any lesions that would impact normal respiration. The neck should be palpated for masses, such as swollen lymph nodes or an enlarged thyroid, that could cause airway obstruction from extrinsic compression.

The pulmonary examination should be fairly detailed. Before auscultation, inspection may reveal signs of increased respiratory effort, such as retractions or nasal flaring. A child with chronic obstructive disease may have a barrel chest. The physician may be able to observe the respiratory pattern when the child is asleep and awake. Irregular respirations, periodic breathing, or any prolonged pauses in respiration should be noted. Auscultation may reveal grunting indicative of increased respiratory effort. Wheezing on expiration implies intrathoracic obstruction, and stridor on inspiration implies extrathoracic, usually tracheal, obstruction. Consolidation of pulmonary parenchyma caused by pneumonia or interstitial edema may result in rales.

The cardiac examination should document rate and rhythm. The character of the heart tones and any associated murmurs, rubs, or gallops should be noted. Preductal and postductal pulses (right arm and leg, for example) should be palpated and compared. In addition to rales as noted earlier, the physician may see hepatomegaly or dependent edema in the presence of congestive heart failure.

Digital clubbing may accompany chronic pulmonary disease and also may be seen in chronic hypoxemic states, such as the obstructive sleep apnea syndrome.

The neurologic examination should be detailed and should carefully document mental status, muscle tone, and strength after the event. Cranial nerve function should be systematically evaluated with special attention paid to the airway protective reflexes, such as cough and gag.

A thorough history and physical examination should greatly narrow the scope of the differential diagnosis. This information can then be used to develop an approach to the patient designed to provide a definitive diagnosis and management plan.

Approach to the Patient

The approach to the infant with apnea is directed toward elimination of immediate life-threatening situations, determination of specific causes and treatment if they exist, and ongoing observation in the absence of a specific diagnosis.

If an infant has ongoing apnea or ineffective respiratory effort, cardiopulmonary resuscitative measures should be instituted without delay. Similarly, when confronted with a septic-appearing infant, cultures of blood, urine, and cerebrospinal fluid should be obtained immediately and broad-spectrum antibiotics administered promptly.

The majority of patients with apnea do not present *in extremis* but rather present shortly after an ALTE. The physician can best determine the severity of the apneic event in these patients by the neurologic examination at the time of presentation. A blood gas determination immediately on presentation objectively establishes the severity of the event. In a stressful situation where seconds of apnea may have seemed like hours, an immediate blood gas that shows no metabolic acidosis can reassure both parents and physicians.

If the history is that of a prolonged apnea, in addition to acidosis on a blood gas the examiner may see hypoxic injury to organ systems as evidenced by elevation of blood urea nitrogen and creatinine with renal impairment or elevation of transaminases with liver injury.

If apnea is recurrent and chronic as seen in the obstructive sleep apnea syndrome, severity can be determined by carbon dioxide retention on a blood gas, polycythemia from chronic hypoxia seen on a blood count, or evidence of right ventricular hypertrophy (reflecting long-standing pulmonary hypertension) noted on a 12-lead electrocardiogram.

Once the patient is out of immediate danger and the severity of the episode has been gauged, the next task is to determine the specific event that led to the apnea. To this end the history and physical examination are truly the most useful tools. Only rarely do ancillary studies establish a specific diagnosis that was not suspected after a detailed history and physical examination. The most common approach uses a combination of laboratory, radiographic, and polysomnographic studies. Occasionally, endoscopic examination of the airway and/or upper gastrointestinal tract is also useful. Three typical scenarios are now addressed—the infant with an ALTE, the patient with classic obstructive apnea, and the patient with classic central apnea.

Infants presenting immediately after an ALTE should be hospitalized and placed on a cardiorespiratory monitor in the hopes of capturing an event. Every infant with an ALTE should have a blood gas determination to look for evidence of chronic hypoventilation or hypoxemia. The value of an immediate blood gas and bicarbonate value in determining severity of an event was discussed previously. A blood count

to look for anemia, polycythemia, and leukocytosis in the case of infection also should be obtained for all infants.

If any respiratory distress or abnormalities on the pulmonary examination exist or if the spell was accompanied by choking or gagging, a chest radiograph should be obtained to look for evidence of pneumonia, bronchiolitis, or aspiration.

If a history consistent with GER is obtained, an esophageal pH probe can be coupled with a pneumogram to determine whether apnea occurs and whether it can be correlated with episodes of acid reflux into the esophagus.

Spells associated with tachycardia or hypertonia are suspicious for seizures and should be investigated further with an electroencephalogram (EEG). An EEG should also be obtained when spells are associated with convulsive movements of the extremities or glassy, open-eyed stares or are followed by a postictal period. In addition to an EEG, any infant with a suspected convulsion should have rapid determinations of electrolytes (specifically sodium), glucose, calcium, and magnesium.

Abnormal heart rates during a spell or any abnormalities on the cardiac examination should prompt an immediate electrocardiogram (ECG). In addition to looking for obvious dysrhythmia, hypertrophy, or signs of ischemia, the clinician should carefully calculate the corrected QT interval (see Fig. 12-3) and look for a delta wave (Fig. 13-2) as evidence of a predisposition to ventricular or supraventricular tachycardia respectively. Any patient with a pathologic cardiac murmur or an abnormal ECG should be referred to a pediatric cardiologist for further testing, such as echocardiography or electrophysiologic studies.

Infants with developmental delays, persistent lethargy, impaired growth, dysmorphic features, recurrent vomiting, or unexplained acidosis require more extensive metabolic testing, including amino and organic acid studies and serum ammonia, lactate, and pyruvate determinations. In cases of suspected metabolic disease, immediate consultation with an appropriate specialist is prudent.

Many patients with purely obstructive apnea have an easily identifiable lesion on physical examination. Nasal secretions, choanal atresia or stenosis, and tonsillar hypertrophy account for the majority of obstructive apnea. These lesions can be diagnosed on physical examination alone. Dynamic obstruction or obstruction caused by lesions below the oropharynx requires more invasive evaluation. Lateral neck films and magnified anteroposterior views of the tracheobronchial tree give an indication of adenoidal size and show obvious soft tissue lesions. Radiopaque foreign bodies are also detected in this manner. Barium-enhanced esophagrams may show episodes of aspiration of material into the airways and may show lesions involving both the airway and the gastrointestinal tract, such as tracheoesophageal fistulas. Further delineation of the airways is possible using laryngotracheobronchoscopy. MRI of the chest is ideal for showing lesions extrinsic to the airway that cause obstruction by compression. The approach to patients with purely obstructive apnea should begin with simple procedures, such as suctioning

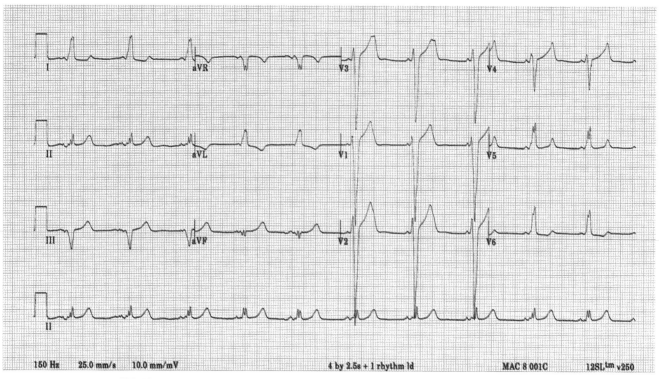

FIG. 13-2 Rhythm strip showing the delta wave of Wolff-Parkinson-White syndrome.

of the nares and attempting to pass a feeding tube through each nostril. When simple procedures fail to yield a diagnosis, the examiner should progress to the more invasive tests, usually in consultation with an otolaryngologist.

In addition to the testing outlined for the patient with an ALTE, the patient with confirmed central apnea should undergo imaging of the brain (CT or MRI) with close attention to the posterior fossa structures. Because seizures may cause unusual outward manifestations, an EEG should be obtained in the patient with central apnea.

Occasionally, despite careful attempts at obtaining a history, the physician is unable to determine whether an apneic event is central, obstructive, or mixed. In these cases even close clinical observation may be misleading. There are many varieties of polysomnographic studies that can clarify this situation. These studies involve simultaneous recording of ECG, respiratory effort (as evidenced by impedance plethysmography detecting chest wall movement), and respiratory airflow (as evidenced by a nasal thermistor). Depending on the clinical situation, other channels may be added, including pulse oximetry, transcutaneous capnography, esophageal pH, electroencephalography, and even electromyography and ocular movements (to determine sleep staging). The basic level of testing is very useful in the primary care setting, but the more involved levels are best reserved for specialists in apnea. Examples of multiple-channel pneumograms are shown in Fig. 13-1.

If repeated attempts at documentation of an event fail and by history the event is recurring in the home situation, direct

confrontation regarding the diagnosis of Munchausen syndrome by proxy may be necessary. This is a very delicate situation and should be carried out only after meticulous medical workup and exclusion of other possibilities. A psychologist, social worker, or psychiatrist familiar with this syndrome should be involved in the diagnostic phase of the patient's care.

The long-term approach to patients with a defined cause for apnea involves correction of the underlying lesion to whatever extent possible. This may involve surgical procedures, such as tonsillectomy and adenoidectomy to relieve airway obstruction, or medical intervention, such as institution of prokinetic and antacid therapy for GER. Methylxanthines, such as theophylline and caffeine, are occasionally used in children with recurrent central apnea, but they have no proven efficacy for disease states other than apnea of prematurity. In children with chronic hypoventilation from any cause, a variety of respiratory supports are available, ranging from simple oxygen delivery systems to home ventilators.

One of the most difficult questions faced by physicians dealing with recurrent (often idiopathic) apnea is whether an infant should have home-based cardiopulmonary monitoring. Although this remains a very individualized decision, some clinical guidelines for monitoring are listed in Boxes 13-1 and 13-2. These guidelines are based on the 1986 NIH consensus conference on apnea and home monitoring. The goal is to establish a subset of patients at highest risk for sudden death caused by recurrent apnea. A pneumogram should not be the sole test used to determine whether or not to discontinue monitoring. This decision should be based on clinical criteria. An infant with apnea of infancy can be taken off of the monitor after 2 to 3 months with no significant alarms. As a general rule the caregivers for any child on a monitor should be instructed in proper monitor use and event reporting and should also take a class in infant and/or child cardiopulmonary resuscitation (CPR).

SUMMARY

Apnea in a child, whether associated with a true apparent life-threatening event or not, often provokes fear and anxiety in both parents and physicians. This fear stems from the perceived relationship between apnea and sudden death. Although certain groups of patients are at high risk for sudden death, the majority are not. With a good grasp of the range of differential diagnostic possibilities, a careful history and physical examination often lead to a specific diagnosis. In the absence of any clues from the history and physical examination, a variety of physiologic recording techniques are available to document the events that lead to apnea. When a specific cause for apnea is found, treatment is directed to the underlying disorder. Respiratory supports are available for the child with recurrent apnea. In some cases apnea is idiopathic, and the descriptive term *apnea of infancy* is invoked. In these cases optimal management consists of continued close observation, including home monitoring and supportive care.

ILLUSTRATIVE CASES

Case 1. A 2-month-old boy was brought to the emergency room after he "stopped breathing" according to his mother. She fed him just before lying him on his back in the crib for a nap. She looked in on him about 15 minutes later and found him with perioral cyanosis. She did not think he was breathing but could not tell whether he was making any respiratory effort. She immediately shook him, blew a mouth-to-mouth breath into him, and slapped him on the back. He then took a deep gasp and began to cry. His mother called the paramedics, and by the time they arrived, they found him fussy but pink and active.

Physical examination in the emergency department revealed a bright, contented boy in no distress. His vital signs were normal, and a complete physical examination was unremarkable.

A CBC and capillary blood gas were quickly obtained, and both subsequently returned normal as did a set of electrolytes with a bicarbonate and glucose.

Further history reveals him to be a term infant with no medical illnesses. He is on no medications and has no known allergies. He has not been ill in any way of late, including no history of fever, vomiting, cough, or cold symptoms. The only notable history is that after some of his feedings in the last 3 weeks, he has spit up a mouthful of undigested formula. The emesis was not projectile.

Given the history of the event, including the perceived need for rescue breaths, he is admitted to the hospital. Because the nature of the apnea (length, central versus obstructive) is unclear, a pneumogram is performed simultaneously with an esophageal pH probe. It shows obstructive apnea correlated with acid reflux into the esophagus. There is no central apnea or bradycardia. The child is started on a prokinetic agent (metoclopramide) and discharged. Parents are instructed in infant CPR, and a home monitor is arranged before discharge. After 2 apnea-free months, the monitor is discontinued. The metoclopramide is continued for 6 months total and then discontinued with no recurrence of the reflux.

Case 2. A nurs aide in the normal nursery finds a 1-day-old who is pale and cyanotic. He is immediately examined and found to be asleep with face-mask oxygen in place. His skin is now pink, and capillary refill is 3 seconds. Examination of the head, eyes, ears, nose, and throat shows a flat fontanelle, normally shaped head, reactive pupils, and patent nares with no oropharyngeal lesions noted. Cardiac and pulmonary examinations are unremarkable. His abdomen is benign. Extremities show full range of motion without clubbing. Neurologic examination reveals slightly decreased tone but vigorous movement of all extremities. Deep tendon reflexes are normal. He awakens to painful stimuli and cries. His suck is somewhat weak.

Further history reveals a term newborn delivered by planned caesarian section because of breech presentation.

There were no antenatal complications and no maternal fevers or signs of chorioamnionitis.

While transferring the infant to the neonatal intensive care unit, he has a prolonged apnea with cyanosis and bradycardia. No respiratory effort is noted. He recovers and begins to cry after five breaths of bag-valve-mask ventilation with 100% inspired oxygen.

A sepsis workup is performed, and he is started on broad-spectrum antibiotics. A CBC and spinal fluid analysis are unremarkable. Cultures subsequently prove negative. Because of recurrent, severe, central apnea, a head CT is performed 36 hours later and shows cystic transformation of the fourth ventricle. A diagnosis of Dandy-Walker malformation is made, and neurosurgical consultation is obtained for shunt placement.

Case 3. A 9-year-old boy presents immediately after an episode of severe respiratory distress and apnea. He was in his usual state of health until 2 days before this episode. He developed a diffuse headache along with mild abdominal pain and a low-grade fever. The day before admission he complained of a mild sore throat and some swollen glands in his neck. He fell asleep reclining on the family sofa, and his parents noted noisy, raspy breathing and retractions. He then had an episode where his mouth was held agape, but no breathing was noted. The apnea lasted for "what seemed like 5 or 10 minutes," but his parents aren't sure of the exact timing. They shook him and yelled his name, and he awoke sluggishly. No convulsive movements were noted. He had no vomiting with the episode. Afterward, he was drowsy but otherwise back to his baseline of the previous 2 days.

The child is awake and alert, and the examiner immediately notices the sonorous, raspy inspiration phase that the parents described. The child is moderately obese and has a temperature of 38° C, a heart rate of 70 beats per minute, and a respiratory rate of 16, with no obvious respiratory distress. On further examination nearly "kissing" tonsils with white exudates are noted. He has soft, mildly tender adenopathy in the anterior cervical chain bilaterally. His lungs are clear, and his cardiac examination is normal. His abdomen is benign, and on neurologic examination he is awake and alert, with normal cranial nerve testing and a nonfocal examination.

While awaiting a blood count, blood gas, and rapid streptococcal antigen swab, further history is obtained. Past history is notable for recurrent episodes of tonsillitis (about three per year over the past 4 years) and recurrent ear infections, prompting myringotomy and tube placement. He snores "louder than his father." He has frequent morning headaches. He was an above-average student in first and second grades but now receives slightly below-average report cards. His teachers have commented on his falling asleep in class.

His streptococcal test returns positive. The CBC is normal with the exception of mild leukocytosis, and the blood gas shows pH, 7.36; pco_2, 48; po_2, 59; and HCO_3, 30. A diagnosis of the obstructive sleep apnea syndrome is made, and an ECG is obtained and shows mild right ventricular hypertrophy. He is treated with intramuscular benzathine penicillin G and observed overnight. He has one 16-second obstructive apnea. Late the next day his tonsils are slightly diminished in size and less erythematous. ENT consultation is obtained, and a tonsillectomy and adenoidectomy are scheduled for the next week.

ANNOTATED BIBLIOGRAPHY

Apnea (infantile) and home monitoring: report of a consensus development conference, NIH 87-2905, Bethesda, Md, 1986, US Department of Health and Human Services.

The "official word" on apnea monitoring. This report is the basis for many sets of guidelines and position statements. Fairly dense reading but well researched and authoritative.

Brooks JG: Apparent life-threatening events and apnea of infancy, *Clin Perinatol* 19:809-838, 1992.

A wonderful overview and review of the topic, this article gives clinically relevant recommendations that are well substantiated by review of scientific studies, as well as guidelines for choosing the most useful literature.

Keens TG, Davidson Ward SL: Apnea spells, sudden death, and the role of the apnea monitor, *Pediatr Clin North Am* 40:897-909, 1993.

This article presents a scientific look at a topic pervaded with dogma and anecdotal practice. Anyone prescribing monitors would benefit from this paper. Although the apnea/SIDS area is a rapidly evolving field, this reference remains relevant.

BIBLIOGRAPHY

Arens R, Gozal D, et al: Prevalence of medium-chain acyl-coenzyme A dehydrogenase deficiency in the sudden infant death syndrome, *J Pediatr* 122:715-718, 1993.

Ariagno R, Guilleminault C, Korobkin R, et al: "Near-miss" for sudden infant death syndrome in infants: a clinical problem, *Pediatrics* 71:726-730, 1983.

Bennett MJ, Powell S: Metabolic disease and sudden unexplained death in infancy, *Hum Pathol* 25(8):742-746, 1994.

Brazy JE, Kinney HC, Oakes WJ: Central nervous system structural lesions causing apnea at birth, *J Pediatr* 111:163-175, 1987.

Coleman J, Mammec M, Reardon C: Hypercapneic ventilatory responsiveness of infants at high risk of sudden infant death syndrome, *Pediatr Pulmonol* 3:226-230, 1987.

Guilleminault C, Peraita R, Souquet M, et al: Apneas during sleep in infants: possible relationship with sudden infant death syndrome, *Science* 190:677-679, 1975.

Guilleminault C, Stoohs R: Obstructive sleep apnea syndrome in children, *Pediatrician* 17:46-51, 1990.

Irgens LM, Skjaerven R, Peterson DR: Prospective assessment of recurrence risk in sudden infant death syndrome siblings, *J Pediatr* 104:349-351, 1984.

Potsic WP, Wetmore RF: Sleep disorders and airway obstruction in children, *Otolaryngol Clin North Am* 23:651-663, 1990.

Reiterer F, Fox WW: Multichannel polysomnographic recording for evaluation of infant apnea, *Clin Perinatol* 19:871-889, 1992.

Roloff DW, Aldrich MS: Sleep disorders and airway obstruction in newborns and infants, *Otolaryngol Clin North Am* 23:639-650, 1990.

Samson H, Mendelson L, Rosen JP: Fatal and near fatal food anaphylaxis reactions in childhood, *New Engl J Med* 327:380-384, 1992.

Shannon DC: Prospective identification of the risk of SIDS, *Clin Perinatol* 19:861-869, 1992.

Steinschneider A: Prolonged apnea and the sudden infant death syndrome: clinical and laboratory observations, *Pediatrics* 50:646-654, 1972.

Stevens L: Sudden unexplained death in infancy, *Am J Dis Child* 110: 243-247, 1965.

Van der Hall A, Rodriguez A, Sargent C, et al: Hypoxic and hypercapneic arousal response and predictors of subsequent apnea in apnea of infancy, *Pediatrics* 75:848-854, 1985.

Veereman-Wauters G, Bochner A, Van Caille-Bertrand M: Gastroesophageal reflux in infants with a history of near-miss sudden infant death, *J Pediatr Gastroenterol Nutr* 12:319-323, 1991.

Willinger M, Hoffman HJ, Hartford RB: Infant sleep position and the risk for sudden infant death: report of a meeting held January 13 and 14, 1994, *Pediatrics* 93:814-819, 1994.

14

Chronic Cough

BASIL J. ZITELLI

Key Points

- Chronic cough is defined as cough persisting for 3 weeks or longer and represents a common problem for office-based pediatricians or family practitioners.

- Recurrent viral infections and reactive airway disease are common causes of chronic cough in all age groups, although congenital anomalies may cause cough in infants.

- Careful history and physical examination frequently give clues to the diagnosis, and appropriate therapy is successful in eliminating cough in 80% of cases.

Chronic cough in children is a frequent and challenging clinical problem for the pediatrician. More than 1 in 20 pediatric office visits are for persistent cough, with nearly 4.3 million children seeking care every year for this complaint. It is the fifth most common problem seen by office-based pediatricians. The definition of *chronic cough* is somewhat arbitrary, but most investigators consider a cough persisting more than 3 weeks worthy of further investigation. This period allows ample time for most simple, uncomplicated viral upper respiratory tract infections to resolve. The nonspecific nature of the cough and the anxiety it produces in patients, parents, and pediatricians create the diagnostic and therapeutic challenge. With an understanding of basic pathophysiology, knowledge of common age-related differential diagnoses, and a meticulous history and physical examination, most causes can be elucidated and a satisfactory result obtained.

Pathophysiology

Cough is an important defense mechanism that protects the airway by removing secretions, foreign bodies, and irritating substances. Cough occurs infrequently during health; the natural ciliary clearance mechanisms are responsible for removal of small, superficial substances from the airway. The normal cough reflex usually develops during the first month of life in full-term infants but varies depending on factors such as prematurity and mechanical ventilation.

The cough reflex arc consists of the following five components: (1) cough receptors, (2) afferent nerves, (3) medullary cough center, (4) efferent nerves, and (5) the musculoskeletal system effecting cough. Cough receptors are located in many areas of the respiratory tract from the pharynx to the terminal bronchioles and are concentrated within the larynx, carina, and bifurcation of large- and medium-sized bronchi. No receptors are found within terminal bronchioles or alveoli. Four types of receptors are most likely to exist in these areas: slowly and rapidly adapting fibers at the level of the carina and larger bronchi that respond to mucosal tactile stimulation, C-fiber endings from the pharynx to bronchioles that respond to chemical and mechanical stimulation, pulmonary stretch receptors in the smooth muscle of the respiratory tree that respond to mechanical stimuli, and irritant receptors located between and beneath columnar epithelial cells that react to chemical and mechanical irritants. Afferent fibers from these areas are generally carried by the vagus, glossopharyngeal, and trigeminal nerves. Other receptors can be found in the external auditory canal (hence the frequent reflex of coughing while the child's ear is being cleaned), tympanic membrane, pleura, stomach, pericardium, diaphragm, and esophagus.

Most afferent impulses travel via the vagus nerve to the cough center located diffusely in the medulla. This center integrates and coordinates efferent impulses through the vagus, phrenic, and spinal motor nerves, causing a coordinated response from the larynx, tracheobronchial tree, intercostal muscles, diaphragm, abdominal wall, and pelvic floor.

The cough mechanism is divided into three phases that permit high expiratory flow rates and decrease cross-sectional area of the airway essential for an effective cough. The initial phase is a sudden, deep inspiration that fills the lungs with

BOX 14-1

Complications of Cough

Musculoskeletal
Chest pain
Rib fracture
Rupture of abdominal muscle
Disk herniation

Hemorrhagic
Hemoptysis
Subconjunctival hemorrhage
Head and neck petechiae

Barotrauma
Pneumomediastinum
Pneumothorax

Cardiac
Bradycardia
Syncope

Constitutional
Apnea
Fatigue
Headache
Vomiting and dehydration
Anorexia/failure to thrive
Social stigma

air and increases the diameter of the bronchi. The second (compressive) phase begins with tight closure of the larynx primarily effected by approximation of the false cords. The false cords, or ventricular bands, have a flat inferior surface that more evenly distributes high pressures from the trachea and act as a one-way valve, preventing egress of air. The true vocal cords, however, offer no resistance to air pressure from below but can withstand up to 140 mmHg from above. Contraction of muscles (intercostals, diaphragm, abdomen, and pelvic floor) producing expiration creates tremendous intrathoracic pressures up to 300 mmHg.

The actual cough occurs during the third (expiratory) phase. Sudden opening of the glottis associated with continued muscular contraction produces marked acceleration of airflow, with peak airflows reaching roughly 2 vital capacities per second in children. This initial high expiratory flow (the "bechic blast") is associated with narrowing of the cross-sectional area of the trachea up to 80%. Air velocities approach 25,000 cm/sec, nearly three fourths the velocity of sound. The narrowing of the trachea and large bronchi (the "tussive squeeze") decreases dead space; offers more resistance to airflow, holding smaller airways open; and creates turbulence that vibrates and shakes loose mucous secretions.

With such sudden, massive pressure changes occurring dramatically, a variety of complications may occur, particularly with recurrent or chronic cough. Persistent cough may lead to irritation of the mucosa in the larynx and tracheobronchial tree, posttussive emesis, and failure to thrive as a result of reduced caloric intake and exhaustion (particularly with pertussis infections). Other complications are listed in Box 14-1.

Inadequate cough mechanics can be found in patients who have disturbances of the inspiratory or expiratory phases of cough or both. Patients who experience severe pain with thoracic movement (e.g., postthoracic surgery or rib fractures) or neuromuscular weakness (e.g., spinal muscular atrophy or muscular dystrophy) have limited thoracic excursions. Central nervous system depression, such as coma or some sedating drugs, interferes with the cough reflex. Any process producing reduced expiratory flow rates (extrinsic compressive masses, bronchial strictures, foreign body, or bronchospasm) reduces cough effectiveness.

Literature Review

Numerous reviews of chronic cough in children emphasize the diverse differential diagnosis and the prevalence of certain disorders at different ages. Mellis, Eigen, Urbach, and others generally considered disorders within certain age groups, then analyzed historic, physical, and laboratory information leading to a particular evaluation and diagnosis. Information helpful in the evaluation included timing of the cough (time of the year and time of day), nature of the cough, and quality of the sputum produced. Other reviews summarized pathophysiology and a general approach to chronic cough.

Few studies actually summarize clinical pediatric practice experience with chronic cough. Movsowitz surveyed 256 private pediatric patients who had cough of at least 3 weeks' duration in South Africa. This retrospective survey included children from 3 months to 15 years of age. Of the 256 patients, 129 (50%) were asthmatic, 71 (28%) had recurrent upper respiratory tract infections, and 56 (22%) had pertussis or pertussis syndrome. Also, single cases of pulmonary tuberculosis, bronchiectasis, and right middle lobe syndrome were diagnosed.

Holinger and Sanders reported their experience with 72 children under 16 years of age referred to the Ear, Nose, and Throat Clinic for chronic cough of at least 4 weeks' duration with a normal chest radiograph. The average delay from onset of symptoms to evaluation by the specialist was 13 months. Patients were stratified according to age, and the most common diagnoses were determined by an extensive evaluation protocol. In the 32 patients from birth to 18 months of age, aberrant innominate artery, cough-variant asthma (CVA), and gastroesophageal reflux (GER) were the most common causes of cough. Endoscopy barium esophogram and a therapeutic trial of bronchodilators were the most helpful diagnostic modalities in this group.

In children from 18 months to 6 years of age, sinusitis was the most frequent diagnosis (50%); CVA was second most frequent (27%). Sinus radiographs and a trial of bronchodilators were most helpful in this group.

Older children from 6 to 16 years of age had a variety of disorders, including CVA (45%), psychogenic cough (32%), and sinusitis (27%). Notably, 18% of all children in the study had more than one diagnosis, and when specific therapy was initiated, 83% of children had complete resolution of their cough and another 7% were subjectively improved.

Major Causes of Chronic Cough According to Age

Infant	Toddler/Young School-Age	Older School-Age/Adolescent
Anomalies	—	—
Vascular ring		
Innominate artery compression		
Tracheoesophageal fistula		
Pulmonary sequestration		
Subglottic stenosis		
Gastroesophageal reflux	*Gastroesophageal reflux*	*Gastroesophageal reflux*
Infections	*Infections*	*Infections*
Recurrent viral/bacterial infections	Recurrent viral infections	Recurrent viral infections
Respiratory syncytial virus	Sinusitis	Sinusitis
Pertussis, pertussis-like syndromes	Tuberculosis	Tuberculosis
Cytomegalovirus		*Mycoplasma* species
Chlamydia trachomatis		
Pneumocystis carinii		
Ureaplasma urealyticum		
Tuberculosis		
—	*Inhaled foreign body*	—
Interstitial pneumonia	*Interstitial pneumonia*	—
Desquamative interstitial pneumonitis	Desquamative interstitial pneumonitis	
Lymphocytic interstitial pneumonitis	Lymphocytic interstitial pneumonitis	
—	—	*Psychogenic cough*
Reactive airway disease	*Reactive airway disease*	*Reactive airway disease*
Asthma	Asthma	Asthma
Cough-variant asthma	Cough-variant asthma	Cough-variant asthma
Pollutants (passive cigarette smoking)	Pollutants (active/passive cigarette smoking)	Pollutants (active/passive cigarette smoking)
Suppurative lung disease	*Suppurative lung disease*	*Suppurative lung disease*
Cystic fibrosis	Cystic fibrosis	Cystic fibrosis
Ciliary dyskinesia syndromes	Bronchiectasis	Bronchiectasis
Immunodeficiency	Right middle lobe syndrome	Immunodeficiency
	Ciliary dyskinesia syndromes	

Differential Diagnosis

The differential diagnosis of chronic cough encompasses a diversity of pathophysiologic processes and a large number of disease entities. Because different age groups have different prevalences of disease processes, stratification of the differential diagnosis according to age might be helpful. Although significant overlap exists, infants, preschoolers, and older children may have different illnesses that clinicians must keep in mind (Box 14-2). In addition, evaluating the nature and timing of the cough, as well as any sputum produced, helps determine the origin of the cough.

Infants

The most frequent cause of chronic cough in infants is viral respiratory tract infection. Children normally have up to eight infections per year, with most of them clustered during the winter months. If each infection lasts 7 to 14 days, it is not surprising that recurrent viral respiratory tract infections can lead to persistent cough. Lower respiratory tract disease is commonly caused by viral agents, including respiratory syncytial virus (RSV), parainfluenza, and influenza. RSV may cause cough, wheezing, or apnea without significant fever, and the cough may persist long after the acute illness resolves. Parainfluenza is commonly associated with laryngo-tracheobronchitis (croup), and influenza may produce both upper and lower respiratory tract disease.

Bacterial infections also can cause protracted cough. Pertussis infection is recognized by its characteristic paroxysms of cough of long duration. Patients usually have had a nonspecific prodromal stage similar to an upper respiratory tract infection with cough and rhinorrhea. Diagnosis is usually made during the paroxysmal stage when severe bouts of coughing can lead to cyanosis, apnea, pneumothorax, pneumomediastinum, or even intracranial hemorrhage. Other organisms can mimic the paroxysmal cough of pertussis, including *Bordetella parapertussis, Bordetella bronchiseptica,* adenovirus, *Chlamydia trachomatis,* and cytomegalovirus (CMV).

Chlamydial infections generally are perinatally acquired, with maternal–newborn transmission rates approaching 50%. Conjunctivitis occurs in half of colonized infants, and pneumonia develops in 5% to 13% of infected infants. Infants who develop pneumonia often have a chronic afebrile course with diffuse lung involvement. Infants can have a characteristic staccato-like cough that may help differentiate pneumonia from pertussis infection.

Perinatally acquired CMV has also been associated with pneumonitis in infants under 4 months of age. Diffuse interstitial pneumonitis and hypoxemia are common. Diagnosis may be difficult, depending on inferential data from serologic tests and urine CMV cultures.

Ureaplasma urealyticum and *Pneumocystis carinii* have also been implicated in infantile lower respiratory tract disease and may produce cough without fever. Diagnosis rests with nasopharyngeal culture for the former and bronchoalveolar lavage for the latter.

The incidence of tuberculosis infection is increasing in the United States, and infants and children are especially susceptible if they have close contact with infected and contagious individuals. A 5-TU intradermal tuberculin test with an appropriate control test for anergy is the best and easiest diagnostic method for high-risk individuals.

Reactive airway disease (RAD) is one of the most common causes of chronic cough in all age groups. Although wheezing is a common manifestation of RAD, it is not a necessary component. CVA, or RAD without wheezing, was initially described in 1972 by Glauser. Since then, CVA has been described as a cause of chronic cough in children and adults of all ages. Movsowitz found that 50% of private patients had asthma as an explanation for chronic cough, and Holinger and colleagues found that CVA was the most common diagnosis in 72 children referred to an otolaryngologist for cough. Many of these children were incorrectly diagnosed because physicians did not consider the diagnosis or because the diagnosis was discarded after an inadequate trial of bronchodilator therapy.

Cloutier and Loughlin summarized findings in 15 children with cough. Most had normal baseline pulmonary function tests but developed mild bronchospasm after exercise. Children improved on bronchodilator therapy. Similarly, Hannaway and Hopper evaluated 32 children with chronic cough who were thought to have CVA. The cough universally worsened with respiratory infections, generally was nonproductive and nocturnal, and worsened with exercise and cold air exposure. More than half of all patients have a family history of atopy and frequently have a personal history of atopy as well. Exposure to certain drugs, such as angiotensin-converting enzyme inhibitors and beta-adrenergic receptor blockers, may exacerbate bronchial hyperreactivity and stimulate cough from RAD. Local pollutants can also stimulate RAD, with passive cigarette smoking being one of the most common offenders.

GER is relatively common in infants and may cause a wide variety of respiratory complications; GER may be caused by various respiratory disorders. Reflux may cause respiratory distress by occlusion of the airway with aspirate. During reflux the airway becomes narrowed by induction of mucus, edema, or bronchial smooth muscle contraction. Irritation of the upper airway by acid material may cause vagal-mediated bronchoconstriction even with overt aspiration. Similarly, acid reflux into the esophagus without aspiration induces bronchospasm and increases airway resistance. Children who have swallowing dysfunction because of local anatomic or neuromuscular disease or because of central nervous system disorders are at high risk for GER and secondary pulmonary complications with chronic cough.

Cystic fibrosis may cause protean manifestations, including chronic cough. Infants may have meconium ileus; rectal prolapse; recurrent pneumonia; poor growth; foul-smelling, malabsorptive stools; and wheezing that may lead the physician to perform a sweat test, using the pilocarpine-iontophoresis method. Other disorders that mimic cystic fibrosis in causing infantile suppurative lung disease include ciliary dyskinesia syndromes and primary and secondary immunodeficiency states.

Congenital anomalies causing chronic cough usually present in infancy. Vascular rings (Fig. 14-1) and innominate artery compression cause cough by stimulating mechanical receptors in the trachea. Tracheoesophageal fistula is associated with choking or gagging during feedings and recurrent pneumonia (Fig. 14-2). Pulmonary sequestration may present as recurrent pneumonia or infiltrates, particularly in the left lower lobe. It represents an embryologic accessory lobe of the lung that is neither attached to the normal lung tissues nor aerated. The systemic circulation rather than the pulmonary vasculature provides its blood supply and it is almost always located between the diaphragm and inferior surface of the left lung. Other anomalies associated with chronic cough and often best diagnosed by bronchoscopy include subglottic stenosis, tracheomalacia, and bronchogenic cysts.

Uncommon causes of infantile chronic cough include the interstitial pneumonias, such as desquamative interstitial pneumonitis, lymphocytic interstitial pneumonia associated with human immunodeficiency virus (HIV) infection, and bronchiolitis obliterans. These disorders require extensive evaluation, including bronchoscopy and lung biopsy, for proper diagnosis.

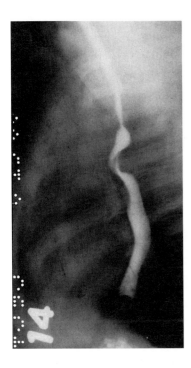

FIG. 14-1 Infant with a double aortic arch and retroesophageal impingement on the trachea, causing cough. A barium swallow demonstrates the retroesophageal indentation.

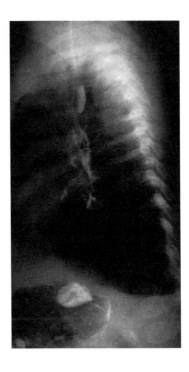

FIG. 14-2 A water-soluble contrast esophagram (lateral view) demonstrates aspiration of contrast into the trachea through an H-type tracheoesophageal fistula.

Preschool and Young School-Age Children

Children from about 18 months to 6 or 7 years of age are susceptible to the same disorders that affect younger children. Recurrent viral infections, RAD and CVA (especially on exposure to pollutants), and inhaled foreign bodies are common causes of chronic cough. Pulmonary tuberculosis, cystic fibrosis, and GER are less common but should be considered along with some unusual causes of suppurative lung diseases.

Particulate matter from wood-burning stoves or chemical pollutants from industrial airborne waste have been associated with chronic cough. More commonly, however, passive cigarette smoking has been associated with a 30% increase in hospitalizations for infants with pneumonia and lower respiratory tract disease. In addition, upper respiratory tract infections are twice as common in children with smoking mothers, including up to a 36% increase in middle ear effusions attributable to passive cigarette smoke inhalation. Chronic cough was positively associated with parental smoking in children under 11 years of age. Most symptoms exhibited dose-response curves, with symptoms increasing as the number of individuals who smoked and the number of cigarettes smoked increased.

Sinusitis may complicate 5% to 10% of upper respiratory tract infections in children, with two common clinical presentations. The most common presentation is a persistent upper respiratory tract infection lasting longer than 10 days. Cough may be present during the day but is often worse at night, and malodorous breath may be noted by parents. Character of the nasal discharge is not diagnostic, and complaints of headache, facial pain, and swelling are uncommon. A less common presentation of acute sinusitis is a severe upper respiratory tract infection accompanied by temperature greater than 39° C and purulent nasal discharge. Patients with sub-

acute or chronic sinusitis (symptoms not improving by 30 days) have protracted respiratory symptoms, nasal congestion, and cough. Fever and nasal discharge are uncommon. Physical examination usually is not specific for sinusitis. Confirmation of the clinical diagnosis can be made by standard radiographs in the anteroposterior, lateral, and occipitomental views. In symptomatic children older than 1 year of age, radiographic findings of diffuse sinus opacification, mucosal thickening of at least 4 mm, or an air-fluid level suggest sinus inflammation. Usual infecting organisms are *Streptococcus pneumoniae*, *Haemophilus influenzae*, and *Moraxella catarrhalis*. Adenovirus, parainfluenzae virus, influenza virus, and rhinovirus can be recovered in about 10% of cases.

Diagnosis of an inhaled foreign body may be particularly difficult if parents do not recall coughing or choking, or it may not be considered until coughing, wheezing, fever, or pneumonia develop. Inspiratory and expiratory chest radiographs (Fig. 14-3), chest fluoroscopy, and ultimately bronchoscopy (Fig. 14-4) may yield a diagnosis.

Suppurative lung diseases other than cystic fibrosis are uncommon in this age group. Bronchiectasis, right middle lobe syndrome, and the ciliary dyskinesia syndromes may cause recurrent pneumonia and cough. Bronchiectasis may be secondary to localized anomalies, such as bronchial stenosis, or the result of systemic disease, such as immunodeficiency (e.g., agammaglobulinemia with recurrent pneumonia). Right middle lobe syndrome is characterized by recurrent pneumonia generally confined to the right middle lobe because of stenosis or compression of the right main stem bronchus. Abnormal, uncoordinated ciliary movement produces ineffective clearance of mucus and debris, sometimes associated with an abnormal ultrastructure of the ciliary cytoskeleton. About half

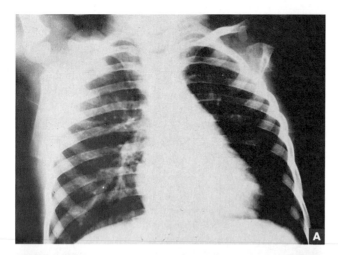

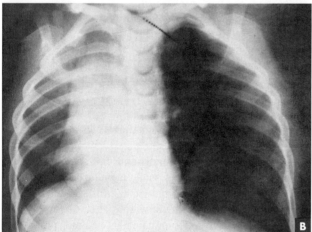

FIG. 14-3   Inspiratory *(A)* and expiratory *(B)* chest radiographs demonstrate airtrapping from a ball-valve effect of a foreign body in the left main stem bronchus.

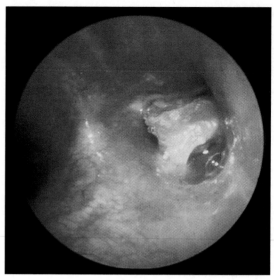

FIG. 14-4   Foreign body (carrot) lodged in the right main stem bronchus seen at bronchoscopy.

of patients with ciliary dyskinesia syndrome also have dextrocardia and abdominal situs inversus, known as Kartagener syndrome. This rare autosomal recessive disorder occurs in about 1 in 20,000 children. Serial radiographs documenting location of infiltrates and clearing of pneumonia are important in these suppurative lung diseases. Thin-cut chest computerized tomography (CT) (1.5 to 3 mm) in the involved area of lung may be helpful in detecting small, localized parenchymal lesions or determining extent of disease. Biopsy of respiratory tract ciliated columnar epithelium with electron microscopic examination could identify patients with ciliary dyskinesia syndromes. Findings include uncoordinated ciliary sweeping motion viewed under the dissecting microscope or absence of dynein arms or central spokes.

Tuberculosis in children in the United States has increased almost 40% from 1986 to 1991. This is in part related to exposure to adults coinfected with HIV and *Mycobacterium tuberculosis,* immigration of people from countries with a high incidence of tuberculosis, and the decline of public health services and access to care in many communities, which hinders identification, treatment, and contact investigation. Most

children with intrathoracic tuberculosis are asymptomatic, but infants and children are more likely to have fever, cough, and other respiratory signs and symptoms, as well as weight loss. Chest radiographs may demonstrate hilar adenopathy with or without parenchymal infiltrates or atelectasis. The standard of diagnosis is the Mantoux tuberculin skin test, applied intradermally. Criteria for a positive Mantoux test are as follows: (1) 5 mm of induration or more if the patient has contact with infected individuals, has evidence of clinical disease, or is immunosuppressed; (2) 10 mm of induration or more in an infant or child at high risk (i.e., foreign-born from high-prevalence countries, poor and medically indigent, or exposed to high-risk adults); and (3) 15 mm of induration or more in a child with no risk factors.

Older School-Age Children and Adolescents

Children in this age group similarly are affected by recurrent upper respiratory tract infections, acute and chronic sinusitis, RAD, cystic fibrosis and other suppurative lung diseases, tuberculosis, and some other disorders that may be more prevalent. *Mycoplasma* sp. infections, cigarette smoking, and psychogenic cough should also be considered in these children.

Mycoplasma pneumoniae infection may occur at any age but is more common in the older child. Infection may begin as a nonspecific upper respiratory tract syndrome but then progress to fever, chills, malaise, and cough. Cough has been reported to persist for 3 to 4 weeks in half of patients with pneumonia and for as long as 3 to 4 months in some patients. Radiographic findings may be striking, with infiltrates extending from the hilum and affecting one or more lobes. Despite the clinical symptoms and x-ray film changes, surprisingly few signs may be detected by physical examination. *Mycoplasma* titers, immunofluorescent techniques, and specific DNA probes have been used to diagnose *Mycoplasma* sp. infection.

TABLE 14-1

Clinical Evaluation of Chronic Cough

Characteristic	Diagnosis
Prematurity, neonatal respiratory distress	Bronchopulmonary dysplasia, RAD
Cough beginning shortly after birth	Congenital anomalies
Cough associated with feeding	Swallowing incoordination, tracheoesophageal fistula, GER
Malodorous stools, poor weight gain	Cystic fibrosis
Conjunctivitis	Chlamydia, adenovirus, *H. influenzae*
Weakness, neuromuscular disease	Swallowing incoordination, poor mucous clearance, aspiration
Family members with lung disease	Cystic fibrosis, tuberculosis, alpha$_1$-antitrypsin deficiency, asthma
Exposure to pollutants, cigarette smoke	RAD
Productive cough	Upper or lower respiratory tract disease
Unremitting cough	Suppurative lung disease
Brassy cough	Tracheal, large airway lesion
Paroxysmal cough	Pertussis, chlamydia, CMV, adenovirus, cystic fibrosis, foreign body
Bizarre cough	Psychogenic cough
Seasonal cough	Allergies
Morning cough	Sinusitis, smoker's cough, suppurative lung disease
Nighttime cough	CVA, GER
Green/yellow sputum	Inflammatory cells in sputum
Blood-tinged sputum	Suppurative lung disease, tuberculosis, pertussis, influenza, aspergillosis, coccidiomycosis, vasculitis, pulmonary embolus

Cigarette smoking is increasingly prevalent in preteens and adolescents. It induces ciliary stasis and a productive cough. Among adults, cigarette smokers have the highest prevalence of cough, and cessation of smoking is the most effective mechanism for alleviating the cough. Of patients who stopped smoking, 77% had complete disappearance of cough, over half within 1 month. Another 17% noted considerable improvement in the cough after cessation of smoking.

Psychogenic cough is most frequent during adolescence. The cough usually begins during the school year and persists for weeks or months. There may be no antecedent respiratory infection. The cough is isolated and explosive rather than repetitive spasms associated with infection. Often the cough is described as honking, barking, or bizarre and may occur as frequently as every 5 seconds. However, a hallmark of this disorder is the absence of cough during sleep. Psychogenic cough worsens with attention or stress and may be associated with school avoidance or psychologic disorders. Although the vocal component of Gilles de la Tourette syndrome must be considered as part of the differential diagnosis, psychogenic cough is not associated with other tics, such as grunting, snorting, or facial and body movements.

History

With a meticulous history and careful physical examination, the physician can often narrow the differential diagnosis and tailor further investigation through appropriate laboratory studies (Table 14-1).

Characterization of the illness includes questions as to when the cough began; if it is associated with any respiratory infection, fever, dyspnea, or chest pain; if respiratory symptoms include other areas of the respiratory tract, such as otitis media or acute or chronic sinus disease; how frequently the cough occurs; the nature and timing (vide infra) of the cough; if exposure to other persons with cough occurred; if exposure to pollutants or tobacco smoke occurred; if vomiting or spitting occurs in infants or epigastric or substernal chest pain occurs in older children, pointing to GER; and if there are associated systemic or constitutional symptoms, such as chills, fatigue, malaise, or weight loss.

A complete review of systems, including general state of health; growth and development; feeding history, especially in infants and toddlers; and symptoms of fever, headache, conjunctivitis, nasal congestion, rhinorrhea, sore throat, retractions, chest pain, choking, emesis, abnormal stools, or neuromuscular weakness, can focus the direction of the evaluation.

Past medical history should include a perinatal history looking for evidence of early onset respiratory disorders that may impact later years, such as respiratory distress syndrome, bronchopulmonary dysplasia, or congenital pneumonias. Previous hospitalizations, especially for respiratory symptoms, should be noted, and any radiographs or laboratory data from those evaluations should be reviewed. A history of known or suspected allergies, current medications, immunization status, environmental exposures (including industrial waste, tobacco smoke, and household pets) may yield important clues. Family history of atopy, asthma, cystic fibrosis, tuberculosis, recurrent infections, or chronic lung disease should be obtained. A careful psychosocial history may reveal prolonged school absences or stressors within the family, pointing to psychogenic cough.

The nature and timing of the cough, as well as the character of any sputum, are central to establishing a diagnosis. A loose or productive cough suggests mucoid or purulent upper or lower respiratory tract disease. Suppurative lung disease or chronic postnasal drip from sinuses, adenoids, or nasal passages produces a moist cough. Bacterial pneumonias produce purulent sputum, and unremitting coughs suggest cystic fibrosis, immunodeficiency, ciliary dyskinesia syndromes, or bronchiectasis. Chronic, recurrent aspiration in patients with neuromuscular disorders and swallowing incoordination may cause a productive cough and wheezing. Tobacco smoke classically produces a wet cough.

In contrast a dry, "brassy" cough is characteristic of tracheal or large airway origins, classically described with measles infection. Mechanical receptors can be stimulated by a mass exerting pressure on the trachea, such as innominate artery compression; other disorders, such as subglottic stenosis, and surgical repair of esophageal atresia and tracheoesophageal fistula also cause a dry, brassy cough.

Paroxysmal coughing, frequently associated with pertussis, can be heard with other disorders as well. The infant with pertussis looks well between episodes of cough but then launches into a dramatic episode of coughing, gagging, and choking that may be associated with apnea. Even when these severe episodes abate, infants may exhibit "the 100-day cough," a persistent cough lasting weeks or months. Other disorders to be considered include chlamydia, adenovirus, CMV, foreign body aspiration, and suppurative lung diseases, such as cystic fibrosis.

The bizarre cough of psychogenic origin is often most notable when attention is drawn to it. It frequently is disturbing to anyone around the patient, and although parents and patient may exhibit high levels of anxiety, some children may appear indifferent to the cough (belle indifférence).

Timing of the cough also may provide important information for diagnosis. The infant who coughs shortly after birth may have a congenital anomaly. After 6 months of age, foreign body aspiration becomes more prevalent, and after the child enters daycare or school, viral infections become more common. Seasonal cough, especially in spring and summer, might suggest atopy, and fall and winter may be associated with RAD or CVA and frequent viral infections. The cough of CVA usually occurs at night and during exercise. The cough of postnasal drip is usually worse at bedtime and on arising when mucous clearance is less efficient. Other causes of morning cough include cystic fibrosis, suppurative lung diseases, and active or passive smoking. Coughing during or shortly after meals in infancy suggests GER, tracheoesophageal fistula, or an abnormal swallowing mechanism.

Young children do not "produce" sputum well but rather swallow it, occasionally leading to emesis. However, if a child can give a sputum sample (not saliva) for analysis, it may provide an indication of pathology and the microbiologic cause. Clear sputum may be devoid of white cells or contain a few eosinophils. Green or yellow sputum contains the breakdown products of inflammatory cells and may be seen in suppurative lung disease and even bronchospasm once the airway obstruction is relieved. Older children may complain of a foul, metallic taste and have fetor oris as a result of purulent sputum. Hemoptysis most frequently results from bleeding within the oropharynx. When no apparent source is found on examination, pulmonary causes should be considered, including suppurative lung disease and foreign body aspiration. Infections noted for producing hemoptysis include tuberculosis, pertussis, influenza, aspergillosis, and coccidiomycosis. Rare disorders causing bloody sputum are pulmonary hemosiderosis, pulmonary emboli, and pulmonary vasculitis caused by systemic lupus erythematosus, Goodpasture syndrome, and Henoch-Schönlein purpura.

Physical Examination

The physical examination should be complete and meticulous. General appearance, growth measurements over several years, and vital signs should be obtained. Fever may indicate infection or systemic inflammation, and an increased respiratory rate may indicate elevated minute ventilation, which is sensitive for pulmonary disease in the young child. A careful head and neck examination for upper airway disease and a thorough cardiac examination for evidence of cor pulmonale (jugular venous distension, enlarged liver, tachypnea, or gallop) should be accomplished.

Examination of the chest includes inspection for breathing patterns, chest wall deformities, asymmetry, or unequal expansion. Palpation of the chest may reveal areas of increased vocal fremitus, indicating underlying parenchymal consolidation. Percussion may be difficult in young infants but may help determine areas of increased resonance associated with airtrapping or dullness found with pleural thickening, pleural effusions, consolidation, or masses. Auscultation compares both sides of the chest when listening for quality and equality of breath sounds, prolongation of expiration, and adventitious sounds, such as rhonchi, wheezing, and rales. Clubbing and cyanosis should be noted on extremity examination. The neuromuscular examination includes mental status, gag reflex, muscle tone and strength, and swallowing coordination.

More peripheral findings that may be helpful, especially noting the presence of atopic disease, may include allergic shiners (dark circles under the eyes caused by engorged venous plexus under the lower eyelid resulting from nasal or sinus mucosal swelling); Dennie Morgan lines (accessory transverse crease of the lower eyelid extending one half to two thirds the width of the palpebral fissure) (see Fig. 15-6); pale blue, boggy nasal mucosa with a clear nasal discharge (see Fig. 15-3); the allergic salute (turning the nose upward with the palm of the hand to increase nasal airflow, resulting in a transverse nasal crease; cobblestone lymphoid follicles on the palpebral conjunctivae;

eczema; and urticaria. Patients with cystic fibrosis often have poor growth, barrel chest, and clubbing. Nasal polyps have been found in children with aspirin-sensitive asthma, cystic fibrosis, and ciliary dyskinesia syndromes.

Approach to the Patient

Most children with chronic cough have recurrent or persistent viral infections or RAD and require no further evaluation other than a careful history and physical examination. If further laboratory studies are deemed necessary, they should be planned to identify the diagnosis as quickly and directly as possible with minimal physical, psychologic, and economic trauma to the patient. How aggressive the evaluation should be depends on the severity of symptoms, the degree of interference with a normal lifestyle, and the potential morbidity of the most likely diagnosis.

Laboratory tests should be directed toward a specific diagnosis suggested by the history and physical examination. A complete blood count and differential may show anemia of chronic disease or polycythemia of chronic hypoxemia, leukocytosis of infection or more specifically lymphocytosis of pertussis, eosinophilia of atopy, or lymphopenia of immunodeficiency. A chest radiograph (posteroanterior, lateral views) may show infiltrates, effusions, masses, atelectasis, or airtrapping. If hypoxia is suspected, hemoglobin oxygen saturation can be measured using pulse oximetry or more directly blood gas analysis. A 5-TU Mantoux tuberculin skin test is assuming more importance in the diagnosis of chronic cough because of the rising incidence of tuberculosis.

Infants may have anomalies causing cough that may be best diagnosed radiographically with a barium swallow. More specialized imaging studies, including chest CT, magnetic resonance imaging (MRI), or even angiography may be necessary. Because infections are most likely to produce chronic cough, specific cultures for pertussis and viral pathogens, as well as Chlamydiazyme, may yield a specific diagnosis. The sweat test performed by pilocarpine iontophoresis may be diagnostic for cystic fibrosis, and more recently specific identification of gene mutation can be diagnostic when the sweat test cannot be performed.

GER can be confirmed by using a barium swallow with small bowel follow-through and extended 18- to 24-hour esophageal pH probe monitoring. If RAD is suspected, a trial of bronchodilators, including antiinflammatory agents, such as cromolyn sodium or steroids, may be diagnostic and therapeutic.

Toddlers and younger school-age children may undergo an evaluation similar to that of infants with some important additional considerations. Because foreign body aspiration should be considered, inspiratory and expiratory chest radiographs or chest fluoroscopy may be helpful in demonstrating airtrapping caused by the ball-valve effect of the foreign object. Bronchoscopy is diagnostic and therapeutic. Sinus radiographs in children older than 1 year of age may demonstrate findings consistent with infection and congestion. Suppurative lung diseases may require the more sophisticated imaging studies cited previously and selective bronchography. Pulmonary function testing before and after bronchodilator therapy or after exercise may be revealing in children with RAD or CVA. The use of a peak flowmeter can be helpful diagnostically and therapeutically. Baseline values can be obtained over several days at different times of the day, and then a response to bronchodilators can be observed. Improvement in peak flow suggests bronchodilator-responsive RAD. Sputum, if obtained, should be sent for Gram stain and culture; examination may reveal eosinophils, crystalline material, and protein spirals (Curschmann spirals) in patients with RAD.

Older children and adolescents may undergo similar examination if necessary, and they may be more cooperative with certain imaging studies and pulmonary function testing. Other diagnostic tests, such as MRI, $alpha_1$-antitrypsin levels, ciliary biopsy (Fig. 14-5), and immunologic evaluation, may be suggested in the appropriate clinical setting. These tests should be used when clinically indicated or to confirm results of preliminary evaluations.

Therapy

Once a diagnosis is established, specific therapy usually is successful in eliminating the cough in over 80% of cases. Because recurrent viral infection is the most common cause of chronic cough in all age groups, the cough is usually self-limited and spontaneously resolves with time. Cough suppressants have potential side effects and generally limited efficacy. They should not be used in diseases involving the lower respiratory tract. Dextromethorphan and codeine are two commonly used cough suppressants, particularly for a dry, irritative cough of the upper respiratory tract. Both drugs act on the central cough center. In a placebo-controlled study of cough of less than 14 days' duration associated with upper respiratory tract infection, neither codeine nor dextromethorphan was superior to the placebo in treating the night cough. Cough suppressants generally should not be used routinely in children. Physicians should reassure and educate the child and family and explain the limited benefits of these medications.

RAD and CVA are the most common diagnoses, other than viral infection, in all age groups. Treatment should be directed toward relieving underlying inflammation and bronchospasm using selective beta$_2$-agonist inhalation therapy and cromolyn sodium with possible short bursts of steroids when indicated. Some experts do not consider therapy a failure until a course of oral steroids (oral prednisone 1 mg/kg/day in two daily doses) has been attempted. Theophylline and cromolyn sodium may be effective for around-the-clock therapy. Failure of therapy may be more related to undertreatment or noncompliance rather than an incorrect diagnosis. Sinusitis and GER may act as potentiators of CVA and should be treated con-

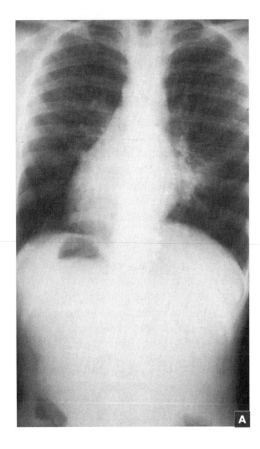

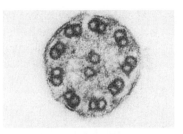

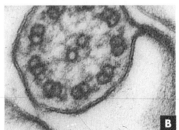

FIG. 14-5 *A,* Chest radiograph of a patient with Kartagener syndrome demonstrating dextrocardia and situs inversus. *B,* Electron micrograph of cilia from the same patient with abnormal cilia on the top missing dynein arms from the outer doublets. A normal cilia is on the bottom.

currently if found. Theophylline, via its relaxation of the lower esophageal sphincter, may exacerbate GER.

Infections such as tuberculosis, sinusitis, mycoplasma, and the afebrile pneumonias of infancy require specific therapy. Drug-resistant tuberculosis may be prevalent in certain areas of the United States, and therapy depends on the specific sensitivity of prevalent strains of mycobacteria within the community. Pneumococcus, *H. influenzae,* and *M. catarrhalis* frequently cause sinusitis and can be effectively treated with the same antibiotics used to treat otitis media, including amoxicillin, amoxicillin/clavulanate, erythromycin/sulfisoxazole, trimethoprim/sulfamethoxazole, cefaclor, and cefuroxime axetil. Macrolide antibiotics, including erythromycin, are effective in treating *Mycoplasma* sp. respiratory infections in older children, although the cough may linger beyond the acute disease for weeks.

Specific diagnosis of the afebrile pneumonias of infancy prompts directed therapy. Ribavirin is recommended for high-risk infants with prematurity or chronic lung or heart disease with RSV infection. Erythromycin is effective for *U. urealyticum* and chlamydia, and *P. carinii* can be treated with trimethoprim/sulfamethoxazole. Specific therapy should be directed toward opportunistic infections in AIDS patients, and steroids may be beneficial in lymphocytic interstitial pneumonia.

Medical therapy for GER may be quite successful and includes thickened feedings; position changes enhancing a prone, head-up posture; and histamine H_2 antagonists or prokinetic agents. Rarely a fundoplication may be necessary when medical therapy fails. Anatomic anomalies causing chronic cough (i.e., tracheoesophageal fistula, vascular rings, and innominate artery tracheal compression) may also require surgical intervention.

Psychogenic cough has been successfully treated in some instances using the bedsheet technique as described by Cohlan and Stone. A bedsheet is tightly wrapped around the patient's chest because the chronic cough supposedly has weakened the chest muscles and the sheet helps strengthen the chest and alleviate the cough. Cough has disappeared in some patients within 24 hours. Others find that simple reassurance and a conscious effort to voluntarily suppress the cough also works well. Occasionally, patients and families may require psychologic counseling.

On occasion, consultation or referral may be desirable for the patient with chronic cough (i.e., the physician is uncomfortable proceeding with a diagnostic or therapeutic plan; the diagnosis is not apparent after reasonable evaluation; the child has not responded to simple therapeutic modalities; or the diagnostic evaluation requires subspecialty technical expertise, such as pH probe monitoring, pulmonary function testing, bronchoscopy, or other specialized testing).

SUMMARY

Chronic cough in children is a common and sometimes perplexing disorder. However, viral infections are the most common cause of persistent cough in all age groups, and reactive airway disease is frequently associated with chronic cough. Infants and toddlers should be examined for anomalies and aspirated foreign bodies respectively as the origin for their cough. Generally a meticulous history and physical examination yield most clues necessary to make an appropriate diagnosis. More than two thirds of children recover when appropriate and specific therapy is provided.

ILLUSTRATIVE CASES

Case 1. *A 6-week-old infant was seen for coughing associated with feedings. The prenatal course, labor, and delivery were uncomplicated, and the child tolerated initial feedings of breast milk well. Once the mother's breast milk supply was established, the patient coughed, choked, and gagged with cyanosis during feedings. As the breast emptied and the velocity of milk letdown slowed, she nursed well. Physical examination, including growth parameters, was normal. Her pediatrician suspected either GER or an anomaly. A barium swallow was obtained, revealing H-type tracheoesophageal fistula, which was successfully surgically corrected.*

This case demonstrates that infants with early onset of coughing may have structural disorders causing cough. A barium swallow was diagnostic in this case, although bronchoscopy sometimes may be necessary to demonstrate a fistula.

Case 2. *An 8-year-old boy has a chief complaint of nighttime cough over the past 4 months. He does not cough during the day, although his mother reports he has slightly decreased exercise tolerance. The mother has never heard any wheezing. The patient has no other symptoms and has continued to eat well, grow, and gain weight. The cough is dry and nonproductive. Family members have eczema and seasonal rhinitis. Physical examination is normal. Blood count and differential and chest radiographs are normal. Pulmonary function tests are normal before and after bronchodilators but show evidence of bronchospasm with exercise. Treatment with a $beta_2$-agonist and cromolyn sodium eliminated the cough and increased exercise tolerance.*

This child demonstrates a classic presentation of CVA with only nighttime cough and normal physical examination. Pulmonary function tests generally are normal except after exercise or possibly with methacholine challenge.

Case 3. *A 10-year-old girl is evaluated for a 6-week history of cough, occurring every 3 to 5 minutes during the day. The child has missed 3 of the first 5 weeks of school. She has no fever, chills, weight loss, headache, or nasal congestion. The cough is nonproductive. She has had no exposure to anyone with chronic cough or other illnesses. The child is described as an excellent student who likes school. Physical findings are confined only to a "goose-honk" type of cough that worsens when the physician directs questions*

to her but lessens when questions are directed to parents. The parents are puzzled as to why the cough disappears at night. Otolaryngologic evaluation, including sinus and chest x-rays, are normal. A diagnosis of psychogenic cough was made, and physicians recommended the child have a bedsheet wrapped around her chest until "her chest was stronger and the cough lessened." The patient refused the bedsheet but accepted a wide elastic bandage. Within 48 hours the cough significantly improved; however, the patient complained that her arms hurt and she still refused to go to school.

This patient had a psychogenic cough with a bizarre quality that disappeared at night. When suggestive therapy relieved the cough, this patient developed a new symptom to replace the psychogenic cough. The patient and family ultimately were referred for psychiatric counseling.

ANNOTATED BIBLIOGRAPHY

Fielding JE, Phenow KJ: Health effects of involuntary smoking, *N Engl J Med* 319:1452-1460, 1988.
This is an excellent review of the profound effects of second-hand smoke on the health of children.

Johnson D, Osborn LM: Cough variant asthma: a review of the clinical literature, *J Asthma* 28:85-90, 1991.
This is an excellent review of cough variant asthma and its associated clinical correlates.

Kamei RK: Chronic cough in children, *Pediatr Clin North Am* 38(3):593-605, 1991.
This classic article is an excellent review of chronic cough in all age groups.

BIBLIOGRAPHY

Cloutier MM, Loughlin GM: Chronic cough in children: a manifestation of airway hyperactivity, *Pediatrics* 67:6-12, 1981.

Cohlan SQ, Stone SM: The cough and the bedsheet, *Pediatrics* 74:11-15, 1984.

Dworsky ME, Stagno S: Newer agents causing pneumonitis in early infancy, *Pediatr Infect Dis* 1:188-195, 1982.

Eigen H: The clinical evaluation of chronic cough, *Pediatr Clin North Am* 29(1):67-78, 1982.

Glauser FL: Variant asthma, *Ann Allergy* 30:457-459, 1972.

Hannaway PJ, Hopper DK: Cough variant asthma in children, *JAMA* 247:206-208, 1982.

Holinger LD, Sanders AD: Chronic cough in infants and children: an update, *Laryngoscope* 101:596-605, 1991.

Irwin RS, Rosen MJ, Braman SS: Cough: a comprehensive review, *Arch Intern Med* 137:1186-1191, 1977.

Kravitz H, Gomberg RM, Burnstine RC, et al: Psychogenic cough tic in children and adolescents, *Clin Pediatr* 8:580-583, 1969.

Mellis CM: Evaluation and treatment of chronic cough in children, *Pediatr Clin North Am* 26(3):553-564, 1979.

Movsowitz L: Chronic cough and cough mixtures in a private paediatric practice, *S Afr Med J* 71:573-574, 1987.

Orenstein SR: Gastroesophageal reflux, *Curr Prob Pediatr* 21:193-242, 1991.

Reisman JJ, Canny GJ, Levison H: The approach to chronic cough in childhood, *Ann Allergy* 61:163-171, 1988.

Starke JR: Childhood tuberculosis in the 1990s, *Pediatr Ann* 22:550-560, 1993.

Taylor J, Novak A, Almquist J, Rogers J: Efficacy of cough suppressants in children, *J Pediatr* 122:799-802, 1993.

Urbach AH, Bloom MD, Mendelsohn MJ, et al: What's behind that chronic cough? *Contemp Pediatr* 10(3):106-127, 1993.

Wald ER: Sinusitis, *Pediatr Rev* 14:345-351, 1993.

15

Chronic Nasal Obstruction and Rhinorrhea

SARA C. McINTIRE

 Key Points

- Allergic disorders and sinusitis account for the majority of cases of chronic nasal obstruction and rhinorrhea.
- Chronic nasal obstruction and/or rhinorrhea in the newborn mandates an investigation for structural anomalies.
- Persistent unilateral nasal discharge of any character, but especially if it is foul or bloody, is highly suggestive of a foreign body in the nose.

Although nasal obstruction and rhinorrhea are discrete symptoms and often occur independently, they are often linked as outcomes of a single process. Together they constitute common complaints in the primary care setting. Upper respiratory tract infection, the most common cause of acute nasal obstruction with rhinorrhea, is the most prevalent outpatient complaint but usually poses no diagnostic uncertainty. Persistent nasal obstruction and/or rhinorrhea, however, pose a greater challenge. In this chapter a strategy for the clinical and diagnostic evaluation of patients with chronic nasal obstruction and rhinorrhea is proposed. The reader is also referred to Chapter 14 for other information germane to this discussion.

Physiology and Pathophysiology

A basic understanding of the normal anatomy, physiology, and immunology of the nose and sinuses aids the approach to disorders of these structures. The nose conducts and humidifies inhaled air, adjusts air temperature, protects the lower air-

ways from particulate and infectious matter, and elaborates IgA antibody locally to fight infection. The turbinates provide an additional surface area to catch particulate matter. The nasal mucociliary apparatus traps and expels foreign matter anteriorly or posteriorly into the nasopharynx. Blowing the nose, sneezing, coughing, and swallowing help complete the removal of nasal secretions.

Nasal neural control is largely autonomic. The "nasal cycle," which refers to alternating patency and airflow between the two nasal passages, is driven by sympathetic outflow. As a consequence, for other reasons discussed later, nasal obstruction and rhinorrhea may arise as normal rather than pathologic states, and patients may thus experience symptoms with or without any objective findings.

The nasal mucosa reacts to stimuli with a limited number of symptoms, including obstruction, rhinorrhea, sneezing, itching, and less frequently, pain and epistaxis. Obstruction (generally referred to as *congestion* or *stuffiness* by patients) arises from mucosal swelling, secretions, deformities, or masses. Rhinorrhea may result from mere obstruction of the passage by normal secretions or increased volume of secretions provoked by irritants, allergens, or infections. Sneezing and itching ensue from the release of histamine (and other chemical mediators) and from nerve stimulation.

Understanding nasal and sinus anatomic relationships aids comprehension of sinus infections. The nose is divided into two passages by a midline septum. The lateral nasal walls contain the superior, middle, and inferior turbinates. The sinuses are four paired air spaces lined by pseudostratified ciliated columnar epithelium in continuity with the nasal mucosa (Fig. 15-1). The maxillary and frontal sinuses and the anterior ethmoid air cells drain into the nose via the middle meatus. The sphenoid sinuses and posterior ethmoid air cells drain via the superior meatus. The inferior meatus drains the lacrimal duct. The mucociliary apparatus sweeps secretions

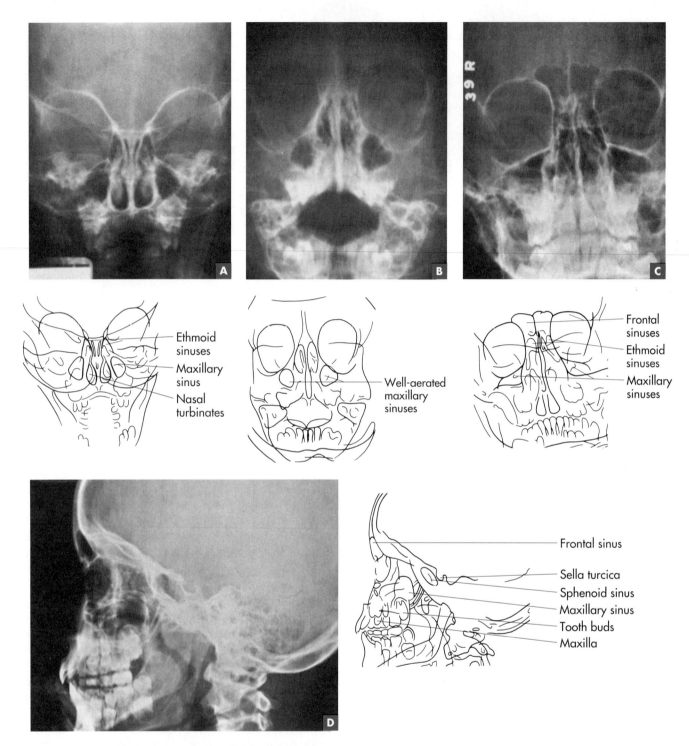

FIG. 15-1 Normal sinus radiographs. *A,* Anteroposterior Caldwell view demonstrates clear ethmoid sinuses. *B,* Waters view demonstrates clear maxillary sinuses. *C,* Posteroanterior Caldwell view (used
in older children) demonstrates clear ethmoid and frontal sinuses. *D,* Lateral view demonstrates the
frontal and sphenoid sinuses in an 8-year-old child.

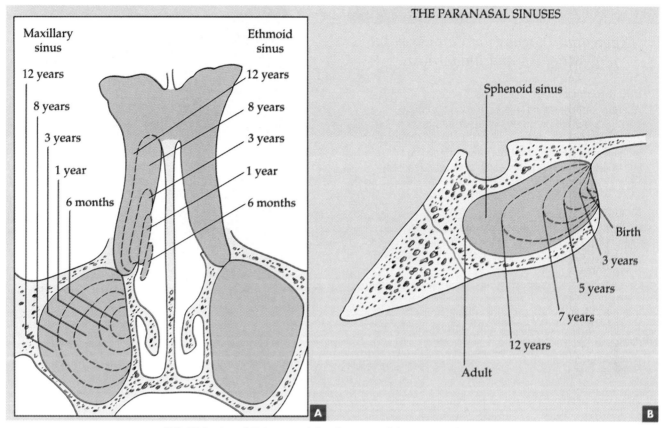

FIG. 15-2 *A* and *B,* Temporal development of the paranasal sinuses.

through the meatuses, into the nares, and then posteriorly into the nasopharynx. The maxillary and ethmoid sinuses are present, albeit in rudimentary form, at birth. The sphenoid sinuses emerge in early childhood, and the frontal sinuses are first seen by school age and develop fully by late adolescence (Fig. 15-2).

Recent literature on sinusitis has emphasized the importance of the osteomeatal complex (OMC), the area of confluent drainage of the maxillary, frontal, and anterior ethmoid sinuses (see references by Wald, Wegenmann, and Yousem). Because of the close proximity of structures in the OMC, relatively small changes in this area can produce obstruction and create the potential for multiple sinus cavity infection.

Differential Diagnosis

The list of differential diagnoses of chronic nasal obstruction and rhinorrhea is substantial, but for the pediatrician or family practitioner a firm grasp of the main classes of nasal disease and the most common entities within each is sufficient for the diagnosis and management of most children. The main classes discussed in this chapter are inflammatory,

structural, and drug-induced (Box 15-1). This chapter devotes particular attention to allergic rhinitis and chronic sinusitis.

Inflammatory

Allergic Rhinitis

Allergic rhinitis (AR) causes a complex of symptoms (nasal obstruction, rhinorrhea, sneezing, and itching) that result from an IgE-mediated hypersensitivity response to inhaled antigens. The *sine qua non* of this disorder is the rapid onset of symptoms after allergen exposure. Culprit allergens include wind-borne pollens from grasses, weeds, and trees; animal dander; dust mites; mold spores; and foods. Exposure of IgE-bearing mast cells in or on the nasal mucosa to allergens results in cellular degranulation and release of chemical mediators. Eosinophils are delivered into the nasal mucus in large numbers, and their presence frequently indicates allergic disease.

As in asthma, an early reaction and a late-phase inflammatory response occur in AR. Studies of the late-phase nasal reaction suggest that it accounts for the chronicity of AR. Repeated exposures lead to heightened sensitivity, a phenomenon called *priming.* As a result, even though the pollen count

BOX 15-1

Differential Diagnosis of Chronic Nasal Obstruction and Rhinorrhea

Inflammatory
Allergic rhinitis—rapid onset, sneezing, itching
NARES (*nonallergic rhinitis with eosinophila syndrome*)—no atopy, similar to allergic rhinitis
Sinusitis—persistent mucopurulent rhinorrhea
Other infectious rhinitides—*S. pyogenes*, adenoiditis, chlamydia, pertussis, syphilis

Structural
Choanal atresia/stenosis—obstruction from birth
Craniofacial malformation syndromes—fetal alcohol syndrome, Treacher Collins syndrome, Crouzon syndrome
Gliomas and CNS malformations—chronic obstruction, possible CSF leak
Trauma—deviated septum, septal hematoma
Foreign body—foul, bloody, mucopurulent unilateral discharge
Benign and malignant masses—loss of facial sensation, hearing, vision

Drug-Induced
Rhinitis medicamentosa—overuse of topical decongestants
Substance abuse or withdrawal—cocaine, antihypertensives, oral contraceptives

Miscellaneous
Pregnancy
Hypothyroidism
NANIR (*nonallergic, noninfectious rhinitis*) syndrome

CNS, Central nervous system; *CSF,* cerebrospinal fluid.

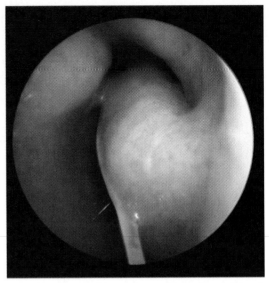

FIG. 15-3 Watery nasal secretions observed on the pale and swollen inferior turbinate of a patient with AR.

door inhalant allergens, such as dust, dust mites, animal dander, feathers, molds, and some insect antigens. Surprisingly, certain foods act as inhalant antigens; peanuts, eggs, and milk are the most prominent examples. The symptoms of PAR are the same as SAR, but because the exposure is continuous, the characteristic seasonal onset of symptoms is lacking.

A careful history of exposures is critical to the diagnosis and subsequent management of AR. There is usually a family history of allergy. In addition to typical nasal symptoms and equally critical is a detailed general physical examination, with special attention to the head and neck, including a search for other signs of atopy, such as eczema or wheezing. Nasal smears and other laboratory studies are discussed later in the chapter.

Nonallergic Rhinitis With Eosinophilia
Nonallergic rhinitis with eosinophilia syndrome (NARES) was first described in adults but has also been reported in children. Patients with NARES are clinically similar to those with AR and may demonstrate striking eosinophilia on nasal smear during symptomatic episodes but have normal serum IgE levels and no other evidence of atopy. The presumed pathogenesis involves the release of histamine or other chemical mediators that are not moderated by IgE. As would be expected, patients with NARES do not respond to antihistamines but may respond to topical or oral steroids.

Sinusitis
Although the common cold accounts for most cases of acute infectious nasal obstruction and/or rhinorrhea, bacterial infection of the sinuses is the most common cause of chronic infectious nasal symptoms. Sinusitis is acute or chronic. Distinguishing between acute recurrent episodes and chronic infection is arbitrary; Wald suggests that symp-

declines as the season goes on, smaller amounts of allergen cause equally severe symptoms.

Symptoms of AR are not always confined to the nose; other symptoms include postnasal drip (Fig. 15-3); pruritus of the conjunctivas, throat, palate, and ears; injection of the conjunctivas; puffy eyelids; watery discharge from the eyes; and epistaxis. Patients also may report more systemic complaints, such as fatigue, malaise, poor sleep, headache, and exacerbation of lower respiratory tract symptoms, particularly cough, wheezing, and shortness of breath.

The pattern of AR occurrence may be seasonal or perennial. Symptoms of seasonal allergic rhinitis (SAR) occur during discrete periods when wind-borne pollens, such as ragweed, are plentiful. Symptomatic AR that lasts all or most of the year is termed *perennial allergic rhinitis* (PAR). The symptoms of PAR are the same as those of AR. Unlike SAR, in which symptom onset bears a direct temporal relationship to exposure to outdoor allergens, PAR is usually caused by in-

Risk Factors and Complications of Sinusitis

Risk Factors	Complications
Recurrent upper respiratory tract infection	Mucoceles
	Polyps
Allergic and nonallergic rhinitis	Orbital cellulitis
Cystic fibrosis	Orbital abscess
Asthma	Cavernous sinus
Nasal polyps	thrombosis
Septal abnormalities	Meningitis
Rhinitis medicamentosa	Brain abscess
Trauma	
Diving	
Immunodeficiency	
Immotile cilia syndromes	
Wegener granulomatosis	

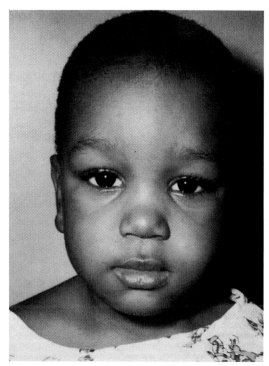

FIG. 15-4 Periorbital and infraorbital swelling in a child with fever, cough, scanty nasal discharge, and opacification of the maxillary sinuses.

toms persisting 10 to 30 days be considered acute and symptoms beyond 30 days be considered chronic. Acute sinusitis presents as a prolonged cold or a more toxic process with temperature greater than 39° C and purulent nasal discharge. Chronic sinusitis presents as obdurate nasal symptoms with cough.

The development of sinusitis involves a cascade of events initiated by an acute inflammatory response in the nose to an infectious (e.g., viral) or allergic (e.g., ragweed) agent. The response consists of nasal mucosal swelling and secretions. Because of the continuity of the nasal and sinus mucosa, the acute response blocks the sinus ostium; the sinus cavity, now filled with secretions and under reduced oxygen tension, constitutes an ideal medium for proliferation of bacteria. A similar series of events occurs with impediments to ostial drainage from nasal septum deviation, spurs, polyps, tumors, or foreign bodies.

The usual culprit pathogens in acute and chronic sinusitis in the normal host consist of *Haemophilus influenzae* (nontypable), *Streptococcus pneumoniae,* and *Moraxella catarrhalis; Staphylococcus aureus* and anaerobic bacteria ought to be considered in very prolonged cases. Patients with cystic fibrosis and chronic sinusitis most commonly have infection with *Pseudomonas aeruginosa, H. influenzae,* and alphahemolytic streptococci. In the immunosuppressed patient, chronic sinonasal infections are caused by common organisms and opportunistic invaders, such as *Candida* and *Aspergillus* species.

Risk factors for acute recurrent or chronic sinusitis include recurrent upper respiratory tract infections, AR, asthma, rhinitis medicamentosa, cystic fibrosis, AIDS and other immunodeficiencies, immotile cilia syndromes, foreign bodies, trauma, diving, and congenital anatomic disorders (Box 15-2). A rare condition regularly associated with re-

current or chronic sinus disease is Wegener granulomatosis, with sinus, pulmonary, and renal involvement.

Cough and nasal discharge are the most common symptoms of sinusitis. The cough is often worse at night and in the early morning. Nasal secretions need not be purulent and may be of any character. Except in cases of severe disease, fewer than half of patients have significant fever. Headache and facial pain are helpful clues but occur infrequently. Eyelid and nasal bridge swelling (Fig. 15-4), sore throat, postnasal drip, and foul-smelling breath are other findings sometimes seen in patients with sinusitis. Older children and adolescents may complain of loss of smell. In adults a history of maxillary toothache and failure to improve with nasal decongestants greatly increases the likelihood of acute sinusitis if accompanied by purulent secretions and abnormal sinus transillumination. The same parameters cannot be applied equally well to children. The prolonged duration of relatively mild symptoms is often the dominant patient complaint, but the significance of these symptoms must not be underestimated.

The physical examination of the child with uncomplicated sinusitis is generally benign; the examiner expects to find a nontoxic appearance, no or low-grade fever, nasal mucosal changes of pallor or hyperemia and swelling, and nasal discharge of any kind. Visualization of purulent discharge from the middle meatus is highly correlated with sinusitis but often impossible because of swollen turbinates. Use of a topical decongestant to shrink the turbinates may improve visualization. The presence of polyps is important to determine because they may be associated with cystic fibrosis, asthma, or allergies. Percussion of the frontal and maxillary sinuses is indicated to elicit facial pain. Accurate transillumination of the maxillary sinuses requires patient cooperation and thus may be difficult in the younger patient. Frontal and maxillary sinus transillumination in the older child or adolescent may confirm the diagnosis of sinusitis if light transmission is totally absent on one side. The voice may be normal, hoarse, or nasal in quality if the adenoids are enlarged. Facial edema and hyperemia of the throat and posterior pharyngeal secretions also may be seen. Pneumatic otoscopy is mandatory to detect the presence of middle ear disease.

A careful general survey for signs of long-standing illnesses or associated disorders is indicated as well. Is there growth failure suggesting an underlying disorder, such as cystic fibrosis? Does the child have allergic "shiners" (Fig. 15-5), infraorbital or transverse nasal creases (Fig. 15-6), or eczema or other emblems of atopy? An increased anteroposterior diameter of the chest and clubbing point to chronic pulmonary disease. A loud pulmonic component of the second heart sound is associated with cor pulmonale from chronic upper airway obstruction. Absent lymph nodes and tonsils or generalized lymphadenopathy with hepatosplenomegaly point to an immunodeficiency, as does oral candidiasis in an older child.

In most children, sinusitis is a relatively uncomplicated illness that responds promptly to appropriate antimicrobial therapy. Mucocele formation is a comparatively benign sequela of chronic sinus disease. These mucous retention cysts grow slowly over months to years, are often discovered incidentally by sinus radiography, and may obstruct nasal passages or expand into the orbits. Nasal polyps are herniations of hypertrophied mucosa originating from the nares or the maxillary and ethmoid sinuses. The role of sinus disease in polyp development is unclear, although patients with chronic sinusitis, allergies, or cystic fibrosis are clearly at higher risk for nasal polyps (Fig. 15-7). Whatever the cause of polyps, once they form, they obstruct sinus ostia, and sinusitis occurs. Serious or life-threatening complications of sinusitis include orbital cellulitis or abscess, osteomyelitis, brain abscess, cavernous sinus thrombosis, and meningitis (Box 15-2). Orbital involvement is the most common serious complication of sinusitis and deserves careful investigation whenever a child with sinusitis has progressive swelling and erythema of the periorbital tissues. Diagnostic imaging is discussed later in this chapter.

Streptococcosis

Group A streptococci *(S. pyogenes)* cause an indolent nasopharyngitis in children younger than 3 years. Streptococcosis is not characterized by sore throat in the absence of cough and nasal discharge as is classic group A streptococcal pharyngitis; rather, patients manifest obvious congestion, purulent nasal discharge that often excoriates the nostrils, cervical adenopathy, and low-grade fever lasting for weeks to

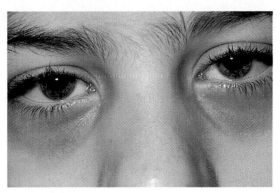

FIG. 15-5   Patient with AR and classic "allergic shiners."

months. Nasopharyngeal or throat cultures are positive for group A beta-hemolytic streptococci.

Adenoiditis

Chronic infection of the adenoids is another source of lasting nasal symptoms. Features include congestion, a nasal voice, mouth-breathing, postnasal drip, sore throat, and purulent nasal discharge. Abnormal facial development is postulated to ensue from long-standing upper airway obstruction; a long, narrow face with a retrognathic jaw is classically associated with "mouth-breathers" (Fig. 15-8). The examiner should suspect adenoiditis when other causes have been excluded, particularly if the nasal passages are patent.

Other Infections

Other infectious agents cause prolonged nasal but not sinus symptoms. *Chlamydia trachomatis, Bordetella pertussis,* and congenital *Treponema pallidum* infection all have prominent nasal congestion and rhinorrhea.

C. trachomatis is a cause of an afebrile pneumonia in early infancy that is typically preceded by conjunctivitis, nasal congestion, and rhinorrhea. The onset of respiratory distress with a staccato cough, tachypnea, and rales but no wheezes associated with prominent nasal symptoms and conjunctivitis with copious mucopurulent discharge is strongly supportive of infection with *C. trachomatis.*

B. pertussis infection in young infants, like that of *C. trachomatis,* has a distinctive clinical presentation that evolves over several weeks consisting of a long prodrome of nasal congestion and rhinorrhea followed by the onset of severe paroxysms of cough. The prodromal, or catarrhal, phase is nonspecific and resembles a typical viral upper respiratory tract infection; generally the diagnosis is made during the paroxysmal phase.

Since 1985, there has been a large increase in the number of cases of congenital syphilis. The newborn with a rash that includes the palms and soles, petechiae, lymphadenopathy, hepatosplenomegaly, anemia, leukopenia, low platelet count, jaundice, hepatitis, and cerebrospinal fluid (CSF) pleocytosis is easily recognized and probably infected

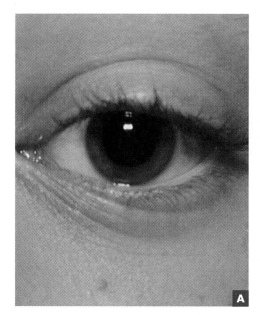

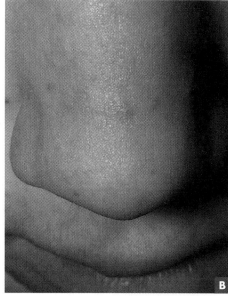

FIG. 15-6 *A,* Infraorbital creases, or Dennie-Morgan lines, in a patient with AR. *B,* The transverse nasal crease or "allergic salute" sign.

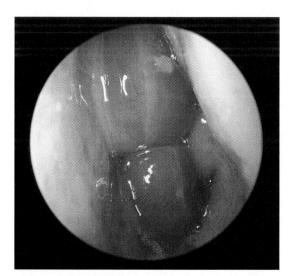

FIG. 15-7 A large polyp in the left nostril of a 2-year-old girl with cystic fibrosis.

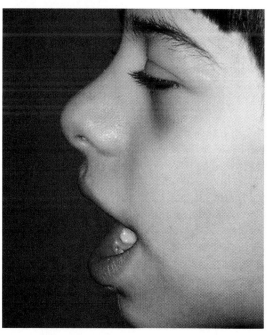

FIG. 15-8 "Mouth-breather," or adenoidal, facies in a patient with chronic AR.

with *T. pallidum.* However, infected infants may be completely asymptomatic at birth. In 1990, Dorfman and Glaser reported seven such infants who presented for the first time between 3 and 14 weeks of age; rhinitis, or "snuffles," was present in four cases, including the two oldest infants, and was the only other physical sign in a 7-week-old infant with hepatomegaly. The nasal discharge of syphilis is initially watery and becomes thick and purulent. Perforation of the nasal septum and saddle nose deformities are late manifestations of untreated syphilis.

Structural

Congenital

Congenital abnormalities of the nose are rare but potentially devastating because of the neonatal dependency on nasal respiration. Obstruction may be unilateral or bilateral and complete or partial. The primary symptom in the neonate is respiratory distress that is either overt or manifests during feeding or with upper respiratory tract infections. Congenital problems may present as isolated anomalies or as part of a syndrome. For example, choanal atresia (Fig. 15-9), the most

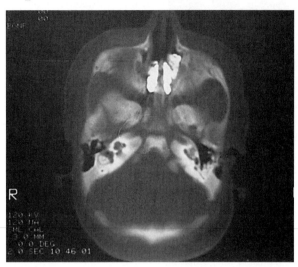

FIG. 15-9 Complete choanal atresia revealed by CT scanning. Radiopaque dye placed in the nares does not pass into the nasopharynx in complete obstruction.

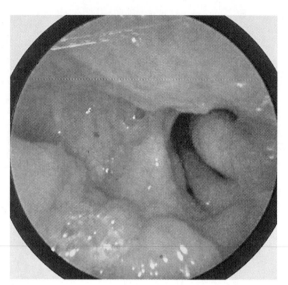

FIG. 15-10 Unilateral right-sided choanal atresia.

common congenital nasal anomaly, occurs in isolation but is frequently associated with a complex of anomalies known as the *CHARGE association* (*c*oloboma, *h*eart disease, *a*tresia choanae, *r*etarded growth and development and/or central nervous system anomalies, *g*enital hypoplasia, and *e*ar anomalies and/or deafness). Unilateral choanal atresia may cause rhinorrhea alone or obstructive symptoms when the patent choana is occluded during an upper respiratory tract infection (Fig. 15-10).

Syndromes of abnormal craniofacial development in which congenital nasal obstruction occurs include fetal alcohol syndrome, Treacher Collins syndrome, Crouzon disease, and Antley-Bixler syndrome. Central nervous system malformations, such as gliomas, meningoencephaloceles, and encephaloceles, may cause nasal obstruction and sometimes an obvious mass on or near the nasal bridge (Fig. 15-11). Extranasal gliomas are firm and do not change in size with crying. Rhinorrhea accompanying these malformations may be purulent, from secondary infection, or clear. Clear fluid in this setting is highly suspicious of CSF egress into the nares. Congenital anterior nasal occlusion is a rare anomaly that causes severe respiratory distress when the obstruction is complete or mild to moderate distress and cyanosis with feeding when the obstruction is partial.

Acquired

Trauma. Nasal obstruction from trauma may affect patients of any age, including the newborn in whom vertex or face presentation alone or delivery with forceps is associated with nasal injury. Severe nasal injury in the obligate nasal breather results in obstruction and respiratory distress. Careful examination of the nose may reveal traumatic septal deviation or even septal hematoma (Fig. 15-12). At any age, nasal

obstruction and epistaxis after trauma point to the possibility of a septal hematoma. This is a crucial determination because the complications include septal abscess and/or perforation and subsequent abnormal nasal growth and function.

Foreign Bodies. Nasal foreign body is especially pertinent to the pediatrician or family practitioner. All manner of things have found their way, by accident or design, into the nose. Common items include peanuts, beads, raisins, buttons, sponges, and seeds. Button batteries are uniquely noxious foreign bodies, causing mucosal burns and other symptoms.

Diagnosis of a nasal foreign body is challenging because the history of insertion is usually absent. The combination of nasal obstruction with unilateral, purulent, foul-smelling or serosanguinous discharge, and halitosis is highly correlated with the presence of a foreign body (Fig. 15-13). Epistaxis arises when the object has penetrated the mucosa. Vasomotor reaction to the material induces mucosal swelling and rhinorrhea that may obscure the object; only radiopaque objects are identified by plain radiographs.

Under most circumstances, consultation with an otolaryngologist for location and removal is indicated. Complications of a retained foreign body include recurrent epistaxis, sinusitis, palatal perforation, battery fluid burns, rhinoliths (calcified foreign bodies), and pyogenic granulomas.

Tumors. Benign and malignant tumors of the nose, paranasal sinuses, and nasopharynx are important considerations in the patient with chronic nasal obstruction, rhinorrhea, or unilateral recurrent epistaxis. Associated cardinal signs of serious pathology include loss of facial sensation, vision, or hearing; otalgia; and progressive enlargement of the nose, cheeks, or periorbital areas. Most nasal tumors in children are benign. Common benign tumors include polyps, papillomas, gliomas, and dermoids. Overall, malignant tu-

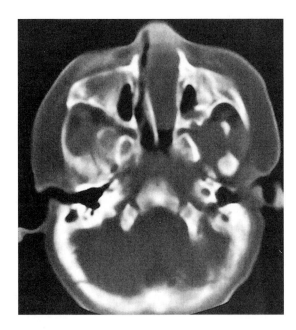

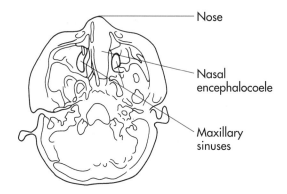

FIG. 15-11   A CT scan shows a nasal encephalocele completely occluding the left nasal passage and causing partial obstruction on the right side via septal deviation.

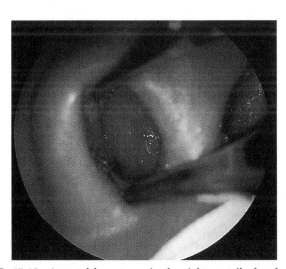

FIG. 15-12   A septal hematoma in the right nostril after facial trauma. This requires emergent drainage to avoid subsequent nasal deformity and dysfunction.

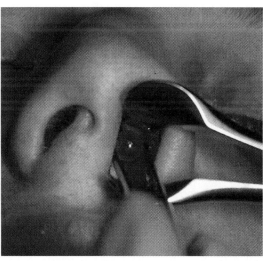

FIG. 15-13   A red bead was removed from the nostril of this patient who had classic symptoms of foul, unilateral nasal discharge.

mors are rare. Important lesions to consider are lymphomas, rhabdomyosarcomas, and carcinomas.

Juvenile nasopharyngeal angiofibroma is a benign tumor histologically but is locally invasive and recurs frequently after resection. It is largely a disorder affecting adolescent boys with nasal obstruction and intermittent epistaxis. As the tumor spreads, it may cause cheek swelling and proptosis. On examination the tumor can be seen in the nasopharynx.

Drug-Induced: Rhinitis Medicamentosa

Overuse of topical decongestants induces worsening nasal congestion. Marked congestion, pale or red mucosa, and scanty mucus are prominent. Improvement is effected by

withdrawing the offending agent, adding alternative therapy for the original condition that led to the overuse, and changing to systemic or topical corticosteroids. Illicit drugs, such as cocaine, also induce rhinitis; narcotic withdrawal can present as a "cold." Other medications that cause persistent nasal symptoms include antihypertensive agents and oral contraceptives.

Miscellaneous

A number of other processes are associated with persistent nasal symptoms in the absence of allergies, infections, drugs, or mechanical obstruction. Pregnancy and hypothyroidism are both associated with persistent nasal symptoms, particu-

TABLE 15-1

Key Clinical Features of Chronic Nasal Obstruction and Rhinorrhea

History or physical finding	Diagnosis
Neonatal presentation, symptoms worse with feedings or URI	Anomalies, GER
Seasonal or perennial nasal symptoms	Allergies
Persistent nasal symptoms after URI, cough worse at night	Sinusitis
Unilateral obstruction, discharge, halitosis	Foreign body
Polyps	CF, allergies
Wheezing	Allergies, CF
Mouth-breathing, snoring	Enlarged adenoids and/or tonsils
Poor growth, abnormal stools	CF
Nasal trauma	Septal hematoma

CF, Cystic fibrosis; *GER*, gastroesophageal reflux; *URI*, upper respiratory tract infection.

larly congestion. NANIR (*nonallergic noninfectious rhinitis*) syndrome is not a single diagnostic entity but rather represents chronic rhinitis without an allergic, structural, or systemic explanation. Another name for this condition is *vasomotor rhinitis*. Symptoms occur in response to environmental catalysts. The history and physical findings are the same as for AR. Nasal smears do not show eosinophilia, serum IgE levels are normal, and skin tests are negative.

History

The key to most disorders, even those that are chronic, remains a scrupulous history and a complete physical examination. These tools either are sufficient alone for diagnosis or direct the physician's investigation further (Table 15-1).

The age of onset and temporal association of symptoms are important; cyanosis and apnea in the neonate may stem from congenital nasal anomalies. Do symptoms of obstruction arise only while the infant is feeding or has a cold, suggesting partial obstruction in an obligate nasal breather? Infants who reflux oral or gastric secretions into the nasopharynx may experience obstructive symptoms only while feeding. Toddlers are especially likely to insert foreign bodies into the nose. Older infants, children, and adolescents are more at risk for sinusitis and allergies than are very young infants. Did the symptoms persist after a typical viral upper respiratory tract infection, suggesting sinusitis? Children who

are symptomatic after exposures to pollens or certain animals but are otherwise well are likely to have seasonal allergies. Did trauma precede the onset of nasal symptoms with pain and epistaxis, suggesting a septal hematoma? Asking the family what precipitates or aggravates symptoms is crucial.

The frequency and duration of symptoms are important leads to pursue. Unremitting obstruction in the newborn implies a structural abnormality. Persistent malodorous discharge signifies the presence of a foreign body. Persistent nasal itching, sneezing, congestion, and rhinorrhea without a seasonal component point to PAR, and episodic symptoms are the hallmark of SAR. Persistent daytime cough that intensifies at night suggests sinusitis. Worsening nasal obstruction accompanies rhinitis medicamentosa and enlarging masses.

Characterization of the nasal discharge may be helpful. Is the discharge always from one side, suggesting a foreign body or other mass lesion? Children with allergies typically have clear watery or mucoid discharge. CSF rhinorrhea is clear and watery unless there is associated infection. Congenital syphilis produces copious amounts of watery or mucopurulent secretions. The discharge of sinusitis may be thin, thick, clear, or colored. Foul-smelling, purulent secretions develop with foreign bodies. Infected septal hematomas (septal abscess) release bloody purulent fluid. Intermittent unilateral epistaxis is typical of juvenile angiofibroma.

The nature and pattern of associated symptoms help identify the primary illness. Does the patient have seasonal onset of nasal symptoms mingled with sneezing, itching, and coughing, as expected in SAR? Does the child typically react to certain foods, animals, plants, or places? Where does the child feel best? Do symptoms arise only after exposure to perfume, cigarette smoke, or spicy foods, indicative of NANIR (vasomotor) syndrome? An indispensable question is whether there are associated lower respiratory tract symptoms or signs; chronic sinusitis and recurrent wheezing and/or pneumonia are found in patients with asthma, cystic fibrosis, and immotile cilia syndromes.

Information about other head and neck symptoms must be obtained. Allergies and sinusitis are associated with morning headaches. Is there periorbital swelling in the morning that improves or disappears after the patient gets up? Have any changes in facial appearance been observed? Parents may notice subtle widening of the nasal bridge or proptosis as early signs of enlarging nasal, sinus, or central nervous system masses. Similarly, mechanical or inflammatory obstruction of the lacrimal duct leads to increased tearing. Is there itching or inflammation of the eyes? Does the patient snore, mouth-breathe, or have a muffled voice, suggesting chronic adenoidal enlargement? Chronic postnasal drip produces sore throat and cough. Middle ear disease is a fellow traveler in patients with allergies, chronic sinusitis, immunodeficiency, and immotile cilia syndromes.

Lower respiratory tract symptoms, such as cough, shortness of breath, and wheezing with colds, exercise, or allergen exposures, implies coexistent asthma. The meaning of the production and the character of sputum is discussed in Chapter 14. The triad of sinus disease, hemoptysis, and hematuria points to Wegener granulomatosis. In many patients, gastrointestinal involvement is a hallmark of cystic fibrosis; malabsorption leads to growth failure and loose, malodorous stools. Swollen glands, easy bruising, and pallor suggest lymphoreticular malignancy. Questions directed at changes in vision, hearing, facial movement, or sensation are relevant in patients with suspected nasal, sinus, orbital, or nasopharyngeal lesions.

Finally, even though the patient may complain of only localized nasal symptoms, a careful general review of systems is mandatory. Is the child basically healthy or "always sick"? How has the patient grown, and are there any recent changes in growth velocity or weight loss? Constitutional symptoms suggest a more generalized process; fever, anorexia, weight loss, and disproportionate fatigue are companion symptoms of immunodysfunction. Is there a pattern of recurrent, serious, or unusual infections to indicate an immunodeficiency?

The past medical history must include complete information about immunizations, allergies, illnesses, surgeries, and hospitalizations. The medication history is crucial. Does the patient use nasal sprays or other medications known to cause nasal symptoms? What has been the response to prior treatments, and is the patient immunosuppressed by infection, drugs, or malignancy? Review of all previous records and studies is required. A detailed family history of allergies, asthma, eczema, cystic fibrosis, and other disorders is imperative. Risk factors for tuberculosis and human immunodeficiency virus (HIV) infection should be explored.

Physical Examination

The physical examination must be complete and include measurement of growth parameters and vital signs. Particular attention is directed to the head and neck. The physician should inspect the face for dysmorphic features, asymmetry, proptosis, masses, and abnormal nasal alignment. The insignias of atopy include allergic "shiners," infraorbital (Dennie-Morgan lines) and transverse nasal creases, and eczema. Other features of allergy include swollen eyelids and erythematous conjunctivas. The ears should be inspected for evidence of active or chronic inflammation, perforations, and scars. The examiner should note whether the child breathes through the mouth and has "adenoidal facies," implying continuous obstruction. The symmetry and size of the tonsils and any associated injection or exudate should be recorded. A bifid uvula is frequently associated with a submucous cleft that can be palpated as a V-shaped notch at the junction of the hard and soft palates rather than the normal rounded U shape. The examiner should note the presence of cervical lymphadenopathy. Finally, is there any evidence of impaired cranial nerve function, such as decreased smell, hearing, sensation, or extraocular muscle movement?

Examination of the nose, inside and out, is of the utmost importance. A bulging or broad nasal bridge may signify a glioma, dermoid tumor, or an encephalocele. The physician should look for evidence of trauma. A wide nasal speculum attached to a pneumatic otoscope permits inspection of the nares, septum, turbinates, mucosa, and secretions. Are the nares patent and symmetric? Is the septum straight or deviated and intact or perforated, and is there a septal hematoma or abscess? Foreign bodies, masses, and polyps may be evident if the mucosal surfaces are not swollen. Swollen, boggy, and pale nasal mucosa with clear or mucoid secretions are characteristic of AR, NARES, and vasomotor rhinitis. Whereas the secretions of chronic sinusitis may be of any description, those of adenoiditis and streptococcosis are purulent. What is the color of the mucosa, and is it swollen? The examiner may apply a topical vasoconstrictor to swollen tissues to improve the view if necessary. Edema of the nose and a transverse crease across the nasal bridge may be seen in children with AR.

The skin should be inspected for evidence of poor nutrition and eczema. The chest should be assessed for evidence of acute or chronic respiratory disease. The examiner should look for an increased anteroposterior diameter and listen for rhonchi, wheezes, or other adventitious sounds. In the same vein the nailbeds should be checked for clubbing and cyanosis. The physician should evaluate the possibility of cor pulmonale from obstructive tonsils and/or adenoid tissue with a chest examination. Either absent or diminished lymph nodes and tonsils or generalized adenopathy are found in children with immunodeficiencies.

Approach to the Patient

After a complete history and physical examination, most patients with chronic nasal obstruction and rhinorrhea are diagnosed with an inflammatory process, most commonly AR or sinusitis. In many cases treatment can be accomplished without further investigation. In other instances simple office measures and laboratory tests are indicated before or concurrently with treatment; the minority of children require more advanced study and subspecialty care.

In a patient with suspected allergies, a positive nasal smear for eosinophils, an elevated total IgE level, and peripheral eosinophilia support this diagnosis. To collect nasal secretions the physician should have the patient blow his or her nose into clear plastic wrap or waxed paper; a Wright stain of the secretions will reveal the presence of eosinophils. However, these are screening tests of low sensitivity and specificity and thus are neither indicated nor helpful in all children with suspected AR. Children with mild to moderate symptoms and easily identified allergens may be managed by their primary practitioners with education about avoiding allergens and simple medications. Children who fail initial therapy, have severe symptoms, or whose allergens are uncertain are properly referred to a pediatric allergist.

Children with uncomplicated acute or chronic sinusitis merit an initial trial of therapy without additional study. Nasal culture is not useful for diagnosis. Maxillary sinus aspiration, which is not indicated in uncomplicated cases, should be done only by experienced personnel. Children with refractory or complicated sinusitis may require sinus imaging. However, the examiner must consider which specific studies to order based on the limitations of the imaging procedures selected.

Plain radiographs of the sinuses, although no longer the gold standard for sinus imaging, still play an important role in the evaluation of children with chronic or refractory sinusitis. The small size of the maxillary and ethmoid sinuses in children under 1 year of age precludes the use of plain films; in children older than 1 year of age, radiographs may be obtained for the initial diagnosis (Fig. 15-1). They should include (1) a posteroanterior (Caldwell) view to evaluate the ethmoid air cells, (2) an occipitomental (Waters) view to evaluate the maxillary sinuses, and (3) a lateral view to judge the sphenoid and frontal sinuses. Findings most consistent with sinusitis include air-fluid levels, unilateral opacification, and mucosal thickening greater than 4 mm. Unfortunately, some asymptomatic children with upper respiratory tract infection or allergies demonstrate radiographic sinus opacification that is not representative of true infection. Imaging of the sinuses is mandatory if there is a known or suspected complication of sinusitis, such as orbital abscess; if there is concern for a mass lesion or other structural deformity as the cause of sinus disease; or if surgery is contemplated. For most purposes, coronal computed tomography (CT) scanning is the preferred imaging study. Consultation with radiologists and other subspecialists is indicated to select the best views and to decide if contrast administration is necessary. Magnetic resonance imaging (MRI) is also indicated if a tumor is suspected as the source of sinus ostium obstruction with secondary infection.

Children with suspected streptococcosis should have a nasopharyngeal culture for group A beta-hemolytic streptococci and treatment with antibiotics if the culture is positive. The clinical impression of enlarged adenoids may be confirmed by plain radiography (Fig. 15-14); antimicrobial therapy is indicated if adenoid infection is assumed to be present. Children with chronic obstruction from enlarged adenoids should be referred for consideration of adenoidectomy.

Infants with presumed pertussis infection typically have an elevated white blood cell count with an absolute lymphocytosis. They need no supplementary screening tests unless there is confusion about the diagnosis, but the cause should be confirmed by nasopharyngeal culture on Bordet-Gengou media, the gold standard for bacteriologic confirmation. Treatment of family members to prevent further spread is an important result of confirmation of the diagnosis of pertussis. For the same reason, efforts to confirm chlamydial infection are important before treatment is started. Congenital syphilis is a diagnosis that must be definitively proven or excluded. A comprehensive discussion of the diagnosis of syphilis is be-

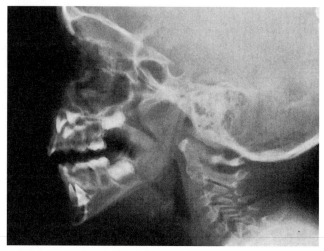

FIG. 15-14 Note the enlarged adenoid shadow that impinges on the nasal airway.

yond the scope of this chapter, and the reader is referred to the references.

Ciliary dyskinesia syndromes are diagnosed by ciliary biopsy when the patient is free of infection. A screening evaluation for immunodysfunction is indicated in the patient with recurrent, serious, or unusual infections; Stiehm recommends a complete blood count with white cell differential, erythrocyte sedimentation rate, quantitative immunoglobulins (IgG, IgA, IgM), antibody titers to tetanus, diphtheria and pneumococcal immunizations, delayed hypersensitivity skin tests (*Candida* sp., tetanus toxoid, *Trichophyton* sp.), and chest and sinus radiographs. More specific tests can be obtained initially if there is reason; for example, recurrent *Staphylococcus aureus* infections in a young boy are an indication to test for chronic granulomatous disease by doing a nitroblue tetrazolium dye reduction test. HIV testing is mandatory for an infant born with congenital syphilis or other known risk factors for HIV infection.

The minority of children have mechanical obstruction as the basis of their symptoms. Many of these patients eventually require the services of pediatric otolaryngologists or neurosurgeons, but simple office measures and studies confirm or support the initial diagnosis and guide the patient to the correct imaging modality and subspecialty service.

In the neonate or young infant with suspected mechanical obstruction, the easy passage of a catheter transnasally eliminates complete nasal occlusion and choanal atresia. However, the examiner may miss a relatively mild but clinically significant stenosis. CT scanning is the modality of choice to identify choanal atresia or stenosis. In the older child or adolescent with suspected adenoidal hypertrophy, plain radiographs will identify an enlarged adenoid shadow. Children with nasal polyps deserve definitive testing for cystic fibrosis.

If masses are seen or suspected, an imaging study is indicated. Plain radiographs are fruitless in this situation because soft tissue masses may be obscured by bone, and more pre-

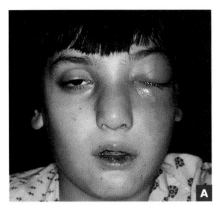 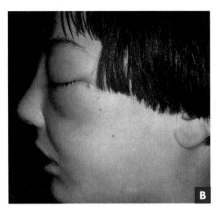 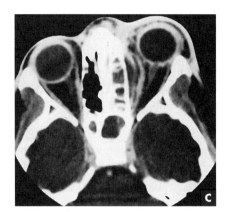

FIG. 15-15 CT scan of the orbits shows a typical orbital abscess.

cise information about anatomic detail and relationships is required. Contrast-enhanced CT scanning and MRI are useful alone or in conjunction for localization, diagnosis, and treatment design. Clearly these children must be referred to pediatric surgical subspecialists in otolaryngology and/or neurosurgery.

SUMMARY

The investigation of chronic nasal obstruction and rhinorrhea is a challenge to clinicians, but an accurate diagnosis leads to effective therapy and relief of symptoms for most patients. The majority of patients have allergies or sinusitis as the explanation of their symptoms; far fewer children suffer from immunodeficiencies, tumors, or other serious disorders. A careful history and meticulous physical examination combined with selected tests and imaging procedures ultimately solve the puzzle in most cases or indicate the correct focus of the subsequent evaluation.

ILLUSTRATIVE CASES

Case 1. A 15-year-old previously healthy white boy had a 3-week history of nasal discharge and cough without fever. Three days before presentation, he developed high fever, headache, pain over the left eyebrow, and purulent nasal discharge. There was a history of seasonal allergies but no sinus disease or other illnesses. On physical examination he was febrile, awake, alert, and in pain. The left forehead was swollen just above the medial border of the eyebrow and exquisitely tender to touch. The left eyelid was swollen with mucopurulent discharge from the conjunctiva. Visual acuity, pupillary reactivity, and fundi were normal, but the left eye failed to adduct completely, and the patient complained of severe globe pain with any movement. Nasal turbinates were swollen, and purulent discharge was present in both

nares. Sinus films revealed an air-fluid level in the left frontal sinus and bilateral maxillary and ethmoid sinus opacification. CT scans revealed a left orbital abscess (Fig. 15-15) and fluid in the frontal, maxillary, and ethmoid sinuses. After parenteral antibiotics were started, he was taken to the operating room for incision and drainage of the left frontal sinus and left orbital abscesses. He rapidly became afebrile and had normal eye movements the second day after surgery. Cultures grew anaerobic streptococci sensitive to penicillin and clindamycin. He was treated with 5 days of parenteral antibiotics and 22 days of oral clindamycin. He was well after treatment, with a normal examination and sinus films.

This case demonstrates that patients with nasal allergies are at risk for bacterial sinusitis and its complications. Sinus films in this case were diagnostic for sinusitis, although CT scanning was required to confirm the clinical impression of an orbital abscess.

Case 2. A 4-year-old boy, with a complaint of persistent bad breath, was referred by an urgent care center to a dentist. The dentist obtained a history of halitosis for several weeks that continued despite good tooth care and unilateral purulent nasal discharge. Suspicious of a foreign body, the dentist referred the child to an otolaryngologist. The child was well and denied putting anything in his nose. Nonetheless a piece of sponge was extracted from the left nostril and the symptoms resolved rapidly.

In this case the classic history of unilateral purulent nasal discharge and halitosis directed the dentist to the correct diagnosis, and an appropriate referral was made.

Case 3. A 7-year-old boy was brought in by his parents who were concerned about a persistent cold lasting for several weeks and recent onset of right eye enlargement. There was no sneezing, itching, or cough and no history of aller-

gies, asthma, otitis media, sinusitis, recent fevers, other constitutional symptoms, or epistaxis. Physical examination revealed a healthy child with proptosis of the right eye and a question of a mass in the right nostril. The remainder of the examination was normal. A CT scan of the head revealed a large soft tissue mass involving the right nostril, maxillary sinus, and floor of the orbit on the same side. Tissue biopsy was consistent with a rhabdomyosarcoma.

Until the development of proptosis, this child was considered to have a typical upper respiratory tract infection by his parents. This case demonstrates the mild and nonspecific nature of nasal complaints that accompany tumors and that more overt signs are delayed until the lesion is quite large.

ANNOTATED BIBLIOGRAPHY

Druce HM: Allergic and nonallergic rhinitis. In Middleton E, Reed CE, Ellis EF, et al, editors: *Allergy: principles and practice,* vol 2, ed 4, St Louis, 1992, Mosby–Year Book.
This text is a comprehensive review of all categories of rhinitis.

Wald ER: Sinusitis in children, *N Engl J Med* 326:319-323, 1992.
This article is a superb review on the pathophysiology, microbiology, diagnosis, and treatment of sinusitis in children.

Yousem DM: Imaging of sinonasal inflammatory disease, *Radiology* 188:303-314, 1993.
This article beautifully clarifies the anatomic relationships vital to understanding sinus disease and its evaluation.

BIBLIOGRAPHY

Connell JT: Quantitative intranasal pollen changes. III. The priming effect in allergic rhinitis, *J Allergy* 43:33-44, 1990.

Diament MJ: The diagnosis of sinusitis in infants and children: x-ray, computed tomography, and magnetic resonance imaging, *J Allergy Clin Immunol* 90:442-444, 1992.

Dorfman DH, Glaser JH: Congenital syphilis in infants after the newborn period, *N Engl J Med* 323:1299-1302, 1990.

Dvoracek JE, Yunginger JW, Kern EB, et al: Induction of nasal late-phase reactions by insufflation of ragweed-pollen extract, *J Allergy Clin Immunol* 73:363-368, 1984.

Fireman P: Diagnosis of allergic disorders, *Pediatr Rev* 16:178-183, 1995.

Fireman P: Diagnosis of sinusitis in children: emphasis on the history and physical examination, *J Allergy Clin Immunol* 90:433-436, 1992.

Gentry S: Allergic rhinitis: always in season, *Contemp Pediatr* 8:88-108, 1991.

Kovatch AL, Wald ER, Ledesma-Medina J, et al: Maxillary sinus radiographs in children with nonrespiratory complaints, *Pediatrics* 73:306-308, 1984.

Naclerio RM: Allergic rhinitis, *N Engl J Med* 325:860-869, 1991.

Pagon RA, Graham JM, Zonana J, et al: Coloboma, congenital heart disease and choanal atresia with multiple anomalies: CHARGE association, *J Pediatr* 99:223-227, 1981.

Powers GF, Boisvert PD: Age as a factor in streptococcosis, *J Pediatr* 25:481-504, 1944.

Rupp GH, Friedman RA: Eosinophilic nonallergic rhinitis in children, *Pediatrics* 70:437-439, 1982.

Shapiro ED, Milmoe GJ, Wald ER, et al: Bacteriology of the maxillary sinuses in patients with cystic fibrosis, *J Infect Dis* 14:589-593, 1982.

Skinner DW, Chui P: The hazards of "button-sized" batteries as foreign bodies in the nose and ear, *J Laryngol Otol* 100:1315-1318, 1986.

Stiehm ER: They're back: recurrent infections in pediatric practice, *Contemp Pediatr* 7:20-40, 1990.

Wald ER: Microbiology of acute and chronic sinusitis in children, *J Allergy Clin Immunol* 90:452-460, 1992.

Wegenmann M, Naclerio RM: Complications of sinusitis, *J Allergy Clin Immunol* 90:552-554, 1992.

Williams JW, Simel DL: Does this patient have sinusitis? diagnosing acute sinusitis by history and physical examination, *JAMA* 270:1242-1246, 1993.

Zenker PN, Berman SM: Congenital syphilis: trends and recommendations for evaluation and management, *Pediatr Infect Dis J* 10:516-522, 1991.

Noisy Breathing

BASIL J. ZITELLI

 Key Points

- Noisy breathing results from turbulent airflow in the airway and affects most children at some time in their life.

- The quality and character of the noisy respirations helps to locate the source of the obstruction. Hoarseness affects the larynx near the vocal cords, stridor may affect the extrathoracic airway, and wheezing results from intrathoracic airway obstruction.

- Age of onset, associated symptoms, and careful history and physical examination often suffice to determine the cause of the noisy respirations. However, at times selected imaging procedures (ranging from static films to fluoroscopy or even computed tomography or magnetic resonance imaging) may be required to delineate the cause of the obstruction.

Noisy breathing of some kind affects most children at some time in their life. Clinicians must decide why the breathing is abnormal, whether it seriously impairs respiration, where the lesion is located, and how to approach the disorder diagnostically and therapeutically. Abnormal sounds from the respiratory tract may emanate anywhere along the entire pathway from the nose to nasopharynx; oropharynx; supraglottic, glottic, and subglottic areas; trachea; bronchi; and bronchioles. Lesions causing obstruction may be intrinsic to the airway or cause extrinsic airway compression. Because nasal obstruction has been discussed in another chapter, lesions from the oropharynx to bronchioles are presented (see Chapter 15).

Pathophysiology

Abnormal sounds during the passage of air arise from turbulence created by partial obstruction. Obstruction within the nasopharynx resulting from enlarged tonsils, abscesses, or masses muffles sounds, creating a "hot potato" voice. Hoarseness is the breathy, harsh, or husky sound of the voice caused by disorders involving the larynx. Intensity of the voice is related to air pressure maintained against glottic resistance; hence obstructive lesions preventing generation of adequate pressure produce a weak voice. Careful attention to the quality of sounds of hoarseness can help to localize the lesion. Low-pitched, coarse, fluttering sounds suggest supraglottic or hypopharyngeal obstruction, and a more high-pitched, cracking sound, or aphonia, points to vocal cord involvement.

Stridor is a harsh sound produced by air moving across a partial airway obstruction, creating vibrations of surrounding tissues. Stridor generally is an inspiratory sound, although abnormal sounds can be produced during expiration as well. To understand and possibly help localize adventitious sounds, a review of the mechanics of air movement through the airways is necessary. Any linear movement of gas is associated with a decrease of pressure from that gas in a direction perpendicular to the direction of flow (Venturi principle). Hence pressure is decreased on the walls of the airway during respiration. In the small, flexible airway of the young child, the decreased lateral airway pressure causes brief collapse and partial obstruction of the airway, which then reduces flow and releases pressure. The airway opens again, and the whole cycle is repeated rapidly, producing a musical sound of stridor or wheezing. The pitch of the sound is due to the thickness of the wall; duration is dependent on the respiratory effort to maintain air movement in the airway. Anatomically fixed lesions tend to create reproducible sounds, and foreign bodies and mobile mucous plugs that migrate produce variable sounds that can be evanescent.

Loosely supported structures of the tongue, pharynx, and supraglottic area can be drawn in toward the airway during respiration. Patients with partial obstructions of the supraglottic area often generate high pharyngeal pressures during respiratory distress. As air traverses the diseased area, the Venturi effect narrows the airway even further, producing inspiratory stridor. Expiration forces the supraglottic airway open, so obstructive lesions involving the pharynx and supraglottic structures tend to produce inspiratory stridor only.

The vocal cords and subglottic region of the extrathoracic trachea are strongly supported structures. The vocal cords are supported by the vocal ligament, and the cricoid ring supports the subglottic region. As a result these structures are not significantly affected by the Venturi principle. Airflow is more dependent on lumen size, and when partial obstruction occurs, a biphasic stridorous sound is produced. Critically small airways in this region require enormous effort to force air through the obstruction on both inspiration and expiration; patients tire easily, and respiratory failure usually is imminent.

Expiration creates positive intrathoracic pressure from contraction of the thorax. Extraluminal positive pressure is applied to bronchi, tending to narrow small airways. The Venturi principle adds to the narrowing effect. Any obstruction of intrathoracic airways results in expiratory sounds, which are musical in quality and less harsh than stridor. These sounds are called *wheezes.*

Retractions occur with increased negative intrapleural pressures during inspiration. Soft tissues in the neck and suprasternal area, sternum, and costal cartilages are drawn in by the negative pressure. The severity of retractions is related to the degree of negative pressures generated and the compliance of the thorax.

Literature Survey

The broad field of airway obstruction encompasses a wide range of topics. The literature is replete with specific articles and reviews. However, for a comprehensive overview of pediatric airway disorders, standard texts give a succinct summary of pathophysiology and differential diagnosis. Perhaps one of the best overall texts is *Pediatric Otolaryngology* edited by Bluestone and Stool. Individual chapters cover common pediatric airway disorders with excellent review of airway physiology and differential diagnosis. Review articles of oropharyngeal obstruction, especially disorders of tonsils and adenoids, have been published by Denny and Deutsch. Kenna, a pediatric otolaryngologist, summarizes hoarseness in children in a simple, yet complete review. An excellent review of acute upper airway obstruction was published in 1981 but remains timely even today. Review articles of asthma often present a differential diagnosis of wheezing.

Differential Diagnosis

Oropharyngeal Obstruction

Obstruction of the oropharynx may be due to congenital lesions, inflammatory disorders, or neoplastic diseases (Box 16-1). Congenital disorders with micrognathia, such as Pierre Robin syndrome (Fig. 16-1) or Treacher Collins syn-

---

BOX 16-1

Some Common Causes of Oropharyngeal Obstruction

Congenital Disorders
Micrognathia
  Pierre Robin syndrome
  Treacher Collins syndrome
Macroglossia
  Down syndrome
  Beckwith-Wiedemann syndrome
  Lymphangioma
  Hemangioma
  Lingual thyroid

Inflammatory Disorders
Tonsillitis/hypertrophy
  Bacterial
    Streptococcus pyogenes
    Staphylococci
    Anaerobic infections
  Viral
    Epstein-Barr virus
    Coxsackievirus
    Adenovirus
Uvulitis
Peritonsillar abscess
Retropharyngeal abscess
Parapharyngeal abscess

Tumors
Hemangioma
Lymphangioma
Ranula
Lymphoma
Lymphosarcoma
Rhabdomyosarcoma
Fibrosarcoma
Epidermoid carcinoma

Other
Adenoidal hypertrophy
Palatal hypotonia
Obesity

---

drome (Fig. 16-2), may cause relative obstruction from glossoptosis, resulting in respiratory embarrassment. Macroglossia is seen in Down syndrome, Beckwith-Wiedemann syndrome, and infiltrative disorders, such as lymphangiomatosis.

Probably the most common cause of inflammatory obstruction in the oropharynx is tonsillopharyngitis resulting from bacterial or viral infection. The tonsils and adenoids are usually small in early infancy and increase in size as lymphoid tissue develops during childhood. The evaluation of tonsillar size is aided by using a standardized grading system (Fig. 16-3). Infections from group A beta-hemolytic streptococci, adenovirus, coxsackieviruses, and Epstein-Barr virus commonly produce pharyngitis and may be associated with tonsillar hypertrophy and inflammation. Streptococcal infections often produce fever, headache, abdominal pain, tonsillar erythema (with or without exudate), and enlarged, mildly tender cervical lymph nodes. Epstein-Barr virus infection produces fever, malaise, exudative tonsillitis, generalized adenopathy, splenomegaly, and mild hepatitis. Coxsackievirus pharyngitis may be associated with ulcerative lesions of the soft palate and tonsillar pillars. These common infectious disorders may produce tonsillar enlargement severe enough

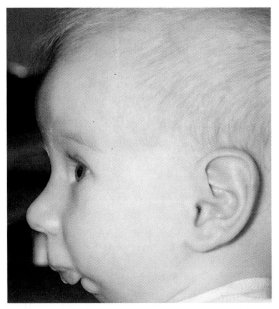

FIG. 16-1 Pierre Robin syndrome is characterized by severe micrognathia and cleft palate. Posterior displacement of the tongue resulted in airway obstruction necessitating tracheostomy. (Courtesy Dr. Wolfgang Loskin, Children's Hospital of Pittsburgh.)

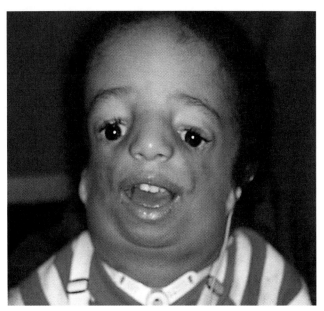

FIG. 16-2 Treacher Collins syndrome. Note the marked craniofacial abnormalities creating airway obstruction leading to tracheostomy.

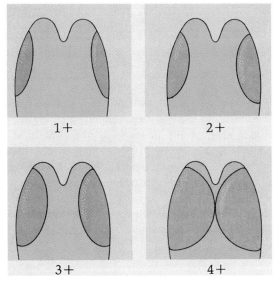

FIG. 16-3 Grading of tonsillar size. (Modified from Feinstein AR, Levitt M: Role of tonsils, *N Engl J Med* 282:285-291, 1970.)

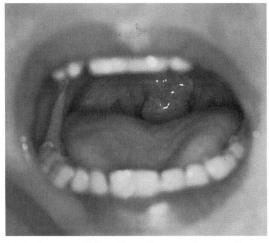

FIG. 16-4 Acute uvulitis with erythema, edema, and petechiae in this case caused by *Streptococcus pyogenes*.

to cause partial airway obstruction. Frequently a muffled or "hot potato" voice is associated with markedly enlarged tonsils. Enlarged adenoids can cause nasopharyngeal obstruction as well, leading to chronic mouth-breathing, snoring, or even sleep apnea. Chronic airway obstruction from tonsils or adenoids may lead to complications, such as apnea, chronic hypoxemia, failure to thrive, right heart failure, and postobstructive pulmonary edema, when they are removed. Palatal hypotonia caused by cerebral palsy or excessive palatal tissue

caused by marked obesity may also cause obstruction and noisy breathing. Uvulitis can rarely cause airway obstruction from marked edema (Fig. 16-4). *Streptococcus pyogenes*, *Haemophilus influenzae* type B, Epstein-Barr virus, and other viral agents have been reported to cause acute uvulitis.

Peritonsillar abscess or cellulitis usually occurs in older children who typically have a history of an antecedent pharyngitis. Unilateral deviation of the tonsil or palatal soft tissue associated with fever, toxic appearance, and torticollis

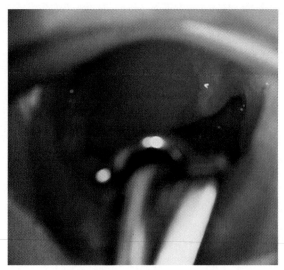

FIG. 16-5 Peritonsillar abscess with an intensely inflamed soft palatal mass that obscures the tonsil and deviates the uvula.

Some Common Causes of Hoarseness

Neonatal	Older Child
Laryngomalacia	Viral infection (laryngitis, croup)
Webs	Postnasal drip
Subglottic stenosis	Epiglottitis
Cystic lesions	Other bacterial infections (diphtheria, tetanus, tuberculosis)
Excessive secretions (fistulas, gastroesophageal reflux)	Recurrent voice abuse (cord polyps, nodules)
Vascular tumors (hemangioma, lymphangioma)	Sicca syndromes (ectodermal dysplasia, collagen-vascular disorders, cystic fibrosis, dry environment, drugs)
Cri du chat syndrome (5p-chromosome syndrome)	Neoplasia (papilloma, hemangioma, lymphangioma)
Vocal cord paralysis	Trauma (postsurgical, intubation)
Myasthenia gravis	Metabolic (Gaucher disease, mucopolysaccharidosis)
Cord trauma	Syndromes (Williams, Cornelia de Lange)
Metabolic disorders (hypothyroidism, hypocalcemia, Farber disease)	Conversion reaction

provides clues for the diagnosis (Fig. 16-5). A retropharyngeal abscess may obstruct the airway by anterior displacement of prevertebral soft tissues, usually occurring in children under 3 years of age. A gurgling, stridorous sound often is heard because the child may have difficulty swallowing secretions. Erythematous swelling of the posterior pharyngeal wall may deviate the uvula and ipsilateral tonsil.

Tumors of the pharynx (benign or malignant) may cause obstruction and noisy breathing. Infiltrative benign lesions, such as hemangioma and lymphangioma, are among the more common disorders. Ranula, a large lateral retention cyst of the floor of the mouth, usually results from an obstructed sublingual salivary gland duct. Malignancies include lymphoma or lymphosarcoma affecting Waldeyer ring, rhabdomyosarcoma, fibrosarcoma, and epidermoid carcinoma. Children with a unilaterally enlarged tonsil who lack evidence of acute infection may have a tonsillar lymphoma, and a careful examination for other adenopathy or pharyngeal masses is imperative. Excisional biopsy usually is diagnostic. These lymphomas are uncommon, however, comprising only 5% to 10% of all oral tumors in childhood.

Hoarseness

The Neonate

The neonate with hoarseness must be examined carefully for congenital abnormalities of the larynx (Box 16-2). Typically the common lesions of laryngomalacia and subglottic stenosis do not cause hoarseness but rather are associated with stridor and alternations in intensity of the voice. Low-pitched, fluttering, coarse sounds arise from the loose structures of the hypopharynx and supraglottic region, and high-pitched, cracking sounds generally indicate vocal cord involvement.

Cysts of the larynx can partially obstruct the airway and produce hoarseness. Most are retention cysts of seromucinous glands, generally located in the valleculae and aryepiglottic folds. Laryngeal webs frequently are simple folds of mucosa located at the anterior commissure at the glottis. Rarely, complete obstruction occurs, causing severe and immediate life-threatening respiratory distress at birth.

A lingual thyroid represents failure of the thyroid to completely descend from the foramen cecum of the tongue to its proper position anterior to the thyroid cartilage. It commonly presents as a mass at the base of the tongue and usually is asymptomatic unless it becomes enlarged from inflammation, infection, or disorders of thyroid function. Resection is not recommended because this may be the only thyroid tissue.

Excessive secretions can cause chronic or recurrent laryngeal irritation and hoarseness. Tracheoesophageal fistula often is associated with chronic aspiration of secretions and hoarseness. Radiographic contrast studies or endoscopy can define the fistula. Gastroesophageal reflux with or without aspiration may be associated with chronic erythema and swelling of supraglottic structures and consequent hoarseness.

The cri du chat syndrome consists of an unusual and abnormal cry associated with other anomalies, including microcephaly, mental retardation, and hypotonia. The cry is

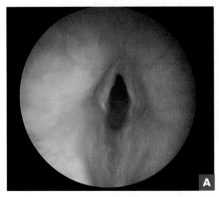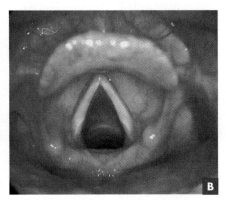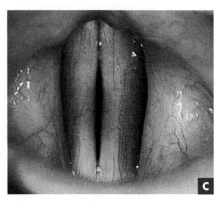

FIG. 16-6 Bilateral vocal cord paralysis. The marked narrowing of the opening between the cords *(A)* occurs because of loss of ability to abduct the cords on inspiration. Normal cord functioning, with opening during inspiration *(B)* and closing during expiration *(C)*.

high-pitched and weak and sounds like the meow of a cat. The larynx is narrow and abnormally shaped and allows escape of air during expiration.

Vocal cord paresis or paralysis produces an abnormal cry that ranges from hoarseness with unilateral involvement to very weak cry with bilateral disease (Fig. 16-6). Injury to the motor vagus nerve, from the nuclei to peripheral locations, can alter vocal cord function, leading to hoarseness, difficulty swallowing, and recurrent aspiration of secretions. Injury to the recurrent laryngeal nerve, including pressure on the nerve from a double aortic arch, abnormal subclavian artery, enlarged left atrium in heart failure, and mediastinal masses can cause hoarseness. The Arnold-Chiari malformation involves elongation and herniation of the cerebellar tonsils through the foramen magnum, applying pressure and stretching the vagus nerve. Hoarseness and stridor can be seen with this anomaly. Myasthenia gravis may affect the larynx, causing respiratory distress and hoarseness as part of the global presentation of profound neuromuscular weakness.

Trauma from intubation or overzealous pharyngeal suctioning of secretions may cause hoarseness in the neonate. Traumatic intubation may cause arytenoid cartilage dislocation.

Metabolic disorders of the neonate causing hoarseness include hypothyroidism, hypocalcemia, and Farber disease (lipid storage disease with accumulation of ceramide).

The Older Child

Hoarseness in the older child commonly occurs with inflammatory disorders of the larynx (Box 16-2). Acute laryngitis is often associated with a viral respiratory tract infection, is transient in nature, and generally has full recovery. Laryngotracheitis (croup) may cause hoarseness along with the characteristic "barking seal" cough of subglottic edema. Secretions from chronic sinusitis and postnasal drip may cause hoarseness that is frequent in the morning. Acute epiglottitis is rapidly declining in incidence because of immunization programs against *H. influenzae* type B but may cause hoarse-

ness early in its clinical course. Rarely, diphtheria, tuberculosis, or tetanus may affect the larynx, causing a weak or husky voice. Inflammation of the cricoarytenoid joint with juvenile chronic arthritis produces hoarseness and dysphagia and if not recognized can result in permanent ankylosis.

Recurrent trauma, particularly with voice abuse, can lead to a vocal cord nodule, polyp, or keratosis. Hoarseness tends to progress as the abuse continues. Fluctuation in severity occurs as the patient rests his or her voice and may worsen by the end of the day. The sicca syndromes, whether from ectodermal dysplasia, cystic fibrosis, collagen-vascular disorders, dry environments, or drug therapies, create hoarseness that often can be relieved with frequent sips of water.

Rapidly progressive hoarseness implies a neoplastic disorder. Laryngeal papillomas are most common between 1 and 4 years of age. Respiratory distress with airway obstruction may occur with hoarseness as these lesions progress in size. Hemangioma and lymphangioma often are progressive lesions that may be life-threatening if they involve the airway. Stabilization of the airway is essential, and different treatment modalities for hemangiomas range from systemic steroids, intralesional steroid injection, laser therapy, and interferon alpha-2b to embolization.

Hoarseness after surgical procedures is a common result of trauma to the cords during intubation. However, any procedure involving the neck or mediastinum may inadvertently cause injury to the recurrent laryngeal nerve. Thyroid surgery, tracheoesophageal fistula repair, and cardiac surgery involving the aortic arch have been associated with laryngeal nerve damage.

A variety of metabolic disorders in older children are associated with hoarseness, which often results from storage material deposited within the cords or neurologic involvement. Gaucher disease may cause a pseudobulbar palsy and laryngospasm; mucolipidosis II (I-cell disease) and lipid proteinosis are storage disorders that cause hoarseness, as is amyloidosis. Williams syndrome and Cornelia de Lange syndrome both have a husky voice as part of typical findings.

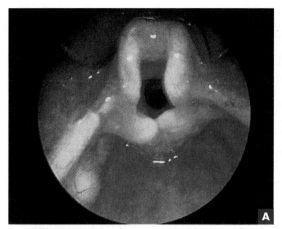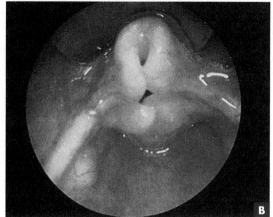

FIG. 16-7 Laryngomalacia. *A,* Note the omega-shaped epiglottis and elongated arytenoid cartilages. *B,* During inspiration the laryngeal structures collapse to the laryngeal inlet, causing obstruction and stridor.

BOX 16-3

Some Common Causes of Stridor

Neonatal
Laryngomalacia
Subglottic stenosis
Webs
Laryngeal cysts
Tracheal stenosis
Tracheomalacia
Tracheal cartilage
  ring defect
Laryngeal/tracheal
  ring calcification
Vascular ring
Pulmonary sling
Innominate artery
  tracheal compression
Vocal cord paralysis
  (Arnold-Chiari malfor-
  mation, Dandy-Walker
  cyst, recurrent laryngeal
  nerve injury)
Tumor (papilloma, heman-
  gioma, lymphangioma)
Trauma (intubation, ther-
  mal, corrosive, gastric
  secretions)

Older Child
Oropharyngeal infec-
  tion (peritonsillar
  abscess, retropha-
  ryngeal abscess,
  tonsillitis, parapha-
  ryngeal abscess)
Viral infections
  (croup, spasmodic
  croup)
Acute epiglottitis
Bacterial tracheitis
Aspirated/swallowed
  foreign body
Tumor (hemangioma,
  lymphangioma,
  fibroma, rhab-
  domyosarcoma)

Conversion reactions associated with hoarseness may be difficult to diagnose without endoscopy. Cords are not adducted during speech but are opposed during glottic closure with coughing.

Stridor

Stridor, the musical inspiratory sound produced by partial obstruction of the extrathoracic airway, may be caused by many of the same disorders that cause oropharyngeal obstruction and hoarseness (Box 16-3). Expiratory stridor more frequently occurs in lower airway obstruction, and biphasic stridor implies midtracheal involvement. Respiratory obstruction tends to occur more frequently and generally is more severe in younger children for the following three reasons: (1) the larynx is smaller in young infants, (2) submucous connective tissue is loose in the supraglottic area, and (3) the subglottic area is encircled by the cricoid cartilage. The infant's triangular-shaped glottic opening is approximately 7 mm long and 4 mm wide at its base with an area of 14 mm²; 1 mm of edema reduces its dimensions to 5 mm by 2 mm, with an area of 5 mm². A reduction to 35% of original area produces severe distress in the infant. The same 1 mm of edema reduces the area in a 1-year-old child to 50% of original area but reduces the area only to 85% of the original area in an adult, who might experience only hoarseness. Soft tissues are affected by external atmospheric pressure and decreased intraluminal pressures generated by the Venturi effect. Edema of the subglottic area impinges on the airway because of the rigid airway cartilage.

Congenital lesions causing stridor are often present at birth or shortly thereafter. Laryngomalacia is the most common cause of persistent stridor in infants, accounting for 60% of cases. Flaccid laryngeal structures, particularly the epiglottis and arytenoid cartilages, collapse toward the airway during inspiration (Fig. 16-7). Infants usually have mild inspiratory stridor that is positional (worse when the infant is excited or lying supine and improved when lying prone or when the neck is mildly hyperextended). Stridor is usually inspiratory, consists of a fluttering sound, and may be associated with sternal retractions. Diagnosis is made by direct observation of collapse of supraglottic structures into the airway during inspiration. Usually, stridor is mild and self-limited and gradually resolves as the child grows.

Subglottic stenosis may result from a congenital narrowing of the cricoid cartilage or injury caused by previous intubation. Recurrent stridor often develops even with mild upper respiratory tract infections, and severe or prolonged obstruc-

TABLE 16-1

Croup Scoring System

Sign	0	1	2	3
Stridor	None	Mild	Moderate at rest	Severe, on inspiration and expiration; or none with markedly decreased air entry
Retraction	None	Mild	Moderate	Severe, marked use of accessory muscles
Air entry	Normal	Mild decrease	Moderate decrease	Marked decrease
Color	Normal	Normal (0 score)	Normal (0 score)	Dusky or cyanotic
Level of consciousness	Normal	Restless when disturbed	Anxious, agitated when undisturbed	Lethargic, depressed

Modified from Taussig LM, et al: Treatment of laryngotracheobronchitis (croup): use of intermittent positive pressure breathing and racemic epinephrine, *Am J Dis Child* 129:790-793, 1975.

tion occurs with croup. Although over half of these children improve with age, nearly 40% develop serious airway obstruction with infections, requiring tracheostomy.

Laryngeal webs generally occlude the anterior commissure and produce stridor and/or hoarseness. The presence of hoarseness localizes the lesion to the cordal area. Stridor may be biphasic, indicating critical airway obstruction. Laryngeal cysts are generally mucous retention cysts that enlarge and obstruct the airway.

Tracheal stenosis, tracheomalacia, absence of or defect in the tracheal cartilaginous rings, or calcification of laryngeal or tracheal rings can be associated with stridor. Tracheal stenosis may occur after repair of a tracheoesophageal fistula. Tracheomalacia is associated with marked increased mobility of the posterior tracheal wall to the point where anterior and posterior tracheal walls may touch. Usually, tracheomalacia spontaneously improves between 12 to 18 months of age. Abnormal tracheal rings may provide poor support, leading to collapse of soft tissue structures while edema of the rigid calcified airway impinges on the airway lumen.

Vascular compression of the trachea may cause stridor. Complete vascular rings encircle and compress the trachea and esophagus (see Fig. 14-1) often with a right aortic arch or possibly a ligamentum arteriosus. An anomalous subclavian vessel, double aortic arch, or pulmonary artery in the pulmonary vascular sling may impinge on the trachea, producing stridor. The innominate artery, arising more distally than usual from the aorta, crosses the trachea posteroanteriorly and obliquely from left to right. Endoscopic visualization demonstrates a pulsatile obstructive lesion compressing the trachea anteriorly.

Unilateral vocal cord paralysis often is a result of a peripheral nerve lesion and produces a weak cry, hoarseness, and stridor but no respiratory distress unless a supervening respiratory infection occurs. Left-sided paralysis may be associated with cardiovascular or pulmonary disorders, but right-sided paralysis is usually an isolated finding. Bilateral

vocal cord paralysis is a life-threatening condition associated with stridor, respiratory distress, and cyanosis. The vocal cords cannot abduct on inspiration. Aspiration frequently occurs because of concomitant depressed cough reflex. Arnold-Chiari malformation with compression and stretching of the motor portion of the vagus nerve often causes bilateral cord paralysis.

Tumors of the airway include laryngeal papillomas and vascular tumors, such as hemangiomas and lymphangiomas. These latter disorders were discussed previously. Papillomatosis occurs when a viral infection affects the cords, producing multiple benign papillomas. Hoarseness and stridor develop. Excision is frequently followed by recurrence, and tracheostomy has been associated with seeding and growth of papillomas in the distal tracheobronchial tree.

Repeated trauma from intubation, dislocation of arytenoid cartilage, thermal or corrosive injury to the supraglottic tissues, or repeated aspirations caused by gastroesophageal reflux may produce stridor resulting from soft tissue inflammation and edema.

Acute infections from a variety of causes and locations produce stridor. Peritonsillar abscess, retropharyngeal abscess, or acute tonsillitis from bacterial or viral causes can produce stridor and a muffled voice. Croup, or laryngotracheobronchitis, is a common infection in childhood usually caused by parainfluenza and influenza viruses and less commonly caused by measles and varicella. The illness more frequently occurs in younger children under 3 years of age. Usually, after a prodrome of low-grade fever and upper respiratory tract symptoms, sudden respiratory distress develops with loud inspiratory stridor; a characteristic barking, seallike cough; and hoarseness. Symptoms wax and wane and are often worse at night, and the disease course is variable and unpredictable. Stridor, retractions, decreased air entry, color, and level of consciousness form the basis of a numeric clinical scoring system (Table 16-1). Severe airway obstruction may cause minimal stridor, and fatigue may decrease

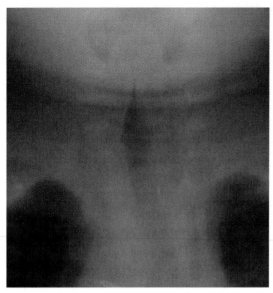

FIG. 16-8 Steeple sign in croup. The subglottic airway is narrowed from edema, producing a pointed appearance rather than a symmetric squared-off shoulder.

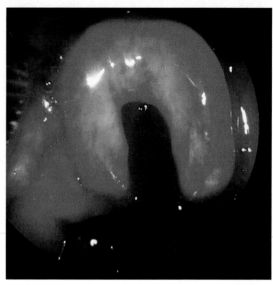

FIG. 16-9 Acute epiglottitis with marked erythema and swelling.

respiratory effort, leading to imminent respiratory failure. Diagnosis is largely clinical, although typically the anteroposterior radiograph of the airway demonstrates subglottic edema manifested as the steeple sign (Fig. 16-8). Cool mist (from the night air) or warm mist (from the steamy bathroom shower) improves the stridor in mild cases. Aerosolized racemic epinephrine, nebulized budesonide, and intravenous dexamethasone have been used with some success in the treatment of croup.

Spasmodic croup may be a mild, often recurrent variant of viral croup characterized by sudden onset without a prodrome of an upper respiratory tract infection. Spasm of the larynx appears to be the major pathologic process. Vomiting or cool mist often enhances resolution of symptoms.

Acute epiglottitis is less frequent now than it was before the introduction of immunization to *H. influenzae* type B. Peak age of presentation is between 1 and 7 years. It is characterized by sudden onset and rapid progression with high fever, toxicity, acute respiratory distress, stridor, drooling, and dysphagia. The child may assume a characteristic posture (sitting up with the neck extended to enhance opening of the airway). When a child presents in this typical fashion, the most expeditious course is to transport the child to the operating room, where experienced anesthesiologists, otolaryngologists, or pulmonologists can intubate the child and secure the airway safely. The epiglottis is often found to be swollen and erythematous (Fig. 16-9). Cultures of the epiglottis may show *H. influenzae* type B, pneumococci, streptococci, or rarely staphylococci. Antimicrobial therapy should be instituted, and the epiglottis should be visualized in 24 to 72 hours before extubation.

Bacterial tracheitis often is characterized by symptoms of croup followed by sudden progression of respiratory distress and airway obstruction similar to epiglottitis. Emergency intubation and airway stabilization often are necessary. The trachea may be severely inflamed with erythema, edema, and copious purulent secretions. Cultures of tracheal secretions may grow staphylococci, pneumococci, or streptococci. Some investigators postulate that this disorder is a secondary bacterial infection occurring after a primary viral infection.

Aspirated or swallowed foreign bodies can cause airway obstruction and stridor. Mobile toddlers are at highest risk, and foods such as nuts, seeds, popcorn, raw vegetables, and hot dogs are common offending agents (see Fig. 14-4). Portions of toys, buttons, and other small objects can lodge in the larynx. Initially the patient coughs and chokes in an attempt to clear the object, but a silent period may follow, lasting hours to days or weeks. Cough, stridor, wheezing, or respiratory distress may then follow. Radiographs may reveal the presence of radiopaque objects. If the object creates a ball-valve effect, pulmonary airtrapping can occur on expiration, resulting in unilateral hyperinflation and mediastinal shift (see Fig. 14-3). Ultimately, atelectasis and/or pneumonia may develop. Many patients, however, may have no radiographic abnormalities despite a history consistent with aspiration of a foreign body. Endoscopy of the airway is indicated in these patients as well. Foreign objects lodged in the esophagus may compress the trachea and create respiratory symptoms in addition to emesis and dysphagia. Radiographs and endoscopy are warranted in these patients.

Wheezing

Wheezing is the musical sound created by partial obstruction, usually of intrathoracic bronchi. Most often it is an ex-

BOX 16-4

Some Common Causes of Wheezing

Infant	Older Child
Vascular ring	Asthma
Tracheoesophagel fistula	Aspiration (reflux, foreign body)
Gastroesophageal reflux	Epiglottitis
Asthma	Laryngotracheobronchitis (croup)
Viral infection (bronchiolitis, upper respiratory tract infection)	Cystic fibrosis
	Hypersensitivity pneumonitis
Pertussis	Tuberculosis
Cystic fibrosis	Tumor
Bronchopulmonary dysplasia	Alpha$_1$-antitrypsin deficiency
Congenital heart disease	Vocal cord dysfunction

piratory sound because positive thoracic pressures during expiration along with decreased intraluminal pressures from the Venturi effect exaggerate obstruction of the airway. Severe obstruction can also produce inspiratory wheezing. Wheezes usually are higher pitched, less harsh sounds than stridor.

Although the phrase "all that wheezes is not asthma" is true and forces pediatricians to generate a differential diagnosis, most wheezing in children is a result of asthma (Box 16-4). Asthma is a leading cause of morbidity and increasing mortality in children in the United States, with onset usually before 5 years of age. Children have repeated episodes of respiratory distress, a tight cough, airtrapping, adventitial lung sounds, rales, rhonchi, and expiratory wheezes. In markedly severe cases of respiratory obstruction or extreme patient fatigue, when airflow diminishes across the obstruction, wheezes may not be heard. This is an ominous sign of impending respiratory failure. Asthma may be due to hypersensitivity to environmental allergens, or it may be seasonal or exacerbated by changes in weather. Family history frequently is positive, with first-degree relatives having similar symptoms. Pathophysiology of obstruction involves bronchospasm, inflammation, edema, and increased mucous secretion. Therapy is aimed at the bronchoconstrictive and inflammatory components.

Infections of the lower respiratory tract may produce wheezing through bronchiolar edema, inflammatory secretions, and mucus. Reactive airway disease can also contribute to symptoms. Bronchiolitis, usually caused by the respiratory syncytial virus, frequently causes wheezing in the infant. Low-grade fever may be present, often with copious rhinorrhea. Bronchitis and pneumonitis may have fever as part of the clinical presentation along with poor response to bronchodilators.

Aspiration of a foreign body often causes sudden onset of respiratory distress with cough, stridor, or wheezing. Auscultatory signs, particularly wheezing, may be unilateral. A silent period lasting hours to days may follow aspiration before new symptoms of fever, cough, or respiratory distress develop.

Bronchopulmonary dysplasia frequently has wheezing as part of the chronic respiratory distress it produces. A history of prematurity with neonatal respiratory distress syndrome and perhaps prolonged ventilation point to this diagnosis.

Gastroesophageal reflux may have wheezing and respiratory symptoms as complications. Overt aspiration of gastric contents can occur with recurrent aspiration pneumonia. In addition, nonregurgitant reflux (intraesophageal reflux without emesis) may occur, stimulating vagal afferents that can produce reflexive bronchospasm in the absence of aspiration. Neurologically impaired children or those with bulbar palsies, cleft palate, or rarely familial dysautonomia may have swallowing difficulties leading to aspiration and wheezing. Tracheoesophageal fistula with aspiration also can produce wheezing.

Congenital abnormalities compressing airway structures frequently present early in life with respiratory distress. Bronchial stenosis causes repeated lower respiratory tract infections and wheezing. Bronchomalacia can cause airway collapse on expiration, and redundant structures can be seen with tracheobronchomegaly, causing recurrent infections. Lobar emphysema occasionally presents with wheezes over the affected lobe, or the emphysematous lung may compress otherwise normal lung tissue. Pulmonary sequestration commonly causes recurrent infection and sometimes wheezing.

Congenital heart disease may cause pulmonary symptoms of tachypnea and possibly wheezing. Wheezing is the result of compression of airway structures by anomalous vessels or an enlarged heart or left atrium. Pulmonary congestion with wheezes occurs with large left to right shunts or overt left-sided heart failure.

Children with cystic fibrosis and recurrent lung infections frequently wheeze with pulmonary exacerbations. A history of meconium ileus at birth, failure to thrive, steatorrhea, and chronic cough may lead the clinician to perform a sweat test or deoxyribonucleic acid (DNA) analysis for common cystic fibrosis mutations.

Extrabronchial masses that impinge on the airway and cause wheezing include infected or enlarged lymph nodes resulting from tuberculosis, sarcoidosis, lymphoma, and metastatic tumors. The right middle lobe syndrome of recurrent right middle lobe pneumonia and atelectasis frequently is caused by enlarged hilar nodes compressing the right main stem bronchus. Cysts and mediastinal masses can obstruct bronchi, leading to retained secretions, infection, and wheezing.

Hypersensitivity pneumonitis, allergic bronchopulmonary aspergillosis, visceral larval migrans, pulmonary vasculitis, ciliary dyskinesia syndromes, and alpha$_1$-antitrypsin deficiency are rare disorders that have wheezing as part of the symptom complex.

TABLE 16-2

Key History Questions in the Evaluation of Noisy Breathing

Disorder characteristics	Causes
Oropharyngeal obstruction	
Presence of craniofacial anomalies	Micrognathia, macroglossia, cleft palate
Cutaneous abnormalities	Hemangioma, lymphangioma, neurofibroma
Fever, sore throat, headache	Streptococci, Epstein-Barr virus, other viral infection, diphtheria
Muffled voice	Tonsillar enlargement, tumor
Neurologic symptoms	Cerebral palsy, palatal hypotonia
Hoarseness	
Sound changes with position	Mobile lesion (cyst, polyp)
Present since birth	Congenital lesions (web, stenosis, cysts, vocal cord paralysis)
Neurologic disorders (hydrocephalus, Arnold-Chiari malformation)	Vocal cord paralysis
Loud crying/screaming	Vocal cord nodules, polyps
Acute onset, fever	Infection
Sinusitis	Postnasal drip
Trauma	Hematoma, arytenoid dislocation
Previous surgery	Recurrent laryngeal nerve injury
Stridor	
Perinatal trauma	Recurrent laryngeal nerve injury
Method of delivery	Neck injury
Present at birth	Laryngomalacia, subglottic stenosis, vocal cord paralysis, vascular ring
Worsens in supine position	Laryngomalacia
Feeding difficulties	Cricopharyngeal achalasia, gastroesophageal reflux, tracheoesophageal fistula, vascular rings
Previous intubation	Subglottic stenosis
Gradual onset	Neoplasia (hemangioma, papilloma)
Acute onset, fever	Croup, epiglottitis, tracheitis
Acute onset, no fever	Aspirated/swallowed foreign body
Wheezing	
Prior lung disease, poor growth	Bronchopulmonary dysplasia, cystic fibrosis, immunodeficiency
Mental retardation, cerebral palsy	Recurrent aspiration
Poor response to therapy	Cystic fibrosis, structural abnormalities
Heart murmur	Heart failure, great vessel abnormalities
Acute onset, no fever	Foreign body

Conversion disorders manifested by functional disorder of the vocal cords may mimic asthma. These patients respond poorly to usual asthma therapy.

History

A careful and detailed history often leads the clinician to the appropriate portion of the airway that is causing noisy breathing (Table 16-2). General questions as to age and time of onset, duration of symptoms, rate of progression of symptoms, associated signs or symptoms, exposure to infections, measures that cause exacerbation or relief, and degree of respiratory effort and distress give the historian a foundation upon which to work.

Oropharyngeal obstruction resulting from congenital causes may be apparent on physical examination. Respira-tory distress from micrognathia, craniofacial syndromes, or macroglossia can be anticipated if these abnormalities are apparent. However, questions about the presence of hemangiomas might lead the clinician to vascular obstructive lesions elsewhere in the body, especially the head or neck. Inflammatory conditions are frequently signaled by fever, sore throat, and perhaps headache and malaise. Slowly progressive voice changes, especially a muffled voice, may suggest tonsillar hypertrophy or perhaps a tumor of the oropharynx. Neurologic symptoms might implicate cerebral palsy with palatal hypotonia.

Hoarseness always indicates obstruction, but factors such as size and location of the lesion may produce differing sounds in different patients. Hoarseness may be an early sign resulting from a small lesion close to the vocal cords. Conversely, hoarseness may occur late if the lesion is farther away from the cords. If hoarseness changes with position, a mobile lesion, such as a cyst or polyp, should be considered. If hoarseness is present at birth, congenital lesions are more likely. Neurologic symptoms suggest that supranuclear lesions, such as hydrocephalus or brainstem involvement caused by an Arnold-Chiari malformation, Dandy-Walker cyst, or meningocele, might be a primary cause of hoarseness. Older infants and children may have a history of vocal cord abuse, with loud crying or screaming, leading to polyps or nodules. Acute onset and fever suggest an infectious cause, and chronic postnasal drip indicates possible sinusitis. Trauma or previous surgery may lead to discovery of a hematoma, arytenoid dislocation, foreign body, or nerve injury.

History related to congenital stridor should begin with questions about perinatal events. Was the infant in an abnormal position in utero, especially with a hyperextended neck, that may have caused injury? How was the infant delivered, and was delivery assisted by forceps or excessive neck traction? Were any anomalies present to suggest defined syndromes or involvement of the airway that could cause stridor? Was respiratory distress or stridor present at birth, or did it evolve with time? Stridor present at birth suggests laryngomalacia, subglottic stenosis, vocal cord paralysis, or vascular ring. Bilateral vocal cord involvement implies a central nervous system abnormality, such as Arnold-Chiari malformation or hydrocephalus. Onset of symptoms may be delayed for 1 to 2 months until significant intracranial pressure forces the brainstem through the foramen magnum, stretching the vagus nerves.

If stridor increases with stress or is worse in a supine position but improved in a prone position with the neck extended, congenital laryngomalacia should be suspected. Rarely does stridor from laryngomalacia interfere with eating. Stridor of vocal cord paralysis may be positional and generally is not as prominent when the child is asleep. If the child lays on the side of the affected cord, gravity allows the cord to drop away from the midline of the larynx, opening the glottis and relieving stridor. Congenital cysts and other mobile lesions behave in a similar fashion. Feeding difficulties, coughing, choking, cyanosis, and regurgitation may suggest cricopharyngeal achalasia, gastroesophageal reflux, or tracheoesophageal fistula. Children with vascular rings may have feeding difficulties because esophageal obstruction can be caused by anomalous vessels. Unilateral vocal cord paralysis (frequently from a peripheral recurrent laryngeal nerve injury) can cause coughing and choking with feedings because the paralyzed cord cannot protect the airway from aspiration.

A history of previous intubation might suggest acquired subglottic stenosis. Small degrees of obstruction may be inapparent for years or may be heralded by repeated episodes of croup with upper respiratory tract infections.

Gradual, progressive stridor suggests a neoplastic process, either benign or malignant. Half of infants with hemangiomas of the airway have cutaneous lesions as well. Usually, symptoms begin between 3 and 6 months of age, and papillomas develop somewhat later, after 1 year of age. Other tumors should be suspected as well, especially if peripheral cranial nerve involvement also occurs.

Acute onset of stridor, often with low-grade fever and a prodrome of upper respiratory tract infection, suggests viral laryngotracheobronchitis. The barking seal cough is characteristic. Little or no prodrome before sudden onset of high fever, toxicity, and drooling with stridor suggests acute epiglottitis; combination of these presentations (i.e., prodromal upper respiratory tract infection before sudden toxicity and airway obstruction) indicates possible bacterial tracheitis.

Acute onset of stridor without constitutional symptoms but possible coughing and choking may indicate an aspirated foreign body. Apnea and aphonia may be symptoms of a laryngeal foreign body or an object lodged in the upper esophagus, compressing the trachea. A high index of suspicion for foreign body must be maintained even in a neonate because innocent older siblings can place foreign bodies in the neonate's mouth with subsequent aspiration.

Causes of wheezing in the younger child often can be determined from a careful history. Background information of previous pulmonary disease might be helpful. The child who was premature and ventilated might have bronchopulmonary dysplasia. Mental retardation and/or cerebral palsy may have recurrent aspiration as part of the clinical picture. Recurrent episodes of wheezing might suggest asthma or bronchiolitis, but if other associated features of failure to thrive and recurrent pneumonias are also present, cystic fibrosis, immunodeficiencies, and ciliary dyskinesias should be considered. Early onset of wheezing, especially if wheezing is constant with poor response to usual therapy, suggests structural anomalies, such as aberrant vessels, large lymph nodes, cardiomegaly, bronchomalacia, and other disorders. Acute onset of wheezing in an older infant or toddler with no constitutional features of infection might indicate foreign body aspiration. Similar to croup, the severity of asthma can be assessed by a scoring system, applying 0 to 3 points for color, retractions, air entry, inspiratory/expiratory ratio, level of consciousness, and wheezing (Table 16-3).

Physical Examination

The initial assessment of any child with noisy breathing should be the adequacy of oxygenation and ventilation (Table 16-4). Ensuring a stable airway must take precedence over any diagnostic studies. Quick assessment includes general appearance. Is the child alert, anxious, fatigued, or obtunded? Anxiety and restlessness are early signs of hypoxia and precede more ominous signs of cyanosis and obtundation. Cyanosis indicates the need for urgent intervention. Respiratory rate and quality of breaths are helpful. Tachypnea is common in patients with respiratory distress; hyperpnea is seen in patients with acidosis; shallow breaths are frequent in lower airway disease, such as asthma; slower, more

---

TABLE 16-3

Asthma Scoring System

Sign	0	1	2	3
Color	Normal	Normal (0 score)	Normal (0 score)	Dusky or cyanotic
Retraction	None	Mild intercostal only	Moderate intercostal to generalized	Generalized, with marked use of accessory muscles
Air entry*	Normal	Slight to mild decrease	Moderate decrease	Severe decrease to nearly absent breath sounds
I/E ratio	1.5 : 1	<1.5 : 1 but >1 : 2	1 : 2 to 1 : 3	>1 : 3
Level of consciousness	Normal	Restless or agitated only when disturbed	Restless or agitated when undisturbed	Lethargic, tiring, or depressed
Wheezing	None, with good air entry	Scattered or mild generalized wheezes with mild decrease of air entry	Moderate generalized wheezing with moderate decrease of air entry	Severe generalized or absent wheezing with poor air entry

*If air entry is asymmetric, the worst area should be scored.

measured breaths sometimes are noted in upper airway obstruction.

Pulse oximetry is a useful part of the initial evaluation to determine adequacy of oxygenation. Previously healthy patients with a hemoglobin saturation less than 95% require supplemental oxygen, and saturations less than 90% indicate the need for aggressive intervention.

If the patient is not in severe distress, a complete physical examination may give clues to the underlying process of noisy breathing. Vital signs and the respiratory rate may indicate stress, infection with tachycardia, or fever. Growth parameters might indicate growth failure, suggesting chronic airway obstruction, hypoxemia, or chronic illness, such as cystic fibrosis or immunodeficiencies.

Examination of the skin, lips, and nails for cyanosis is essential, and the presence of clubbing should alert the clinician for chronic hypoxemia. A careful cardiac evaluation looking for pathologic murmurs, abnormal pulses, or asymmetric blood pressures could lead to a cardiac cause for noisy respirations.

Careful examination of the respiratory system is essential. Examination of the head and neck for congenital anomalies, however minor, might give clues to more serious malformations leading to abnormal breathing. The tongue should be symmetric, move in all directions, and be free of any masses. The palate should be intact with a normal uvula. A bifid uvula may indicate a submucous cleft, which is found by palpating a V-shaped notch in the hard palate at the junction with the soft palate. Tonsils should be symmetric without touching. The palate should rise symmetrically, and a brisk gag reflex should be present. The neck should be free of masses or external fistulas, and the trachea should be midline. Examination of the chest begins with inspection, look-

ing for chest wall movement and symmetry, presence and severity of retractions, increased anteroposterior chest diameter, use of accessory muscles (indicating severe obstruction), mouth-breathing, nasal flaring, or grunting respirations. Palpation of the chest, particularly eliciting vocal fremitus, could indicate areas of consolidation with pneumonia or decreased fremitus with pleural effusions. Percussion can determine dullness of fluid, consolidation of a mass, or the hyperresonance of airtrapping.

The careful listener should be able to distinguish among the different sounds of muffled voice, hoarseness, stridor, and wheezes and differentiate them from lung adventitious sounds of rhonchi and rales. A muffled voice or hyponasal speech is found in significant oropharyngeal or adenoidal obstruction respectively. Hypernasal speech can be seen with cleft palate or submucous cleft palate. Supraglottic lesions may have quiet, moist stridor as compared with loud noises of subglottic obstructions. Supraglottic lesions often cause a muffled voice, whereas hoarseness is more characteristic of subglottic disorders. Children with epiglottitis frequently sit upright with the neck extended and head held forward, whereas children with a retropharyngeal abscess adopt an opisthotonic posture. A peritonsillar abscess characteristically causes the patient to tilt the head toward the affected side. A low-pitched, coarse, fluttering quality to hoarseness suggests supraglottic or hypopharyngeal obstruction; involvement of the cords produces a high-pitched, cracking, or aphonic voice. Associated stridor suggests glottic or subglottic involvement. Inspiratory stridor generally implies a supraglottic obstruction; however, biphasic stridor usually is generated in the extrathoracic trachea and often indicates severe obstruction, requiring tremendous effort to breathe. Auscultation of the chest may be required to hear wheezing. Sym-

TABLE 16-4

Key Findings on Physical Examination

Finding	Diagnosis
General	
Anxiety, fatigue, lethargy	Hypoxia
Cyanosis	Hypoxia
Tachypnea	Respiratory distress, acidosis
Hyperpnea	Acidosis
Shallow breaths	Lower airway obstruction
Slow, deep breaths	Upper airway obstruction
Pulse oximeter <95%	Need for supplemental oxygen
Pulse oximeter <90%	Need for aggressive intervention
Poor growth	Chronic airway obstruction, hypoxemia, chronic illness
Clubbing	Chronic hypoxemia, chronic illness
Cardiac examination	
Heart murmur	Congenital heart disease, heart failure, vascular ring
Head and neck	
Congenital anomalies	Craniofacial syndromes, macroglossia, micrognathia
Bifid uvula	Submucous cleft palate
Enlarged tonsil(s)	Tonsillar hypertrophy, infection, tumor
Neck mass	Thyroglossal duct cyst, branchial cleft cyst, adenitis, tumor
Thorax/lungs	
Asymmetric chest expansion	Poor air entry in one lung
Retractions	Airway obstruction
Increased anteroposterior chest diameter	Airtrapping, emphysema
Use of accessory muscles	Impending respiratory failure
Mouth-breathing	Nasal obstruction
Grunting, nasal flaring	Severe respiratory distress
Abnormal vocal fremitus	Consolidation of lung, bronchial obstruction, pleural effusion
Abnormal percussion	Airtrapping, consolidation, pleural effusion, mass
Abnormal sounds/posture	
Muffled voice	Oropharyngeal obstruction
Hyponasal speech	Adenoidal obstruction
Low-pitched, fluttering sound	Supraglottic or hypopharyngeal obstruction
High-pitched, cracking sound, aphonia	Vocal cord involvement
Hypernasal speech	Cleft palate
Quiet, moist stridor	Supraglottic lesions
Loud stridor	Subglottic lesions
Inspiratory stridor	Supraglottic obstruction
Biphasic stridor	Midtracheal obstruction
Symmetric wheezes	Bronchiolitis, asthma
Asymmetric wheezes	Foreign body obstruction, structural lesion
Upright posture, neck extended	Epiglottitis
Opisthotonic posture	Retropharyngeal abscess
Torticollis	Peritonsillar abscess

metric, diffuse wheezes suggest a generalized process, such as bronchiolitis or asthma, whereas asymmetric and localized wheezes imply structural abnormalities or a foreign body.

Approach to the Patient

After a careful history and physical examination, the examiner should have a good idea of where the obstruction is and per-

haps even the pathogenic mechanisms producing the abnormal sound. Evaluation of the patient should be directed toward determining the effects of the obstruction and delineating exactly where the obstruction is and what is causing it.

Initial laboratory evaluation should examine adequacy of oxygenation and ventilation. Although pulse oximetry is an excellent screening and monitoring tool, venous or arterial blood gases provide specific information about the presence of hypercapnia or hypoxemia. A complete blood count may indicate infection or other processes, such as malignancies (leukemia), that lead to obstructive lesions.

Imaging studies frequently are helpful in determining the location, extent, and possible complications of obstructive lesions. The clinical suspicion of where the lesion may be can determine which imaging procedure is used. Plain neck and chest radiographs are good screening tests for intrinsic airway abnormalities, foreign bodies, vascular rings (abnormal aortic arch), neck or mediastinal masses, and parenchymal abnormalities. The ball-valve effect of some foreign bodies lodged in major bronchi can be demonstrated with inspiratory and expiratory films (see Fig. 14-3). The optimal plain film view of the airway is a filtered high-kilovoltage (kV) magnified radiograph. If fluoroscopy is coupled with this technique, the clinician may be able to get a dynamic assessment of the larynx, epiglottis, vocal cords, trachea, and bronchi. Filtered high-kV magnified airway fluoroscopy separates fixed from variable airway narrowing. A barium swallow can reveal intrinsic abnormalities of the esophagus, such as achalasia, stenosis, or foreign body. It also may demonstrate displacement or compression of the esophagus by a mass or vessel but may not define what the extrinsic mass is. Magnetic resonance imaging (MRI) allows multiplanar definition of intrinsic and extrinsic lesions, especially when masses or vascular rings are suspected. Drawbacks include the static nature of the films and the sedation that younger patients frequently require, which may be dangerous with airway obstruction. Computed tomography (CT) is better than MRI for parenchymal lung disease and can easily evaluate the airway and mediastinum. Unlike MRI, CT can produce dynamic images. It produces images only in an axial plane, however, and like MRI frequently requires sedation.

At times, direct visualization of the airway is essential for diagnosis and possible therapy. Flexible fiberoptic endoscopy is a valuable tool for assessing the dynamic mechanics of the airway. It offers the advantages of avoiding general anesthesia and allows the study of airway dynamics during regular tidal breathing. Fiberoptic bronchoscopy is especially useful for evaluation of hoarseness, stridor, unexplained cough or wheeze, or suspected airway malformation and obtaining specimens from the respiratory tree for culture or pathologic examination. Use of rigid tube bronchoscopy, however, is still preferable if a foreign body is suspected because of better ability to control the airway and remove the object.

The therapeutic approach to the patient with noisy breathing depends largely on the location, severity, and cause of the obstruction. Some lesions with mild obstruction, such as tonsillar hypertrophy or mild laryngomalacia, may not require any intervention except careful observation as the child grows and the obstruction lessens. Tonsillectomy or adenoidectomy may be indicated if chronic obstruction produces failure to thrive, chronic hypoxia, or swallowing difficulties. Acute laryngotracheobronchitis often transiently responds to racemic epinephrine, although rebound obstruction may occur. Dexamethasone, in a dose of at least 0.6 mg/kg intramuscularly also seems beneficial. Nebulized budesonide has been reported to reduce severity of symptoms. Acute epiglottitis represents a medical emergency, and a well-designed protocol should be followed when a patient arrives at a local hospital to allow rapid assessment, minimal or no laboratory tests, and safe transportation to the operating room. In the operating room the anesthesiologist, otolaryngologist, or pulmonologist can safely stabilize the airway under controlled conditions. At that time, diagnostic tests, including cultures of the epiglottis, can be obtained.

Because most wheezing in infants and children results from reactive airway disease, therapy should be directed toward bronchodilation with beta-agonists and reduction of the inflammatory component of obstruction with antiinflammatory drugs, such as cromolyn sodium or steroids. Acute onset of wheezing without a prior history or asymmetric wheezing suggests a foreign body, and radiographs and possible endoscopy should be considered. Chronic fixed wheezing, which responds poorly to usual medications, should prompt an evaluation for compression of intrathoracic airways by mass lesions or vessels.

SUMMARY

Noisy breathing in children results from obstruction of the airway from the nose and oropharynx to the bronchi. The characterization of the sound, whether muffled, hoarse, stridorous, or wheezing, helps locate the site of obstruction. A careful history, physical examination, and selective laboratory tests define the site and cause of the narrowing. The approach to the patient should initially be toward assessing the adequacy of respiration and severity of obstruction, providing for and stabilizing the airway if necessary before any potentially delaying diagnostic tests are undertaken.

ILLUSTRATIVE CASES

Case 1. A 2-month-old infant girl is seen because of noisy breathing since birth. The mother relates that the child had an inspiratory noise beginning shortly after birth, which is worse when she cries and less prominent but still present when she sleeps. She is formula fed and frequently chokes with feeds, causing the mother to temporarily stop feeding. The mother denies cyanosis or other color change. Physical examination reveals a pleasant, alert, pink, stridorous infant whose growth is in the 5th percentile for age, down from the 50th percentile at birth. The respiratory rate is 46 per minute with inspiratory stridor and sternal retractions. Stridor does not change with position. The chest is clear of adventitial sounds, and the remainder of the examination is normal. Pulse oximetry reveals hemoglobin oxygen saturation of 97% in room air. Plain radiograph of the chest demonstrates a right aortic arch. A barium swallow shows bilateral indentation of the esophagus also compressing the trachea, causing the stridor.

This case demonstrates the early onset of stridor from congenital lesions. Lack of variation of stridor with posi-

tion changes suggested a more fixed lesion rather than laryngomalacia. Plain radiographs suggestive of abnormalities of the great vessels were confirmed by a barium esophagram. An MRI would also delineate the anatomy.

Case 2. A 2-year-old boy developed a hacking cough 2 days before being seen in the emergency room. The mother thought he had an upper respiratory tract infection and gave him an over-the-counter cough preparation. Cough continued, and 1 day before admission he developed temperature to 102.8° F. The patient also began drooling, and the mother noted difficulty swallowing, poor eating, and increasing irritability. The voice sounded muffled and soft. On examination in the emergency room, the patient was drooling and irritable, and he tilted his head to the right. Retractions were not noted. Audible breath sounds were apparent without the stethoscope. The chest was clear to auscultation. Examination of the oropharynx revealed an enlarged, inflamed right tonsil that deviated the palate and uvula to the left. A peritonsillar abscess was suspected. Neck radiographs surprisingly showed a straight pin lodged in the right tonsillar area. The child was admitted, begun on antibiotics, and taken to the operating room where a tonsillectomy was performed with drainage of the peritonsillar abscess.

This child had a muffled, soft voice indicating oropharyngeal obstruction. Fever and the child's age suggested a peritonsillar abscess. Despite making a different diagnosis, physicians were surprised to find a pin in the tonsil causing the infection. This case emphasizes that children of this age should always be suspected of ingesting or aspirating a foreign body.

Case 3. A 12-year-old boy was referred for evaluation of asthma refractory to therapy. He had a history of recurrent bronchiolitis as an infant and has been admitted 3 times over the past 4 years for pneumonia, each documented to be in different areas of the lung fields. The patient has been on beta$_2$-agonists, cromolyn sodium, ipratropium bromide, systemic and inhaled steroids, and antibiotics. Allergy testing in the past revealed only minor reactions to dander. Symptoms consist of chronic cough occurring all day but worse in the morning on arising and chronic tightness in his chest with wheezes. Family history is positive for seasonal allergies. Physical examination revealed a small, thin boy whose height was at the 10th percentile for age and weight was less than the 50th percentile for age. Respiratory rate was 30 per minute. The patient was afebrile. He was pink in room air. Chest examination demonstrated increased anteroposterior diameter with mild intercostal retractions. Hyperresonance was generalized over the thorax. Auscultation of the lungs revealed scattered wheezes, occasional shifting rhonchi, and rales in the bases. He had 2+ clubbing. Hemoglobin oxygen saturation was 86% in room air. Plain radiographs of the chest showed hyperexpansion with prominent pulmonary mark-

ings and peribronchial cuffing. Sputum culture grew heavy pseudomonades (two types) and normal flora. Sweat test was positive with sweat chloride 88 mEq/L and 94 mEq/L on two occasions.

Although asthma is the most common cause of wheezing, chronic wheezing that is refractory to usual therapy may indicate another disease. This patient was labeled as asthmatic early in life. Despite poor response to therapy and development of other physical signs, such as clubbing, the diagnosis of cystic fibrosis was not considered until late in childhood.

ANNOTATED BIBLIOGRAPHY

Bluestone CD, Stool SE, editors: *Pediatric otolaryngology,* ed 2, Philadelphia, 1990, WB Saunders.
This is a comprehensive, excellent text that includes several chapters on disorders of the pediatric airway.

Kenna MA: Consultation with the specialist: hoarseness, *Pediatr Rev* 16(2):69-72, 1995.
This is an excellent review of the causes of hoarseness in children.

Quinn-Bogard AL, Potsic WP: Stridor in the first year of life, *Clin Pediatr* 16:913-919, 1977.
This is an old, but thorough review of causes of stridor in infants.

BIBLIOGRAPHY

Bissett GS III, Strife JL, Kirks DR, et al: Vascular rings: MR imaging, *Am J Radiol* 149:251-256, 1987.

Brouillette RT, Ferbach SK, Hunt CE: Obstructive sleep apnea in infants and children, *J Pediatr* 100:31-40, 1982.

Davis HW, Gartner JC, Galvis AG, et al: Acute upper airway obstruction: croup and epiglottitis, *Pediatr Clin North Am* 28(4):859-880, 1981.

Denny FW, Jr: Tonsillopharyngitis 1994, *Pediatr Rev* 15:185-191, 1994.

Deutsch ES, Isaacson GL: Tonsils and adenoids: an update, *Pediatr Rev* 16:17-21, 1995.

Ferguson CF: Congenital abnormalities of the infant larynx, *Otolaryngol Clin North Am* 3(2):185-200, 1970.

Gartner JC, Jr: Acute laryngotracheobronchitis. In English GM: *Otolaryngology* (looseleaf series), Scranton, Penn, 1991, Harper & Row.

Goldenhersh MJ, Rachelefsky GS: Childhood asthma: an overview, *Pediatr Rev* 10:227-233, 1989.

Larsen GL: Asthma in children, *N Engl J Med* 326:1540-1545, 1992.

Oh KS, Newman B, Bowen A, et al: Pediatric airway disorders: practical approaches to imaging evaluation, *Curr Probl Diagn Radiol* 18:199-233, 1989.

Putnam PE, Orenstein SR: Hoarseness in a child with gastroesophageal reflux, *Acta Pediatr* 81:635-636, 1992.

Sofer S, Duncan P, Chernick V: Bacterial tracheitis: an old disease rediscovered, *Clin Pediatr* 22:407-411, 1983.

Weber AL, Grillo H: Tracheal lesions assessment by conventional films, computed tomography, and magnetic resonance imaging, *Isr J Med Sci* 28:233-240, 1992.

Gastrointestinal

17

Constipation

ANDREW H. URBACH

Key Points

- The majority of patients with constipation do not have a major organic disease but rather chronic idiopathic constipation.

- Hirschsprung disease is rare (1 in 25,000 births); 90% of those affected are boys, and stool retention is almost always present in the newborn period. These children are rarely incontinent and often have other features of the disease, such as failure to thrive, abdominal distension, and a chronically ill appearance. Clinical features are usually present and distinguish this entity from chronic idiopathic constipation.

- Encopresis is often emotionally devastating to the child. Careful history and direct questioning about bowel patterns are often necessary to uncover this problem. Appropriate diagnosis and management often results in a successful outcome.

Never put off until tomorrow what you can do the day after tomorrow.

MARK TWAIN

Constipation is an extremely common and generally benign symptom in the pediatric age group. Despite the fact that it is rarely a marker for significant organic pathology, a great deal of energy is spent making children "regular." Although fecal continence may be an evolutionary adaptation to assist humans in the avoidance of predators that track by scent, this function has become secondary in modern times. Perhaps more than any other bodily function, maintaining continence defines human beings socially. The uncontrolled passage of feces rapidly alienates an individual from peers and evokes ridicule. As a result, constipation and the commonly associated problem of encopresis are important entities for the pediatrician to manage appropriately. (Encopresis is the repeated voluntary or involuntary passage of stool into clothing or other places not

intended for that purpose, occurring in children 4 years of age or older, for at least 1 month's duration. The term *soiling* is used interchangeably with encopresis.) Furthermore, constipation is a starting point, a symptom, not a final diagnosis. The search for an organic cause in the child with constipation is often fruitless, but this should not deter the clinician from a thoughtful and methodical approach. Should this evaluation prove to be negative, a label of idiopathic functional constipation is justified.

Despite the fact that constipation accounts for 10% to 20% of gastroenterology clinic referrals, approximately 3% of outpatient general pediatric clinic visits, and 3% to 6% of psychiatric referrals, a consistent definition does not exist in pediatrics. Therefore to understand what should be considered abnormal, a review of normal stool appearance, consistency, and frequency is necessary. Normal stools begin in infancy as meconium, which is odorless, viscous, and greenish-black in color. Typically these stools are passed until the third or fourth day of life. Transitional stools begin at this time and are yellowish-brown to greenish-brown in color with a thin, slimy appearance and may contain occasional milk curds. After 1 week of age, breast-fed babies develop yellow, pasty, mushy stools that may absorb into the diaper. Early constipation in exclusively breast-fed babies is the exception, with some breast-fed infants stooling as often as each feeding. Cow's milk formula feedings result in stools that are puttylike or firm in consistency and pale yellow in color. Infants who are fed cow's milk formula pass stools that are smaller and harder than stools of breast-fed babies. Although the adult brown stool color doesn't appear until the introduction of weaning (Beikost) foods, the stools of breast-fed and cow's milk formula feeders turns brown or green when exposed to air.

Meconium stools are passed at a frequency of 4 to 5 times each day. Delayed passage of meconium for greater than 24 to 48 hours is a "red flag" for a variety of problems, such as Hirschsprung disease and intestinal obstruction caused by stenosis or atresia. Of newborns, 95% pass meconium within the first 24 hours. During the first week of life, 97% of infants have daily stool output of between one and nine stools. By 16 weeks the average number of stools per day is two. In a study of 350 preschool children ranging in age from 1 to 4 years, 96% were found to have bowel movements in the range of 3 times per day to 3 times per week. Adolescent and adult studies indicate that 94% to 98% of individuals evacuate between 3 times per day to 3 times per week, which is remarkably similar to childhood data. These data represent healthy subjects from industrialized countries; diet, disease, and medications may modify this pattern. The size and consistency of stools may be affected by these same factors, with amount of fiber playing a key role in the volume of residue presented to the large intestine. Stool volume of infants per bowel movement ranges from less than 5 ml to more than 40 ml, with most children averaging 25 ml. Adult stools range between 50 to 300 g/day, averaging 140 g/day. Mean intestinal transit time increases with age. At 1 to 3 months of age, transit time is 8½ hours; at 4 to 24 months, 16 hours; and from 3 to 13 years, 26 hours. In young adults the range is from 30 to 48 hours.

Wide variation in stool character precludes uniform stool description, but low-residue diets appear to result in smaller, less frequent stools than high-fiber diets. The consistency of most stools in childhood is soft, but with age an increasing number of children produce hard stools. This is particularly true in children with less than one bowel movement per day. Furthermore, data from Weaver suggest that infrequent bowel movements are associated with hard and at times bloody stools. In summary, constipation may be defined by stool frequency, size, and consistency and ease of elimination. Infrequent bowel movements alone do not indicate constipation. Rather, stools also must be dry and hard and contain minimal water. A history of difficulty or pain on defecation, sometimes severe enough to cause crying, is often reported and usually prompts a visit to the physician.

Pathophysiology

Fecal continence is achieved in the presence of a functional colon, adequate stool consistency, and intact internal and external anal sphincters. Failure of any of these components may cause involuntary expulsion of stool. The colon serves as a reservoir for fecal material and removes water, creating a solid, formed consistency. The muscles of the pelvic floor and the internal and external sphincters regulate defecation by controlling the passage of gas, liquid, or solids.

Normal defecation occurs when a bolus of stool passes into the rectum and results in rectal distension. The presence of as little as 15 ml of stool may cause a relaxation of the internal sphincter and eventual contact with the anal canal's sensory nerves, resulting in the urge to defecate. Effective defecation then comes under conscious control. The child must voluntarily relax the external anal sphincter, tense the muscles of the pelvic floor, and enlist the Valsalva maneuver, increasing intraabdominal pressure. Failure to allow this

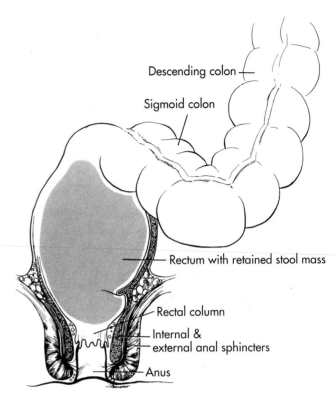

FIG. 17-1 Accumulation of a retained mass of stool in the rectum. As a child repeatedly withholds stool, liquid stool leaks around the functional stool obstruction with resultant soiling.

process to proceed by voluntarily contracting the external anal sphincter and buttocks results in stool movement in a proximal direction, relieving the body's natural urge to defecate. If this process of stool withholding occurs repeatedly, a large volume of stool is retained in a dilated colon. Eventually this stool is passed (often with much difficulty), or liquid, semi-formed stool leaks around the hard mass of retained feces (Fig. 17-1). Though the child frequently tries to resist the passage of stool by closing the external sphincter, this mechanism is limited by the child's ability to concentrate or simple exhaustion of the external sphincter muscle.

A significant build-up of stool in the colon results in a loss of sensitivity in the rectum and a loss of the critical sense of fullness that accompanies stool in the rectum. Once this stage is reached, the self-perpetuating cycle of constipation and encopresis is difficult to break. If most stools that are passed are hard, voluminous, and associated with rectal fissures, the child begins to associate defecation with discomfort. Additional "discomfort" may be a function of negative early toilet training experiences. As the maintenance of bowel continence slips out of the child's control, the child assumes a casual attitude to the problem, which is often at odds with the intense frustration of the family. The socially ostracizing odor and the peer ridicule that predictably follows intensify this already sensitive problem. The child therefore becomes hopelessly trapped by the decrease in rectal sensation of an overly dilated colon and the pain that is felt with the passage of a large, hard bowel movement. Anal fissures add to this dilemma.

Literature Survey

Several large series of children with constipation have helped to better define the nature of this population. Abrahamian and Lloyd-Still evaluated 192 children with constipation who were seen over a period of 7 years. Only six (3%) of these patients were noted to have major organic conditions, such as mental retardation, multiple congenital anomalies, anterior anus, sacral spine defect, and Hirschsprung disease. The majority of children (97% in this study) have chronic idiopathic constipation. The authors reported presenting complaints as follows: soiling, encopresis, constipation, "rule out" Hirschsprung disease, "diarrhea" (actually soiling with liquid feces), and rectal bleeding (secondary to fissures). Many of these patients had already been evaluated with complete blood counts, urine studies, thyroid function tests, and barium enemas. When indicated, these studies were performed (if not already done), and nine patients had rectal biopsies performed, all of which were normal. The boy/girl ratio was 1.6:1.0 with a mean age of onset between 1 and 3 years of age. Of note, 27% of patients had onset of symptoms before 12 months of age. Only 12% developed constipation after age 6 years, and none had onset of symptoms after 10 years.

A wide range of clinical features was reported. Large stools were reported in 85%, with 16% having stools large enough to cause toilet blockage. Most patients had a bowel movement every 3 to 5 days. A history of soiling was present in 71%, frequently associated with parental punishment despite the physiologic data indicating that soiling is often out of the child's control. Furthermore a family history of constipation was elicited in 55% of patients. Many families believed that a clear event heralded the onset of the problem. These factors included weaning from breast milk (to formula or cow's milk), introduction of solid foods, dehydration, hospitalization, onset of toilet training, school or housing change, birth of a sibling, divorce, travel, or anal fissures.

Additional data from this series indicate that urinary tract infection and enuresis may accompany the symptom of constipation. A history of anal fissures was present in 22% of children, abdominal pain in 7%, and rectal prolapse in 3%. Although these children were generally healthy and well grown, in the majority rectal examination revealed copious stool, and often an abdominal mass was palpated. Notably *absent* was evidence of primary psychiatric disease. Rather, any emotional concerns seemed to result from the burden of this problem and the inevitable teasing encountered. This seems to contradict the commonly held belief that constipation and subsequent soiling may be psychogenic in origin. Further reassuring is the fact that none of the children described in this study continued to have constipation after 12 years of age.

Another large series of nearly 200 patients (3 years of age or older) referred to a "constipation clinic" reported findings similar to those mentioned earlier. Encopresis again dominated the clinical picture. Many parents reported that their child hid soiled underwear to avoid confrontation. Typically, stooling occurred in the late afternoon or evening. In some a cyclic pattern developed in which the family noted increased soiling, anorexia, and decreased physical activity followed by the passage of a large bowel movement. This led to temporary relief with improved appetite, less soiling, and an improved sense of well-being. Again, little evidence for primary emotional problems was found. Resolution or improvement often occurred once the encopresis disappeared.

Differential Diagnosis

The symptom of constipation has many causes. With this said, the majority of children with constipation do not have an identifiable cause and fall into the category of chronic idiopathic functional constipation. As with any chronic symptom a detailed history and physical examination are the starting point. Extensive laboratory and diagnostic evaluation is usually unnecessary and unhelpful. One exception to this rule is the newborn or young infant (Box 17-1).

Newborns and Young Infants

Because 95% of newborns pass meconium within 24 hours, failure of this occurrence is a marker for significant underlying organic pathology. Intestinal obstruction by meconium or meconium ileus is most commonly a feature of cystic fibrosis (CF) (Fig. 17-2). Though 90% of patients with meconium ileus are diagnosed with CF, 10% do not have the disease. Typically, symptoms begin at 24 to 48 hours of age with abdominal distension, emesis (at times bilious), and decreased oral feeding but may present earlier, particularly if intestinal perforation is present. Physical examination may reveal an abdominal mass, and imaging studies may demonstrate dilated bowel loops, air-fluid levels, and microcolon secondary to disuse (Fig. 17-3). Another entity, meconium plug syndrome, may have features of intestinal obstruction. These infants pass a sticky, whitish mucous plug, which is eventually followed by gas and liquid meconium. This entity occurs particularly in premature infants, and Hirschsprung disease should be considered. Functional ileus also occurs most commonly in the premature infant and presents as intestinal obstruction. It is a result of a significant systemic illness, such as sepsis, pneumonia, respiratory distress syndrome, electrolyte imbalance, or metabolic disorder. Small left colon syndrome also mimics intestinal obstruction and reflects abnormal peristalsis. Presentation is much the same as that of meconium plug syndrome, with the passage of a plug of meconium then gas and liquid meconium. Maternal diabetes mellitus is often present.

Intestinal obstruction resulting from congenital intestinal anomalies may be heralded by maternal polyhydramnios before delivery and abdominal distension and emesis in the neonatal period. A wide range of anatomic abnormalities, including volvulus, webs, stenosis, and atresia, must be con-

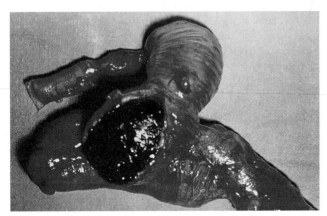

FIG. 17-2 Gross appearance of the thick, tarlike meconium found at laparotomy in meconium ileus.

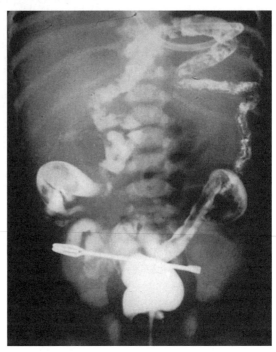

FIG. 17-3 Barium enema in a newborn with meconium peritonitis and evidence of a small, unused distal colon (note small extraluminal calcifications).

BOX 17-1

Constipation in Neonates and Young Infants

Meconium ileus	Anorectal anomalies	Maternal medications
Meconium plug syndrome	Imperforate anus	Magnesium
Functional ileus of the newborn	Anal stenosis	Opiates
Small left colon syndrome	Anterior ectopic anus	Ganglionic blocking agents
Congenital intestinal anomalies	Anterior anal displacement	Inadequate nutrition/fluids
Volvulus	Hirschsprung disease	Excessive cow's milk consumption
Web	Acquired aganglionosis	Absence of abdominal musculature
Stenosis	Tumors (intrinsic or extrinsic)	(i.e., prune-belly syndrome)
Atresia	Dysraphic states (myelodysplasia)	Hypertonic states (e.g., cerebral palsy)
Acquired intestinal stricture	Hypothyroidism	
(i.e., necrotizing enterocolitis)		

sidered. Failure to pass meconium is more common with a low obstruction but at times is also a feature of high obstruction. Atresia and obstruction should be considered more likely in the presence of other congenital anomalies and in the premature infant. Residual effects of acquired disorders, such as necrotizing enterocolitis, also cause constipation.

Anorectal anomalies reportedly occur in 1 in 2500 live births (not including Hirschsprung disease), necessitating careful evaluation of the anorectal area. Anal stenosis is diagnosed by the presence of a very small, tight anus and the passage of very small-caliber stools. Anal stenosis may be congenital (very rare) or acquired as a result of previous surgery. Anterior anal displacement and anterior ectopic anus are other entities to consider. Anterior anal displacement and anterior ectopic anus can be diagnosed when the anal position index (determined by calculating the ratio of the anus-fourchette distance to coccyx-fourchette distance for girls and anus-scrotum distance to coccyx-scrotum distance for boys) is less than 0.46 in boys and less than 0.34 in girls. In anterior ectopic anus the anal canal and the internal sphincter exit anteriorly to the anatomically correct location. The external sphincter, however, is located separately in the anatomically correct posterior location. In anterior anal displacement, normal structures are simply located anteriorly. In

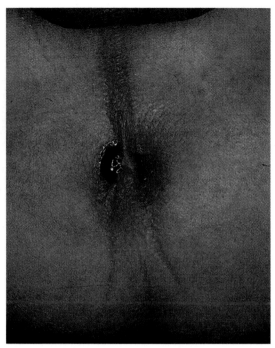

FIG. 17-4 A spot of meconium is visible beneath a "bucket-handle" bridge of skin in an infant with a low imperforate anus.

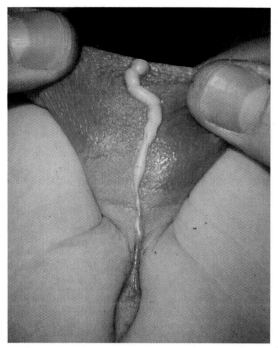

FIG. 17-5 In boy infants, white mucus or black meconium may pass through a perineal fistula, from a low imperforate anus, into the scrotal raphe.

both of these entities, girls predominate. Constipation, often evident in the newborn, is caused by the sharp angulation of the anus in an anterior direction. The presence of a "posterior shelf" on rectal examination can assist in diagnosis. At the other end of the spectrum of anorectal anomalies is imperforate anus, which is easily diagnosed by the absence of a normal anal opening. Although an anal dimple is usually present, stool exits through a fistulous tract, perineum or vulva in girls, urethra in boys (Figs. 17-4 and 17-5).

Could the cause be Hirschsprung disease? When evaluating the child with constipation, this disorder causes more consternation to clinicians than any other diagnostic entity. Hirschsprung disease, or congenital aganglionosis, occurs in 1 in 25,000 live births, with a 90% male predominance. Familial occurrence is well documented, and Down syndrome accounts for 2% of all cases. The cause is an absence of ganglion cells in the distal rectum, with varying degrees of involvement of proximal bowel. Functional obstruction is produced because tonic, uninhibited contraction prevents bowel relaxation. Most often (80%) the rectosigmoid alone is involved. Rarely, ultrashort segment disease of the very distal rectum does occur, and 5% of the time the entire colon and portions of the small bowel are involved (Fig. 17-6). Definitive diagnosis can be made by rectal biopsy, which demonstrates both absence of ganglion cells and abnormal neuronal staining.

The majority of patients present within the first week of life, and some authors suggest that 100% of patients have

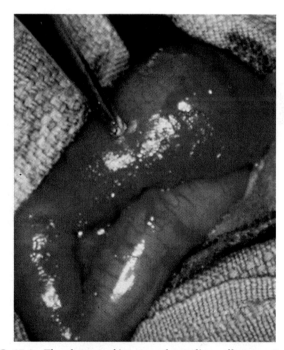

FIG. 17-6 The absence of intramural ganglion cells prevents intestinal peristalsis through segments affected by Hirschsprung disease, causing a functional bowel obstruction. The involved segment appears narrow when compared with the distended, obstructed proximal bowel, which possesses normal ganglion cells.

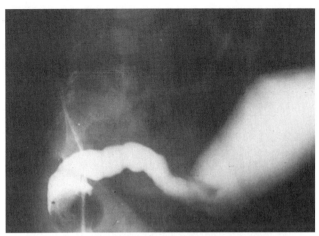

FIG. 17-7   Barium enema outlines the transition zone between the contracted (aganglionic) rectosigmoid lying distal to the obstructed but normally innervated colon. To demonstrate this sign the examination must be conducted in an unprepped patient who has undergone neither enemas nor digital rectal examination.

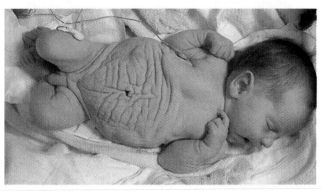

FIG. 17-9   A newborn with prune-belly syndrome shows the characteristic wrinkled and redundant skin covering the abdominal wall. On palpation, no abdominal muscular tissue or muscular tone could be detected.

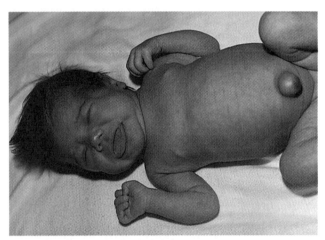

FIG. 17-8   A child with cretinism. (Courtesy Dr. T.P. Foley, Jr., Pittsburgh.)

onset of symptoms *before* 1 month of age. Conversely, 97% of constipated children with negative rectal biopsies (no evidence of Hirschsprung disease) develop onset of symptoms *after* 1 month of age. The diagnosis of Hirschsprung disease can be suspected with delay in or failure to pass meconium and marked stool infrequency. Associated features include vomiting (at times bilious) and abdominal distension. Half of children with Hirschsprung disease develop enterocolitis manifested by diarrhea, protein-losing enteropathy, hypoproteinemia, and evidence of systemic toxicity. Should the diagnosis escape detection in infancy, features of failure to thrive, anemia, severe constipation, a tympanitic abdomen, peristaltic waves, prominent abdominal veins, and foul-smelling, "ribbon" stools may suggest the diagnosis. Palpation of the abdomen may reveal a mass, and rectal examination is remarkable for a tight, narrow anus devoid of stool. Evacuation of the colon may follow digital manipulation, but does not rule out the diagnosis. Plain radiographs of the abdomen may show distension, and barium enema may reveal a dilated proximal bowel and a transition zone (Fig. 17-7). With a detailed evaluation, most children with typical Hirschsprung disease are detected. The exception to this may be the child with ultrashort segment disease. Symptoms in these children may indeed mimic those of idiopathic constipation. Table 17-1 outlines the major differences between Hirschsprung disease and idiopathic chronic constipation (dysfunctional stool retention).

Rarely, acquired aganglionosis has been reported as a result of anoxic injury. In one case report the sicker of monozygotic twins (smaller and suffering respiratory distress, necrotizing enterocolitis, and prolonged umbilical artery catheterization) was diagnosed with aganglionosis, but the sibling was normal. Additional entities that may present with decreased stooling in infancy include intrinsic or extrinsic tumors, hypothyroidism (Fig. 17-8) (prolonged jaundice, depressed body temperature, umbilical hernia, and lethargy), dysraphic states (myelodysplasia) (see Fig. 2-5), and maternal medications in the immediate neonatal period (magnesium, opiates, and ganglionic blocking agents). Inadequate nutrition or fluid intake, excessive cow's milk consumption, and absence of abdominal musculature (i.e., prune-belly syndrome) (Fig. 17-9) complete the differential diagnosis. These entities are summarized in Box 17-1.

Older Infants and Children

Constipation continues to be a common problem in older children. Issenman reported that 16% of parents of 22-month-old

TABLE 17-1

Comparison of Aganglionic Megacolon and Chronic Dysfunctional Stool Retention

Characteristic	Aganglionic megacolon	Stool retention
Prevalence	1 in 25,000 births	1.5% of 7-yr-old boys
Gender ratio	90% boys	86% boys
Retention as newborn	Almost always	Rare
Problems with bowel training	Rare	Common
Late onset of symptoms (after 2 yr)	Rare	Common
Toilet avoidance	Rare	Common
Incontinence	Rare	Common
Stool size	Often thin "ribbons"	Often large caliber
Frequency of defecation	Greatly diminished	Variable
Abdominal pain	Rare, except in obstruction	Common, especially in cases of recent onset
General appearance	Often chronically ill	Usually healthy
Failure to thrive	Common	Rare
Obstruction	Common	Rare
Abdominal distension	Common	Variable
Stool in ampulla	Often diminished	Often increased
Plain roentgenograms	Narrow rectum	Often dilated, distended rectum
Barium enema	Localized constriction with proximal dilation may be seen	Often diffuse megacolon

Modified from Francoeur TE: Constipation. In Hoekelman RA, editor: *Primary pediatric care*, St. Louis, 1992, Mosby–Year Book.

children consider their children constipated. Idiopathic chronic constipation and Hirschsprung disease often top the list of possibilities in the minds of most clinicians. However, in Sondheimer's series of 200 patients ages 3 years and older with chronic constipation, Hirschsprung disease had not been "missed" in any. Rather, in this series the diagnoses of sacral agenesis, ectopic anus, and unsuspected mental retardation were uncovered. The clinician therefore should remember that idiopathic constipation is more common than any other diagnosis. Loening-Baucke also reported that in the Encopresis Clinic at the University of Iowa, 95% of patients have functional constipation.

No single mechanism appears to cause idiopathic constipation, but it may result from inherited, constitutional, psychologic, intrinsic slow motility or pain with passage of bowel movements. Despite the fact that few patients have a definable organic cause, a thorough search for an organic cause is necessary. The differential diagnosis of constipation in the older infant and child is quite broad but can be managed more easily if divided into several categories (Box 17-2). The division of these entities into physiologic causes, voluntary withholding, neurogenic disorders, endocrine and metabolic disorders, and miscellaneous disorders may be helpful.

Physiologic Causes

Breast-fed babies initially have frequent bowel movements. However, at around 6 weeks of age the daily frequency may decrease substantially, and bowel movements may occur every other day or even less frequently. Cow's milk and the casein curd that it contains is also known to result in constipation. Lack of fiber and bulk in the diet also leads to a similar clinical scenario. Alterations in fluid balance caused by decreased fluid intake or increased fluid losses result in stools that are devoid of adequate water and may cause constipation. Additional situations include fever, excessive insensible losses, or iatrogenicly induced imbalance resulting from inadequate intravenous fluids. Constipation may also occur in the immobilized patient as a result of injury, surgery, or orthopedic casting. In the adolescent child, eating disorders, such as anorexia nervosa, can produce the same result.

Voluntary Stool Withholding

Voluntary stool withholding with or without encopresis is a common cause of constipation in the preschool-age child. These "stool hoarders" typically begin their pattern between the second and third birthdays. Although parents may be aware of a problem, it is typically brought to medical attention when fecal soiling develops. Encopresis is reported to occur in 2.8% of 4-year-olds, 2.2% of 5-year-olds, 1.9% of 6-year-olds, 1.5% of 7- to 8-year-olds, and 1.6% of 10- to 11-year-olds. As alluded to earlier, a huge mass of stool develops and stool leakage around this obstruction results in liquid or claylike stool spilling into underwear. Anorexia, enuresis, and urinary tract infection are symptoms seen in these otherwise developmentally normal children. A wide

BOX 17-2

Causes of Constipation in the Older Infant and Child

Physiologic Causes
Dietary
  Breast milk
  Cow's milk
  Low roughage
Deficient fluid intake
  Fever
  Heat
  Inadequate intravenous fluids
  Immobility
  Anorexia nervosa

Voluntary Stool Withholding
Megacolon with or without
  encopresis
Painful defecation
  Anal fissure
  Perianal dermatitis or irritation
  Hemorrhoids
Behavioral issues
Mental retardation
Depression

Neurogenic Disorders
Hirschsprung disease
Intestinal pseudoobstruction
Cerebral palsy
Myelomeningocele
Spinal cord injury
Transverse myelitis
Sacral agenesis
Diastematomyelia
Spinal dysraphism
Neurofibromatosis
Muscular weakness
  Myopathies
  Rickets
  Prune-belly syndrome

Endocrine and Metabolic Disorders
Hypothyroidism
Diabetes mellitus
Pheochromocytoma
Hypokalemia
Hypercalcemia
Hypocalcemia

Endocrine and Metabolic Disorders—cont'd
Diabetes insipidus
Renal tubular acidosis
Porphyria
Amyloidosis
Lipid storage disorders

Miscellaneous Disorders
Anal or rectal stenosis
Anteriorly placed anus
Dolichocolon
Appendicitis
Celiac disease
Scleroderma
Lead poisoning
Viral hepatitis
Salmonellosis
Infantile botulism
Tetanus
Chagas disease
Drugs

range of causes has been suggested. Early colonic inertia may begin at a young age, leading to straining to withhold or release stool. This sets up a negative association with stooling, and if intense parental reaction occurs (perhaps in the form of rectal manipulation) the problem is exacerbated. A stressful family situation coincident with toilet training may also set up a functional megacolon. If there is a death, separation, loss, birth of a sibling, or other emotional trauma during this time interval, toilet training may be interrupted. The literature also provides examples of fortuitous toilet avoidance. Children become frightened by the prospect of drowning or falling into the toilet. One report indicts a television commercial in which a toilet bowel turns into a monster and the seat cover makes biting motions. At times, children avoid a secondary toilet outside of the home, such as a nonprivate toilet at school or other public setting. Children with attention-deficit disorder may not be persistent enough with the task of defecation and only partially evacuate. Eventually this pattern may lead to constipation or encopresis. "Voluntary" stool withholding may also represent a response to disturbed family relationships, such as divorce, abuse, or neglect. Lastly, anorectal surgery earlier in life may carry emotional "baggage" that interferes with normal bowel habits, even when physiologic competence can be demonstrated.

Regardless of what initiates the constipation/encopresis cycle, the final effect on a child's self-esteem is devastating. There is the enormous burden of the "secret" being discovered, and if this occurs, peer ridicule, name-calling, and emo-

tional trauma will soon follow. These children often isolate themselves and show signs of dependency. They remain perplexed by their apparent inability to understand why they are unable to control their stools. Adults, on the other hand, have little difficulty assigning blame and labeling the child as lazy, forgetful, and otherwise incompetent.

Other causes of voluntary stool withholding include perianal conditions, such as hemorrhoids, anal fissures (Fig. 17-10), dermatitis, or any form of irritation that can result in pain with defecation. Mental retardation also can lead to constipation, and depression can do the same.

Neurogenic Disorders

A wide range of neurogenic entities have been implicated as causes of constipation. As already mentioned, Hirschsprung disease, cerebral palsy, and lesions of the spinal cord are factors. Spinal cord lesions include myelomeningocele, spina bifida occulta, diastematomyelia (a congenital anomaly of the spinal cord with bony spicules, or fibrous bands, splitting the cord into two halves wrapped in dura), neurenteric cysts, intradural lipomata, dermoid cysts, and sacrococcygeal agenesis. Sphincter function may deteriorate as a result of the differential growth patterns of the spinal cord and vertebral column. A loss of previously achieved function may therefore occur, causing the child to lose this milestone as the pathology evolves. Chronic intestinal pseudoobstruction syndrome often presents with constipation (60%). These children have been noted to have intestinal

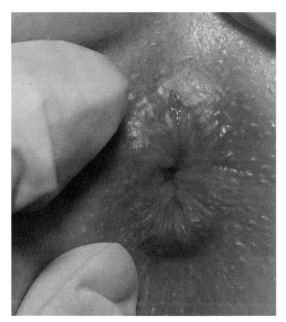

FIG. 17-10 Small tears in the anoderm may bleed, producing small amounts of blood on the stool of healthy infants.

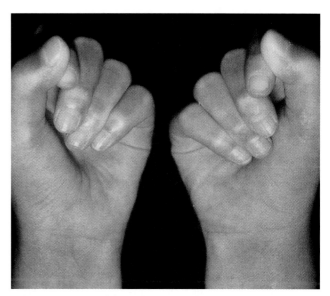

FIG. 17-11 Lack of flexibility in the hands is characteristic of scleroderma.

motility abnormalities that result in recurrent symptoms of bowel obstruction. Vomiting, diarrhea, abdominal distension, and failure to thrive are additional features. Occasionally, urinary tract infection and difficulty voiding are present as well. Although many children have no identifiable cause, some have definable abnormalities of intestinal nerve plexuses and smooth muscle. Neurofibromatosis and muscular weakness (myopathies, muscular dystrophies, rickets, and prune-belly syndrome) may also cause symptoms of constipation.

Endocrine and Metabolic Disorders

As with dehydration, diabetes mellitus, diabetes insipidus, and renal tubular acidosis may lead to decrease in stool water and cause constipation. Hypokalemia, hypercalcemia, and hypocalcemia are also established causes. Although hypothyroidism often comes to mind when constipation is mentioned, other symptoms usually overshadow the gastrointestinal features. Pheochromocytoma typically causes increased blood pressure and heart rate, palpitations, headache, nausea, and vomiting, but constipation is also reported. Porphyria, lipid storage diseases, and amyloidosis are unusual causes as well.

Miscellaneous Disorders

As highlighted in the section on causes of infantile constipation, anal or rectal stenosis and anteriorly placed anus may escape recognition until symptoms appear at an older age. An unusual condition, dolichocolon, is manifested by a particularly long colon, resulting in the excessive removal of water from stool. Infantile botulism, though rare, is an important cause of decreased stooling. Hypotonia, weakness, facial and ocular palsies, autonomic nervous system abnormalities, and respiratory failure may accompany botulism. Lead poisoning

may cause constipation, and a history of pica should be sought. More frequently, elevated lead levels result from the subtle hand-to-mouth behaviors often exhibited by toddlers. Other entities, such as celiac disease (see Fig. 18-4), meconium ileus equivalent, scleroderma (Fig. 17-11), mixed connective tissue disease, systemic lupus erythematosus, viral hepatitis, salmonellosis, tetanus, and Chagas disease (parasitic infection that causes, among other things, destruction of ganglion cells of the myenteric plexus, leading to constipation and megacolon) are rare explanations for constipation in children. Drugs (prescribed, over-the-counter, or illicit) should always be considered as a potential cause. Examples include aluminum (antacids), opiates, calcium channel blockers, anticholinergics, methylphenidate, diuretics, and nonsteroidal antiinflammatory drugs. All of these forms of chemical use should be explored thoroughly.

History

As with most entities in the field of pediatrics, the history is the foundation of the approach. History should start with the child's baseline stooling pattern, beginning at birth (time of first passage of meconium) and progress chronologically to the present pattern. Although the symptom of constipation may not present overtly for months or years, subtle early clues or harbingers of problems can be elicited with a careful history. Partin, who suggests that painful defecation is a critical factor in the development of stool withholding and encopresis, reports that these symptoms are often present in children less than 36 months of age. Timing may also be important for the encopretic patient, with most episodes occurring in the afternoon, during exercise, or while walking home from school. Stool frequency, consistency, and size are basic facts to be established at the outset. Bulky, fatty-appearing stools with a particularly foul odor may be a clue to malabsorption and CF. Stool with streaks of blood may suggest a fissure or hemorrhoid and hence evidence of hard stools and painful defecation. Dietary history is also vital. Excessive cow's milk or limited fiber consumption or occasionally breast-feeding results in constipation. Wide variations in diet make conclusions more difficult, but a change in diet may be a key factor. In addition to a detailed history of stool frequency, information about consistency, soiling, and related behavior should be sought. The nature of soiling, if present, and the time of day are important. Are stools formed, liquid, or scybalous (small, dry, rabbitlike pellets)? What is the evidence for withholding behavior? Some children complain of diarrhea, mistaking overflow incontinence for a completely opposite symptom complex. A number of clues help determine which children have stool retention (Box 17-3). The existence of constipation may be overlooked if incomplete defecation results in a daily bowel movement. This may cause parents to attribute soiling to a wide range of acute events rather than to a preexisting chronic condition.

As the clinician proceeds through this history-gathering process, it is important that he or she keep in mind that constipation is not just decreased stool frequency but also increased firmness and increased difficulty in the passage of fecal material. This might be suggested by squeezing, straining, abdominal pain, or having bowel movements clandestinely. Francoeur points out that the child with legs hyperextended, fists clenched, and a red face may not be trying to pass stool but perhaps to withhold stool. The "urge" to defecate is a critical historic feature in differentiating children with idiopathic constipation from those with Hirschsprung disease. The latter children simply lack this "call to stool" because the stool is retained proximal to the anorectum.

Clarity of language cannot be overemphasized. The accurate use of words for feces, urine, soiling, and bodily anatomy is vital for an accurate history. Sondheimer points this out, using the example of a mother who asks her child, "Did you go to the bathroom?" This question can be interpreted by the child as *asking* if he or she attempted to defecate, rather than the intended "Did you have a bowel movement?" Clear use of language and meticulous detail are important if a successful diagnosis is to be achieved. In addition, parents and children may choose not to communicate or have difficulty communicating about issues as personal and sensitive as the child's bowel movements. If encopresis develops, communication may be further impaired by the heightened emotion this symptom brings. At times a hidden concern about cancer or issues of sexual orientation may be present. Particular attention to the real message facilitates trust and leads to more rapid and accurate diagnosis.

Sondheimer offers an excellent intake database for her Constipation Clinic (Box 17-4). Of note is specific information about any previous evaluations, family history, and social history. An endless array of specific questions about unusual

> ### BOX 17-3
> ### *Possible Clues to Stool Retention*
>
> 1. A period longer than 3 or 4 days without a bowel movement
> 2. A history of blood-streaked stool (fissure)
> 3. Straining with small, hard stools (pellets)
> 4. Occasional presence of very large stools (filling the toilet or requiring mechanical breakup)
> 5. A child's feet suspended in air when having a movement
> 6. A child who stays on the toilet for less than 1 minute at a time
> 7. Enuresis (especially daytime and late onset)
> 8. History of soiling underwear
> 9. History of use of laxatives and enemas
> 10. Onset of recurrent abdominal pain

From Francoeur TE: Constipation. In Hoekelman, editor: *Primary pediatric care*, St Louis, 1992, Mosby–Year Book.

causes of constipation could be offered, but the broadness of the list of differential diagnoses provided limits such exhaustive efforts. Nonetheless a few specific questions are warranted regarding recent illness, bed rest, fever, birth of a sibling, emotional stress, housing move, dehydration, or dietary change. A search for urinary incontinence is often fruitful because a distended rectum may compress the bladder, causing day and night enuresis. Other specific questions can be obtained from the comprehensive list of diagnostic entities provided in Boxes 17-1 and 17-2.

Physical Examination

The focuses of the physical examination in the child with constipation are the abdomen and rectal area. However, as is often the case, a complete and thorough examination often provides the clue that leads to diagnosis. Poor growth may suggest failure to thrive and a diagnosis of CF, celiac disease, or Hirschsprung disease. The detailed neurologic and developmental examination provides a clue to mental retardation, or a detailed skin examination reveals café au lait spots and a diagnosis of neurofibromatosis. Elevated blood pressure may point toward pheochromocytoma, or careful examination of the sacral area may reveal a hemangioma or hair tuft, suggesting occult spinal dysraphism. The child with a relatively short history of constipation, weak cry, and decreased pupillary response may have infantile botulism. Very weak abdominal musculature may suggest muscular dystrophy or prune-belly syndrome. Certainly this list of specific findings is lengthy, but careful examination and thoughtful correlation with a list of differential diagnoses maximize the chances of success.

BOX 17-4

Constipation Data Sheet

Historical Information
Planned pregnancy
Birth weight
Bowel problems in first 6 months

Toilet Training
Age initiated
Age of urinary continence
Age of fecal continence
Problems associated with training

Present Problem
Date of onset
Number of stools/week
Pain or straining
Blood in BM
Description of BM
Fecal soiling
　At home
　At school
　At night

Present Problem—cont'd
Number of episodes/day
　Amount
　Sensation
Abdominal distension
　Vomiting
Psychologic evaluation or treatment
　When
　With whom
Fissures
　Thyroid function studies, result
　BE, result
　Biopsy, result
　UTI, UTI symptoms (dates)
　Enuresis (date of onset)
Other physicians consulted for this
　problem
Past medical therapies with doses, dates,
　and results
Present medical regimen

Family History
Thyroid disease
Bowel disease, constipation
UTI
Psychiatric disease
Seizures

Social History
Parents' marital status
Parents' occupations
Number of homes child has
　lived in since birth
Present school
Grade
School performance
Behavior problems

Modified from Sondheimer JM: Helping the child with chronic constipation, *Contemp Pediatr* 2:12-28, 1985.
BE, Barium enema; *BM,* bowel movement; *UTI,* urinary tract infection.

In the much more common situation of chronic idiopathic constipation, a more focused examination often yields the key to diagnosis. The abdomen should first be inspected for evidence of mild distension. Moderate to severe distension is more typical of an obstructive process, such as celiac disease or Hirschsprung disease. Peristaltic waves are sometimes seen in children with Hirschsprung disease but are not a feature of idiopathic constipation. Anal placement should be normal in children with idiopathic constipation, unlike children with anterior ectopic anus or anterior anal displacement. A careful examination of the perianal area to the level of the mucosa should be performed, looking for fissures, excoriation, diaper rash, dermatitis, and hemorrhoids. Any of these findings could interfere with pain-free defecation.

Palpation of the abdomen may reveal evidence of stool, which is at times dramatic enough to be mistaken for an abdominal tumor. Fecal masses are typically felt in the area just above the pubic symphysis and in the left lower quadrant. Tenderness is not typically present. Because stool is often soft and pasty, enormous amounts of stool may be stored in the bowel, yet escape detection by palpation. Rectal examination, though tempting to defer, should always be an integral part of the examination. Before digital examination is performed, an anal "wink" should be sought. Gentle rubbing of the perianal skin results in reflex contraction of the external anal sphincter. Rectal examination in the child with idiopathic constipation typically uncovers large amounts

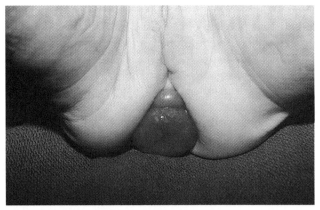

FIG. 17-12 Although the cause of rectal prolapse is unknown in the majority of cases, all infants should undergo an evaluation for cystic fibrosis.

of stool in a cavernous ampulla, and the child with Hirschsprung disease has an empty distal rectal segment. Anal tone is tight and the rectum narrow in the child with aganglionosis. Neither of these features is present in idiopathic constipation. Occasionally a child is excessively fearful and resistant to the rectal examination. Should sensitive attempts at exploration fail, the examination can be deferred. This should be the exception, however. Rectal prolapse (Fig. 17-12) may be a feature of idiopathic chronic constipation but must be considered a possible marker for the child with CF. Rarely, reported findings of potential pseudoverrucous papules have been described in encopretic children as a result of repeated exposure of the perirectal mucosa to liquid stool. There are, however, no pathognomonic perianal signs in childhood constipation.

A search for evidence of stool leakage should be a routine aspect of the evaluation. Soiling may be seen on underpants or in the perianal and buttock area. Stool odor is an unmistakable feature of soiling. Interestingly the patient may be unable to sense this odor because individuals accommodate to their own smells. The conflicts between parents and child that this can produce, if not understood, can be quite dramatic.

Approach to the Patient

General

A detailed history and physical examination should guide any further work-up. Because the majority of children with constipation do not have underlying pathology, this work-up is minimal. Clues from the history and physical examination may necessitate that the clinician check blood studies for calcium, glucose, electrolytes, or evidence of acid-base derangements. Thyroid function tests and studies to evaluate adrenal function may be indicated as well. Urine analysis and culture may prove necessary if enuresis is an associated problem or if diabetes mellitus, diabetes insipidus, or renal tubular dysfunction is suspected. Urinary tract infection is the only significant complication of constipation. It has been suggested that 20% of girls with recurrent urinary tract infections have underlying chronic constipation. Relieving the constipation decreases the frequency of infection.

Radiologic studies are usually unnecessary in straightforward constipation, although a plain abdominal film may assist in the assessment of retained stool and its volume. A granular or rocklike appearance to the stool may be seen. In the unusual circumstance when a rectal examination is not performed or in the case of an obese child, the plain film may answer questions not easily ascertained by physical examination. Spine films are indicated if a dysraphic state is a consideration. It is not likely, however, that spinal cord disease is present if the neurologic examination is normal and urinary findings are absent. Several conditions (e.g., Hirschsprung disease) may warrant barium x-ray studies. A transitional zone between aganglionic bowel and normal bowel is present (Fig. 17-7). In most patients with constipation, these studies are not helpful.

Anorectal manometric evaluation of children may be helpful if Hirschsprung disease is a consideration. Interestingly, children with idiopathic chronic constipation have an increased threshold for rectal distension and decreased rectal contractibility. These abnormalities may persist for years, even after therapy. Should Hirschsprung disease be a consideration, anal manometry, barium enema, and rectal biopsy may be indicated. Rectal biopsy is the most direct method, and often preliminary procedures can be bypassed.

Consultation is rarely needed for uncomplicated chronic constipation. In the unusual event that an underlying organic cause is suspected, subspecialty pediatric or surgical assistance may be required. Conditions such as Hirschsprung disease, anorectal anomalies, dysraphic states, and pheochromocytoma are examples. Some serious organic disorders may require evaluation by a pediatric subspecialist. Cystic fibrosis, celiac disease, hypothyroidism, neurofibromatosis, and myopathies are examples.

Management

The management of chronic idiopathic constipation is relatively straightforward and hinges on education, disimpaction, a bowel maintenance regimen, and the eventual reestablishment of a normal bowel evacuation pattern. Above all, establishing a relationship with the child and family and recognizing the long-term nature of the management of this problem are essential.

Much can be accomplished by simply explaining the pathophysiology of the problem and removing blame, guilt, and any form of punishment. The release of frustration that occurs when a well-educated family begins to embark on a solution can be remarkable. A wide range of agents can be used for "clean-out," including hypertonic phosphate enemas, normal saline enemas (less effective), and oral or nasogastric lavage solutions (i.e., polyethyleneglycol electrolyte). Soapsuds and tap water enemas are dangerous and should be avoided. Once clean-out has been documented, a variety of maintenance therapies are available. These include carbohydrates (Maltsupex, Karo), magnesium salts (Milk of Magnesia), mineral oil, lactulose, senna syrup, and natural fiber. As a successful bowel pattern emerges, a gradual reduction in therapy may be considered. A behavior modification program with emphasis on positive reinforcement must be established. Sitting on the toilet several times a day, especially after meals, is essential so that the gastrocolic reflex can be used. Additional behavioralist assistance may be necessary in some children. A supportive and sensitive approach that does not view cooperation with this program as punishment but rather bowel strengthening or training and a "team and coach" approach is vital. Management of specific organic disorders is quite detailed and beyond the scope of this text.

Algorithm

The complexity of history-taking, behavioral assessment, and physical examination is not easily distilled into a very useful algorithm; however, Altschuler provides a simple and useful guide (Fig. 17-13). He suggests beginning with a careful examination of the rectal area for fistulas, fissures, or pain-inducing findings, such as an abscess. A digital rectal examination should then be performed. If tone is decreased, a po-

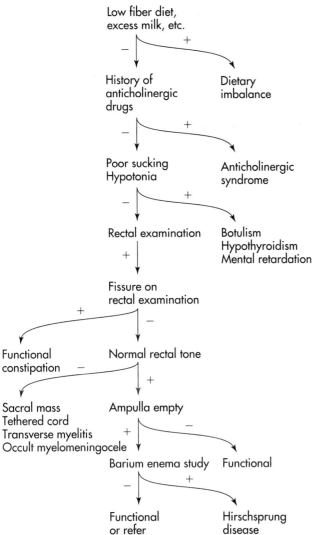

FIG. 17-13 Decision tree for differential diagnosis of constipation. (From Altschuler S: Constipation. In Schwartz MW, editor: *Pediatric primary care: a problem-oriented approach*, ed 2, St. Louis, 1990, Mosby–Year Book.)

tential problem with S2-S4 innervation should be considered, using additional data gathered from the neurologic examination. If neurologic evaluation is normal and the stigmata of Hirschsprung disease are present (Table 17-1), a barium study or rectal biopsy should be performed. A diagnosis of functional constipation can be made if the patient does not have bleeding, is on no medications that cause constipation, and consumes adequate bulk or fiber. Table 17-2 offers key findings paired with possible diagnoses.

SUMMARY

Although the breadth of diagnoses in the child with constipation may be daunting, a careful methodical approach often yields a diagnosis and positively impacts the child's physical and emotional well-being. More than 90% of children have functional constipation and can be managed well by their primary care physician.

TABLE 17-2

Clues to Diagnosis of Constipation

Key findings	Diagnosis
Low fiber, excess milk	Dietary imbalance
Anticholinergic drugs	Anticholinergic syndrome
Delayed passage of stool as a newborn	Hirschsprung disease, cystic fibrosis, anatomic anomalies (stenosis, atresia)
Sacral dimple, hemangioma, hair tuft	Dysraphism
Bilious emesis	Obstructive lesion
Hypotonia or poor suck	Myopathy, infant botulism, mental retardation
Incontinence	Encopresis, dysraphism
Poor rectal tone	Sacral mass, tethered cord, transverse myelitis, occult dysraphic state
Tight rectum	Hirschsprung disease, anal stenosis
Rectal prolapse	Cystic fibrosis, idiopathic chronic constipation

ILLUSTRATIVE CASES

Case 1. L.A. is a 2-month-old boy with a history of difficulty passing stools in the newborn nursery. His first stool was passed at 28 hours. His stools are often spaced 4 to 5 days apart. Abdominal distension has been noted by his mother. Rectal examination revealed an absence of stool, and barium enema showed an area of localized constriction with proximal dilation. Rectal biopsy revealed an absence of Meissner and Auerbach plexuses and increased size of nerve bundles. An increase in acetylcholinesterase was also present.

This case illustrates the presence of early stooling difficulty in children with Hirschsprung disease. Ninety percent of affected children are boys, and associated symptoms are often failure to thrive, a chronically ill appearance, obstruction, abdominal distension, and an absence of stool in the ampulla.

Case 2. J.S. is a 7-year-old boy who had normal bowel movements for the first year of life. Beginning at approximately 1 year of age, he had difficulty passing stools and seemed to grunt with discomfort with each bowel movement. Bowel movements occurred every 3 to 4 days and often had a hard, scybalous appearance. At the 18-month pediatric check-up, a rectal fissure was noted. On one occasion, J.S.'s mother noted that his rectum prolapsed after a bowel movement. Of late, he has been refusing to go to school, and both formed and liquid bowel movements have been discovered in J.S.'s underpants. On several occasions, underwear have been discovered hidden under his bed. Lately, he has appeared more withdrawn. After education, aggressive bowel "clean out," and maintenance with mineral oil, J.S. has reestablished a normal bowel pattern and is regaining his previous personality.

This case illustrates a child with typical functional constipation and encopresis and highlights the value of aggressive pediatric management.

Case 3. *S.N. is a 5-month-old infant who was in excellent health until 1 week ago when her mother noted that she was not feeding as well as she had previously and had developed a weak suck. In addition, her cry had become quieter. On careful questioning, her mother reported that the infant had her last bowel movement 10 days ago and that this bowel movement was quite small. Although she had recently learned to sit up, during the last 3 days she has been unable to do so. Careful physical examination revealed a hypotonic and weak child with a poor gag and decreased pupillary reflex to light. A diagnosis of infantile botulism is suspected and confirmed by stool studies upon admission to the intensive care unit for ventilatory support.*

This case points out the occasional acquired nature of constipation and alerts the pediatrician to this unusual but important diagnosis. Of note, dietary review did not reveal exposure to any of the known causes of botulism (i.e., honey or Karo syrup).

ANNOTATED BIBLIOGRAPHY

Altschuler S: Constipation. In Schwartz MW, editor: *Pediatric primary care: a problem-oriented approach,* ed 2, Chicago, 1990, Year Book.

A fine review on the subject of encopresis, this article provides insight into basic mechanisms of the problem and also covers an approach to therapy.

Sondheimer JM: Helping the child with chronic constipation, *Contemp Pediatr* 2:12-28, 1985.

A basic diagnostic approach to the constipated child, this article focuses on developing a complete database and achieving a diagnosis. Therapy is also covered in some detail.

Tunnessen WW: *Signs and symptoms in pediatrics,* Philadelphia, 1988, JB Lippincott.

This text provides an excellent list of causes of constipation with brief descriptions of each entity and is organized in a logical, clinically useful fashion.

BIBLIOGRAPHY

Abrahamian FP, Lloyd-Still JD: Chronic constipation in childhood: a longitudinal study of 186 patients, *J Pediatr Gastroenterol Nutr* 3:460-467, 1984.

Francoeur TE: Constipation. In Hoekelman RA, editor: *Primary pediatric care,* St Louis, 1992, Mosby–Year Book.

Green M: *Pediatric diagnosis: interpretation of symptoms and signs in infants, children, and adolescents,* Philadelphia, 1992, WB Saunders.

Issenman RM, Hewson S, Pirhonen D, et al: Are chronic digestive complaints the result of abnormal dietary patterns? *Am J Dis Child* 141:679-682, 1987.

Levine MD: Children with encopresis, *Pediatrics* 56:412-416, 1975.

Levine MD: The school child with encopresis, *Pediatr Rev* 2:285-290, 1981.

Loening-Baucke V: Chronic constipation in children, *Gastroenterology* 105:1557-1564, 1993.

Long SS, Gajewski JL, Brown LW, Gilligan PH: Clinical, laboratory, and environmental features of infant botulism in southeastern Pennsylvania, *Pediatrics* 75:935 941, 1985.

Mercer RD: Constipation, *Pediatr Clin North Am* 14:175-185, 1967.

Murphy MS: Constipation. In Walker WA, Duriel PR, Hamilton JR, et al, editors: *Pediatric gastrointestinal disease,* Philadelphia, 1991, BC Decker.

Nolan T, Oberklaid F: New concepts in the management of encopresis, *Pediatr Rev* 14:447-451, 1993.

Partin JC, Hamill SK, Fischel JE, Partin JS: Painful defecation and fecal soiling in children, *Pediatrics* 89:1007-1009, 1992.

Pettei M, Davidson M: Constipation. In Silverberg M, Daum F: *Textbook of pediatric gastroenterology,* Chicago, 1988, Year Book.

Pilapil VR: A horrifying television commercial that led to constipation, *Pediatrics* 85:592-593, 1990.

Reisner SH, Sivan Y, Nitzan M, Merlob P: Determination of anterior displacement of the anus in newborn infants and children, *Pediatrics* 73:216-217, 1984.

Rosenberg AJ: Constipation. In Wylie R, Hyams JS, editors: *Pediatric gastrointestinal disease: pathophysiology, diagnosis, management,* Philadelphia, 1993, WB Saunders.

Vargas JH, Sachs P, Ament ME: Chronic intestinal pseudo-obstruction syndrome in pediatrics, *J Pediatr Gastroenterol Nutr* 7:323-332, 1988.

Weaver LT: Bowel habit from birth to old age, *J Pediatr Gastroenterol Nutr* 7:637-640, 1988.

Weaver LT, Ewing G, Taylor LC: The bowel habit of milk-fed infants, *J Pediatr Gastroenterol Nutr* 7:568-571, 1988.

Weaver LT, Steiner H: The bowel habit of young children, *Arch Dis Child* 59:649-652, 1984.

18

Chronic Diarrhea

J. CARTON GARTNER, Jr.

Key Points

- Age of onset and dietary history are crucial in the diagnostic approach to chronic diarrhea.

- Early-onset diarrhea (less than 3 months of age) must be treated carefully to prevent chronic protracted diarrhea, which often becomes a primary nutritional disease.

- Chronic nonspecific (toddler's) diarrhea has several dietary relationships, such as excessive carbohydrate or fluid ingestion in the form of juices.

Acute gastroenteritis is one of the most common illnesses in pediatric patients. Less common, but perhaps more difficult to manage, is persistent diarrhea that lasts for weeks or months. Although there is no widely accepted definition of chronic diarrhea, a minimum period of abnormal stools is 2 weeks. Most authors would accept a period of 1 month as truly chronic. The stool pattern may include an increase in volume, fluid, or frequency compared with the patient's previous pattern. Causes may range from serious, congenital abnormalities of villous development to minor abnormalities of gut transport. As a world health problem, persistent diarrhea is now beginning to receive the attention previously focused on acute diarrhea and oral rehydration therapy. The deadly cycle of diarrhea, malnutrition, and chronic diarrhea is well recognized. In this chapter the emphasis is on more common problems that require office diagnosis and management, but the differential diagnosis and discussion include problems that are worldwide in scope.

Pathophysiology

It is useful to review the normal stool pattern in childhood. For the first 4 to 6 months, breast-fed infants' stools are frequent and yellow, with a pH of 5. Many breast-fed infants

have a period of "physiologic constipation," with stools every few days. Formula-fed infants (4 to 6 months of age) have less frequent (1 to 3 per day), firmer, yellow to yellowish-brown stools, with a pH of 7. Infants older than 6 months have firmer stools, usually 2 to 3 per day. After 1 year the stool pattern is similar to that of adults.

A detailed review of normal intestinal absorption can be found in several texts and review articles. However, a brief review here helps the reader understand the later discussion of stool examination. Carbohydrate is composed of sugars and starches. Both salivary and pancreatic amylase split larger molecules into polymers and disaccharides. Glucoamylase is a brush border enzyme that splits polymer linkages. The brush border disaccharidases (sucrase-isomaltase, glucoamylase, and lactase) hydrolyze disaccharides and oligosaccharides, and then transport across the brush border occurs via specific carrier molecules for glucose or galactose and fructose. The majority of dietary fat is triglyceride (glycerol with three molecules of fatty acid, called *neutral fat*). Lipolysis is the first step in fat digestion, using mostly pancreatic lipase. This process yields fatty acids (called *split fat*) and glycerol. The second step is micelle formation, which requires bile acids. Pancreatic bicarbonate enhances lipase activity, and additional pancreatic enzymes aid digestion of cholesterol esters, fat-soluble vitamins, and phospholipids. Micelles allow the products of lipolysis to diffuse across the mucosa into the enterocytes, where significant resynthesis occurs, and then junction with apolipoproteins. The final release form is as chylomicrons, which reach the circulation via the lymphatics and thoracic duct. Bile acids are reabsorbed in the distal ileum, and recirculation then occurs. Protein digestion begins with formation of oligopeptides from larger molecules through the action of pancreatic proteases. These pancreatic enzymes are activated by enterokinase, a brush border enzyme. Peptidases in the brush border then form dipeptides, tripeptides, and amino acids from the oligopeptides. Active transport of amino acids and peptides then takes place across the brush border of enterocytes. Abnormal absorption of carbohydrate may occur as an isolated problem, but mal-

247

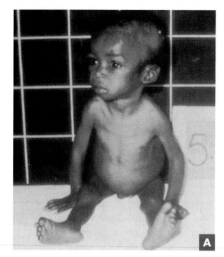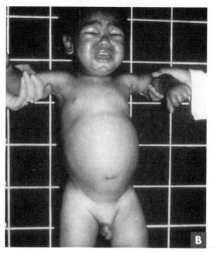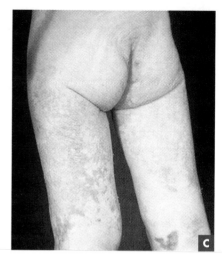

FIG. 18-1 *A,* Marasmus. Note profound wasting and sparse hair, producing a characteristic simian appearance. *B,* Kwashiorkor. This patient has a typical "sugar baby" appearance with generalized edema. Note the periorbital and limb edema. *C,* The rash of kwashiorkor is scaly and erythematous and may weep, especially in edematous areas. This is a typical rash of malnutrition.

absorption of fat and protein is usually part of a more generalized malabsorption.

The intestine also absorbs water and electrolytes. Water generally diffuses across the intestinal lining in response to an osmotic gradient created by sodium-coupled pump(s).

Multiple mechanisms may be responsible for diarrhea, and often several different mechanisms may be present in the same patient. However, it is useful to classify the mechanisms as osmotic, secretory, mucosal damage, and abnormal intestinal motility. Osmotic diarrhea occurs when solutes that cannot be absorbed are present in the gut lumen, resulting in an osmotic gradient. The usual stool osmolality is approximately 280 mOsm ($2 \times [Na^+ + K^+] = 280$ mOsm. In osmotic diarrhea the product of the ion concentrations is less than 280 because the nonabsorbed solute accounts for a portion of the osmolality. A classic example of this mechanism is carbohydrate malabsorption, such as lactose, with the sugar as the osmotic agent. Secretory diarrhea occurs when active sodium-coupled transport is blocked and chloride transport into the lumen is enhanced, usually by cyclic adenosine monophosphate (second messengers), which may be increased by toxins, such as cholera toxin or *Escherichia coli* enterotoxin. Characteristically, secretory diarrhea does not improve rapidly when the patient takes nothing by mouth. Mucosal damage may result in diarrhea caused by loss of surface area (e.g., celiac disease) or diffuse damage to enterocytes from an infectious or inflammatory enteropathy. Motility disturbance is often a secondary phenomenon in the cause of diarrhea, but either decreased motility, which may predispose to bacterial overgrowth, or increased motility (short-bowel syndrome, drugs, infection, etc.) may lead to diarrhea. Multiple mechanisms are often present in patients with chronic diarrhea, and the initiating event, such as rotavirus gastroenteritis, may have little to do with the persistence of loose bowel movements. Some knowledge about mechanisms may be helpful in differential diagnosis and treatment.

Literature Survey

Reviews of chronic diarrhea emphasize mechanisms and differential diagnosis. Discussion of causative factors also occurs in textbooks and review articles dealing with malabsorption in childhood. It may be useful to divide the topic by age of onset. The term *chronic protracted diarrhea* is reserved for those infants who have onset of symptoms early, generally before 3 months of age. In this group the illness is potentially life-threatening, and the diagnostic possibilities include familial villous atrophy and more treatable conditions, such as milk-protein allergy. Secondary malnutrition is a major factor in this group of disorders, and attention to nutrition is mandatory. Some authors indicate that the onset of symptoms before 1 year of age changes the diagnostic possibilities. Another categorization emphasizes normal growth, which is generally associated with common and more treatable conditions, and failure to thrive, which is often seen with serious and uncommon conditions (Fig. 18-1). Blood in the stool is a clue to certain diagnoses, and it helps exclude more benign conditions, such as nonspecific diarrhea or toddler's diarrhea. Other stool patterns, such as watery versus fatty stools, are used by several authors in an attempt to aid differential diagnosis. There are no prospective studies of chronic diarrhea, but three reviews offer excellent differential diagnosis and approaches based on various categorizations as discussed previously.

The other large and rapidly expanding subject of literature on diarrhea is the topic of chronic nonspecific diarrhea. This is the most prevalent condition in older infants and preschool-age children, and controllable dietary factors may play a major role in its pathogenesis.

TABLE 18-1

Differential Diagnosis of Chronic Diarrhea

Cause	Age of presentation	Cause	Age of presentation
Allergic		**Endocrine**	
Milk	2, 3	Adrenal insufficency	2
Soy	2, 3	Hyperthyroidism	2-4
Eosinophilic gastroenteritis	2, 3	Hypoparathyroidism	2
Food	3		
		Immunodeficiency	
Anatomic/Surgical		Immunoglobulin deficiency	3, 4
Hirschsprung disease	2, 3	HIV/AIDS	2-4
Malrotation/volvulus	2, 3	Severe combined immunodeficiency	2, 3
Short-bowel syndrome	2, 3	Common variable immunodeficiency	3, 4
Blind loop syndrome/	2, 3		
bacterial overgrowth		**Inborn Errors**	
Pseudoobstruction	2, 3	Galactosemia	2
		Tyrosinemia	2
Bile/Biliary Tract		Abetalipoproteinemia	2
Cholestasis	2, 3	Wolman disease	2, 3
Bile-acid induced	2, 3		
		Infectious/Postinfectious	
Carbohydrate/Enzymatic		Bacterial	2-4
Lactase/sucrase deficiency	1-4	Viral	2-4
(primary and secondary)		Parasitic	2-4
Monosaccharide intolerance	1-3		
Enterokinase deficiency	2	**Inflammatory**	
		Regional enteritis	4
Congenital/Genetic		Ulcerative colitis	4
Villous atrophy	1		
Chloridorrhea	1	**Pancreatic**	
Acrodermatitis	2	Cystic fibrosis	2-4
Celiac disease	3, 4	Shwachman-Diamond syndrome	2, 3
		Chronic pancreatitis	3-4
Dietary			
Overfeeding	2, 3	**Psychogenic/Functional**	
Carbohydrate overload	3	Encopresis	3-4
Chronic nonspecific	3	Munchausen syndrome by proxy	2, 3
Malnutrition	2, 3	Factitious	4
		Laxative abuse	4
Drug-Related			
Antibiotic induced	2-4	**Tumor**	
C. difficile	2-4	Neuroblastoma/ganglioneuroma	2, 3
Laxatives (see also	2-4	Gastrinoma	2-4
Psychogenic/Functional)		Zollinger-Ellison syndrome	2-4

1, Birth; *2*, 0 to 3 months; *3*, 3 months to preschool; *4*, school-age/adolescence.

Differential Diagnosis

A logical approach to the extensive differential diagnosis of chronic diarrhea is to start with the age of the patient. A helpful categorization is time of onset defined as follows: (1) birth or immediately after first feedings, (2) less than 3 months, (3) 3 months to preschool, and (4) school age to adolescence. Although not precise, this approach highlights the most frequent causes. The next helpful step is to group the disorders into broad categories (which may overlap at times) to be certain that possible diagnoses are not overlooked. Tables 18-1 and 18-2 can be used in conjunction with the text to review diagnostic categories, age of onset, and clues to the diagnosis.

TABLE 18-2

Diagnostic Clues in Chronic Diarrhea

Finding	Characteristic
History	
Age of onset	Early onset—congenital/genetic
Onset	Previous normal stool pattern important
Stool	Blood, mucus suggest infection, colitis
Diet	Introduction of new food/formula, changes made and results, caloric intake critical
Growth	Key; poor growth with adequate calories suggests malabsorption, normal growth suggests more benign illness
Family history	Allergy; genetic, metabolic, or inborn error
Secretory	Suggests mucosal damage to small bowel
Osmotic	Enzyme deficiency (especially carbohydrate malabsorption)
Systemic symptoms	Infection, inflammation, tumor, immunodeficiency
Physical Examination	
Poor growth	Younger child—malabsorption; older child—Crohn disease
Hypertension	Tumor
Fever	Infection, inflammation
Jaundice	Cholestasis, inborn error
Rash	Malnutrition, zinc deficiency, allergy
Erythema nodosum	Inflammatory bowel disease
Pyoderma gangrenosa edema	Protein loss, malnutrition
Clubbing	Celiac disease, cystic fibrosis, Crohn disease
Crackles, wheezing	Cystic fibrosis, allergy, immunodeficiency
Abdominal mass	Tumor, fecal impaction
Organomegaly	Inborn error, immunodeficiency, infection, tumor
Abnormal genitalia	Adrenal insufficiency, abuse
Perianal tags	Crohn disease
Rectal impaction	Encopresis
Ataxia, ↓dtr's	Vitamin E deficiency, abetalipoproteinemia
Laboratory Screen	
Stool	Neutral fat—maldigestion; split fat—malabsorption; carbohydrate, leukocytes, good screen for malabsorption

↓ *dtr's,* Diminished deep tendon reflexes.

Onset Before 24 Hours of Age

Several major, serious illnesses cause early onset of diarrhea. Infants with congenital villous atrophy, which is often familial, never have normal stools or even meconium. The cause is believed to be abnormal differentiation of the epithelial cells lining the gut mucosa. The diarrhea is secretory and profuse. These children require parenteral nutrition and may eventually be helped by small bowel transplantation. Congenital chloride diarrhea, in which there is an abnormality of ion transport, also has an immediate onset, and polyhydramnios may be present. Rarer and more recently described is a defect in sodium transport. Diarrhea from congenital lactase deficiency and glucose or galactose malabsorption starts after the first feedings.

Surgical conditions, such as Hirschsprung disease, may present in the first day with symptoms of obstruction rather than diarrhea.

Early Onset, Before 3 Months of Age

Before discussing individual disorders with early onset in the first months of life, the entity termed *chronic protracted,* or *intractable diarrhea* should be mentioned. First described by Avery and others in 1968, this illness has many causes, both medical and surgical. However, in the majority of cases the precise cause cannot be determined. More common causes include postinfectious and allergic disorders. There is a cycle of continued diarrhea and nutritional deficiency. The essential factors in the management of this condition are nutritional support and repletion. Although the mortality was high in the initial series, modern nutritional methods have markedly improved the outlook.

Allergic disorders usually have onset of symptoms after several weeks of exposure to the allergen, most commonly cow's milk or soy protein. This condition is overdiagnosed (crying or colicky babies often undergo a formula change) but important to recognize early. Diarrhea with mucous and blood streaks, fretfulness, and emesis are presenting complaints. Leukocytes may be present in the stools (with a negative culture). Change to a hydrolyzed protein formula is mandatory. Proteins in the maternal diet may be present in breast milk and may trigger an allergic response. Eosinophilic gastroenteritis mimics protein allergy in many ways but often does not respond to elimination of the allergen. Frank colitis with eosinophilic infiltration may be present, and therapy with corticosteroids or other immunomodulators, such as cromolyn, may be necessary.

Anatomic and surgical conditions should be considered in the young infant. Pediatricians often consider such disorders late, when obstruction, sepsis, and electrolyte abnormalities have made management quite difficult. Hirschsprung disease (see Fig. 17-7) may cause diarrhea before the onset of severe enterocolitis. Short-bowel or blind loop syndromes may complicate neonatal surgery or be late sequelae of necrotizing enterocolitis. Intestinal malrotation with recurrent volvulus may cause emesis and diarrhea. Chronic intestinal pseudoobstruction may have a neonatal onset, with constipation, intestinal stasis, and recurrent diarrhea. Diagnosis of this condition is often quite delayed, allowing years of incorrect treatment. A clue to this condition is its association with urologic obstruction. Intestinal lymphangiectasia is probably best categorized as an "anatomic" disorder because there is obstruction of lymphatic flow and protein loss through the gut. Edema is often a presenting sign.

Disorders of bile and the biliary tract may cause prolonged diarrhea as a result of several different mechanisms. Cholestasis leads to diminished bile flow, abnormal micelle formation, and secondary fat malabsorption. Disorders such as hepatitis and biliary atresia fall into this category. Fat-soluble vitamin deficiencies may be a major problem for patients with these conditions. Bacterial overgrowth (stasis and blind loop syndrome) may lead to deconjugation of bile salts, fat malabsorption, and abnormal bile acids. Bile acids in the large bowel cause watery diarrhea, which may be seen when the terminal ileum is absent (resection) or abnormal and fails to reabsorb bile acids.

Carbohydrate or enzymatic disorders begin in the first few months of life. The most common of these is secondary lactase deficiency, which follows a prolonged enteritis, usually of an infectious cause. Fermentation of unabsorbed lactose in the colon leads to the classic elevation of breath hydrogen in this disorder, which also is associated with watery, acidic, sugar-containing stools. This is the typical osmotic diarrhea. Less common is monosaccharide intolerance. Apart from the immediate congenital disorder, monosaccharide malabsorption often accompanies chronic diarrhea and loss of villous surface area. Constant drip feedings or substitution of glucose polymers may be beneficial. Intestinal enterokinase deficiency is a rare disorder that leads to malabsorption of protein, diarrhea, and hypoproteinemia.

An example of a congenital or genetic condition with early onset is acrodermatitis enteropathica, which results from an inability to absorb zinc. Diarrhea, poor growth, dermatitis in the perioral and perianal areas, and irritability are common. This condition has also been reported in breast-fed infants with inadequate zinc intake (Fig. 18-2).

Dietary causes of chronic diarrhea are unusual at this young age. Overfeeding may occur, and solid foods introduced before pancreatic amylase activity is sufficient may lead to malabsorption. Carbohydrate in juices (including the sugar alcohol sorbitol) may lead to dramatic increases in stool volume. Malnutrition itself leads to villous atrophy and pancreatic dysfunction, a vicious cycle that produces chronic diarrhea and secondary nutrient deficiencies and is a true global problem.

Drug-induced diarrhea is most commonly related to the use of antibiotics. There are several mechanisms, including alteration in normal flora, direct competition for absorption, and overgrowth of *Clostridium difficile*, which produces a toxin associated with pseudomembranous colitis. It has been known for years that stools of normal infants contain this organism, although the colonization rate drops sharply after 1 year of age. The toxin is less frequently present but may be found in the stools of asymptomatic infants. Nonetheless, colitis occurs, and there is some evidence that chronic, relapsing diarrhea may be caused by *C. difficile*.

Endocrine disorders usually have other, more prominent associations than diarrhea. However, congenital adrenal hyperplasia (and adrenal insufficiency later in childhood) has prominent enteric symptoms—emesis and diarrhea. Usually, abnormalities of the genitalia and fluid or electrolyte disturbance are the presenting symptoms. Neonatal hyperthyroidism and occasionally hypoparathyroidism may be associated with the passage of frequent, watery stools.

Immunodeficiency diseases may cause diarrhea and failure to thrive. The most frequent disease in this category at this time is acquired immunodeficiency syndrome (AIDS), which may be accompanied by a multitude of signs and symptoms, including infections with multiple organisms, skin rashes, adenopathy, and hematologic abnormalities. Severe combined immunodeficiency syndrome may have a somewhat similar presentation, and agammaglobulinemia may be accompanied by chronic enteric infection and diarrhea. IgA deficiency is usually associated with recurrent respiratory tract infections, but diarrhea may be present as well.

Inborn errors of metabolism rarely cause only diarrhea, but it may be a dominant clinical feature. Abetalipoproteinemia, a disorder of fat transport, causes early onset of loose, fatty stools and failure to thrive. The late, untreated course is characterized by visual and neurologic symptoms resulting from nutrient deficiency, largely vitamin E related. Similarly, Wolman disease (acid esterase deficiency) has a clinical onset with diarrhea. Later, characteristic hepatosplenomegaly and adrenal calcification develop. Both galactosemia and tyrosinemia, disorders that may now be diagnosed by many neonatal screening programs, cause gastrointestinal symptoms. Sepsis from *E. coli* is also seen in galactosemia, possibly secondary to decreased leukocyte function.

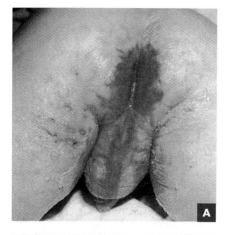
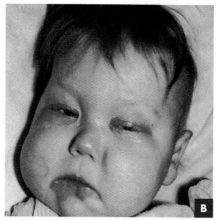
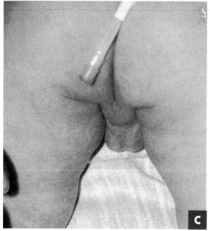
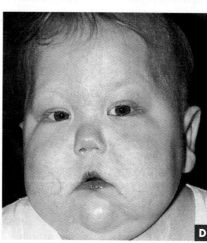

FIG. 18-2 Biotin deficiency (mimicking zinc deficiency). *A* and *B,* This child on chronic hyperalimentation developed dermatitis in perianal, perioral, and lid areas along with some thinning of hair. *C* and *D,* The rash has cleared dramatically after 4 days of biotin. Findings are similar to those of zinc deficiency.

Infectious and postinfectious causes of diarrhea are frequent at all ages. Viral causes, of which rotavirus, Norwalk virus, adenovirus, and other enteroviruses are the best examples, are most common. The illness is often brief, with rapid recovery unless there is underlying malnutrition or severe villous injury. These complicating factors may lead to generalized malabsorption or specific dietary intolerances, such as lactose. Bacterial agents cause enteritis in several different ways, including direct invasion, toxin production, and adherence to epithelial cells. Fever, crampy abdominal pain, and blood and mucus in the stool are common symptoms of bacterial infection (*Salmonella* or *Shigella* organisms, *Campylobacter jejuni, Yersinia enterocolitica, C. difficile,* or *Plesiomonas shigelloides*). The dominant features of *Yersinia* species infection may be fever, pain, low albumin level, and more chronic symptoms. Each of the bacterial agents may lead to a more prolonged course. Parasitic infection may resemble bacterial dysentery (as in *Entamoeba histolytica* infection) or be dominated by loose, watery stools similar to those in viral enteritis (as in infection with *Giardia lamblia* or *Cryptosporidium* organisms). Routine stool analysis may be insufficient, especially when *Giardia* species is suspected, and duodenal intubation may be necessary.

Noninfectious inflammatory causes in infants less than 3 months of age are unusual. Ulcerative colitis in this period is usually related to protein allergy.

Pancreatic disorders may cause early onset of abnormal stools; the most common is cystic fibrosis, with accompanying respiratory symptoms and failure to thrive. The Shwachman-Diamond syndrome includes neutropenia and chronic pancreatic insufficiency. The clinical course may be dominated by infectious illness. Other causes of chronic pancreatitis, such as those related to anatomic abnormalities, present later in childhood.

Psychogenic causes of diarrhea in early infancy are related to child abuse or Munchausen syndrome by proxy. The loose stools may be factitious or real, caused by laxatives administered by the caretaker. The latter children are in danger, and the possibility of abuse must be openly discussed by the physician.

Tumors in childhood may produce diarrhea by secretion of substances such as vasoactive intestinal polypeptide. Frequently accompanying the watery diarrhea are hypokalemia and achlorhydria, hence the acronym WDHA. The substance may be secreted by several tumors, including neuroblastoma, ganglioneuroma, and pheochromocytoma. In addition, both the Zollinger-Ellison syndrome and medullary carcinoma of the thyroid may be associated with hormone-induced diarrhea.

Onset 3 Months to Preschool Age

The cause of chronic diarrhea in this age group may include many of the disorders discussed previously, but a number of disorders that start later in infancy or in the preschool years are also possibilities. These additional diagnostic entities are highlighted here.

Allergic disorders in this group begin to include true food allergies beyond milk and soy protein. The introduction of new foods may be associated with true anaphylaxis and systemic symptoms or a more subtle increase in stools. Blinded food challenge is the best diagnostic test to clarify the role of foods in the child with chronic diarrhea. Several long-term studies demonstrate that many food reactions cannot be confirmed by blinded or even open challenge testing and that true anaphylaxis is rare. Food reactions blamed on allergy may represent intolerance, as in the case of fruit or fruit juices. Elimination diets without knowledge of specific allergens may lead to poor nutrition and failure to thrive or may even mask the diagnosis of celiac disease.

Anatomic or surgical disorders, especially blind loop syndrome after previous surgery, may present later in infancy. Rarely, Hirschsprung disease comes to medical attention because of symptoms of mild enterocolitis, chronic diarrhea, and failure to thrive.

Secondary carbohydrate intolerance, most commonly lactase deficiency, may occur after infectious diarrhea at any age. Primary, genetic lactose intolerance may have its onset between 5 and 6 years of age.

In the category of genetic disorders, the major diagnosis in late infancy and preschool ages is celiac disease. Gradual onset of loose, malodorous stools and failure to gain weight are common symptoms. Occasionally, anorexia and emesis are prominent. The older child may have only short stature. Typical histologic alterations of the small bowel mucosa and a dramatic clinical and histologic response to the elimination of gluten are characteristic. Because of the late risk of malignancy, it is important to make an accurate and lifelong diagnosis of celiac disease (Fig. 18-3).

Perhaps the most common and vexing cause of loose stools in the preschooler is chronic, nonspecific diarrhea, or toddler's diarrhea, a disorder that fits best in the category of dietary causes. Most frequently this entity begins late in the first year of life after an episode of gastroenteritis. Several large, liquid stools per day are passed, and there may be some undigested food in the stool. If allowed to take a regular diet, these children gain weight normally. Detailed evaluation, including culture, stool analysis, and malabsorption studies, is normal. Several factors have been implicated, including excessive fluid and carbohydrate intake (fruit juices), decreased fat consumption (fat slows intestinal motility), increased intestinal motility, and elevated prostaglandins. It is

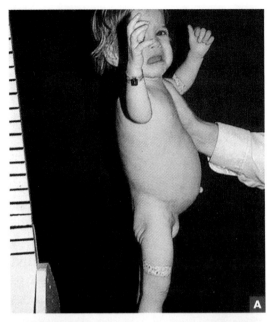

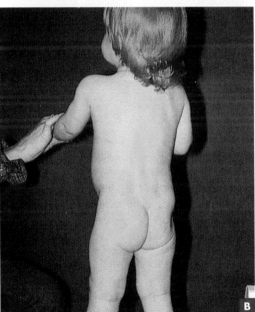

FIG. 18-3 Celiac disease. *A,* This child had a potbelly, vomiting, and weight loss as her major symptoms and was originally thought to have psychosocial failure to thrive. When celiac disease was suspected, the child was placed on a gluten-free diet. Note the protruding abdomen and wasted buttocks. *B,* After 10 weeks on the diet the improvement is obvious.

essential to keep these patients on a regular diet as much as possible and follow growth.

Drug-induced diarrhea in this age group must include the possible administration of laxatives by a caretaker as a form of child abuse (Munchausen syndrome by proxy). Closer scrutiny of the situation often yields other clues to the diagnosis.

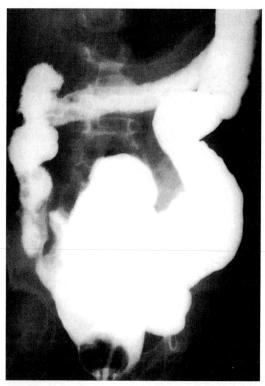

FIG. 18-4 X-ray findings in ulcerative colitis. There is narrowing and loss of haustral markings, especially in the transverse colon. Mucosal irregularities are prominent in the right colon.

Immunodeficiency may present in late infancy or preschool-age patients. Acquired immunodeficiency through perinatal transmission may cause enteric symptoms and growth failure. Patients with immunoglobulin or common variable immunodeficiency may develop chronic diarrhea from infectious causes, such as *Giardia* organisms.

Pancreatic disorders, of which cystic fibrosis is the major category, may present late in infancy. The physician should consider more unusual presentations, such as protein-losing enteropathy with edema (usually seen in infants on soy or breast milk), recurrent wheezing (with digital clubbing), and fat-soluble vitamin deficiency.

A common psychogenic or functional cause of loose stools in this age group is overflow around impacted stool in a chronically constipated child. Encopresis should be evident when the history suggests stool withholding as the primary problem.

Onset in Later Childhood and Adolescence

Most of the disorders that cause chronic diarrhea have been discussed. Many of them can occur in the older child and represent the most common causes (infectious or postinfectious, dietary, etc.). Several categories are unique, however.

Inflammatory bowel disease, which generally includes regional enteritis (Crohn disease) and ulcerative colitis, generally has its earliest onset in the school-age child. Rectal symptoms, such as diarrhea with mucus and blood, tenes-

mus, and urgency, are more prominent in ulcerative colitis. Crohn disease often has a more indolent presentation, with fever, weight loss, diarrhea, and poor growth. Perianal disease and fistulas are common. Extraintestinal manifestations are common in both disorders. Radiographic studies, endoscopy, and biopsy may be necessary to make the diagnosis (Fig. 18-4, see Fig. 1-1 and 1-2).

Under the category of psychogenic or functional causes, factitious diarrhea should be considered, especially in the adolescent patient. Use of laxatives, especially in those with eating disorders, is characteristic. Patients seeking medical attention may even add water to their own stools, causing an extremely low osmolality when compared with material aspirated during endoscopy.

Differential diagnosis, age of onset, and diagnostic clues are presented in Tables 18-1 and 18-2.

History

The obvious first step in evaluating a child with persistently abnormal stools is a thorough history. Major clues and the necessity for a detailed diagnostic evaluation may be determined from the history and later examination of the patient. Of first concern is the age of onset. From the previous section on differential diagnosis it is evident that a number of disorders may present at any age, whereas several have an early onset and several a late onset. The timing and description of the last normal stools are important. In confusing situations it is useful to explore the pattern of stooling from birth so that it can be determined if and when an abnormal pattern began.

Dietary manipulations and their effect on the stooling pattern are important. In infants, what formula changes were made? What effect did the elimination of certain dietary constituents have? Another important aspect, especially in infants, is the effect of a period without oral intake. Patients with osmotic diarrhea (e.g., carbohydrate malabsorption) usually improve when they do not eat. Secretory diarrhea continues unabated. The relationship of stool production to eating is important. The details of the diet are also important to assess the child's growth and weight gain. A key decision is whether there has been sufficient caloric intake for growth. Unfortunately, often the child's failure to thrive is iatrogenic, resulting from dietary manipulations. In other situations there may be excellent caloric intake without growth, which is strongly suggestive of malabsorption. Careful calculation of intake or use of a 3-day dietary record may prove extremely useful.

Although descriptions of the stool are often inaccurate, they may offer clues to the diagnosis. Parents are quite clear when frank blood is present, as in severe allergic, infectious, or inflammatory conditions. It is more difficult to decide about fatty (malodorous, less dense) or watery stools. Some authorities feel there is a useful distinction between small and large bowel diarrhea. Small bowel stools are more voluminous and watery, whereas large bowel stools are usually smaller and more likely to be accompanied by blood or mucus and increased frequency, urgency, and tenesmus.

Exposures and travel history should be evaluated next. Al-

to ill contacts and possible sources of infection are critical.

The presence of systemic symptoms, such as fever, weight loss, rashes, and joint complaints is important. Major infectious, immunodeficiency, and inflammatory conditions may be accompanied by such symptoms.

Family history is also important. Siblings or other family members may have similar problems, such as milk intolerance. Certain illnesses, such as celiac disease, have a racial or ethnic predisposition. Social history, which is often neglected, may be critical in determining the seriousness of the illness or assessing the possible role of caretakers in producing or exaggerating symptoms. Useful information about water supply, preparation of meals, general sanitation, and pet or animal exposures may be obtained.

The examiner should finish the history with a solid database that includes at least age of onset, frequency, pattern, type of stool, dietary manipulations and caloric content, growth and weight gain, exposures, systemic symptoms, and family and social situations. Most diagnoses are made based on the history, with confirmation by examination and laboratory findings.

Physical Examination

A thorough examination of the patient begins with close observation of general nutrition and growth. Review of past growth points and plotting on a standard are mandatory. If there is a fall-off, the timing is critical. Did it occur early as part of the disease process or only later when the infant or child was placed on a restricted diet? Was it related to the introduction of new foods into the diet? In some conditions, such as celiac disease or Crohn disease, deceleration in growth velocity may occur without obvious change in the stool pattern initially. Careful recording of vital signs may be helpful. Elevated blood pressure may suggest a hormone-secreting tumor, such as a neuroblastoma. Tachycardia and low blood pressure may indicate dehydration. Fever suggests infection, immunodeficiency, or inflammatory bowel disease.

The general appearance is important. A healthy, well-nourished infant or child usually indicates that the diarrhea is not a symptom of generalized malabsorption. The potbelly and wasted buttocks of malnutrition are much more worrisome. The examiner should search carefully for edema in dependent areas; this finding strongly suggests severe malnutrition or loss of protein in the diarrheal fluid from a number of possible disorders, malabsorptive and inflammatory. Occasionally, edema may initially mask underlying marasmus by giving the patient a "well-fed" appearance (Fig. 18-1).

Pallor is important because anemia may be part of a generalized process involving the bowel or suggestive of blood

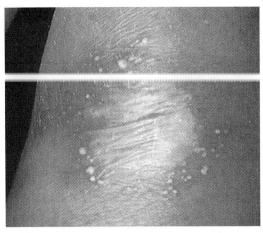

FIG. 18-5 Pyoderma gangrenosum associated with inflammatory bowel disease. Initial papulopustules coalesce to form a deep necrotic lesion.

loss in the stools. Jaundice may be seen in infants with galactosemia, tyrosinemia, or cholestatic disorders or in occasional older children with inflammatory bowel disease. Skin and hair changes should be noted. Rashes may be caused by malnutrition or may suggest specific nutritional deficiencies, such as zinc (Fig. 18-2). Erythema nodosum, pyoderma gangrenosum, and maculopapular rashes may be seen with inflammatory bowel disease (Fig. 18-5). Eczema in an infant suggests an allergic cause of the diarrhea. Clubbing of the digits (see Fig. 1-3) may be a clue to underlying gut disease (celiac or inflammatory bowel disease) or suggest chronic hypoxia (cystic fibrosis). Ocular (Bitot spots with vitamin A deficiency) and oral changes (aphthous ulcerations with Crohn disease) should be sought. Adenopathy should be assessed; is it normal or suggestive of chronic infection? Chest examination should include determination of shape and a search for adventitious findings (crackles or wheezing) suggestive of infection or atopic disease. The abdominal examination is critical and should be done carefully and repeated, if necessary, when the child is quieter or even sleeping so that subtle findings may be appreciated. Degree of distension, tympany, bowel sounds, tenderness, masses, visible or palpable bowel loops, and stool retention should be assessed. Organomegaly, which suggests a chronic infectious or even malignant process, should be evaluated. Genital examination should not be neglected; hyperpigmentation suggestive of adrenal insufficiency or signs of child abuse (infants) or sexual activity (older children) may be found. The perianal area should be inspected closely. Skin tags and fistulas suggest Crohn disease in the older child. Rectal prolapse is characteristic of cystic fibrosis. Rectal examination should be considered in most cases because the type of residual stool may be directly observed and a specimen obtained. Occasionally the examiner finds a palpable mass. Joint examination may reveal evidence of chronic inflammation associated with inflammatory bowel disease. In older children, flexibility of the spine should be assessed. Neurologic examination should include a search for ataxia, diminished deep tendon reflexes, and proprioception seen with vitamin E deficiency (cholestasis, fat malabsorption, and abetalipoproteinemia).

At the conclusion of the examination, an overall impression of nutrition and general health should be made. A normal examination favors a period of watchful waiting and reassessment. Abnormalities suggest specific diagnostic possibilities or at least indicate that the causes of malnutrition must be carefully sought during further investigation.

Office Laboratory

Macroscopic and limited microscopic examination of the stool should be part of the routine evaluation of patients with chronic diarrhea. More sophisticated testing can be referred to the hospital laboratory. Examination of a typical stool is important. A fresh sample is necessary for certain simple tests, such as carbohydrate content, but a sample brought in by parents can be of value. A single stool per day, although not usually described as diarrhea, may be sufficient to indicate malabsorption, as in celiac disease. Frequent small, liquid stools may suggest starvation or even nonspecific diarrhea. The consistency, color, bulk, odor, and greasiness should be compared with the examiner's knowledge of normal-appearing stools. Vegetable fibers are often found in normal stools because of poor chewing and are not a good clue to malabsorption (which can be discovered only through frequent observation). Testing for occult blood is easy and should be done even when the stools appear to have gross blood. Other foods may impart a red color (Jell-O, beets, etc.). Fresh liquid stool, either obtained directly or aspirated from the rectum with a syringe and small feeding tube, should be tested for carbohydrate by mixing 2 drops of stool with 10 drops of water and adding a Clinitest tablet. Sucrose malabsorption may be detected only by acidifying and boiling the liquid stool before using the tablet.

It is even more important to test the stool for fat—neutral fat (triglyceride) or split fat (fatty acids, after action of pancreatic lipase). Infants may excrete 10% to 15% of dietary fat, but after 1 year of age the figure is about 5%. Triglyceride suggests pancreatic insufficiency. Examination of a stool smear under a coverslip after 2 drops of water are added is abnormal if it reveals more than 6 to 8 globules/hpf ($\times$40). Split fat is a bit more difficult to see in a water preparation because it appears as thin crystals, or it is invisible because it is in the form of solid "soap." To enhance the ability to see split fat, 2 drops of acetic acid (36%) may be added to the stool smear, which is then boiled using a match or lighter. This allows the fatty acids to be released from soaps and assume a nonionized form as globules. Once again, more than 6 to 10 globules/hpf ($\times$40) is abnormal. Fat stains, such as Sudan III or Oil Red O, enhance the fat globules, but a water preparation is often sufficient.

If available, a stool smear with 2 drops of water and 1 drop of methylene blue is a useful test for leukocytes. Fresh stool can be sent to the laboratory if this test is unavailable in the office. More than 2 to 4 white blood cells/hpf is considered abnormal.

Approach to the Patient

At this point the history, physical examination, and simple stool examination have been completed, and a decision about further evaluation may be made. The differential diagnosis should be approached in a logical fashion by asking several key questions. What was the age of the patient at the onset of symptoms? This information significantly narrows the possible causes. It is critical that the physician act quickly when treating the youngest infants because chronic protracted diarrhea starts before 3 months of age and may occur after multiple initial insults to the gut mucosa, such as infection, milk-protein allergy, and malnutrition. A trial of an elemental formula before embarking on an extensive investigative process may be the most important therapy. What is the effect of the illness on general health, growth, and weight gain? A very large number of infants and children thrive despite loose stools, which makes detailed, often expensive investigation unnecessary. Caloric intake must be assessed; if it is normal, reassurance is important. If, on the other hand, increased caloric intake is documented along with borderline growth, malabsorption may be present. Decreased caloric intake must be prevented, especially in infants, because secondary malnutrition itself causes gut mucosal and pancreatic atrophy, leading to worsening of diarrhea. Malabsorption generally is confirmed by finding excessive fat in the stools because disturbances in fat digestion and absorption are prominent in most disorders that involve generalized malabsorption.

In the majority of older infants and preschool-age children the initial assessment confirms that there is no major problem with gut function and that the diarrhea truly represents "looser than normal stools" or even parental misperception of stool quantity. Time spent in discussion about normal growth and nutrition is important in this situation and further investigation is unnecessary. A similar statement may be made about the older child who is growing well and has no signs of inflammatory bowel disease or an eating disorder. A detailed dietary history in these healthy children often uncovers a source of loose stools, such as excessive fruit juice consumption, sorbitol in gum, excessive water intake, or even a deficiency of fat content. Appropriate advice may be rewarded with a distinct change in the stool character.

Screening tests should be considered for children who have suspicious histories or physical examination findings. Such children may have a slight fall-off in growth, poor appetite, or slightly increased fat in the stool. Several studies are appropriate for this group, including electrolytes, blood urea nitrogen, total carbon dioxide (screen for stool losses and acidosis), stool culture, stool screen for ova and parasites, complete blood count (CBC), sedimentation rate (especially as a screen for inflammatory bowel disease), serum total protein and albumin levels (screen for nutrition and protein loss), and occasionally a sweat chloride test. Normal results on these screens allow for a period of observation and re-assessment.

Children, especially infants, who have chronic symptoms and failure to thrive should undergo thorough investigation, starting with further testing for malabsorption, such as D-xylose absorption, breath hydrogen, pancreatic function tests, 72-hour fecal fat, and perhaps endoscopy and biopsy, especially of the small bowel. In older infants, antibodies against gluten components (IgG and IgA antigliadin and more specifically antiendomysial antibody) may be very helpful in the diagnosis of celiac disease. A specific cause should be determined in these most severe cases by following a logical progression.

SUMMARY

Careful history and physical examination, followed by office stool examination, and on occasion a few screening tests should lead to an organized and useful approach to the patient with chronic diarrhea. Classification by time of onset, seriousness of associated nutritional problems, and systemic symptoms should allow investigation of only those children who are more likely to have true underlying disease and/or malabsorption.

ILLUSTRATIVE CASES

Case 1. A 5-week-old, breast-fed infant was thriving with a normal pattern of 4 to 5 stools per day until 4 days before an office visit. She became fussier, and stools increased in frequency to 8 per day with some mucus and frank blood. She remained afebrile and continued to nurse well without emesis. There were no known exposures. Both parents are well. Family history is remarkable for milk allergy in the mother as an infant.

On examination the infant appears well, with good weight gain and normal vital signs. General physical examination is unremarkable. Fresh stool demonstrates streaks of blood (confirmed by testing) and mucus. Microscopic examination reveals increased leukocytes and mucus without fat globules.

Stool is sent for culture. While awaiting the results, the examining physician considers possible diagnoses. The diarrhea appears to have a large bowel origin with mucus and blood. There are no exposures. Further family history reveals that the mother breast-fed for multiple reasons, one of which was her family's milk intolerance, which included symptoms of eczema and "colic." She now tolerates milk and dairy products, which she has taken daily. The examiner elects to remove these from the mother's diet. The baby steadily improves. Stool culture is normal.

This case illustrates typical milk-induced colitis. Certain dietary proteins pass through breast milk. Occasional cases of colic may have a similar cause.

Case 2. At 12 months of age a boy developed diarrhea, with an increase in stool frequency to 4 times per day, from a previous number of 1 to 2 times per day. Stools were brown and watery, and undigested fibers were present. Appetite remained good, although decreased from several months ago. He had been on regular formula until 10 months of age and initially tolerated cow's milk. He underwent several dietary changes, initially restricting milk and then wheat, which resulted in a slight reduction in stool volume. Studies performed by his family doctor (stool culture, stool screen for ova and parasites, CBC, electrolytes, carbon dioxide, and serum albumin level) were normal.

At 14 months of age the child still has loose stools. Parents have additionally restricted fat because a grandfather has coronary artery disease. On examination the child appears well. Growth parameters show a slight fall-off for weight from the 50th to the 25th percentile over 3 months; length and head circumference are in the 50th percentile. Examination is normal. Fresh stool is brown and slightly watery, with undigested vegetable fibers. Fat stain is normal.

This child is well; however, calculation of caloric intake is suboptimal at about 70 kcal/kg/day. On further questioning the parents admit that the exclusion of milk has been difficult and that the child (previously weaned from the bottle) has been taking juices from a bottle again and prefers juice to the soy-based formula substituted by the family doctor.

The first approach to this healthy-appearing child is to increase caloric intake and reinstitute a regular diet for a period of time. Fat intake should be normal, and fruit juices should be decreased and then eliminated. Two months later the boy still has slightly loose stools but has gained weight back to the 50th percentile.

This is a very typical history of chronic nonspecific diarrhea. Motility may play a role, but excessive fluid and fruit juices and diminished fat in the diet can be changed. Most toddlers improve over months to several years.

Case 3. At 5 months of age an infant girl began to vomit frequently and have occasional loose stools. The mother eventually stopped breast-feeding and switched to regular formula and a regular infant diet. The child's weight dropped from the 50th to the 5th percentile over the next 5 months, with a decrease in height from the 50th to the 25th percentile. She had an extremely poor appetite, and the mother became increasingly frustrated with mealtime. She is admitted (at age 10 months) in an attempt to control her diet and work with the family in a different environment. The emesis is now infrequent and stools occur once a day and are formed.

Additional history reveals that there is a handicapped sister who has seizures that are aggravated by this infant's noisy behavior. There are social and some financial stresses.

Examination reveals a slightly wasted, irritable child who clings to her mother. During a structured hospitalization the child begins to feed slightly better and gains 120 g. Routine laboratory tests (CBC, electrolytes, carbon dioxide, serum albumin levels, stool culture, stool screens for ova and parasites, and sweat test) are normal or negative. She is followed as an outpatient with close calorie counts. She now consumes 125 to 150 kcal/kg/day but gains no weight as an outpatient. She is readmitted for failure to thrive.

On first review this case could be considered psychosocial, which was the initial diagnosis. However, the early growth failure and poor weight gain as an outpatient despite recorded adequate caloric intake are disturbing. Several important basic steps were neglected. The stool was not checked for fat because of the infrequent stools. When stained later, fat globules were greatly increased. D-Xylose testing showed minimal absorption, and small bowel biopsy confirmed celiac disease. Although unavailable at the time of this child's presentation, antigliadin and antiendomysial antibody titers would likely have been quite elevated. Response to gluten elimination was dramatic. Remember that symptoms began at about the time solids (cereals) were introduced into the diet.

ANNOTATED BIBLIOGRAPHY

Baldassano RN, Liacouras CA: Chronic diarrhea: a practical approach for the pediatrician, *Pediatr Clin North Am* 38:667-686, 1991.

This is an excellent overview with a discussion of mechanisms, most common and least common disorders, and a useful algorithm for planning investigation.

Rossi TM, Albini CH, Kumar V: Incidence of celiac disease identified by the presence of serum endomysial antibodies in children with chronic diarrhea, short stature, or insulin-dependent diabetes mellitus, *J Pediatr* 123:262-264, 1993.

This is one of a number of papers defining the usefulness of newer antibody techniques in the diagnosis of celiac disease. The incidence will likely rise with newer screening techniques, especially in patients with atypical presentations (i.e., short stature, late-onset diarrhea).

Sondheimer JM: Office stool examination: a practical guide, *Contemp Pediatr* 7:63-82, 1990.

This article provides a useful description of techniques (along with photomicrographs) to define abnormal and normal findings in stools. Accurate use of these screening techniques will help to guide further investigation of chronic diarrhea.

BIBLIOGRAPHY

Avery GB, Villavicencio O, Lilly JR, et al: Intractable diarrhea in early infancy, *Pediatrics* 41:712-722, 1968.

Berezin S, Schwarz SM, Glassman M, et al: Gastrointestinal milk intolerance of infancy, *Am J Dis Child* 143:361-362, 1989.

Bock SA: Prospective appraisal of complaints of adverse reactions to foods in children during the first 3 years of life, *Pediatrics* 79:683-688, 1987.

Boyne LJ, Kerzner B, McClung HJ: Chronic nonspecific diarrhea: the value of a preliminary observation period to assess diet therapy, *Pediatrics* 76:557-561, 1985.

Colin AA, Wohl ME: Cystic fibrosis, *Pediatr Rev* 15:192-200, 1994.

Davidson GP, Cutz E, Hamilton JR, et al: Familial enteropathy: a syndrome of protracted diarrhea from birth, failure to thrive, and hypoplastic villus atrophy, *Gastroenterology* 75:783-790, 1978.

Fekety R, Shah AB: Diagnosis and treatment of *Clostridium difficile* colitis, *JAMA* 269:71-75, 1993.

Fitzgerald JF, Clark JH: Chronic diarrhea, *Pediatr Clin North Am* 29:221-231, 1982.

Gryboski J: The child with chronic diarrhea, *Contemp Pediatr* 10:71-97, 1993.

Hutt PJ, Tunnessen WW: Very important passages, *Contemp Pediatr* 11:97-99, 1994.

Hyams JS, Etienne NL, Leichtner AM, et al: Carbohydrate malabsorption following fruit juice ingestion in young children, *Pediatrics* 82:64-68, 1988.

Lifshitz F, Coello-Ramirez P, Gutierrez-Topete G, et al: Monosaccharide intolerance and hypoglycemia in infants with diarrhea. I. Clinical course of 23 infants, *J Pediatr* 70:595-603, 1970.

Lloyd-Still JD: Chronic diarrhea of childhood and the misuse of elimination diets, *J Pediatr* 95:10-13, 1979.

Lo CW, Walker WA: Chronic protracted diarrhea of infancy: a nutritional disease, *Pediatrics* 72:786-800, 1983.

O'Gorman M, Lake AM: Chronic inflammatory bowel disease in childhood, *Pediatr Rev* 14:475-480, 1993.

Schmitz J: Malabsorption. In Walker WA, Durie PR, Hamilton JR, et al, editors: *Pediatric gastrointestinal disease: pathophysiology, diagnosis, and management*, Philadelphia, 1991, BC Decker.

Whitington PF, Whitington GL: Eosinophilic gastroenteropathy in childhood, *J Pediatr Gastroenterol Nutr* 7:379-385, 1988.

19

Jaundice

MIRIAM D. BLOOM

Key Points

- The cause of jaundice is best considered within two broad categories—conjugated and unconjugated hyperbilirubinemia—and then by age group—the neonate and the older child.

- Unconjugated jaundice generally is the result of the liver's inability to handle a bilirubin load (excess production or enzymatic deficiency). Conjugated jaundice often denotes hepatocellular injury or underlying abnormal hepatic and/or biliary structures.

- The management of jaundice is evolving. Significant developments include altered thresholds of intervention in the healthy full-term infant, new techniques to identify and manage metabolic disorders, advances in therapy for the complications of chronic jaundice, and improved surgical interventions for obstructive jaundice.

When jaundice appears in the newborn period, the challenge to the pediatrician is to determine if a child requires further investigation. When jaundice appears in the older child, the question is not whether to investigate but rather how best to tailor the investigative process. As with other chronic problems in pediatrics, the keys to unlocking the diagnosis are a thorough history and physical examination combined with a basic understanding of the pathophysiology. The subject of jaundice is best considered within two broad categories—conjugated and unconjugated hyperbilirubinemia—and then by age group—the neonate and the older child.

Pathophysiology

Jaundice in the newborn period results from an imbalance between the production of bilirubin and its mechanisms of excretion. The increased load of bilirubin to the system is explained by several additive factors, such as the shortened half-life of fetal red blood cells, polycythemia, increased enterohepatic circulation of bilirubin, extravascular blood, and hemolysis. Hemolysis may be exaggerated to varying degrees by fetal-maternal blood group incompatibility (ABO and Rh) and erythrocyte disorders (spherocytosis, glucose-6-phosphate dehydrogenase, and the hemoglobinopathies). The metabolic route that takes heme to bilirubin is detailed fairly well. The pathways that enable bilirubin to be transported, accepted into the liver, conjugated, and excreted into the biliary tract are not as well understood. Many of the diseases that result in jaundice can be related to specific errors in the process of excretion. For example, specific enzymatic defects or deficiencies are associated respectively with Crigler-Najjar syndrome and physiologic jaundice of the newborn.

Bilirubin production begins with the conversion of heme by heme oxygenase and then biliverdin reductase to create bilirubin. Unconjugated bilirubin is transported to the liver by albumin on three binding sites, although bilirubin is usually bound tightly to one primary, high-affinity site. The availability of binding sites is important clinically because many compounds can compete with bilirubin for these sites, for example, sulfonamides, salicylates, and fatty acids. Changes in the cellular milieu caused by hypoglycemia, hypoxia, and acidosis can also decrease binding by albumin. This results in diminished transfer of bilirubin to the liver for excretion and increased free lipid-soluble bilirubin in the serum, which may cause neurotoxicity. Kernicterus is the pathologic state characterized by unconjugated bilirubin staining and necrosis of neurons in the basal ganglia, hippocampal cortex, and subthalamic nuclei of the brain. Clinically, bilirubin encephalopathy manifests as a wide spectrum of symptoms ranging from reversible changes in brainstem auditory evoked potentials and lethargy to the classic description of kernicterus (lethargy, rigidity, opisthotonos, high-pitched cry, fever, convulsions, and death). True kernicterus is a rare entity in modern neonatal care units. Risk factors for kernicterus, identification of a specific toxic bilirubin threshold, and correlation between serum bilirubin concentrations and neurologic sequelae are still not clearly elucidated.

Once the unconjugated bilirubin is presented to the liver, the subsequent metabolic mechanisms are less clearly understood. A series of cellular transport steps involving membrane kinetics, membrane binding sites, and carrier proteins, such as ligandin, deliver bilirubin to the hepatocyte endoplasmic reticulum. Within the endoplasmic reticulum, the enzyme uridine diphosphate (UDP) glucuronyl transferase conjugates bilirubin to either a monoglucuronide or diglucuronide. The capacity of the enzyme system for diglucuronide formation in vitro appears to be considerably lower than that for monoglucuronide synthesis. This becomes important in explaining the types of bilirubin found in the bile of newborns and patients with certain genetic abnormalities that result in jaundice. Adult human bile may contain 80% to 90% bilirubin diglucuronide, 10% to 20% monoglucuronide, and 1% or less of unconjugated bilirubin. Neonates may have 50% or more bile pigment in the form of monoconjugates. Patients with Gilbert syndrome and Crigler-Najjar type II syndrome also have an increased percentage of monoconjugates. Phenobarbital is known to induce glucuronyl transferase activity, increasing the conjugation of bilirubin.

The mechanisms by which bilirubin conjugates are transferred from the endoplasmic reticulum to the biliary canalicular membrane are not well defined. Secretion of bilirubin into the bile is considered to be the rate-limiting step in the overall process of transporting bilirubin from blood to bile. Errors in this final step are presumed to be primarily responsible for the hyperbilirubinemia associated with hepatocellular disorders. Defects in the hepatic transport of conjugated bilirubin and transferral across the canalicular membrane have been implicated in Dubin-Johnson syndrome and familial intrahepatic cholestasis, or Byler disease. Phenobarbital is a known choleretic, increasing bile flow. Bile acid flow has a direct positive correlation with bilirubin output.

Enterohepatic circulation is another source of increased serum bilirubin concentration in the neonatal period. The newborn is particularly at risk because of a transient absence of intestinal bacteria that break bilirubin into polar nonabsorbable compounds. Instead, gut lumen beta-glucuronidase hydrolyzes conjugated bilirubin to unconjugated bilirubin, which then diffuses across the enterocyte membrane and is transported back into the portal blood flow. The hepatocyte must absorb and reconjugate the bilirubin to be excreted into the bile once more. Any structural pathology that prolongs neonatal intestinal transit time, for example, intestinal obstruction, escalates serum bilirubin levels.

Differential Diagnosis

The numerous disorders of bilirubin metabolism that result in jaundice originate from one or a combination of the key metabolic processes. Generally, hyperbilirubinemia is divided into two broad categories—unconjugated and conjugated.

Common causes of both types of hyperbilirubinemia are seen in the neonate (Box 19-1).

Neonatal Indirect Jaundice

Two nonpathologic causes of hyperbilirubinemia in the neonate are physiologic jaundice and breast milk jaundice (BMJ). Physiologic jaundice is a self-limited clinical state that usually appears on the second or third day of life and resolves in 7 to 10 days in the full-term infant but may last 2 to 3 weeks in the premature infant. About 50% of all neonates have clinically apparent jaundice with unconjugated bilirubin levels that peak on average between 5 to 6 mg/dl. Multiple mechanisms, such as increased production of bilirubin overwhelming the hepatic metabolic pathways, decreased hepatic uptake thought to be related to maturation of hepatic ligandin, decreased activity of glucuronyl transferase, and increased enterohepatic circulation, have been proposed to be responsible for physiologic jaundice in the newborn.

BMJ is another form of physiologic jaundice, occurring in 0.5% to 2% of otherwise healthy breast-fed infants. Serum unconjugated bilirubin levels begin to rise on the fourth day of life, and with continued breast milk feedings, jaundice may persist for 3 to 16 weeks. The cause of BMJ is still debated. Various theories include competitive inhibition of glucuronyl transferase by long-chain fatty acids within the breast milk, a glucuronidase present in the breast milk, increased absorption from the gastrointestinal tract, and altered bile acid metabolism. BMJ must be differentiated from "breast-feeding" jaundice, which causes early increased bilirubin secondary to decreased caloric intake and decreased stool output.

Neonatal jaundice is considered pathologic when jaundice is noted within 36 hours of birth, the total bilirubin level is greater than 12 mg/dl in the full-term or greater than 15 mg/dl in the premature infant, or the direct bilirubin level is greater than 1.5 mg/dl or 20% of the total bilirubin and jaundice persists for more than 8 days. Results of long-term outcome studies of neonatal jaundice have sought to redefine pathologic jaundice in the well-appearing full-term infant. The idea of a broader range of physiologic unconjugated bilirubin levels is generally accepted. The aforementioned guidelines serve as a point at which to begin reevaluating an infant.

The most common causes of pathologic unconjugated hyperbilirubinemia are the more severe cases of bilirubin overproduction described earlier (increased hemolysis from Rh/ABO incompatibility, hemoglobinopathies, erythrocyte membrane defects, extravascular blood collection as with cephalohematoma, polycythemia, and increased enterohepatic uptake). There are also three genetic causes of pathologic unconjugated hyperbilirubinemia, each associated with some degree of decreased hepatic UDP-glucuronyl transferase activity. The syndromes are distinguished on the basis of the plasma bilirubin level, the presence or absence of bilirubin glucuronides in bile, and the response to phenobarbital

BOX 19-1

Differential Diagnosis of Neonatal Jaundice

Nonpathologic Causes
Physiologic
Breast-feeding
Breast milk

Pathologic Causes
Unconjugated hyperbilirubinemia
Bilirubin overproduction
  ABO/Rh incompatibility
  Hemoglobinopathies
  Erythrocyte membrane defects
  Polycythemia
  Extravascular blood
Increased uptake
  Increased enterohepatic uptake
  Intestinal obstruction
Genetic
  Crigler-Najjar types I and II
  Gilbert syndrome
Miscellaneous
  Hypothyroidism
  Sepsis, urinary tract infection
  Hypoxia, acidosis
  Hypoglycemia
  Maternal diabetes mellitus
  High intestinal obstruction
  Drugs
  Fatty acids (hyperalimenation)
  Lucey-Driscoll syndrome

Pathologic Causes—cont'd
Conjugated hyperbilirubinemia
Anatomic
  Extrahepatic
    Biliary atresia
    Bile duct stenosis
    Choledochal cyst
    Bile duct perforation
    Biliary sludge
    Biliary mass (stone or neoplasm)
  Intrahepatic
    Alagille syndrome (arteriohepatic
      dysplasia)
    Nonsyndromic interlobular ductal
      hypoplasia
    Caroli disease
    Congenital hepatic fibrosis
    Inspissated bile
Metabolic/genetic
  Alpha$_1$-antitrypsin deficiency
  Galactosemia
  Hereditary fructose intolerance
  Glycogen storage disease type IV
    (brancher defect)
  Tyrosinemia
  Zellweger syndrome
  Cystic fibrosis

Pathologic Causes—cont'd
Conjugated hyperbilirubinemia—
  cont'd
Excretory defects
  Dubin-Johnson syndrome
  Rotor syndrome
  Summerskill syndrome
  Byler disease
Infections
  TORCH (*toxoplasmosis, other
    agents, rubella, cytomegalovirus,
    herpes simplex*)
  Syphilis
  HIV
  Varicella-zoster virus
  Coxsackievirus
  Hepatitis (A, B, C, D, and E)
  Echovirus
  Tuberculosis
  Gram-negative infections
  Listeria monocytogenes
  Staphylococcus aureus
  Sepsis, urinary tract infections
Miscellaneous
  Trisomies 17, 18, and 21
  Total parenteral nutrition
  Postoperative jaundice
  Extracorporeal membrane
    oxygenation
Idiopathic neonatal hepatitis

administration. Crigler-Najjar type I syndrome is a rare form of hyperbilirubinemia transmitted in an autosomal recessive manner and characterized by a virtual absence of hepatic glucuronide synthesis for bilirubin but less severe for other substrates. Consequently a severe, unconjugated hyperbilirubinemia results with no evidence of hemolysis. Only trace if any bilirubin or bilirubin conjugates are found in the bile. Serum bilirubin levels may range from 25 to 35 mg/dl, and there is a high incidence of kernicterus. There is no clinical response to phenobarbital.

Crigler-Najjar type II syndrome is a milder form of unconjugated hyperbilirubinemia characterized by an autosomal dominant inheritance with variable penetrance, a partial defect in hepatic UDP-glucuronyl transferase activity, and a dramatic response to phenobarbital. Patient serum bilirubin levels are less than 20 mg/dl; kernicterus is rare. The bile contains a preponderance of bilirubin monoglucuronide.

Gilbert syndrome is the third inherited form of unconjugated hyperbilirubinemia, usually presenting in young adulthood. It is a benign, fairly common syndrome, affecting approximately 6% of the population. Hepatic bilirubin clearance is reduced, and activity of hepatic UDP-glucuronyl transferase

is less than one half of physiologically normal levels. Serum bilirubin levels range from normal to 8 mg/dl, most commonly hovering between 2 and 3 mg/dl. Levels may increase during periods of fasting, stress, illness, and fatigue. Gilbert syndrome may be associated with a mild, chronic hemolysis.

Other disturbances in physiology can cause unconjugated hyperbilirubinemia. Hypothyroidism may cause unconjugated jaundice; there is no increased rate of hemolysis, but decreased bile flow has been demonstrated. Sepsis, as well as hypoxia and acidosis, may cause both conjugated and unconjugated hyperbilirubinemia. The pathophysiology is thought to be a combination of impaired transport of bilirubin; decreased hepatic blood flow, inhibiting hepatic uptake of bilirubin; and toxin-mediated hepatocellular necrosis. Hypoglycemia also causes a rise in unconjugated bilirubin because glucose is the substrate needed to form glucuronic acid used in bilirubin conjugation. Maternal diabetes also has been associated with increased and prolonged levels of unconjugated hyperbilirubinemia. The mechanism is not understood but seems to be independent of the severity of maternal disease. High intestinal obstruction is associated with unconjugated bilirubinemia, possibly caused by decreased glucuronyl transferase activity.

Various compounds, such as sulfonamides, salicylates, or fatty acids, can elevate bilirubin levels by competing for albumin binding sites. The Lucey-Driscoll syndrome is a rare cause of unconjugated jaundice. A potent inhibitor of glucuronyl transferase is found in maternal and infant serum but not in maternal milk. Bilirubin levels have been demonstrated as high as 65 mg/dl, and kernicterus has been reported.

Neonatal Direct Jaundice

Conjugated hyperbilirubinemia, or direct jaundice, indicates hepatobiliary disease and has numerous causes. It is defined in the simplest terms as a conjugated bilirubin level of more than 1.5 mg/dl or greater than 10% to 20% of the total bilirubin concentration. Neonatal cholestasis occurs within the first 90 days of life and affects approximately 1 in 2500 births. The neonate in particular may be predisposed to cholestasis for several reasons, including immaturity of hepatic excretory function, inborn errors of metabolism that cause liver dysfunction and are manifest in early postnatal life, and the immature hepatocyte's inherent susceptibility to viral or toxic insult associated with a stereotypic response to such injury.

Any disruption in bile transport, bile formation, or bile flow may result in cholestasis. Errors in each of these steps have been identified. Studies have demonstrated inefficient liver cell transport of bile acids in early life. Enzymatic conjugation of bile acids with glycine and taurine is diminished in the neonatal period. Evidence has also shown a difference in mature and immature bile synthesis. Atypical bile acids in infants suggest the existence of a fetal synthetic pathway and a delay in the establishment of mature synthetic capabilities. It is unknown whether these atypical bile acids have a harmful cytokinetic effect on hepatobiliary structures. Pinpoint errors of bile metabolism may block a step in the excretory pathway. Disturbances in the hepatic environment caused by sepsis, hypoxia, acidosis, or introduction of toxins via medications and nutritional supplementation diminish bile formation and bile flow. Anatomic atresias and strictures block bile flow. Specific damage to hepatocytes caused by accumulation of toxic metabolites as result of an inborn error of metabolism or cell destruction secondary to infection also causes biliary obstruction and conjugated hyperbilirubinemia.

The causes of conjugated or cholestatic jaundice can be grouped into anatomic (i.e., extrahepatic and intrahepatic), metabolic, infectious, and miscellaneous categories. Although the list is extensive, the evaluation leads to a diagnosis of either biliary atresia or idiopathic neonatal hepatitis in approximately 70% to 80% of infants. Identification of extrahepatic biliary atresia is the initial critical element in the overall assessment of cholestatic jaundice. Delay in recognition of extrahepatic biliary atresia significantly increases morbidity and mortality.

Anatomic

Extrahepatic. Biliary atresia is one of the most common extrahepatic causes of neonatal cholestasis. The cause is not

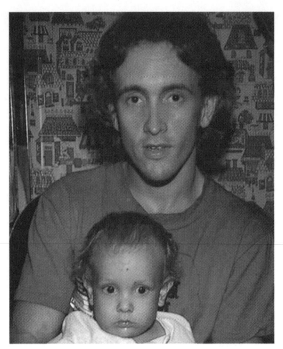

FIG. 19-1 Father and son with Alagille syndrome. Note the characteristic facial features of narrow face and pointed chin. The child also had intrahepatic biliary hypoplasia, butterfly vertebrae, and pulmonic stenosis.

well understood. Early theories regarding failure of recanalization of the biliary tree or congenital insult during the first trimester have fallen out of favor. A more recent theory focuses on the progressive nature of the disorder and suggests that a single process, probably viral in origin, causes neonatal hepatitis, biliary atresia, or choledochal cyst. Reovirus type 3, cytomegalovirus (CMV), and rubella have been implicated.

Choledochal cysts are dilations of the extrahepatic biliary tree. The enlarging cyst produces signs and symptoms of obstruction approximately 50% of the time. More often the cyst is identified incidentally during the ultrasound evaluation for cholestatic jaundice.

Spontaneous perforation of the bile duct is another cause of extrahepatic conjugated jaundice. The site of the perforation is almost always the junction of the cystic and common bile ducts. Other disorders of the extrahepatic biliary system are quite rare and include bile duct stenosis, neoplasm, and cholelithiasis. The extrahepatic biliary tree can also be obstructed by bile plugs or sludge. Patients at risk for increased bile viscosity might include individuals with cystic fibrosis, hemolytic disorders, hepatocellular damage, total parenteral nutrition, extensive ileal resections, and dehydration.

Intrahepatic. The second classification of cholestatic jaundice is intrahepatic biliary disease. Paucity of intralobular bile ducts exists as two distinct entities—the syndromic form, known as *Alagille syndrome* (arteriohepatic dysplasia), and the nonsyndromic form. Alagille syndrome is associated with hypoplastic intrahepatic bile ducts, cholestatic jaundice, a triangular-shaped face with a broad forehead and prominent chin (Fig. 19-1), deep-set eyes, a bulbous nose, persistence of posterior embryotoxon in the eye, pulmonary artery hypoplasia or stenosis, butterfly vertebral defects, growth retardation, developmental delay, hypogonadism, and bone ab-

and the periportal fibrosis is nonprogressive. The cholestasis is most prominent in infancy and often improves with time. Nonsyndromic interlobular bile duct hypoplasia is associated with several disease states and characterized by progressive fibrosis and giant cell transformation on biopsy. Bile duct paucity has been reported in alpha₁-antitrypsin deficiency, congenital rubella or cytomegalovirus infection, hepatitis B, trisomies 17 and 18, Down syndrome, trihydroxycoprostanic acidemia, and graft-versus-host disease.

Rare forms of intrahepatic biliary disease include Caroli disease, or cystic dilation of the intrahepatic bile ducts, and congenital hepatic fibrosis. The cholestasis in these conditions tends to be mild. Bile duct plugs or inspissated bile also can cause obstruction in the intrahepatic biliary tree.

Metabolic and Genetic

Conditions that result in hepatocellular disease can cause obstruction to bile flow and subsequent cholestatic jaundice. Metabolic disorders, genetic abnormalities, infections, and iatrogenic interventions each can lead to conjugated hyperbilirubinemia. One of the more common metabolic disorders is alpha₁-antitrypsin deficiency. Alpha₁-antitrypsin is a protease inhibitor (Pi) for trypsin and several other enzymes. The allele producing normal enzyme concentrations is Pi M. Individuals with Pi MZ phenotype have intermediate levels of the inhibitor enzyme, and those with the Pi ZZ phenotype have enzyme levels between 10% to 15% of normal and are at risk for liver disease. It is estimated that 5% to 10% of infants with neonatal cholestasis are deficient in circulating alpha₁-antitrypsin, though not all infants with alpha₁-antitrypsin become jaundiced.

Two disorders of carbohydrate metabolism often present in the neonatal period with severe jaundice. Galactosemia is classically caused by a deficiency of galactose 1-phosphate uridyl transferase. If breast-feeding or taking a lactose-containing formula, the infant with galactosemia has rapid onset of cholestasis, hepatomegaly, lethargy, emesis, anorexia, cataracts, and growth failure. The second disorder, hereditary fructose intolerance, is the most common metabolic disorder of the fructose pathway. It is caused by a deficiency of fructose 1-phosphate aldolase and results in severe obstructive jaundice and hepatic disease. Glycogen storage disease type IV, a brancher enzyme defect, is the only glycogen storage disease that is associated with neonatal cholestasis.

Hereditary tyrosinemia is a defect in amino acid metabolism that is inherited as an autosomal recessive disorder. The disease affects the liver, kidneys, and pancreas and occurs in two forms. The acute form presents in infancy with severe hepatotoxic injury; exclusionary diet does not seem to protect against progressive liver disease. The chronic form of tyrosinemia is more gradual in onset and less severe in its pre-

sentation. Liver dysfunction and jaundice progress over a period of years.

Specific defects of lipid metabolism and certain peroxisomal disorders are associated with neonatal cholestasis. One associated with a specific defect in bile acid metabolism. Multifaceted disorders, such as hypopituitarism and hypothyroidism, or trisomies 17, 18, and 21 may cause early onset of conjugated jaundice. Cystic fibrosis is a common genetic disorder (occurring in 1 in 2000 live births among caucasians) that can cause cholestasis. Jaundice is rarely the first sign of cystic fibrosis, but meconium ileus with intestinal obstruction or thickened, tenacious bile secretions causing bile plugs may lead to early conjugated hyperbilirubinemia.

Several familial diseases with uncharacterized defects can present in the neonatal period with cholestatic jaundice. Two of the more well-recognized disorders are Dubin-Johnson and Rotor syndromes. Dubin-Johnson is an autosomal recessive syndrome with a nonhemolytic conjugated hyperbilirubinemia. It is often asymptomatic until early adulthood but may present at any time from birth to the fourth decade. Transaminases are normal, hepatomegaly is absent, and pruritus is uncommon. The liver is grossly pigmented, with accumulation of melanotic deposits in the centrilobular hepatocytes. Clinical prognosis is excellent. An excretory defect is suspected though not yet specifically identified.

Rotor syndrome is also an autosomal recessive, nonhemolytic conjugated hyperbilirubinemia. There is no hepatomegaly, transaminases are normal, and the liver biopsy is normal with no pigment deposition. Prognosis is excellent.

Idiopathic recurrent intrahepatic cholestasis has been recognized as an entity with several subtypes. As with Dubin-Johnson and Rotor syndromes, a specific excretory defect is suspected. Benign recurrent intrahepatic cholestasis is a rare disorder also known as *Summerskill syndrome*. It is described as multiple periods of cholestasis lasting months to even years with spontaneous remissions of variable duration. The cholestatic episodes are associated with pruritus and anorexia, but the long-term prognosis is excellent with no residual liver damage. More recent reports have noted that in this group of patients the gamma-glutamyltransferase (GGT) remains normal or low, whereas other laboratory markers for obstruction are elevated during the cholestatic phase. There have been reports of patients with idiopathic recurrent intrahepatic cholestasis, with low GGT, who have had progressive deterioration and a poorer prognosis. This subtype of recurrent cholestasis is believed to be similar to Byler disease. Byler disease is an autosomal recessive, progressive intrahepatic cholestatic disorder. Studies have demonstrated defective excretion of conjugated bile acids and bilirubin across the canalicular membrane.

Infections

Infectious diseases causing hepatocellular destruction can also present in the neonatal period with conjugated hyperbilirubinemia. Any of the numerous causes of perinatal hep-

Differential Diagnosis of Jaundice in the Older Child

Metabolic/Genetic	Infections	Infections—cont'd
Gilbert syndrome	Viral	Bacterial
Dubin-Johnson syndrome	Hepatitis (A, B, C, D, and E)	Sepsis
Rotor syndrome	CMV	Toxic shock syndrome
Cystic fibrosis	Epstein-Barr virus	Lyme disease
Indian childhood cirrhosis	Herpes simplex virus	Rocky Mountain spotted
Wilson disease	Varicella-zoster virus	fever
Tyrosinemia	Adenovirus	Miscellaneous
Alpha$_1$-antitrypsin deficiency	Enterovirus	Visceral larval migrans
	Rubella virus	Schistosomiasis
Anatomic	Arbovirus	Reye syndrome
Caroli disease	HIV	
Congenital hepatic fibrosis	Echovirus	
Choledochal cyst		
Cholelithiasis		
Pancreas and pancreatic duct abnormalities		

atitis can be associated with jaundice, including CMV, rubella, herpes simplex, toxoplasmosis, syphilis, human immunodeficiency virus (HIV), varicella, coxsackievirus, and hepatitis viruses B and C. Tuberculosis can also cause cholestatic jaundice. Bacterial infections with hepatic manifestations may result in obstructive jaundice. Gram-negative pathogens are especially associated with hepatocellular dysfunction and cholestasis. It has been hypothesized that the gram-negative endotoxin may reduce bile flow and cause toxic damage to the hepatocytes. It is important to note that gram-negative sepsis, especially with *Escherichia coli,* has been associated with galactosemia. Gram-positive sepsis is less likely to cause cholestasis. However, *Listeria monocytogenes* and hepatic abscesses caused by *Staphylococcus aureus* may produce conjugated hyperbilirubinemia. Generalized shock from any cause often produces cholestatic dysfunction, but jaundice is not usually the first manifestation of septicemia.

Miscellaneous

Total parenteral nutrition (TPN) cholestasis was first reported in 1971. Since that time, numerous centers have begun investigating the pathophysiology of the association. After 2 or more weeks of TPN, mild hepatomegaly develops with mild to moderate cholestasis and elevation of hepatic enzymes. The basis of the conjugated hyperbilirubinemia is believed to be multifactorial, depending on the degree of prematurity; length of enteric fasting; duration of inadequate nutrition; extent of underlying illness or associated metabolic disturbances, such as acidosis and hyperglycemia; abnormal amino acids; trace element deficiencies; toxic bile acids; cholelithiasis; and any intervening surgeries. Other iatrogenic causes of cholestatic jaundice have been reported in the literature. Postoperative jaundice is a well-documented

entity. Extracorporeal membrane oxygenation (ECMO) has also been associated with transient and occasionally severe direct hyperbilirubinemia.

Approximately one half of the cases of neonatal cholestasis are identified as having extrahepatic biliary obstruction. A small proportion have obvious triggers, such as TPN or ECMO. Only a small percentage of infants have one of the metabolic or genetic abnormalities causing hepatocellular disease and subsequent obstructive jaundice. The majority of neonates with early-onset conjugated hyperbilirubinemia fall into the category of neonatal hepatitis. This disorder should not be confused with hepatitis in a neonate caused by a specific infectious agent. Neonatal hepatitis implies an idiopathic process and accounts for anywhere between 20% to 50% of affected neonates. The liver pathology demonstrates extensive giant cell transformation, inflammation, fibrosis, and increased extramedullary hematopoiesis. The infants with neonatal hepatitis may eventually prove to have specific underlying disease states merely awaiting discovery and recognition. For example, patients with alpha$_1$-antitrypsin were formerly included in the category of neonatal hepatitis. Since the elucidation of the protein inhibitor deficiency, the disease has been recognized as a distinct entity.

Older Childhood Jaundice

The differential diagnosis of jaundice in the older child has some degree of overlap with that of the neonate but expands to include disease states rarely seen in the first 3 months of life. The majority of cases of conjugated and unconjugated jaundice in an older child extend from hepatocellular disease caused by a primary metabolic defect, infectious agent, autoimmune disorder, or infiltrative process (Box 19-2). Hemolysis from any underlying process may also result in jaundice.

BOX 19-3

Drugs Associated With Cholestatic Jaundice

amoxicillin-clavulanate
anabolic steroids
azathioprine (Imuran)
chlordiazepoxide (Librium)
chlorpromazine HCl (Thorazine)
chlorpropamide (Diabinese)
contraceptive steroids
danazol
erythromycin

haloperidol
imipramine
indomethacin
injectable gold compounds
interleukin-2
megestrol acetate (Megace)
methyldopa (Aldomet)
nitrofurantoin (Furadantin)
phenazopyridine HCl (Pyridium)

phenytoin (Dilantin)
sulfonamides
trimethoprim-sulfamethoxazole

Overdose/Abuse

alcohol
acetaminophen

HCl, Hydrochloride.

Few patients have anatomic extrahepatic disorders as the cause of jaundice.

Jaundice in several of the inherited disorders mentioned in the previous section are more common in the older-age child, for example, Gilbert, Dubin-Johnson, and Rotor syndromes and Caroli disease. The cholestatic symptoms of cystic fibrosis usually manifest in early adulthood. Congenital hepatic fibrosis is an autosomal recessive disorder of the interlobular bile ducts that is rarely discovered before late childhood. Indian childhood cirrhosis is an idiopathic familial illness with onset between 6 and 24 months of age and is a major cause of mortality in young children on the Indian subcontinent. Wilson disease is an autosomal recessive disorder that is a rare cause of progressive liver disease. It is associated with low serum ceruloplasmin. Hepatic presentation is more common in the early childhood and adolescent years; older patients with Wilson disease demonstrate hepatic, neurologic, hematologic, and psychiatric symptoms. Wilson disease is unlikely to present before 4 to 6 years of age and usually does not present until the second decade of life. The exact pathophysiology is not well understood, but low ceruloplasmin levels, copper deposition in the tissues, and high urinary excretion of copper are hallmarks of the disorder. The jaundice of Wilson disease occurs either as a fulminant hepatitis with hemolytic anemia secondary to massive release of copper into the serum or as unconjugated and conjugated bilirubin levels that gradually increase with progressive cirrhosis, fibrosis, and a chronic state of hemolysis.

Acute viral hepatitis is a frequent cause of liver disease and jaundice. The causes in childhood are similar but not identical to those in the neonate. Five viruses cause the majority of cases of infectious hepatitis in this age group. Hepatitis A virus (HAV) is an acute illness common in toddlers and young adults. Hepatitis B virus (HBV) is primarily seen in young adults or in the neonate as a result of vertical transmission. It is recognized as causing both acute and chronic disease. Most nonA, nonB hepatitis is now known to be caused by hepatitis C virus (HCV). Hepatitis D virus (HDV),

formerly the delta-virus, is found in coinfection or superinfection with HBV. The fifth agent is hepatitis E virus (HEV) that causes enterically transmitted epidemic and sporadic nonA, nonB hepatitis primarily in developing countries. Other viral causes of hepatitis and jaundice in the older child include CMV, Epstein-Barr virus, herpes simplex virus, varicella-zoster virus, adenoviruses, enteroviruses, rubella virus, and arboviruses. HIV must be in the differential diagnosis of new-onset jaundice and liver disease. Systemic infections of any type can be associated with hepatocellular dysfunction and subsequent jaundice (i.e., sepsis, toxic shock syndromes, Reye syndrome, Lyme disease, leptospirosis, and Rocky Mountain spotted fever). Acute cholangitis is another cause of jaundice. Parasitic infestation, for example, visceral larva migrans, and schistosomiasis can cause jaundice as part of their symptom complex.

Autoimmune disorders, such as systemic lupus erythematosus, and vasculitis, such as Henoch-Schönlein purpura, can be associated with new-onset jaundice. Infiltrative processes of the liver, such as neuroblastoma, Wilms tumor, leukemia, primary hepatic tumors, Hodgkin lymphoma, sarcoid, and amyloidosis, can cause jaundice. States of acute or chronic hemolysis can lead to indirect jaundice and can be seen in sickle cell anemia, spherocytosis, glucose-6-phosphate dehydrogenase deficiency, paroxysmal nocturnal hemoglobinuria, and hemolytic uremic syndrome. Gastrointestinal disorders can affect liver function, as in Crohn disease or ulcerative colitis. Sclerosing cholangitis, whether a primary disorder or associated with chronic inflammatory bowel disease, may cause cholestatic jaundice. Toxic insult to the liver can also result in conjugated and unconjugated hyperbilirubinemia. TPN, alcohol, medication, and drug use have all been associated with jaundice (Box 19-3).

Anatomic abnormalities that cause jaundice in the older child include entities that overlap and expand on those seen in the neonate. Choledochal cysts occasionally are not identified in the neonatal period but are revealed as they gradually expand in size. Cholelithiasis can occur at any time and is

TABLE 19-1

Clues From the History

Clinical finding	Diagnostic considerations
Neonatal	
Family history	
Presence of familial forms of jaundice	Gilbert, Rotor, and Dubin-Johnson syndromes, Crigler-Najjar
Presence of emphysema in an adult	Alpha$_1$-antitrypsin deficiency
Infant deaths	Metabolic disease, infections
Prenatal history	
Infection in pregnancy	TORCH infection, hepatitis
Maternal behavior risk factors	Syphilis, HIV
Medications in pregnancy	Toxic hepatitis
Perinatal history	
Acute hypoglycemia, vomiting, lethargy with feedings	Carbohydrate intolerance—galactosemia, fructosemia
Pernicious vomiting with feedings	Intestinal obstruction
Failure to pass meconium	Intestinal obstruction, cystic fibrosis
Gradual onset of icterus, acholic stools	Biliary atresia
Older Childhood	
Acute illness	Hepatitis A, Epstein-Barr virus, CMV, sepsis
Failure to thrive	Chronic liver disease, metabolic or genetic disorders, cystic fibrosis, neoplastic or infiltrative process
Family history of jaundice	Inherited disorders; Gilbert, Rotor, and Dublin-Johnson syndromes; Wilson disease; hemolytic anemias
Exposure	
Blood products, raw shellfish, travel	Hepatitis A, B, C, D, and E
Drug abuse	Hepatitis B, C, and D; HIV, toxic hepatitis

usually idiopathic but may result from chronic hemolysis or medications. Congenital abnormalities of the pancreas or pancreatobiliary duct anomalies may cause jaundice.

History

A complete history can allow the astute physician to focus the potentially vast differential diagnosis of jaundice (Table 19-1). When dealing with neonatal jaundice, the historic information concerning the family and perinatal period is crucial. Close inspection of the family medical history can elucidate clues to the familial forms of jaundice. Many of these inherited syndromes are autosomal recessive with variable penetrance, and therefore careful questioning is necessary. Adults with mild jaundice at times of illness or stress could have Gilbert syndrome. An older relative with a history of mild jaundice as an infant and current pulmonary problems could have alpha$_1$-antitrypsin deficiency. An infant that died unexpectedly in the perinatal period may have had one of the metabolic disorders associated with neonatal jaundice.

The course of the pregnancy, history of illness, exposure to infection, and any medications taken during the pregnancy itself are important pieces of information. The details of the infant's clinical course are essential to determining the cause of jaundice. If the onset of jaundice is associated with other symptoms, the pattern can be a discriminating factor. For example, a newborn with acute symptoms of vomiting, hypoglycemia, and lethargy after the first formula feedings is likely to have one of the carbohydrate metabolic disorders. Immediate but otherwise relatively asymptomatic vomiting may be a sign of intestinal obstruction. An infant who fails to pass meconium, becomes distended, and vomits may have meconium ileus caused by cystic fibrosis. The neonate with gradual onset of jaundice, failure to thrive, and irritability may have extrahepatic biliary atresia or other anatomic abnormalities.

In the older child the historic questions must include a complete account of the neonatal course and the family background; a benign neonatal course does not eliminate several of the familial disorders. Associated symptoms and the timing and severity of the jaundice may help distinguish among possible causes. At-risk exposures for hepatitis, for example, blood products, raw shellfish, drug use, and travel, are crucial in identifying causes of infection and toxins. Correlating all the necessary background history and information often enables the clinician to distinguish between medical, structural, and surgical causes of jaundice.

Physical Examination

The physical examination holds many keys to the differential diagnosis of jaundice; attention to detail is essential (Table

Clues From the Physical Examination

Healthy, vigorous infant	Physiologic jaundice
Dysmorphic features	Trisomy 17, 18, or 21; Alagille syndrome, Zellweger syndrome
Microcephaly	TORCH infections
Cataracts	TORCH infections, galactosemia
Lethargy, hypotonia	Sepsis, metabolic disease
Neurologic abnormalities	Storage disorder
Bruises, cephalohematoma	Extravascular blood
Edema, anasarca	Massive hemolysis, liver failure
Hepatomegaly	Vascular congestion, cystic disorders, inflammation, storage disease, neoplasia
Ascites	Liver failure with poor albumin synthesis, portal hypertension, Budd-Chiari malformation
Vascular bruits	Vascular malformation
Fever, rash	Acute hepatitis, autoimmune disorders
Skin excoriation	Chronic cholestasis
Kayser-Fleischer rings	Wilson disease
Xanthomas	Chronic liver disease
Arthritis, erythema nodosum, perianal skin tags	Inflammatory bowel disease
Lymphadenopathy	
Generalized	Infection, HIV, neoplasia
Cervical	Epstein-Barr virus

19-2). Description of the jaundice itself may be of use in narrowing the differential diagnosis. A mild, gradual, caudal progression of yellow skin discoloration may be the presentation of a child with physiologic jaundice or breast-feeding jaundice. It is important to remember that racial skin tones may alter the clinical assessment of jaundice, but examination of the sclera, mucous membranes, and palmar aspects of the hands and feet are good indicators of the degree of jaundice. Jaundice is generally clinically apparent at levels greater than 2 to 2.5 mg/dl. Persistent jaundice in a well-appearing breast-fed infant may be consistent with breast milk jaundice. An irritable infant with a greenish-yellow skin tone is more compatible with cholestatic forms of jaundice.

Dysmorphic features in the neonate can identify chromosomal anomalies, some familial disorders, and certain metabolic diseases. Chromosomal trisomies are generally distinct in presentation. Alagille syndrome was described earlier in the chapter. Zellweger, or cerebrohepatorenal syndrome, has a characteristic facial appearance with hypertelorism, high forehead, large fontanelle, and pursed lips (see Chapter 11; Fig. 11-1). Microcephaly, cataracts, and unusual rashes may be indicative of perinatal infection. Clinical instability, lethargy, and hypotonia may be initial signs of sepsis or an acute metabolic disturbance. An abnormal neuromuscular examination should direct the physician to possible storage disorders. Bruising or a cephalohematoma may cause jaundice.

Generalized edema or anasarca with pallor may indicate massive hemolysis as the source of jaundice.

Examination of the liver and abdomen as a whole provides critical information (Fig. 19-2). Hepatomegaly is best defined in regard to liver span; the height in the midclavicular line is measured by dullness to percussion of the upper border and palpation of the lower liver edge. Estimation of normal liver span in different age groups exists in the literature (see Chapter 24; Fig. 24-1). In the healthy full-term neonate the liver span mean has been reported as 5.65 cm and may range from 4.25 to 7.0 cm; in the 5-year-old child, approximate liver span is 7 cm, and at 12 years of age the mean span has been estimated at 9 cm. The consistency of the liver, whether firm, smooth, or nodular, and whether it is tender are clues to underlying pathology. Masses and their position within the abdomen are indicators of disease. Enlargement of the liver and kidneys can be seen in cystic disorders and some common childhood tumors. Hepatosplenomegaly is characteristic of infiltrative disease, certain storage diseases, and conditions that cause vascular congestion. The presence of ascites is a indication of significant liver pathology. Examination of the abdomen should also include auscultation for vascular bruits.

In an older child with jaundice, in addition to the findings described earlier, there may be other clues. Acute onset or a recent history of associated symptoms, such as fever, rash,

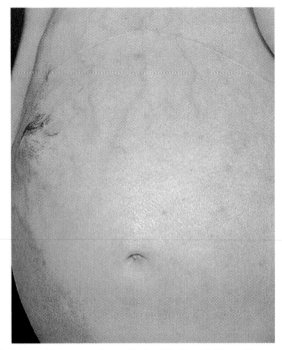

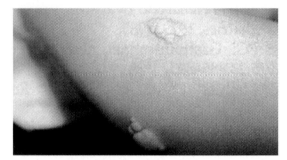

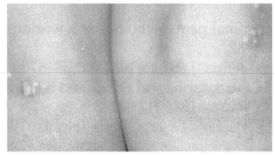

FIG. 19-2   Abdomen of a patient with chronic liver disease and portal hypertension from biliary atresia. Note the prominent abdominal veins surrounding a stoma site.

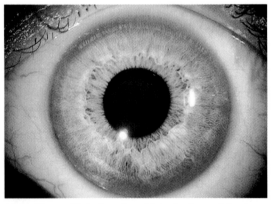

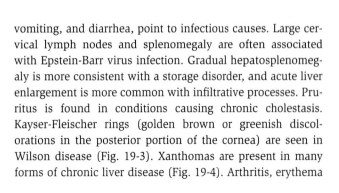

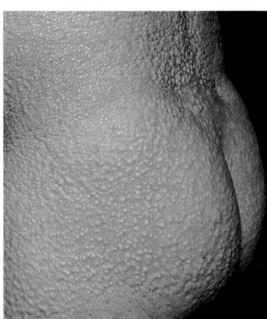

FIG. 19-3   Kayser-Fleischer ring. Note the brownish pigment at the corneoscleral junction, beginning at the superior and inferior poles.

FIG. 19-4   Xanthomas over pressure points in a child with chronic liver disease.

vomiting, and diarrhea, point to infectious causes. Large cervical lymph nodes and splenomegaly are often associated with Epstein-Barr virus infection. Gradual hepatosplenomegaly is more consistent with a storage disorder, and acute liver enlargement is more common with infiltrative processes. Pruritus is found in conditions causing chronic cholestasis. Kayser-Fleischer rings (golden brown or greenish discolorations in the posterior portion of the cornea) are seen in Wilson disease (Fig. 19-3). Xanthomas are present in many forms of chronic liver disease (Fig. 19-4). Arthritis, erythema

nodosum, and perianal skin tags are clues to liver disease secondary to inflammatory bowel disease. A search for physical stigmata of other systemic disorders, such as systemic lupus erythematosus or cystic fibrosis, should be included.

As discussed previously, a meticulous physical examination allows the physician to identify many causes of jaundice. If jaundice is the result of primary liver pathology or an underlying disorder, the physical findings provide essential clues. The information gained from the history and physical helps formulate an appropriate approach to the patient.

Evaluation of Jaundice

Detailed History and Physical Examination

Screening

Complete blood count, platelets, differential, smear
Liver enzyme and function tests
  AST, ALT, GGT, alkaline phosphatase
  Total and fractionated bilirubin levels
  Protein, albumin levels
  PT, PTT
  Clotting factors (if evidence of significant hepato-
    cellular destruction)
Stool color

Assessment

Infection
  Cultures—blood, urine, and cerebrospinal fluid, as
    indicated clinically
  Serologies—toxoplasmosis, rubella, cytomegalovirus,
    herpes, hepatitis panel, syphilis, Epstein-Barr virus
Metabolic
  Alpha$_1$-antitrypsin level and Pi typing
  Thyroid function tests—thyroxine and thyroid stim-
    ulating hormone
  Metabolic screen—urine/serum amino acids
  Sweat chloride test
  Ceruloplasmin, urinary copper excretion
  Toxicology screen
Structural
  24-hour duodenal intubation for bilirubin excretion
  Ultrasound
  Radionuclide or hepatobiliary scan
  Operative cholangiogram
Autoimmune/inflammatory
  ESR
  ANA

Pathologic Diagnosis and Confirmation

Liver biopsy
Red blood cells, bone marrow (identification of
  enzyme deficiency, hemoglobinopathies, and hemolytic anemias)

ALT, Alanine aminotransferase; *ANA,* antinuclear antibody; *AST,* as-
parate aminotransferase; *ESR,* erythrocyte sedimentation rate; *GGT,*
gamma-glutamyltransferase; *PT,* prothrombin time; *PTT,* partial thromboplastin time.

Approach to the Patient

The complete history and physical examination help tailor the evaluation of the child with jaundice. The initial assessment should determine physiologic versus pathologic jaundice, then cholestatic versus noncholestatic jaundice, and from there extrahepatic versus intrahepatic cholestatic jaundice (Box 19-4). Each of these decisions leads to branch points in the course of the evaluation. Unfortunately, especially in the neonate, the evaluation is seldom "neat" or step-by-step. Depending on the age and clinical status of the patient, it is often essential that the physician make several determinations simultaneously.

The age at presentation is one of the key focusing elements of the differential diagnosis and therefore is the appropriate first step in the evaluation. Most well-appearing infants affected with jaundice in the first week of life have physiologic causes of their icterus. Increased hemolysis also causes jaundice at this early stage. The assessment of the jaundiced infant has undergone extensive reevaluation, and new recommendations have been offered by several leading specialists. A more conservative approach to the full-term, well-appearing, bottle- or breast-fed infant has been introduced. In general a blood type, Coombs test, and total bilirubin level are suggested. Other laboratory tests, such as a complete blood count, peripheral blood smear, reticulocyte count, and a direct bilirubin level, should be considered on a case-by-case basis. These screening tests help identify infants with hemolysis and an increased risk of hyperbilirubinemia. The child can then be followed clinically, and additional laboratory testing can be performed as needed. The level at which intervention is recommended is debated. Phototherapy is accepted as a safe, effective means of lowering the indirect bilirubin level. Home phototherapy, when monitored closely by a physician, is also gaining in popularity.

A distinction must be made between the conservative approach to the well-appearing infant and the need for aggressive evaluation and intervention in any neonate with jaundice who has fever, lethargy, poor feeding, vomiting, unusual cry, or abnormal movements. These infants may have jaundice resulting from a more common problem, such as sepsis, or from rare inherited disorders. The ill infant that presents in the first 24 to 48 hours with jaundice should have a full sepsis workup with blood, urine, and cerebrospinal fluid cultures. The evaluation should also include electrolytes, liver function tests, total and direct bilirubin levels, ammonia level, urine testing for reducing substances, and possibly urine metabolic screens. In these patients, rapid intervention can be life-saving and can prevent long-term morbidity. Once the patient is clinically stabilized with appropriate fluids and antibiotics or removal of an offending agent, such as galactose in galactosemia, further testing can proceed as indicated.

The infant with jaundice in the first and second weeks of life requires additional consideration. Breast milk jaundice may last 12 to 16 weeks. In a thriving breast-fed infant, clinical observation and documentation of a pure indirect hyperbilirubinemia may be the only warranted interventions. Sudden onset of jaundice within the first week or sustained jaundice past the second week requires further investigation. Jaundice at this point is no longer physiologic, and differentiation between indirect and obstructive jaundice is crucial. Therefore the first pieces of information to be obtained are the total and direct bilirubin levels. Although there is some degree of overlap, the evaluation of indirect and direct hyperbilirubinemia diverges at this point.

Investigation of indirect jaundice should include chronic hemolysis, and a blood smear should be examined. Hemoglobinopathies can be found by electrophoresis, and red blood cell enzyme defects can be identified by specific assays. Unstable hemoglobins may cause neonatal hemolytic disease and may be diagnosed when a large number of Heinz bodies are seen on a Heinz body slide preparation. The infant's history and examination will point to the possibility of high intestinal obstruction that can be documented by ultrasound or upper gastrointestinal series. Crigler-Najjar syndromes should be suspected in infants with rapidly progressive unconjugated hyperbilirubinemia without evidence of hemolysis; type I may be present in the first 24 hours, and type II presents later in life. Diagnosis can be made via assay of UDP-glucuronyl transferase or by high-performance liquid chromatography of the patient's serum. Patients with Crigler-Najjar syndrome type I have complete absence of bilirubin conjugates; patients with type II deficiency have monoconjugated bilirubin without diconjugates. Treatment of Crigler-Najjar type I in the neonatal period is by exchange transfusions and phototherapy. Phototherapy must continue throughout life. Temporizing measures include phototherapy, a lipid-enriched diet, and cholestyramine. Ultimately, liver transplantation is recommended. Crigler-Najjar syndrome type II can be well controlled, maintaining bilirubin levels around 5 mg/dl through the administration of phenobarbital (3 to 5 mg/kg/day). Gilbert syndrome is benign and is most often diagnosed clinically. Bile aspirated from patients with Gilbert syndrome contains higher proportions of monoconjugated bilirubin. A 24-hour fast raises the bilirubin level 100% to 150%. Bilirubin levels usually range between normal and 5 to 6 mg/dl, and other liver function tests are normal. Liver biopsy is not recommended.

The workup of cholestatic (conjugated, direct) jaundice hinges on the ability to distinguish between intrahepatic and extrahepatic defects. Unfortunately, no one test can absolutely differentiate between the two defects. Clues from the history, hepatic and extrahepatic physical findings, and laboratory evaluations are used. Examination of the stool is a critical part of the decision tree. The presence and persistence of acholic stools is the most characteristic finding in obstructive jaundice. Alagille proposed the following four clinical criteria that were helpful in separating the types of cholestasis: stool color after 10 days, birth weight, age at onset of acholic stools, and clinical features of liver involvement. Physicians may find the data useful, but the degree of overlap between the two groups is significant.

The initial evaluation of obstructive jaundice is broad; the goals are to explore the extent of liver pathology and to screen for causes—infectious, metabolic, and structural. Aspartate aminotransferase (AST, formerly SGOT) and alanine aminotransferase (ALT, formerly SGPT) are markers of hepatocellular damage. Serum alkaline phosphatase (AP) is elevated in both intrahepatic and extrahepatic disease, but higher levels are more common with obstructive disorders. Gamma-glutamyltransferase (GGT) is a membrane-bound enzyme, and 80% to 90% of its activity is found in the biliary tract. Increased GGT is associated with intrahepatic and extrahepatic obstructive biliary disease, including biliary atresia, cirrhosis, alpha$_1$-antitrypsin deficiency, and TPN cholestasis. GGT/bilirubin ratios tend to be higher in intrahepatic cholestasis. Synthetic capability of the liver is assessed with albumin and clotting factors. A decreased albumin in the presence of acute or chronic liver disease is a sign of significant hepatocellular damage. Clotting factors, prothrombin time (PT), and partial thromboplastin time (PTT) should be assayed. Both vitamin K–dependent (II, VII, IX and X) and vitamin K–independent (V) factors can be depressed in acute or chronic liver disease. An infant with significant liver disease may be at risk for a bleeding diathesis and intracranial hemorrhage. Administration of vitamin K can be lifesaving.

Other specific tests can be obtained to rule out a particular disorder. No screening test is perfect, and certain caveats must be kept in mind. A combination of physical findings and blood serologies can pinpoint an infectious disease, such as CMV, rubella, toxoplasmosis, syphilis, and hepatitis B. Physical examination and hormone levels can determine hypothyroidism or panhypopituitarism. Management depends on sufficient hormone replacement and close follow-up. To rule out alpha$_1$-antitrypsin deficiency, serum enzyme levels and protease inhibitor (Pi) typing should be obtained because serum enzyme levels can miss the heterozygote SZ phenotype or may be falsely elevated as an acute phase reactant. Liver biopsy shows characteristic periodic acid–Schiff (PAS)—positive, diastase-resistant cytoplasmic granules. Of affected children, 75% will have resolved their jaundice by 7 months. Persistent, insidious liver damage continues, however, and is clinically evident by early adulthood. Liver transplantation is the only curative intervention.

When testing for reducing substances in the urine to diagnose galactosemia and fructose intolerance, the infant must be receiving the offending dietary substance. If the infant is unable to feed adequately, specific enzyme studies must be obtained on appropriate tissue (i.e., galactosemia [erythrocyte or hepatocyte] and fructose intolerance [hepatic or intestinal mucosal biopsy for aldolase activity]). The characteristic metabolic abnormalities of tyrosinemia alter as the liver disease progresses, and therefore plasma amino acid levels must be obtained early. Treatment of these metabolic disorders is removal of the toxic agent. Prognosis depends on the ability to maintain the diet and the extent of organ system damage before identification of the disorder. Liver transplantation has become the treatment of choice after medical stabilization.

The standard test for cystic fibrosis, pilocarpine iontophoresis (sweat test), has certain pitfalls. It can be falsely negative, or the sample can be inadequate in a very small infant or a patient with edema. False-positive tests may occur in failure to thrive, Addison disease, and hypopituitarism.

Genetic screening with a buccal smear or blood sample can now identify approximately 85% of the more common cystic fibrosis mutations.

The majority of the aforementioned screening tests are obtained, as indicated, as part of a rapid initial evaluation. The remainder of the workup centers on distinguishing other intracellular hepatic disease states (most commonly neonatal hepatitis) from the extrahepatic biliary disorders. In identifying surgical causes of jaundice, many studies have shown that timing is of the utmost importance for prognosis and morbidity. Approximately 80% of infants with biliary atresia who underwent corrective surgery by 60 days of age become anicteric, as compared with 20% to 35% of those who underwent surgery after 90 days of age. Long-term survival rates are also correlated to age at the time of surgery. Advances in radiographic imaging have significantly advanced the capability to determine the patency of the biliary system. However, simpler approaches should not be overlooked. As always, the history and physical examination can give important clues. The appearance of acholic stools, which are grayish-white and chalky, is a critical finding but can occur in both severe neonatal hepatitis and biliary atresia. Conversely the presence of pigmented stools virtually rules out biliary atresia, although bilirubin traversing intestinal epithelium may impart some color to the stool in these infants. Many centers report that if a 24-hour duodenal intubation with serial aspiration reveals bile-stained secretions, biliary obstruction is virtually excluded.

Ultrasonography has become extremely important in the evaluation of the liver and biliary system and is generally recommended as the first imaging procedure. Ultrasonographers with sufficient expertise in infant ultrasound can give crucial information about the liver, including its consistency, presence of the gallbladder, and patency of the biliary tree. Other extrahepatic abnormalities, such as stones, choledochal cysts, and tumors, can be identified as well. Computed tomography (CT) scans and magnetic resonance imaging (MRI) are not usually part of the initial evaluation. High-intensity radionuclide scans often provide key discriminating information. N-substituted iminodiacetates (IDA) labeled with technetium 99 are rapidly taken up by the hepatocytes and secreted into the bile. Abdominal scans are obtained sequentially over a 24- to 48-hour period. Hepatitis characteristically demonstrates slow uptake of the compound and normal excretion into the biliary system. In biliary atresia there is normal uptake of the radioisotope but no excretion into the gut lumen. Two important caveats must be mentioned. First, biliary atresia is believed to be a progressive disorder. Early radionuclide scans may show excretion and presence of isotope in the gut lumen, but when repeated at around 10 weeks of age, they show no excretion. Second, severe hepatitis, even with normal biliary system anatomy, may prevent excretion of the isotope. Therefore it is recommended that oral phenobarbital (5 mg/kg/day) be administered for 5 days before the radionuclide scan to enhance biliary excretion.

Percutaneous transhepatic cholangiography (TC) is an excellent technique to visualize dilated intrahepatic bile ducts.

Unfortunately, TC is not available for most infants because of their small size and the limitations of the instrumentation equipment. Endoscopic retrograde cholangiography (ERC) allows direct demonstration of the extrahepatic biliary system and the major intrahepatic ducts. The procedure requires a high degree of expertise. New, smaller fiberoptic endoscopes allow the use of this technique in infants.

The liver biopsy remains an important component of the diagnostic evaluation. It offers several opportunities that the aforementioned imaging procedures do not. A liver biopsy is recommended in all patients with cholestasis unless extrahepatic obstruction is absolutely identified. Examination of the specimen can show bile duct dilation, bile duct to portal space ratio, bile duct paucity, bile plugs, and giant cell transformation. Special stains and preparations can demonstrate abnormal deposits of iron, copper, glycogen, and lipid; viral inclusion bodies; granuloma; or PAS-positive, diastase-resistant granules. Special assays can identify abnormal enzymatic activity associated with several disorders, including lycogenoses, lysosomal storage diseases, and Criglar-Najjar syndrome.

The entire assessment, including history, physical examination, laboratory studies, radiographic procedures, and biopsy results, distinguishes extrahepatic obstruction in the majority of cases. Treatment is surgical correction. In the case of biliary atresia the Kasai portoenterostomy has become the standard surgical procedure worldwide. Long-term survival rates in Western series vary from 47% to 60% at 5 years, and approximately 30% at 10 years. Patients with biliary atresia represent 35% to 67% of the cases of pediatric liver transplants.

An estimated 20% to 50% of infants with cholestatic jaundice have no specific cause identified after an extensive evaluation. These infants are diagnosed by exclusion with neonatal hepatitis. Liver biopsy demonstrates giant cell transformation and inflammation. Management is supportive. Prognosis is variable because the underlying cause is heterogeneous; estimates of long-term survival range from 60% to 80%.

The assessment of the older child with jaundice shares all the same principles of evaluation as in the neonate. However, there is a shift in focus toward the infectious and metabolic processes more common to this age group. The diagnosis of several of the familial disorders, such as Dubin-Johnson and Rotor syndromes, is made clinically, with confirmation by normal laboratory studies and liver biopsy. Gilbert syndrome is most often a clinical diagnosis, substantiated by normal liver function tests; there is no needed intervention or therapy. Familial disorders, such as congenital hepatic fibrosis and Indian childhood cirrhosis, are identified through history and then laboratory and radiographic evidence. Therapy is supportive, and depending on the progression of the disorder, liver transplantation may be warranted.

Tyrosinemia can present in the chronic form in the older-age child and is evaluated via plasma amino acid screening. Wilson disease can present as either fulminant or chronic liver disease. Important findings in the evaluation are low serum ceruloplasm and high urinary copper excretion. The

TABLE 19-3

Management of Cholestasis

Finding	Treatment
Nutrition	
General principles	Optimize caloric intake, supplement enterally with nighttime or continuous feedings as needed
Malabsorption of dietary long-chain triglycerides	Replace as medium-chain triglycerides in formula or supplement
Malabsorption of fat-soluble vitamins	Replace vitamins A, D, E, and K as recommended with water miscible forms; follow clinical indicators of deficiency and vitamin levels as needed
Water-soluble vitamins	Often deficient, supplement with twice the recommended daily allowance
Micronutrients	Supplement with calcium, phosphorus, zinc; monitor iron, magnesium
Trace elements	Carefully balance to avoid overloading liver's excretional capabilities
Pruritus	
Choleretics	Phenobarbital, ultraviolet light, ursodeoxycholic acid
Bile acid binders	Cholestyramine, colestipol (also binds most other medicines and prevents intestinal absorption)
Miscellaneous	Carbamazepine, rifampin
Ascites/portal hypertension	Salt and water restriction, diuretics, albumin, portacaval shunt
GI bleeding	Ice lavage, balloon tamponade, endoscopic sclerotherapy, variceal ligation, portacaval shunt
Liver failure	Liver transplantation

definitive marker is liver tissue copper content as measured on a liver biopsy specimen. Treatment regimens include low-copper diets and chelating agents to remove excess copper. The drug of choice is penicillamine, which results in dramatic cupruresis. If penicillamine is not tolerated, second-line therapy can be with triethylene tetramine dihydrochloride (trientine). Effectiveness of the chelation can be monitored by the fading of the Kayser-Fleischer rings and improvement in neurologic, hematologic, and hepatic signs and symptoms. Wilson disease is fatal unless treated. Prognosis depends on the timing of the diagnosis and the response to chelation. Screening of the index patient's family members is particularly important because of the often insidious nature of the disorder. Routine liver function tests, slit-lamp examination, and a serum ceruloplasmin level should be obtained in parents and all first-degree relatives over 3 to 4 years of age. Asymptomatic cases should be begun on chelation therapy to prevent the natural evolution of the disease.

Different infectious processes are of primary concern beyond the neonatal period. For example, in the older age groups acute viral hepatitis is more common. The identification of viral serologic markers has made the documentation and staging of viral hepatitis more complete. Treatment is supportive. For chronic hepatitis B and C, interferon alfa-2b has been approved and should be considered in selected patient populations. Prevention has become a major thrust in pediatrics within the last few years since the development of the hepatitis B and hepatitis A vaccines. Serologic testing for

other viral infections, such as Epstein-Barr virus and CMV, are also available.

Acute jaundice from an infection with secondary hepatitis should be approached by treating the inciting infection. Control of sepsis, adequate hydration, and proper nutrition can help diminish the cholestatic effect of the primary infection. Chronic liver disease or jaundice resulting from disorders such as cystic fibrosis, sickle-cell disease, glucose-6-phosphate dehydrogenase deficiency, and autoimmune diseases is best addressed by maintaining adequate control of the underlying disorder. Toxic effects of TPN, medications, drugs, or alcohol are identified through a careful history and elimination of other possible causes as indicated. Elimination of the offending agent as soon as possible along with supportive care allows for gradual normalization of liver function in most cases. Again, in the case of acute, fulminant toxic injury, liver transplantation may be required.

Medical management of chronic liver disease is very challenging (Table 19-3). Patients with acute severe disease or chronic liver disease of any cause should be followed by a physician trained to deal with the complications of hepatic disorders. In cases of fulminant illness the child should be in an intensive care setting, optimally with the resources for liver transplantation. Key issues for the child with chronic liver disease are nutrition and growth. Poor intake because of acute illness, anorexia, and malabsorption are common problems. Caloric supplementation, adequate administration of fat-soluble vitamins as well as water-soluble vitamins, and monitoring of trace minerals are important components of long-term therapy. Control of pruritus is often difficult but can be attempted with phenobarbital, carbamazepine, rifampin, ultraviolet light, ursodiol, and cholestyramine. Ascites, portal hypertension, and gastrointestinal bleeding can be controlled by a combination of medical and surgical interventions, including sodium restriction, diuretics, sclerotherapy, portacaval shunts, and variceal ligation. The ultimate therapy for liver failure is transplantation. Increased surgical experience, advances in immunosuppression, and improved medical management of complications have greatly improved the long-term survival and quality of life of transplant recipients. Two-year survival rates now range between 70% and 80% compared with 35% before 1980. Early diagnosis of the cause of liver disease, whether infectious, metabolic, or toxin-mediated, is the crucial element that allows for effective intervention and possible resolution of hepatic dysfunction.

SUMMARY

Jaundice has a complex biologic and pathophysiologic basis. Teasing apart the clues that ultimately reveal the underlying cause of the jaundice requires a thoughtful step-by-step analysis. Careful, detailed exploration of the patient's history and physical examination enables the physician to develop a meaningful differential diagnosis. Once the differential diagnosis is established, a logical approach to the evaluation provides a specific diagnosis.

The course and treatment of jaundice vary a great deal (close observation and resolution over time, as in breast milk jaundice, or timely intervention required, as in galactosemia or biliary atresia). The care of the infant or child with chronic jaundice is still evolving. Newer diagnostic modalities and therapeutic regimens are under development. Optimizing nutrition and minimizing morbidity remain a challenge. Together, practitioners and subspecialists can provide the full spectrum of clinical care necessary to manage the child with jaundice.

ILLUSTRATIVE CASES

Case 1. 3-week-old infant has jaundice. A careful perinatal history reveals good prenatal care and an uncomplicated pregnancy and delivery. The infant appeared well in the nursery and was discharged home after 24 hours. The mother has been breast-feeding. She remarks that the infant has done very well; is alert, active, and eating vigorously; and has normal yellow, seedy stools and no vomiting. Family history is significant only for prolonged jaundice in an earlier pregnancy; the sibling is now 3 years old and doing well. Growth parameters are normal, and physical examination is unremarkable except for yellow skin tone over the entire body, scleral icterus, and yellow mucous membranes.

This infant has a typical history for breast milk jaundice: a healthy-appearing, breast-fed infant with normal history and physical examination. There is no absolute confirmatory test, but the physician should be certain that it is an unconjugated hyperbilirubinemia and consider checking the peripheral blood count to make sure that chronic hemolysis is not a contributing factor. Total and direct bilirubin levels and a CBC with examination of the smear should be obtained. The infant, followed over time, will continue to do well with gradual resolution of the jaundice over 3 to 16 weeks if breast-feeding is continued. A trial off of breast milk could be initiated; there is usually a rapid fall in bilirubin levels with cessation of breast-feeding. However, in a case in which the infant is thriving, there is no requirement to halt breast-feeding. The mother should be reassured that there is nothing "wrong" with her breast milk, and that breast-feeding her infant is beneficial to her and the baby.

Case 2. A 3-week-old infant has jaundice. The pregnancy and delivery history is unrevealing. The infant had no problems in the nursery and was discharged home in 24 hours. The infant did well initially and was breast-feeding. At 10 days of age a visiting nurse documented good weight gain and normal skin color. Family history is unremarkable. The infant has been alert and active, somewhat more irritable, and breast-feeding well with occasional supplemental formula feedings. The child exhibits no fever, rash, or vomiting. The parents report three to four stools a day and remark that several of the stools have been unusually pale in color. On examination, growth parameters are within normal limits and the infant appears well, with yellowish-green skin color and scleral icterus; otherwise the examination is normal. Stool color is pale and chalky.

This case is characteristic of obstructive jaundice. The evaluation must differentiate between a surgically remediable cause, such as biliary atresia, and a nonsurgical cause, such as neonatal hepatitis. A total and direct bilirubin level is ordered. As suspected, it shows a direct hyperbilirubinemia, and screening studies are obtained. There is no history of infection and no evidence for sepsis or galactose or fructose intolerance. However, some infectious processes are subtle, and screening for reducing substances is simple. Most specialists would obtain a broad initial panel, including CBC, electrolytes, blood urea nitrogen, creatinine, CO_2, glucose, AST, ALT, GGT, alkaline phosphatase, PT and PTT, protein and albumin, thyroid-stimulating hormone, thyroxine, TORCH and hepatitis B titers, urine for reducing substances, $alpha_1$-antitrypsin level, and Pi typing. Further metabolic screening is put on hold. An abdominal ultrasound is performed next; no gallbladder is visualized. The infant had been placed on phenobarbital 5 mg/kg at the outset of the evaluation. A nuclear hepatobiliary scan was ordered after 5 days on the phenobarbital. The scan failed to show excretion of the marker into the intestinal lumen. A liver biopsy is consis-

tent with biliary atresia. An intraoperative cholangiogam confirms the diagnosis. A Kasai portoenterostomy is performed without complication at 5 weeks of age, with subsequent bile drainage and relief of jaundice. The infant is being followed closely by a team of gastroenterologists and surgeons. The family is aware that a liver transplant may be necessary sometime in the future.

Case 3. A 10-year-old boy has jaundice. In the last few weeks he has had fatigue, mild anorexia, nausea, and low-grade temperature. He has has no rash, upper respiratory tract infection symptoms, vomiting, diarrhea, or ill contacts. In the past he has been generally healthy, though he is small for his age. He has had no unusual illnesses, but his mother recalls that he has been jaundiced once before with a viral illness. Perinatal history is unremarkable. Family history is normal. The examination is notable for scleral icterus, diffuse yellow jaundice, mild right upper quadrant tenderness, hepatomegaly with liver edge palpable 4 cm below the costal margin and liver span 10 cm, and no splenomegaly or other masses; neurologic examination is appropriate. The remainder of the examination is normal.

This case points to an infectious cause, although Wilson disease and autoimmune hepatitis should be kept in the differential diagnosis. A total and direct bilirubin level, CBC with differential, platelets, AST, ALT, GGT, and alkaline phosphatase are ordered. Epstein-Barr virus and hepatitis panels are obtained. Liver function tests are moderately elevated, total bilirubin level is 10 mg/dl with a direct level of 3.5 mg/dl. Hepatitis A and Epstein-Barr virus titers return negative. But hepatitis B results are as follows: HBsAg,+; antiHBs, −; antiHBc IgM, −; antiHBc IgG, +++; HBeAg,+; and antiHBe, −. This pattern is consistent with chronic hepatitis B infection. A search for possible sources is negative for blood transfusion or exposure, sexual abuse or sexual contacts, and medication or drug use. The mother's serum screen is found to be that of a chronic carrier as follows: HBsAg,+; antiHBs, −; antiHBc IgG,+++; antiHBc IgM, −; HBeAg, −; and antiHBe,+. The patient is one of the 60% to 90% of infants with perinatally transmitted hepatitis B who go on to have chronic infection. The course can be quite variable—asymptomatic, insidious subclinical hepatic damage; recurrent bouts of clinically active disease, or sustained jaundice rapidly evolving to cirrhosis. His liver biopsy demonstrates periportal necrosis, mononuclear infiltration, and minimal bridging fibrosis. This patient's presentation is most consistent with a chronic active hepatitis with a fluctuating course. He is at risk for cirrhosis and hepatocellular carcinoma. His acute symptoms gradually disappear and his liver function tests returned to normal. He will need to be followed closely for progression of his liver disease. He was referred to a hepatologist and is under consideration for interferon alfa-2b therapy.

ANNOTATED BIBLIOGRAPHY

Gartner LM: Neonatal jaundice, *Pediatr Rev* 15(11):422-432, 1994.
This is an excellent overview of jaundice in the neonatal period, including bilirubin physiology, diagnosis, and management. Focus is on the healthy full-term infant.

Haber BA, Lake AM: Cholestatic jaundice in the newborn, *Clin Perinatol* 17(2):483-506, 1990.
This piece offers complete exploration of cholestatic jaundice, focusing on the newborn, but the disorders presented are relevent to other age groups as well. The article provides a thorough discussion of the evaluation and management of cholestatic jaundice.

Hicks B, Altman R: The jaundiced newborn, *Pediatr Clin North Am* 40:1161-1175, 1993.
This is a general overview of jaundice in the neonatal period with overlap to the older-aged child. It covers in detail the causes of both direct and indirect hyperbilirubinemia and offers concise information on diagnosis, treatment, and prognosis of the various disorders.

BIBLIOGRAPHY

Altman RP, Levy J: Biliary atresia, *Pediatr Ann* 14:481-485, 1985.
Balistreri WF: Neonatal cholestasis, *J Pediatr* 106:171-184, 1985.
Bergman DA: Practice parameter: management of hyperbilirubinemia in the healthy term infant, *Pediatrics* 94:558-562, 1994.
Emblem R, Stake G, Monclair T: Progress in the treatment of biliary atresia: a plea for surgical intervention within the first 2 months of life in infants with persistent cholestasis, *Acta Paediatr* 82:971-974, 1993.
Heubi JE, Daugherty CC: Neonatal cholestasis: an approach for the practicing pediatrician, *Curr Probl Pediatr* 20(5):235-295, 1990.
Krugman S: Viral hepatitis: A, B, C, D, and E—infection, *Pediatr Rev* 13:203-212, 1992.
Krugman S: Viral hepatitis: A, B, C, D, and E—prevention, *Pediatr Rev* 13:245-247, 1992.
Mowat A: The management of metabolic disorders of the liver, *Pediatr Ann* 14:501-507, 1985.
Newman TB, Easterling MJ, Goldman ES, et al: Laboratory evaluation of jaundice in newborns: frequency, cost, and yield, *Am J Dis Child* 144:364-368, 1990.
Newman TB, Maisels MJ: Evaluation and treatment of jaundice in the term newborn: a kindler, gentler approach, *Pediatrics* 89:809-818, 1992.
Noskin GA: Prevention, diagnosis, and management of viral hepatitis: a guide for primary care physicians, *AMA* 1-21, 1995.
Novak DA, Balistreri WF: Management of the child with chronic cholestasis, *Pediatr Ann* 14:488-492, 1985.
Spivak W: Bilirubin metabolism, *Pediatr Ann* 14:451-458, 1985.
Thaler MM: The liver and bile ducts. In Rudolph AM, editor: *Rudolph's pediatrics*, ed 19, Norwalk, Conn, 1991, Appleton and Lange.
van de Bor M, Ens-Dokkum M, Schreuder AM, et al: Hyperbilirubinemia in low birth weight infants and outcome at 5 years of age, *Pediatrics* 89:359-364, 1992.
Watchko JF, Oski FA: Kernicterus in preterm newborns: past, present, and future, *Pediatrics* 90:707-715, 1992.
Yarze JC, Martin P, Munoz SJ, Friedman LS: Wilson's disease: current status, *Am J Med* 92:643-654, 1992.

Persistent Vomiting

BASIL J. ZITELLI

Key Points

- Persistent vomiting in childhood demands an immediate, careful, and thorough diagnostic approach. An understanding of the pathophysiology of persistent emesis helps to establish a differential diagnosis ranging from centrally acting toxins, anatomic anomalies, and migraine headaches to psychogenic vomiting.

- The age of the child helps determine most common diagnostic possibilities. Bilious vomiting often suggests gastrointestinal obstruction, and older children may have cyclic vomiting or a psychologic cause for emesis.

- The hallmark of the evaluation is a careful history and physical examination with emphasis on determining whether intestinal obstruction exists. Selected screening blood chemistries and/or imaging procedures help confirm the clinical impression. Therapy is directed at the specific cause of emesis.

Vomiting is a common symptom in childhood that at sometime afflicts nearly every child. Usually it is part of a benign gastroenteritis and is short-lived. However, when vomiting is persistent, recurrent, develops in the neonatal period, or is associated with abdominal distension, pain, blood, bile, or symptoms of a systemic disorder, the clinician must respond with a thoughtful history, physical examination, and selected laboratory tests to elucidate the cause. Difficulty often arises because the differential diagnosis is so broad, with disorders involving virtually any organ system causing emesis.

Pathophysiology

Nausea, which often precedes vomiting, is an unpleasant sensation referred to the upper abdomen and pharynx and associated with the feeling of a need to vomit. It is accompanied by several autonomic changes, including increased salivation, diaphoresis, mydriasis, tachycardia, and altered respiratory pattern and rate. Duodenal contents may reflux into the stomach.

Vomiting should be differentiated from regurgitation, rumination, and retching. Regurgitation is the effortless return of gastric contents from the stomach and is common in young infants during and shortly after feeding. Rumination involves the regurgitation of food to the mouth where it is rechewed and reswallowed. Rumination may be seen in infants who suffer from disturbed maternal-infant bonding or in neurologically impaired children who practice it as self-stimulatory behavior. Retching, often a precursor to vomiting, is an active process using thoracic and abdominal musculature, including contraction of the diaphragm, but without expulsion of gastric contents. Vomiting is similar to retching; however, forceful but not necessarily projectile ejection of gastric contents occurs.

Both nausea and vomiting are unpleasant but serve useful protective functions. Whereas nausea is difficult to ascertain in animals, the vomiting mechanism is found in virtually all herbivores and carnivores except for rats. Animals constantly expose themselves to various toxins by eating and drinking. Once noxious foods have been ingested, the only mechanism the animal has to rid itself quickly of toxins is emesis or diarrhea. Preabsorptive detectors within the lumen of the upper gut and postabsorptive detectors exposed to the circulation trigger a series of events. The first protective mechanism may be nausea, which stops further ingestion and conditions the animal to avoid ingestion of the substance in the future. A human analogy to such conditioning is the nausea that occurs *before* chemotherapy is administered when previous treatment produced adverse reactions. Gastric relaxation prevents emptying of contaminated food into the intestine, and reverse peristalsis returns food from the upper small bowel to the stomach. Retching and vomiting expel the material from the stomach.

The mechanisms by which these highly coordinated actions occur are complex. Detectors of toxins in the intestine are gut afferents, which compose 80% to 90% of intestinal vagal fibers. When stimulated by either mechanical distension or chemical irritation (acid, alkali, hypertonic solutions, temperature, copper sulfate, and other irritants), these vagal fibers produce emesis within seconds. The indole amine 5-hydroxytryptamine (5-HT) may play a central role in stimulating vagal afferents, especially via a receptor, 5-HT$_3$. These receptors are found on vagal afferents in gastrointestinal mucosa and along vagal afferent nerves in the brainstem vomiting center. Release of 5-HT from enterochromaffin cells by chemotherapy drugs, such as cisplatin, stimulates 5-HT$_3$ receptors on vagal afferents, causing vomiting. 5-HT$_3$ antagonists (e.g., ondansetron) are powerful antiemetics often used for nausea and vomiting caused by such chemotherapeutic agents.

Although vagotomy abolishes emesis induced by intraluminal toxins, it does not ablate emesis from circulating toxins. These circulating toxins cause vomiting by stimulating the area postrema (AP), a U-shaped center in the caudal portion of the fourth ventricle outside of the blood-brain barrier. Polar molecules in blood or spinal fluid have relatively easy access to the AP, making this center ideal as the chemoreceptor trigger zone (CTZ), which is sensitive to circulating emetogenic agents.

Motion sickness induces vomiting by stimulating the vestibular labyrinthine system. Neither vagotomy nor AP ablation prevents motion-induced vomiting, suggesting the presence of other neural connections mediated by histamine H$_1$ receptors. Both antihistamines and scopolamine (acetylcholine muscarinic receptor antagonist) are effective in preventing motion sickness.

Vagal afferents and neural radiations from the AP converge in the nucleus tractus solitarius, which serves as the coordinating center for the emetic action. The motor components of the emetic reflex originate within the dorsal motor vagal nucleus and nucleus ambiguus. During the preejection phase, profound relaxation of the stomach occurs and a retrograde giant contraction originating in the mid-small intestine and under vagal influence travels to the stomach. In the ejection phase with retching, abdominal muscles and the diaphragm contract synchronously, preventing passage of gastric contents into the esophagus. During vomiting, however, the crural diaphragm relaxes, facilitating gastric emptying into the esophagus. Ejecting material from the stomach involves compression of the stomach by the descending diaphragm and contraction of the abdominal muscles.

Literature Survey

The broad topic of vomiting in children often is best covered by textbooks, whether general pediatric texts or specialty texts in emergency medicine or pediatric gastroenterology. These texts give a general overview of the mechanisms of vomiting and include excellent tables of differential diagnosis, which are often organized according to age.

Vomiting in young infants most frequently is functional, and an excellent review of innocent vomiting, nervous vomiting, and rumination was written by Fleisher. However, bilious emesis in the newborn may represent catastrophic illness or a benign disorder. Gastrointestinal surgical emergencies in the newborn are reviewed in most pediatric surgical texts and some review articles.

Older children may have different diagnostic possibilities, including manifestations of cystic fibrosis, malrotation, volvulus, appendicitis, or seizures. Cyclic vomiting remains a poorly understood disorder, occurring in older children who may have psychologic and/or migraine components.

Differential Diagnosis

The differential diagnosis of persistent emesis may be organized in different modes, including mechanism of vomiting, anatomic locus of the stimulus, associated signs and symptoms, or by age. Because most clinicians approach differential diagnosis by age of the patient, diagnostic considerations are presented here according to age.

Young Infants Under 2 Weeks of Age

Any vomiting in a young infant may create concern and raise the possibility of numerous conditions, ranging from benign to life-threatening disorders (Box 20-1). Most infants who vomit do not have serious disorders and often have one of several functional causes of emesis. Innocent vomiting, the most common cause of vomiting, may be seen in nearly half of all infants. Infants vomit easily without nausea, retching, pain, or discomfort as frequently as several times an hour. Innocent vomiting can be distinguished from gastroesophageal reflux (GER) in that it lacks the pathologic features associated with GER, such as hematemesis, apnea, aspiration pneumonia, wheezing, cough, or failure to thrive. Parental reassurance that innocent vomiting spontaneously resolves usually is the only intervention required.

Improper formula preparation (usually too concentrated) as a cause of vomiting can be ascertained easily by history. A can of formula concentrate (13 oz) is properly mixed with a can of water to produce 26 oz of 20-calorie-per-ounce formula. Powdered formula requires 1 measured scoop of powder to 2 oz of water to yield an appropriate concentration. Too little water raises gastrointestinal and renal solute loads, leading to vomiting, diarrhea, obligatory water losses, and dehydration. Aerophagia is common, especially in bottle-fed infants, who tend to gulp formula. Excessive discomfort and flatus may accompany vomiting. Frequent burping or the use of collapsible formula containers may provide some relief. Excessive postcibal handling also may lead to spitting and emesis.

Nervous vomiting, another cause of functional emesis, often accompanies other behavioral manifestations of infant stress, frequently resulting in failure to thrive. Infants may be described as tense or nervous and may also have disturbed sleep patterns. Maternal anxiety causes increased muscle tension that is transmitted to the infant, resulting in increased heart rate and muscle tone. Nervous vomiting may be easily diagnosed as GER, in which vomiting is a primary disorder. Parental anxiety in nervous vomiting can be part of a vicious cycle that leads to and perpetuates emesis in the child. Parental anxiety about other concerns are transmitted to the child, causing vomiting that increases parental distress further, thus increasing the child's emesis even more. Recognizing sources of parental distress and relieving their fears concerning the child's morbidity may interrupt the vicious cycle and allow emesis to resolve. At times, mental health counseling for the parent may be helpful if the role of anxiety is recognized.

GER easily can be confused with nervous vomiting. GER may present as early as the newborn period with nonbilious, effortless emesis without abdominal distension. An extensive review of GER by Orenstein summarizes the manifestations of reflux in infants as follows: regurgitation with loss of calories, apnea, irritability, ruminative behaviors, stridor, lower respiratory tract symptoms, and neurobehavioral abnormalities. Most infants spontaneously improve during the first year of life. Diagnostic evaluation should include a barium swallow and upper gastrointestinal series (UGI) to exclude a partial gastric or high intestinal obstruction. An esophageal biopsy may find evidence of esophagitis with increased papillary height, infiltration of the epithelium by eosinophils, or Barrett esophagitis, resulting in replacement of squamous epithelium with columnar epithelium. The gold standard for diagnosing reflux is 24-hour monitoring of intraluminal esophageal pH. Quantification of the number of acid reflux episodes, average duration of episodes, and the total proportion of time acid is in contact with esophageal epithelium determine a reflux score that is age dependent.

In contrast to functional causes of vomiting, gastrointestinal obstruction may be life-threatening and demands immediate attention. Bilious vomiting often is the presenting symptom of obstruction. Lilien and others found that in the first

---

BOX 20-1

Common Causes of Vomiting in Infants Under 2 Weeks of Age

Functional
  Innocent
  Improper formula preparation
  Aerophagia
  Postcibal handling
  Nervous
Gastroesophageal reflux
Gastrointestinal obstruction
  Esophageal (atresia, stenosis, vascular ring, TEF, cricopharyngeal incoordination, achalasia, hiatal hernia, diaphragmatic hernia)
Torsion of the stomach
Malrotation with or without volvulus
Intestine (atresia, stenosis, meconium ileus with CF, meconium plug)
Webs
Annular pancreas
Paralytic ileus (peritonitis, postoperative, acute infection, hypokalemia)
  Hirschsprung disease
  Imperforate anus
  Enteric duplication
Other gastrointestinal causes (necrotizing enterocolitis, congenital lactose intolerance, milk-soy protein intolerance, lactobeazor, GI perforation, hepatitis, pancreatitis)
Neurologic (increased ICP [subdural, hydrocephalus, edema], kernicterus)
Renal (obstructive uropathy, renal insufficiency)
Infection (systemic infections, pyelonephritis)
Metabolic (urea cycle deficiencies, aminoacidopathies, disorders of carbohydrate metabolism, acidosis, congenital adrenal hyperplasia, tetany, hypercalcemia)
Drugs/toxins (theophylline, caffeine, digoxin)
Blood (swallowed maternal blood, gastritis, ulcers)
Respiratory (pneumonia, wheezing)
Postoperative anesthesia
Dysautonomia

CF, Cystic fibrosis; *GI,* gastrointestinal; *ICP,* intracranial pressure; *TEF,* tracheoesophageal fistula.

72 hours of life, one out of every five infants with bilious emesis required surgical intervention. Diagnoses included malrotation, jejunal atresia or stenosis, jejunal duplication, and myofibromatosis. Nonsurgical obstructions include meconium plug and left microcolon. Over two thirds of the infants with bilious vomiting had idiopathic bilious vomiting with a benign course that led to resolution by 1 week of age. However, another review of bilious emesis in the first week of life by Kao found that more than half of the infants required surgical intervention, with an overall mortality of 8.7%. Risk factors for surgical conditions included green

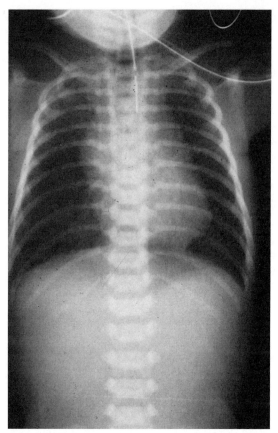

FIG. 20-1 A distended proximal esophageal pouch indicates esophageal atresia. If air is in the intestine (not demonstrated here), a fistula is present between the trachea and distal esophagus.

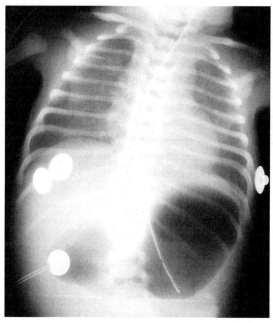

FIG. 20-2 Classic "double bubble" resulting from air in the stomach and proximal duodenum in duodenal atresia.

emesis, abdominal distension, poor feeding, irritability, lethargy, and abdominal tenderness. Those infants who did not have surgical conditions generally lacked lethargy or abdominal tenderness. In both studies, abdominal plain films as a first line examination were helpful if specific findings were noted. Nearly half of infants with specific findings had surgical problems in Lilien's study, and no patient with a normal plain film had a surgical condition in Kao's study. Contrast studies (either UGI or barium enema) are indicated for those patients with signs of complete obstruction, perforation, or peritonitis if plain films are abnormal and the clinical condition does not improve.

Repetitive nonbilious emesis may indicate obstruction proximal to the ampulla of Vater. Esophageal atresia or tracheoesophageal fistula usually present in the newborn period with excessive spitting of mucus from the atretic proximal esophageal pouch. Inability to pass a catheter into the stomach confirms the proximal atresia. Gas in the abdomen indicates a connection of the distal esophagus to the airway (Fig. 20-1). Pyloric stenosis rarely causes emesis in the newborn but is a common cause of nonbilious emesis in the infant 4 to 8 weeks of age. Duodenal atresia (Fig. 20-2) may cause nonbilious emesis if the atretic segment is proximal to the ampulla of Vater, although there may be a communication between the hepatobiliary system and the proximal duodenum.

Postampullary obstructions comprise the majority of obstructions in the newborn and often cause bilious emesis. Duodenal atresia represents 25% of small bowel atresias. Annular pancreas results from fusion of the anterior and posterior segments of the pancreas around the midduodenum. Malrotation, with or without midgut volvulus, can cause obstructive symptoms from the newborn period well into adulthood. Neonates with acute onset of bilious vomiting have a high incidence of malrotation and midgut volvulus. Thick, tenacious meconium causes meconium ileus and obstruction in about 10% of patients with cystic fibrosis (Fig. 20-3). The meconium plug syndrome is characterized by plugs of inspissated meconium occluding the distal colon (Fig. 20-4). Although this condition is not associated with cystic fibrosis, atresias and Hirschsprung disease must be considered. Functional obstruction in Hirschsprung disease is caused by the absence of ganglion cells in the parasympathetic myenteric nerve plexus of the colon and rectum. The aganglionic segment is contracted, with distension of the more proximal colon (see Fig. 17-6 and 17-7). Absence of ganglion cells demonstrated on rectal biopsy with cholinesterase stain is diagnostic.

Other gastrointestinal causes of vomiting in the newborn include necrotizing enterocolitis (NEC). Typically the infant with NEC is premature, possibly has respiratory distress, and

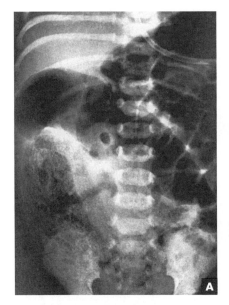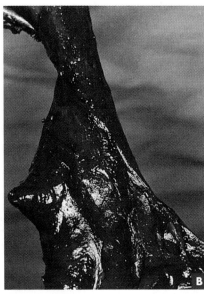

FIG. 20-3 *A,* Meconium ileus seen as large, dilated loops of bowel in the right lower quadrant, with a "soap bubble" appearance. *B,* Thick tenacious meconium removed from the intestine at surgery.

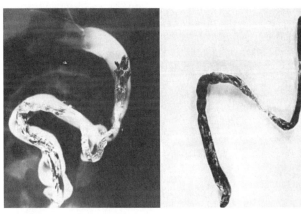

FIG. 20-4 Meconium plug syndrome. Meconium was outlined by barium *(left),* and the plug was removed by Gastrografin enema *(right).*

develops vomiting, abdominal distension, and signs of sepsis and shock. Abdominal radiographs may demonstrate intramural air (pneumatosis intestinalis) or hepatic portal venous gas (Fig. 20-5). Protein intolerance commonly causes inflammatory colitis in infants with blood and mucus in stools, but vomiting also can be seen. As many as 25% of infants who exhibit intolerance to cow's milk protein are also intolerant to soy protein. Treatment consists of offering the infant an elemental formula (or omitting cow's milk from the mother's diet in the case of the breast-feeding infant). Hepatitis resulting from any disorder, ranging from infection to toxic or metabolic causes, may be associated with emesis, and pancreatitis also can cause vomiting, usually coincident with abdominal pain.

Increased intracranial pressure (ICP) caused by subdural effusions, hydrocephalus, cerebral edema, or congenital malformations stimulating the vomiting centers causes vomiting.

The mechanisms by which kernicterus causes emesis are unclear.

Renal disorders, such as obstructive uropathy (see Fig. 1-5), and renal insufficiency of any etiology may cause emesis either by activating afferent vagal nerves or toxins affecting the AP. Systemic infections (e.g., meningitis and sepsis) and localized infections (e.g., pyelonephritis) probably induce vomiting through similar mechanisms as other visceral inflammatory disorders.

A wide variety of metabolic disorders in the newborn may have associated vomiting. Urea cycle enzyme deficiencies with hyperammonemia cause vomiting via toxic stimulation of the AP. Aminoacidopathies, galactosemia, fructose intolerance, glycogen storage diseases, lactic acidosis, disorders of calcium metabolism, and congenital adrenal hyperplasia all may cause recurrent neonatal vomiting by differing mechanisms. Drugs and toxins may produce vomiting either by directly stimulating vagal afferents or by affecting the AP. Blood in the gastrointestinal tract acts as an irritant and often causes vomiting. In the newborn it is important to try to determine the source of blood, whether it is of maternal or infant origin, through the use of the Apt test. Respiratory distress from pneumonia or even bronchospasm may be associated with vomiting. As with GER, bronchospasm may be secondary to reflux or may cause emesis. Postoperative vomiting is common at any age and depends on factors such as which anesthetic agent was used, age of the patient, previous history of postoperative emesis, and the type of surgery performed.

Infants 2 Weeks to 12 Months of Age

Although many of the same causes of vomiting in the young neonate cause vomiting in the older infant, other diagnostic possibilities also must be considered (Box 20-2). In addition to

Common Causes of Vomiting in Infants 2 Weeks to 12 Months of Age

Functional
   Innocent
   Improper formula preparation
   Aerophagia
   Postcibal handling
   Nervous
   Rumination
Gastroesophageal reflux, esophagitis
Gastrointestinal obstruction
   Esophageal (foreign body, stenosis, vascular ring, TEF, cricopharyngeal incoordination, achalasia, hiatal hernia)
   Stomach (bezoar, lactobeazor)
   Intestine (pyloric stenosis, malrotation with or without volvulus, complications of a Meckel diverticulum, intussusception, incarcerated hernia, Hirschsprung disease, appendicitis, duplications)
Other gastrointestinal causes (annular pancreas, paralytic ileus, hypokalemia, *Helicobacter* sp. infection, peritonitis, pancreatitis, celiac disease, viral and bacterial enteritis, lactose intolerance, milk-soy protein intolerance, cholecystitis, gallstones, pseudoobstruction)
Neurologic (increased ICP [subdural, hydrocephalus, edema])
Renal (obstructive uropathy, renal insufficiency, stones)
Infectious (meningitis, sepsis, pyelonephritis, otitis media, sinusitis, pertussis, hepatitis, parasitic infestation)
Metabolic (urea cycle deficiencies, aminoacidopathies, disorder of carbohydrate metabolism, acidosis, congenital adrenal hyperplasia, tetany, hypercalcemia)
Drugs/toxins (aspirin, theophylline, digoxin, iron, ipecac)
Blood
Hydrometrocolpos
Radiation/chemotherapy
Reye syndrome
Postoperative
Psychogenic
Munchausen syndrome by proxy

ICP, Intracranial pressure; *TEF,* tracheoesophageal fistula.

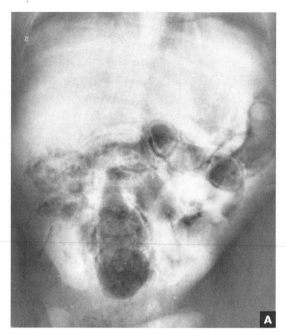

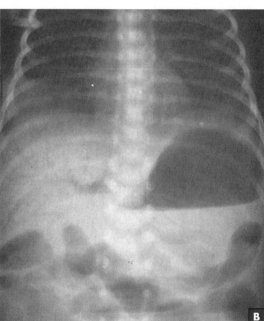

FIG. 20-5 Necrotizing enterocolitis demonstrating intramural air *(A)* and gas within the portal system *(B).*

the causes of functional vomiting previously discussed, rumination can be seen in infants. Rumination is characterized by regurgitation of food, which may be rechewed, reswallowed, or expelled. It usually begins between 3 and 12 months of age, often as a result of a disturbed mother-infant relationship. It has been postulated that the mother does not fulfill a nurturing role, and the infant resorts to internal satisfaction through regurgitation of food. Mentally retarded individuals, on the other hand, use rumination as self-stimulation and self-gratification. Generally these individuals have later onset of rumination at just over 1 year of age. Ruminators often initiate regurgitation with vigorous sucking of fingers, leading to gagging and regurgitation. Later, they may use tongue thrusting or contraction of abdominal muscles. Rumination can be differentiated from GER by the following characteristics: (1) rumination responds poorly to antireflux management; (2) rumination is done with-

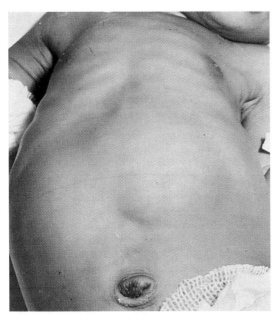

FIG. 20-6 Giant retrograde peristaltic wave marches across the abdomen of a patient with pyloric stenosis.

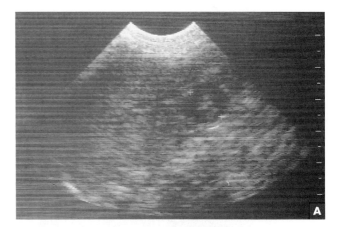

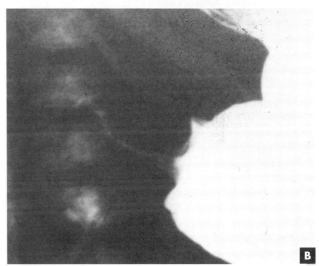

FIG. 20-7 Pyloric stenosis. *A,* Ultrasound demonstrating thickened pyloric muscle, as shown by a lucent ring. *B,* Barium study showing indentation of the gastric antrum by the pyloric mass.

out distress; (3) rumination does not occur during sleep; (4) other self-stimulatory behavior, such as rocking or head rolling, is present; and (5) the parent is unable to nurture the infant.

Various disorders causing gastrointestinal obstruction must be considered. Perhaps the most common cause of intestinal obstruction in this age group is pyloric stenosis. Pyloric stenosis usually affects infant boys, frequently firstborn, with nonbilious emesis presenting between 4 and 8 weeks of age (Fig. 20-6). Palpation of the characteristic olive is virtually diagnostic, but sonography or UGI can be used to confirm clinical suspicion (Fig. 20-7). Torsion of a Meckel diverticulum about its fibrous attachment to the abdominal wall may lead to obstruction, pain, and emesis. Intussusception is a relatively common cause of persistent vomiting, and its peak age of onset is in the latter half of the first year of life. Viral infections, polyps, and rarely tumors provide a lead point for the intussusception. Severe abdominal pain, vomiting, and ultimately the passage of mucousy, bloody stool (currant jelly stool) is the classic triad of symptoms. Often a mass is palpable in the right lower quadrant in the typical ileocolic intussusception (Fig. 20-8). Diagnosis can be made by barium enema (Fig. 20-9), and hydrostatic or pneumatic reduction usually can be performed at the same time. Incarcerated hernias and appendicitis also may have emesis as a presenting sign, although appendicitis in the young infant easily can be missed.

Other gastrointestinal disorders in this age group include viral and bacterial enteritis, *Helicobacter* species infection, celiac disease, cholecystitis, cholelithiasis, and pseudoobstruction. The most common cause of vomiting in children is viral gastroenteritis, with rotavirus enteritis being the proto-

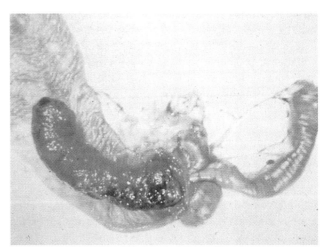

FIG. 20-8 Pathology specimen of ileocolic intussusception with a portion of ileum protruding into the cecum through the ileocecal valve. The normal appendix is to the right.

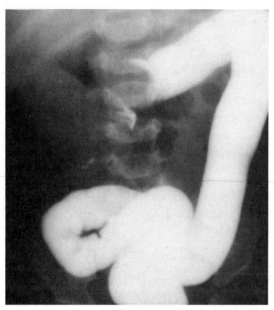

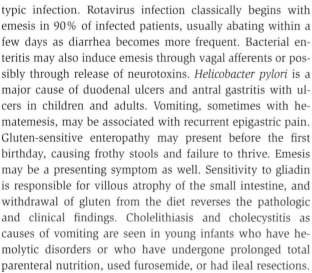

FIG. 20-9 Barium enema in intussusception. The column of barium stops and outlines the intussusceptum.

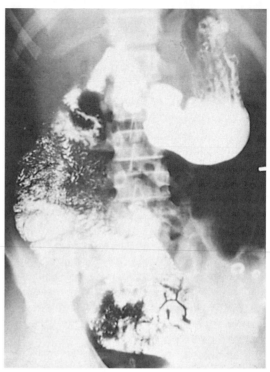

FIG. 20-10 Upper gastrointestinal series in malrotation. The ligament of Treitz is absent or abnormally located, the duodenum is partially obstructed by Ladd bands, and the small intestine lies on the right side of the abdomen. Midgut volvulus may occur, creating complete obstruction.

typic infection. Rotavirus infection classically begins with emesis in 90% of infected patients, usually abating within a few days as diarrhea becomes more frequent. Bacterial enteritis may also induce emesis through vagal afferents or possibly through release of neurotoxins. *Helicobacter pylori* is a major cause of duodenal ulcers and antral gastritis with ulcers in children and adults. Vomiting, sometimes with hematemesis, may be associated with recurrent epigastric pain. Gluten-sensitive enteropathy may present before the first birthday, causing frothy stools and failure to thrive. Emesis may be a presenting symptom as well. Sensitivity to gliadin is responsible for villous atrophy of the small intestine, and withdrawal of gluten from the diet reverses the pathologic and clinical findings. Cholelithiasis and cholecystitis as causes of vomiting are seen in young infants who have hemolytic disorders or who have undergone prolonged total parenteral nutrition, used furosemide, or had ileal resections.

As in young neonates, increased ICP, renal disorders (now including calculi), and infections can produce vomiting in the older infant. Otitis media, perhaps through stimulation of the vestibular nerves, sometimes causes emesis. Sinusitis, with its attendant postnasal drip and mucous drainage, stimulates vomiting. Paroxysms of cough with pertussis infection may stimulate the gag reflex and induce emesis. The older infant, especially with increased mobility, is at risk for ingestion of foreign bodies, although the toddler is at even higher risk. Reye syndrome, now an uncommon disorder, usually be-

gins with pernicious emesis shortly after the resolution of a viral infection. Hyperammonemia, increased ICP, hepatitis, and a variety of metabolites may share in the pathogenesis of vomiting associated with Reye syndrome.

Radiation and chemotherapy are notorious for producing vomiting as a complication. These stimuli are so strong that some patients become nauseated or vomit before repeated therapy is begun, involving higher cortical centers that stimulate the vomiting center in a learned behavioral response. The success of 5-HT$_3$ receptor antagonists (e.g., ondansetron) in the treatment of chemotherapy-induced vomiting has given insight into the mechanisms of anticancer therapy emesis.

Munchausen syndrome by proxy (MSP) should be considered in a child with persistent or recurrent emesis that occurs only in the presence of the mother or cannot be independently substantiated. Emetic drugs, especially ipecac, have been given to infants to feign illness. Finding ipecac in serum or stool or resolution of symptoms when the patient is separated from the mother supports the diagnosis of MSP.

Children Older Than 12 Months of Age

By the time the child reaches the first birthday, most congenital causes of vomiting have been discovered. Gastrointestinal obstructions are usually acquired conditions by this age (Box 20-3). As the child becomes more mobile, the possibility of foreign bodies causing obstruction increases. Swallowed

Common Causes of Vomiting in Children Older Than 12 Months of Age

Gastroesophageal reflux
Gastrointestinal obstruction
 Esophageal (esophagitis, foreign body, corrosive ingestion, hiatal hernia)
 Stomach (foreign body, bezoar, chronic granulomatous disease)
 Intestine (pyloric channel ulcer, intramural hematoma, malrotation with or without volvulus, complications of a Meckel diverticulum, meconium ileus in cystic fibrosis, incarcerated hernia, intussusception, Hirschsprung disease, ulcerative colitis, Crohn disease, superior mesenteric artery syndrome)
Other gastrointestinal causes (annular pancreas, paralytic ileus, hypokalemia, *Helicobacter* sp. infection, peritonitis, pancreatitis, celiac disease, viral and bacterial enteritis, hepatobiliary disease including stones, Henoch-Schönlein purpura, typhlitis)
Neurologic (increased ICP, Leigh disease, migraine, motion sickness, seizures)
Renal (obstructive uropathy, renal insufficiency, stones)
Infection (meningitis, sepsis, pyelonephritis, otitis media, sinusitis, pertussis, hepatitis, parasitic infestation, streptococcal pharyngitis, labyrinthitis)
Metabolic (inborn errors of metabolism, acidosis, diabetic ketoacidosis, adrenal insufficiency)
Drugs/toxins (aspirin, theophylline, digoxin, iron, lead, ipecac, some "recreational drugs")
Torsion of the testis or ovary
Blood
Radiation/chemotherapy
Reye syndrome
Postoperative
Cyclic vomiting
Pregnancy
Psychologic (bulimia, anorexia nervosa, stress, Munchausen syndrome by proxy)

coins may lodge in the esophagus, usually orienting in a transverse position. Prolonged pressure on esophageal mucosa leads to ulceration, stenosis, and even perforation. Ingestion of button batteries can be particularly dangerous because of the size and chemical composition of the battery. In a large review of more than 2300 ingestions of button batteries, 10% of patients were symptomatic, with generally larger-sized batteries (greater than 18 mm) having a greater tendency to become lodged in the esophagus. Also, lithium batteries had disproportionately larger adverse effects because of the greater voltage, and mercury batteries had a greater propensity to fragment and release mercury into the

gut. Perforation of the esophagus caused by button battery ingestion also has been reported.

Chronic granulomatous disease can produce granulmatous inflammation of the antrum, leading to bleeding, anorexia, and vomiting as presenting manifestations. Pyloric channel ulcers may be associated with sufficient edema and pylorospasm to produce emesis, and intramural hematomas may also cause partial obstruction and vomiting. This latter condition can be seen with blunt abdominal trauma (e.g., handlebar injury or child abuse) or Henoch-Schönlein purpura. Inflammatory bowel disease may cause emesis from obstruction because of transmural inflammation, such as in Crohn disease, megacolon associated with ulcerative colitis, or direct inflammation and stimulation of vagal afferents. Pseudoobstruction is a poorly understood disorder of intestinal motility, causing vomiting, diarrhea, constipation, poor growth, and an abnormal UGI, demonstrating poor motility. The superior mesenteric artery (SMA) syndrome may be seen as a secondary phenomenon when the patient has experienced weight loss, has had excessive lordosis, has been in a body cast for a prolonged period, or has had lengthy bed rest or previous abdominal surgery. Proponents of this disorder claim the duodenum is trapped between the aorta posteriorly and the SMA. The existence of this syndrome has been questioned.

Other gastrointestinal causes of emesis overlap significantly with the younger age group. Celiac disease may be more prevalent in the older age group, and patients with malignancies, especially leukemia, can develop typhlitis–ileocecal inflammation sometimes leading to necrosis. Malrotation, with or without intermittent volvulus, can cause symptoms in older children as well. Half of older children and one third of patients with chronic symptoms and/or nonbilious vomiting had midgut volvulus at surgery. Some children were reported to have symptoms of intermittent pain and emesis for as long as 17 years (Fig. 20-10).

A wide variety of drugs (prescription, nonprescription, and "recreational") have emesis as a possible side effect. Torsion of the testis or ovary produces acute, excruciating pain and vomiting rather than persistent emesis. Pregnancy must always be considered in a postpubertal female with persistent emesis.

Psychologic disorders associated with recurrent emesis include stress from virtually any cause in susceptible individuals, anorexia nervosa, and bulimia. Anorexia nervosa and bulimia may coexist, but when they occur separately, patients with anorexia have progressive, relentless weight loss whereas patients with bulimia tend to maintain weight. Subtle signs of chronic self-induced vomiting may include abrasions or callouses on knuckles and eroded enamel of the teeth from gastric acid.

Neurologic causes of vomiting include increased ICP from any cause, often with headache and emesis in early morning hours or upon arising in the morning. Motion sickness occurs through stimulation of the labyrinthine system, which has neural radiations to the medullary vomiting centers. Antihistamines or scopolamine often are effective in reducing nausea and vomiting. Abdominal epilepsy is a rare disorder, with seizures sometimes associated with emesis, abdominal pain, transient disturbances of consciousness, and altered electroencephalographic (EEG) findings. Occipitotemporal seizures, with spread of the electrical activity to limbic structures, cause vomiting in the late stages of the attacks. Often these patients are diagnosed as having migraine-seizure syndromes. Migraine headache frequently has emesis as part of the presentation, and the diagnosis of classic or common migraine usually is not difficult when typical headache pain is associated with emesis.

Ureteropelvic obstruction can cause flank pain or abdominal pain with vomiting as the renal pelvis distends during diuresis (Dietl syndrome). Obstruction occurs because of a relative narrowing of the proximal ureter, commonly at the junction with the renal pelvis; intrinsic narrowing of the ureter; high-riding insertion of the ureter into the renal pelvis; or an anomalous vessel crossing and partially obstructing the ureter. Diagnosis can be confirmed with sonography performed during a crisis, demonstrating a dilated renal pelvis, intravenous pyelogram, or diuretic-enhanced radionuclide renal scan.

Cyclic vomiting is a poorly understood and frustrating problem for patients, parents, and physicians alike. It is defined as bouts of vomiting that recur after intervals of varying lengths and may continue for days or weeks. Other causes of vomiting must be excluded before making this diagnosis. Onset of vomiting usually is sudden and is associated with lethargy. Without intervention, emesis may continue for days or weeks. Headache, abdominal pain, and fever sometimes are associated with the vomiting. Most episodes of cyclic vomiting begin before age 6 and end by age 14, with duration of symptoms ranging from 2 to 13 years. Attacks usually last 4 days or less. Diagnoses to be considered include porphyria, partial ornithine transcarbamylase deficiency, organic acidemias, medium-chain acyl-CoA dehydrogenase deficiency, Addison disease, sinusitis, obstructive uropathy, and gastrointestinal disorders, such as malrotation with intermittent volvulus. Endoscopy should also be considered to exclude mucosal injuries. Causes of cyclic vomiting have ranged from a psychiatric disorder to migraine and epilepsy. Reinhart and colleagues found a high incidence of psychiatric distress with parental and patient anxiety, symbiotic relationships between parent and child, and patients regressing "too easily." Jernigan and Ware found EEG changes that they postulated were evidence for cyclic vomiting being a migraine equivalent, and Hammond found that 20% of pediatric patients had persistent emesis as adults. Treatment generally has been unsatisfactory, although early and aggressive use of intravenous glucose and perhaps the use of prokinetic agents, such as erythromycin or cisapride, may be beneficial.

History

The history and physical examination are essential in guiding the clinician to appropriate diagnostic tests and ultimately the correct diagnosis (Table 20-1).

An important early factor in the evaluation of vomiting is the appearance of the vomitus. Gastric aspirates greater than 20 cc in infants or bilious emesis suggests intestinal obstruction. Maternal polyhydramnios is also an indication of fetal intestinal obstruction. If uncurdled milk is regurgitated, esophageal atresia, esophageal obstruction above the stomach, or esophageal diverticulum might be considered if food is not acted upon by gastric acid. Absence of bile suggests obstruction proximal to the ampulla of Vater or possibly GER, or rumination. Feculent emesis is associated with peritonitis or lower small bowel or colonic obstruction. Blood, an irritating agent, can be found in emesis even if it is not derived from the gastrointestinal tract. Epistaxis or pharyngeal bleeding with swallowed blood may result in characteristic red hematemesis or a coffee-ground appearance of digested blood. Hematemesis from the gastrointestinal tract may come from ulcers anywhere from the esophagus to the pylorus, including erosions of esophageal varices. Corrosive agents to mucosa, such as alkali, theophylline, and iron, may cause bleeding. Bleeding diatheses, vasculitides, and arteriovenous malformations also must be considered.

The character of the emetic act may direct the clinician to a particular mechanism. Innocent vomiting in the young infant occurs without retching or pain and is nonbilious. Overfeeding is a common cause of recurrent emesis, but children experience normal to above-normal weight gain despite recurrent emesis. Innocent vomiting differs from rumination because patients with innocent vomiting do not engage in tongue thrusting or vigorous hand or finger sucking that induces emesis. Also, careful questioning does not reveal evidence of a disturbed maternal-child relationship in innocent vomiting. GER also may be relatively effortless and nonbilious. However, associated symptoms of respiratory distress, wheezing, pneumonia, irritability, poor growth, apnea, hematemesis, or chronic cough often are found with GER. Nervous vomiting is similar to GER, but a detailed history may reveal maternal anxiety and stress in the maternal-infant diad. Questions concerning formula preparation, air gulping, and postcibal handling may be revealing. Projectile or forceful emesis often is seen in gastric-outlet obstruction (e.g., pyloric stenosis) or metabolic disorders.

Vomiting occurring early in the morning may suggest increased ICP, gagging caused by postnasal drip from sinusitis, or possibly pregnancy. Emesis related to meals is found in patients with peptic ulcer disease or psychogenic eating disorders. If specific foods induce emesis, food allergy or intolerance should be suspected, including milk, soy, gluten, or other protein intolerances. Metabolic disorders (e.g., fructose intolerance) also have emesis associated with consumption of specific foods containing the offending agent.

Other gastrointestinal symptoms often are associated with emesis. Nausea usually accompanies and precedes emesis, but lack of nausea may point to increased ICP or intestinal obstruction. Pain on swallowing (odynophagia) or difficulty swallowing (dysphagia) suggests esophageal involvement. Diarrhea most frequently is the result of an infectious disor-

---

TABLE 20-1

Key Historical Questions

Characteristic	Implication
Appearance of Vomitus	
Large volume, bilious	Obstruction, maternal polyhydramnios
Uncurdled milk, undigested food	Esophageal atresia, obstruction, diverticulum
Absence of bile	Preampullary obstruction, GER, rumination
Feculent emesis	Peritonitis, lower bowel obstruction
Bloody, coffee-ground appearance	Respiratory tract bleeding, esophageal bleeding, Mallory-Weiss syndrome, ulcers, gastritis, corrosive ingestions, theophylline, bleeding diathesis, AVM
Character of Emetic Act	
Effortless, nonbilious	Overfeeding, innocent vomiting, GER
Tongue thrusting	Rumination, GER
Finger sucking, gagging	Rumination
Altered maternal-child relationship	Rumination, nervous vomiting
Projectile vomiting	Gastric outlet obstruction, metabolic disorders
Timing of Emesis	
Early morning	Increased ICP, sinusitis, pregnancy
Related to meals	Peptic ulcers, psychogenic
Related to foods	Milk- or soy-protein intolerance, metabolic disorders
Other Gastrointestinal Symptoms	
Lack of nausea	Increased ICP, intestinal obstruction
Swallowing difficulties	Esophagitis, stenosis, obstruction
Constipation	Obstruction, hypercalcemia
Pain	Specific organ involvement
Jaundice	Hepatobiliary disease
Neurologic Symptoms	
Headache	Migraine, increased ICP, abdominal epilepsy
Seizures	Abdominal epilepsy
General	
Well appearing	Functional vomiting, GER, rumination
Ill appearing	Infection, ingestion, inflammation, obstruction
Respiratory distress	Bronchospasm, pneumonia
Travel, animal/pet exposure	Infection
Epidemic/family members ill	Infection
Stress	Psychogenic

AVM, Atrioventricular malformation; *GER*, gastroesophageal reflux; *ICP*, intracranial pressure.

---

der, toxins (e.g., *Clostridium difficile*), or partial obstruction. Conversely, constipation can be found in obstruction or hypercalcemia. Abdominal pain may localize to the involved organ, suggesting inflammation or obstruction. Flank pain suggests renal disease, with infection or obstruction. Jaundice indicates involvement of the hepatobiliary system.

Neurologic symptoms may indicate structural toxic or metabolic disorders. Episodic severe headache in patients who have a family history of severe headache may be caused by a migraine syndrome. Constant headache, worse with Valsalva maneuver and occurring with morning emesis, strongly suggests increased ICP.

General questions give an overall view of the patient and environment. Well-appearing infants may have functional vomiting, GER, or psychologic causes of vomiting. Ill-appearing children may have infections, ingestions, specific organ inflammation (e.g., pancreatitis), or surgical conditions, such as obstruction or appendicitis. Fever suggests inflammation or infection. Respiratory distress might indicate bronchospasm or pneumonia. History of travel, animal or pet exposure, community epidemics, or ill family members may give important clues to infectious causes of vomiting. Separate interviews with parents and the older patient may reveal stress or evidence of psychologic disturbances.

TABLE 20-2

Key Physical Findings

Finding	Implication
Vital Signs	
Tachycardia	Dehydration, infection, fever
Bradycardia	Anorexia nervosa
Tachypnea	Pneumonia, bronchospasm
Fever	Inflammation, infection
Hypotension	Dehydration
Hypertension	Anxiety, renal disease, abdominal masses
Short stature	Chronic illness, Crohn disease
Poor weight gain	Decreased caloric retention, chronic illness
Abdomen	
Distension	Aerophagia, lactose intolerance, ascites, organomegaly, masses, obstruction
Absent bowel sounds	Ileus, toxins, advanced obstruction
Increased bowel sounds	Early obstruction, diarrhea
Pain	Localized organ involvement
Rebound tenderness	Peritonitis
Masses	Duplication, tumor, Crohn disease, intussusception, pyloric stenosis
Genitourinary System	
Adnexal pain	Torsion of ovary, pelvic inflammatory disease
Mass	Ovarian cyst, pregnancy, hydrometrocolpos
Rectal mass	Abscess, inflamed bowel, duplication, tumor
Respiratory tract	Bronchospasm, pneumonia
Neurologic	Migraine, seizures, increased ICP
Renal (flank pain)	Pyelonephritis, obstructive uropathy
Skin	
Rash	Drug reaction, infection
Purpura	Trauma, Henoch-Schönlein purpura

Physical Examination

The physical examination should be meticulous and complete (Table 20-2). Vital signs and growth parameters are basic introductions to the examination. Tachycardia may indicate dehydration, whereas bradycardia can be seen in anorexia nervosa with severe weight loss. Tachypnea indicates respiratory tract involvement, and fever may signal infection or inflammation in general. Hypotension may coexist with dehydration, and hypertension can be associated with anxiety, renal disease, abdominal masses compressing the kidney, or a host of other disorders. Plotting weight over time may give the clinician an indication of severity of emesis, caloric loss, and the estimated time of onset of illness. Linear growth is also important to measure. Inflammatory bowel disease may be relatively silent except for poor linear growth, and emesis may be a later finding.

Careful examination of the abdomen is crucial. Abdominal distension can be seen with excessive air or gas (aerophagia or lactose intolerance), fluid (ascites), organomegaly, masses, or obstruction. High intestinal obstruction may not cause significant distension, although epigastric distension is seen on occasion. Lower bowel obstructions often are associated with distension. Absent bowel sounds occur with ileus, toxins, or advanced obstruction. Increased peristaltic sounds may be heard in early obstruction, including pyloric stenosis. Abdominal pain may help to localize the organ or involvement, and tenderness to percussion or rebound tenderness indicates peritonitis. Palpation may reveal hepatosplenomegaly or nephromegaly. Other masses might indicate duplications, tumors, masses of Crohn disease, intussusception, or pyloric stenosis.

Careful examination of the genitourinary system, especially in girls, might reveal torsion of the ovary, chronic pelvic inflammatory disease, or possibly pregnancy. A rectal examination, examining for perirectal disease seen with Crohn disease (see Fig. 1-2), masses, localized tenderness, or blood in the stool, is imperative for any patient with persistent vomiting.

Examination of the respiratory tract might reveal wheezes, rhonchi, or rales, indicating bronchospasm or pneumonia. The neurologic examination should be complete, particularly examining the fontanelle in infants and fundi in older children for evidence of increased ICP. Costovertebral angle tenderness signals possible pyelonephritis, and the skin may have flushing or rash consistent with toxins or drugs that may cause emesis.

Approach to the Patient

The initial approach to the patient with emesis should be to determine whether or not intestinal obstruction is present. In the neonate, if obstruction is suspected clinically, an abdominal radiograph is indicated, and perhaps decubitus films should be obtained to examine for free air if perforation is suspected. An abdominal sonogram may be helpful, particularly in the gasless abdomen. If plain films are normal and the patient is clinically stable, a UGI may be indicated, particularly using low-osmolality contrast media. Evaluation for sepsis and metabolic disturbances (e.g., hypoglycemia, hypocalcemia, and electrolyte abnormalities) is also indicated. If no obstruction is suspected, the clinician should search for extraintestinal clues. If none point to systemic infections, neurologic disease, renal disease, or cardiopulmonary disorders, then necrotizing enterocolitis, GER, functional vomiting, or other gastrointestinal disorders should be considered.

Obstruction suspected in infants beyond the neonatal period might herald other disorders. A typical history of nonbilious emesis in a firstborn boy 4 to 8 weeks of age might indicate pyloric stenosis, and if an olivelike mass is palpated, perhaps no other diagnostic tests are indicated. However, if no mass is palpated, ultrasound or UGI might be diagnostic. Other obstructive lesions can be determined by plain film or contrast studies. Obstructive lesions of older children can be approached in a similar fashion with plain radiographs, ultrasound, and contrast studies where indicated. Upper endoscopy may be indicated in persistent emesis without obstructive symptoms, especially if the patient has hematemesis. Computed tomography of the abdomen may delineate abdominal masses or intravisceral structural changes. If GER is suspected, esophageal biopsy or possibly 24-hour intraesophageal pH probe might be diagnostic. Renal ultrasound, intravenous pyelography, or radionuclide renal scans help in distinguishing among pyelonephritis, scarring, and obstructive uropathy. Routine hematologic and biochemical screening tests, along with serum aminotransferase levels, amylase, and lipase, are excellent screening tests for abdominal pain with emesis. Urinalysis and urine culture might point to genitourinary disorders causing emesis. Pregnancy testing should be considered in any postpubertal female with persistent emesis. Toxicologic testing is helpful, particularly if extraintestinal symptoms are noted. If stress, anxiety, or evidence of psychiatric illness is found, consultation with a qualified psychiatrist may be indicated.

The approach to the patient must include evaluation for the cause of vomiting, as well as the complications of persistent vomiting (Box 20-4). Vomiting produces several metabolic complications. Dehydration occurs because of the loss of fluids from emesis and the inability to ingest adequate fluids be-

---

BOX 20-4

Complications of Vomiting

Dehydration
Metabolic alkalosis
Hypokalemia
Weight loss, failure to thrive
Hematemesis
Mallory-Weiss syndrome (linear esophageal tears)
Esophagitis

---

cause of anorexia, nausea, or immediate emesis. Metabolic alkalosis occurs as a result of loss of gastric hydrochloric acid and intracellular shift of hydrogen ions secondary to potassium deficiency. Renal wasting of potassium also occurs with renal excretion of bicarbonate when the patient is sodium depleted. Chronic vomiting is associated with caloric loss and weight loss or failure to thrive. Hematemesis occurs because of prolonged, forceful emesis, producing linear mucosal tears at the juxtaesophageal gastric mucosa. These tears are best diagnosed by endoscopy. Esophagitis occurs secondary to repeated and prolonged acid contact with esophageal mucosa.

Therapy for vomiting depends largely on the underlying cause; efforts should be made to treat metabolic and nutritional complications of vomiting. Acutely, frequent small feedings may minimize gastric distension and the stimulus to vomit. If vomiting is due to exogenous chemicals (e.g., drugs or toxins), medications that act on the CTZ may be effective. These drugs include phenothiazines and haloperidol. Prokinetic agents, such as cisapride, metoclopramide, or erythromycin, may be effective in conditions associated with gastric stasis. Central nervous system causes of emesis include anxiety, hence anxiolytic drugs often help. Increased ICP may respond to cyclizine, and vestibular disturbances and motion sickness respond to antihistamines or anticholinergics, such as scopolamine. Chemotherapeutic modalities, including radiation, may best respond to 5-HT$_3$ antagonists, such as ondansetron. Migraine syndromes may be treated by a variety of medications, including common analgesics, antidepressants, propranolol, cyproheptadine, sumatriptan, and others.

Referral and admission should be considered when intensive diagnostic evaluation or acute therapy is undertaken. In addition, if complications of vomiting, such as severe dehydration, hematemesis, aspiration, or metabolic instability exist, hospitalization may be warranted. Any patient in whom a surgical cause of vomiting is suspected, especially acute obstruction, should immediately be referred to an appropriate center for capable surgical consultation.

SUMMARY

Persistent emesis in the child may be the result of a variety of mechanisms stimulating the medullary vomiting center. Circulating drugs and toxins stimulate the chemoreceptor trigger zone; inflammation, irritation, and distension activate vagal afferents; and central nervous system pathways lead to the vomiting center. These several pathways provide the mechanisms of emesis for a large differential diagnosis, ranging from functional causes in the young infant to systemic disorders and intestinal obstruction. The astute clinician uses the history and physical examination to initially determine if obstruction exists and to tailor the appropriate diagnostic and therapeutic approach. Understanding the mechanisms and pathways of emesis allows a more physiologic approach to the treatment of emesis.

ILLUSTRATIVE CASES

Case 1. A 2-week-old infant boy was seen because of recurrent emesis present virtually since birth. The patient was born at 39 weeks gestation (3.7 kg birth weight) after an uncomplicated pregnancy to a 27-year-old primigravida mother. Labor and delivery were uncomplicated, and the mother and child were discharged after 36 hours. The child was breast-fed. Emesis occurred with nearly every feeding, and the mother was concerned that the infant was not gaining weight. Stools were loose, occurring 8 to 10 times per day, without blood or mucus. Vomitus was of curdled milk, without blood or bile. On examination at 2 weeks of age, the infant appeared ill, irritable, and poorly grown. Weight was 3.1 kg. Icterus and decreased subcutaneous tissue were noted. Liver was enlarged to 8-cm span; no spleen was palpable. Laboratory evaluation included a mild anemia to 11.5 gm Hgb, with normal white blood cell count and platelets. Cultures of blood, urine, and spinal fluid were sterile. Aminotransferases were elevated to the 300-IU range, and total bilirubin level was 10.4 mg/dl, with a conjugated fraction of 6.2 mg/dl. Urine was positive for reducing substance, but no glucose was noted. A diagnosis of galactosemia was confirmed by measuring red cell galactose 1-phosphate uridyltransferase activity, and the patient improved on a lactose-free diet.

This patient had early onset of nonbilious emesis, but poor growth was noted, indicating this was not innocent emesis. Hepatomegaly and jaundice suggested liver disease, and a metabolic evaluation found reducing substances in the urine, leading to the diagnosis. Bilious emesis would have led to a surgical evaluation to exclude hepatobiliary obstruction or other gastrointestinal disorders.

Case 2. A 9-year-old girl has had recurrent episodes of abdominal pain and emesis for over 2 years. Episodes occur erratically without periodicity, with sudden onset of severe abdominal pain and emesis that may last hours to 1 to 2 days. Emesis often is green-tinged. No fever, diarrhea, or other symptoms are noted. The patient frequently requires intravenous fluids during episodes. Previous evaluations have included a normal blood count, urinalysis, urine culture, abdominal plain film, and serum electro-lytes. Examination between episodes reveals a well-grown, normal-appearing child. Neurologic examination, including funduscopic examination, is normal. During episodes the abdomen is mildly distended with diffuse tenderness. Aminotransferases, amylase, and lipase are normal. UGI demonstrates an abnormal position of the fourth portion of the duodenum and distension of the proximal duodenum. The small bowel is shifted to the right abdomen, and the cecum is abnormally high.

This patient has typical symptoms and radiographic findings of malrotation. Symptoms of partial or total obstruction from malrotation may occur anytime in childhood, with or without midgut volvulus. Chronic or recurring bouts of emesis, often with abdominal pain and abdominal distension with obstruction, may occur for years before radiographic studies are done to make the diagnosis. The lack of periodicity and the presence of severe abdominal pain helps to distinguish this from cyclic vomiting.

Case 3. A 10-year-old girl was seen for recurrent episodes of emesis occurring almost every 3 to 4 weeks over the past 3 years. Emesis would begin suddenly and persist perniciously, with rapid onset of lethargy. Episodes lasted 1 to 3 days. Attacks would end suddenly, and she would be well between episodes of emesis. No bile was seen in emesis, although on two occasions she did have blood-tinged vomitus. Family history was positive for migraine headache, although the patient never complained of headache during or after episodes. She has undergone an extensive evaluation, including contrast imaging of upper and lower intestinal tracts, renal sonogram, liver and pancreatic tests, metabolic screening for porphyria and medium-chain fatty acid acyl-CoA dehydrogenase deficiency, EEG, MRI of the head, NH_3, and upper endoscopy. All tests were normal. Psychiatric counseling was refused. Early intervention with intravenous fluids seemed to help, but a trial of propranolol for possible migraine did not abort attacks. Erythromycin decreased the frequency and severity of episodes but did not eliminate them.

This patient has the frustrating problem of cyclic vomiting. Numerous theories have been advanced to explain this disorder, with none being entirely satisfactory. Various treatment modalities have also been offered with variable success.

ANNOTATED BIBLIOGRAPHY

Andrews PLR: Physiology of nausea and vomiting, *Br J Anaesth* 69(suppl 1):2S-19S, 1992.
This is an excellent review of the physiology of nausea and vomiting.

Li BUK: Cyclic vomiting: new understanding of an old disorder, *Contemp Pediatr* 13:48-62, 1996.
This article reviews cyclic vomiting and the current thinking of its pathophysiology.

Orenstein SR: Gastroesophageal reflux, *Curr Prob Pediatr* 21:193-242, 1991.

This is a comprehensive review of a common problem in infants that discusses pathophysiology, diagnosis, manifestations, and treatment.

BIBLIOGRAPHY

Belman AB: Ureteropelvic junction obstruction as a cause for intermittant abdominal pain in children, *Pediatrics* 88:1066-1069, 1991.

Bowen A: The vomiting infant: recent advances and unsettled issues in imaging, *Radiol Clin North Am* 26:377-392, 1988.

Fleisher DR: Functional vomiting disorders in infancy: innocent vomiting, nervous vomiting, and infant rumination syndrome, *J Pediatr* 125:S84-S94, 1994.

Gordon AC, Gough MH: Oesophageal perforation after button battery ingestion, *Ann R Coll Surg Engl* 75:362-364, 1993.

Hammond J: The late sequelae of recurrent vomiting of childhood, *Dev Med Child Neurol* 16:15-22, 1974.

Henretig FM: Vomiting. In Fleisher GR, Ludwig S, editors: *Textbook of emergency medicine*, ed 3, Baltimore, 1993, Williams & Wilkins.

Holcomb GW Jr, Holcomb GW III: Cholelithiasis in infants, children, and adolescents, *Pediatr Rev* 11:268-274, 1990.

Jernigan SA, Ware LM: Reversible quantitative EEG changes in a case of cyclic vomiting: evidence for migraine equivalent, *Dev Med Child Neurol* 33:80-85, 1991.

Judd RH: *Helicobacter pylori*, gastritis, and ulcers in pediatrics, *Adv Pediatr* 39:283-306, 1992.

Kao HA: Bilious vomiting during the first week of life, *Acta Paediatr Sin* 35:202-207, 1994.

Lilien LD, Srinivasan G, Pyati SP: Green vomiting in the first 72 hours in normal infants, *Am J Dis Child* 140:662-664, 1986.

Litovitz T, Schmitz BF: Ingestion of cylindrical and button batteries: an analysis of 2382 cases, *Pediatrics* 89:747-757, 1992.

Orenstein SR: Dysphagia and vomiting. In Wyllie R, Hyams JS, editors: *Pediatric gastrointestinal disease*, Philadelphia, 1993, WB Saunders.

Reinhart JB, Evans SL, McFadden DL: Cyclic vomiting in children: seen through the psychiatrist's eye, *Pediatrics* 59:371-377, 1977.

Winter HS: Vomiting. In Dershewitz RA, editor: *Ambulatory pediatric care*, ed 2, Philadelphia, 1993, JB Lippincott.

Urinary Tract

Polyuria, Enuresis, and Urinary Frequency

MARK J. MENDELSOHN ❧ JEAN M. TERSAK

 ## Key Points

- Enuresis is a common problem, affecting 10% of children after 7 years of age. Organic diseases causing enuresis account for less than 1% of cases.

- Polyuria is an inappropriately high urine output for effective circulating blood volume and the serum sodium. It often is associated with underlying neurologic, renal, or metabolic disturbances.

- Functional voiding disturbances have a diverse presentation with urinary and bladder symptoms occurring in the face of normal neurologic and urinary systems. Anatomic and functional studies of the urinary tract are necessary to define the specific functional voiding disorders.

Complaints related to the urinary tract are often expressed by children and their parents during routine office visits. This chapter reviews more common presenting signs and symptoms, including enuresis, polyuria, and urinary frequency. The differential diagnosis for these often persistent signs and symptoms is vast. This chapter is designed to provide an understanding of the pathophysiology of such complaints and to identify key features in the history and physical examination. The information allows for a stepwise approach to the differential diagnosis and subsequent evaluation of the patient with urinary tract complaints.

Pathophysiology

The causes of urinary complaints, such as enuresis, polyuria, and changes in frequency, are diverse. In approaching the patient with such complaints, it is important to understand normal bladder physiology and the mechanism for concentration of the urine.

The normal micturition cycle consists of filling, storing, and voiding phases. Normal urinary control involves coordination of the sphincter and detrusor muscles. The sphincter is a sleeve of striated and smooth muscle surrounding the bladder neck and urethra. The striated portion is under voluntary control. Voluntary control is rare before 18 months of age, although it is common by 3 years. The detrusor muscle surrounds the bladder wall, and detrusor contraction leads to expulsion of urine from the bladder.

The autonomic nervous system is an important component of bladder control. During the filling phase, stimulation of beta-adrenergic receptors allows the detrusor muscle to relax. Concurrently the stimulation of beta-adrenergic receptors increases the muscle tone of the bladder neck and proximal urethral musculature and helps to maintain continence. During the voiding process, the external sphincter relaxes while the detrusor muscle contracts, leading to the passage of urine through the urethra.

Normal evolution of bladder control begins with the completely automatic bladder of the newborn. The urinary tract functions reflexively under control of the lumbosacral spinal cord and involves little conscious sensation. By several months of age the infant begins to experience discomfort with a full bladder and sensation during voiding. There is not any greater control at this point of development but rather more enureses. From infancy to 2 years of age, bladder capacity and urine volume increase, and the number of voids per day decreases. Sensation continues to develop, but continence lags behind sensation. The first step in achieving bladder control involves control of sphincter tone, which is responsible for resistance to flow of urine. The last developmental step is to attain control of the voiding reflex. This involves modulation of the spinal cord reflex center by the central nervous system. By age 4 years, most children are able to voluntarily initiate or inhibit detrusor contraction in coordination with proper contraction or relaxation of the sphincter.

Enuresis

There are several theories as to the pathophysiology of enuresis. Proposed causes have included psychologic disturbances, sleep disorders, outlet dysfunction, and small functional bladder capacity. Recent evidence suggests that in many enuretics, nighttime urine production is equal to or even exceeds daytime production. In the normal individual, urine output has a circadian rhythm, whereby nighttime production is approximately one half of that produced during the day. This may relate to antidiuretic hormone (ADH) production; studies have demonstrated lower levels of nighttime ADH production in enuretics when compared with controls. Alternative theories propose that bladder reservoir function is decreased in patients with nocturnal enuresis. The bladder capacity is therefore exceeded at night, despite normal urine output.

A theory that gained acceptance a few years ago emphasized a psychologic component to enuresis. It suggested that enuresis may be a dynamic mechanism in which there is a split in the ego that may be manifested as sleep disturbance or enuresis. It has also been proposed that enuresis may be related to neurologic defense mechanisms. However, it has not been confirmed that enuretic patients have a different psychologic profile than other children.

A related theory invoked a sleep disorder in enuretic patients in which the arousal mechanism was involved. With the advent of the electroencephalogram (EEG), it became possible to monitor levels of sleep in the enuretic individual. Early studies linked enuresis to the transition from deep sleep to rapid-eye-movement episodes or the amount of time spent in each sleep stage. In a large study involving EEG data on 500 enuretic individuals, no direct relationship between level of sleep or sleep stage and enuresis could be demonstrated.

Polyuria

Understanding the pathophysiology of polyuria requires that one understand the mechanism of production and concentration of urine in the normal individual. Polyuria implies a urine volume that is inappropriately high relative to plasma sodium and effective circulating volume. The volume of urine produced depends on exogenous intake of solute and water, as well as that resulting from intracellular metabolism. The ability to concentrate the urine depends on the presence of ADH and a number of important functions of the nephron, including a hyperosmolar medullary interstitium. Concentration of urine depends on a complex countercurrent system, involving the water-permeable thin descending loop of Henle, passive transport of sodium in the thin ascending loop, and active sodium chloride transport in the thick as-

cending loop. Urea reabsorption takes place in the collecting tubule, leading to a concentration gradient across the tubular lumen.

ADH acts on the cortical and medullary collecting tubules to permit the absorption of water. The neurons that produce ADH are located in the supraoptic and periventricular nuclei of the hypothalamus. Serum osmolality is regulated by osmoreceptors located in and near the supraoptic nucleus of the hypothalamus. The osmoreceptors are able to detect the degree of intracellular dehydration, which results in production and release of ADH along the hypothalamus and posterior lobe of the pituitary gland.

Production of concentrated urine therefore depends on intact osmoreceptors, adequate ADH release, and renal responsiveness to ADH. These mechanisms are absent or ineffective in a number of disease states addressed in this chapter. Alternatively, polyuria may result from abnormal levels of endogenous or exogenous water and solute in the presence of a normal concentrating ability. This topic is also explored in this chapter.

Functional Voiding Disorders

The term *functional voiding disorder* encompasses voiding disorders that occur in children with intact neurologic and urologic systems. The pathophysiology is complex and most often originates in the setting of poor decision making and patterns of behavior surrounding toilet-training habits. It is critical to realize, however, that these nonorganic mechanisms of voiding dysfunction may secondarily lead to urologic pathology. Functional voiding dysfunction over time may lead to significant uropathology, with true deterioration of bladder and/or renal function.

The understanding of the pathophysiology of such disorders has been advanced through use of urodynamic evaluations. Changes occurring in the urologic tract secondary to voiding disorders include a thickened, noncompliant bladder wall and the development of vesicoureteral reflux. The thickened bladder wall may result from sphincter-detrusor dyssynergia, leading to a generalized increase in bladder trabeculation. Noncompliance of this thickened bladder wall then leads to poor emptying, residual urine, and predisposition to infection. Infection is also more likely in these children because of development of vesicoureteral reflux. Voiding dysfunction leads to an abnormal increase in intravesicular pressure, causing reflux of urine and hence predisposition to infection. Finally, in cases of the infrequent voider, urinary tract infection is common because of stasis and inability to completely empty the large, overstretched bladder.

Although the origin is behavioral, the evolution of these disorders involves development of significant pathology.

Background

Enuresis is by far the most common concern related to the urinary tract. The term is derived from the Greek root *enourin,* which means to void urine. The pathophysiology and need for treatment of enuresis has been an area of controversy for hundreds of years. It is an identifiable topic as early as 1550 BC, when the Ebers Papyrus discussed nocturnal enuresis. In 77 AD it was suggested that ingredients such as boiled mice and wood lice added to the food of infants might lead to urinary continence. In the 1800s, various penile bandages were proposed as treatment until complications, including penile gangrene, led to abandonment of this approach. Behavior modification techniques, such as an electric blanket that shocked the wearer when wet, are present in the literature as early as 1881. As Freudian theories became more popular, theories of enuresis became linked to neuroses and patterns of delinquency.

Enuresis is defined as an inappropriate or involuntary voiding of urine at an age when control should be present. Enuresis is primary when the child has never demonstrated urinary continence for a significant amount of time. Secondary enuresis refers to incontinence that recurs after 6 to 12 months of urinary continence and accounts for 25% to 35% of cases. One study examined ages at which children first attained nighttime dryness, defined as one or fewer nocturnal enureses per month for at least 1 month. Approximately 80% were dry by 5 years of age, 90% by 7 years of age, and 95% by 10 years. As many as 1% of adults have primary nocturnal enuresis. Probably most important to the practitioner is the information that detection rates of organic causes of enuresis have been documented to be less than 1%.

Polyuria, although far less common, warrants immediate attention and evaluation in children. It is important to distinguish the polyuric state from urinary frequency, in which there is not necessarily an increase in volume of urine output. Definitions of polyuria are variable and include those based on milliliters of urine per square meter per day. It is important to realize that this definition may be too restrictive. It may be more appropriate for the definition of polyuria to include any situation in which the output of urine is inappropriately high relative to effective circulating volume and serum sodium. In contrast to enuresis, polyuria is commonly associated with an underlying neurologic, renal, or metabolic disorder. The polyuria may be the consequence of either a water or solute diuresis. Topics of discussion include primary polydipsia (compulsive water drinking), central and nephrogenic diabetes insipidus, and metabolic and primary renal causes of polyuria.

A third area of discussion involves the functional voiding disorders of childhood. These disorders consist of a group of diverse symptoms in children with normal neurologic and urinary systems. Symptoms include changes in frequency, abdominal pain, dysuria, and nocturnal enuresis. In contrast to isolated nocturnal enuresis, however, these disorders are accompanied by daytime symptoms as well. Emphasis is on the clinical features that allow one to differentiate the majority of children who have functional voiding disorders from the small percentage who have clinically significant urinary tract or neurologic abnormalities.

TABLE 21-1

Enuresis

Differential diagnosis	Clinical clues
Infection	Urinary frequency, urgency, dysuria, fever, flank pain
Anatomic/surgical	Overflow urinary incontinence, recurrent UTI, weak stream
Nephrolithiasis	Gross or microscopic hematuria, abdominal pain, recurrent UTI
Endocrine	Polydipsia, polyuria, weight loss
Abdominal/pelvic mass	Constipation/fecal impaction, abdominal distension or increased abdominal girth, systemic symptoms (fever, night sweats)

UTI, Urinary tract infection.

Differential Diagnosis

The differential diagnoses of the various urinary complaints are multiple, but they can be organized in such a way as to keep the approach toward the patient logical and organized. For example, polyuria may result from either a water or a solute diuresis. A water diuresis may be related to primary polydipsia or diabetes insipidus. A solute diuresis may be related to such disorders as diabetes mellitus or exogenous solutes given iatrogenically, such as sodium chloride, ammonium chloride, or sodium bicarbonate.

It should be emphasized that enuresis is not a diagnosis but a symptom. Enuresis may be divided into enuresis nocturna, functional voiding disorders, or just one of many complaints related to other complaints, such as polyuria. Finally, dysuria is only a symptom but may be related to a number of disorders caused by infection, foreign body, or metabolic causes. These causes are all discussed in this section.

Enuresis

An organic cause is found in less than 5% of cases of primary enuresis (Table 21-1). In secondary enuresis, less than 1% are found to be organic in origin. The most challenging task for the physician then becomes identifying those individuals with an organic disorder, so that appropriate medical or surgical intervention may be pursued. Alternatively, if the enuresis is believed to be functional in nature, a very different approach is taken with the patient and family. Broad categories that should be considered in the differential diagnosis of the child with enuresis are explored.

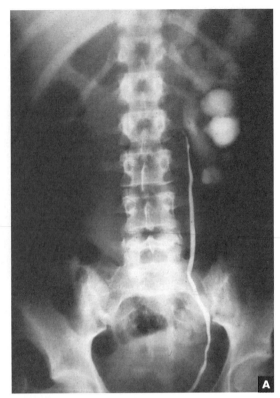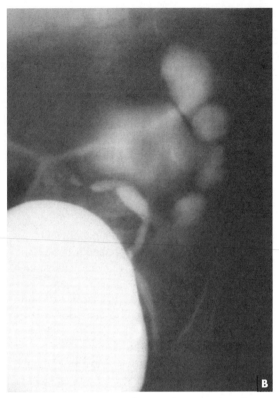

FIG. 21-1   *A,* Retrograde ureterogram defines obstruction at the UPJ. *B,* The coexistence of vesi-coureteral reflux and UPJ obstruction is seen in this voiding cystourethrogram.

Infection

Infection of the urinary tract is a common cause of enuresis. Symptomatic urinary tract infection (UTI) occurs in 1.4 per 1000 neonates, with a slight predominance in boys. Among older children, UTI is much more common in girls. UTI occurs in 1% to 2% of school-age girls, with the most common age between being 7 and 11 years (at 2.5%). Clinical manifestations include urinary frequency with dysuria and often a history of bed-wetting in a previously dry child.

Anatomic/Surgical

There are multiple anatomic or surgical conditions that include enuresis as the presenting symptom. These include lower urinary tract obstruction, occuring in the ureteropelvic junction (UPJ), obstructive ectopic ureter, and posterior urethral valves. Although presenting symptoms are quite variable, overflow urinary incontinence is not uncommon. Overflow incontinence occurs when the bladder becomes overdistended and intravesicular pressure increases, exceeding the urinary sphincter resistance.

UPJ obstruction is the most common obstructive lesion in childhood (Fig. 21-1). It is most often due to congenital stenosis at the UPJ site. Additional symptoms in children include abdominal or flank pain, UTI, or hematuria after minor blunt trauma.

Obstructive ectopic ureter may also lead to lower urinary tract obstruction. The ectopic ureter may occur in any location along the path of the mesonephric duct. It often represents a duplication of the collecting system and may lead to very significant obstruction. Symptoms depend in part on the location at which the ectopic ureter enters the lower urinary tract. Symptoms of UTI and overflow urinary incontinence may occur.

Posterior urethral valves are a congenital anomaly in which abnormal membranous structures act as valves, leading to obstruction of the lower urinary tract (Fig. 21-2). Signs and symptoms include a weak stream, UTI, and overflow incontinence. Urinary incontinence may continue to occur in up to 50% of children after correction of the posterior urethral valves, although this tends to improve with age.

Neurogenic bladder refers to a condition in which bladder dysfunction results from a congenital anomaly, traumatic injury, or disease process involving the brain, spinal cord, or nervous supply to the urinary bladder. In children, neurogenic bladder most often reflects a congenital lesion, such as myelomeningocele or tethered cord (Fig. 21-3), sacral agenesis, or other lesion of the spinal cord. Symptoms are variable and include urinary retention, incontinence, and frequency. Subsequent complications include UTI secondary to inadequate emptying. Spina bifida refers to a specific condition in which there is a defect in closure of the vertebral column. It varies from the occult type, in which there are no clinical symptoms, to a more significant neural tube defect, in which paralysis and bladder dysfunction may occur.

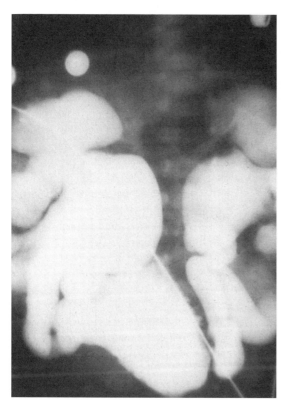

FIG. 21-2 Voiding cystourethrogram reveals posterior urethral valves and severe bilateral vesicoureteral reflux.

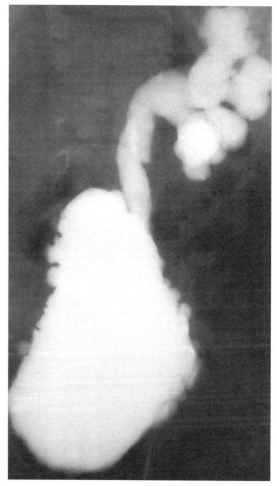

FIG. 21-3 Severe bladder trabeculation and vesicoureteral reflux in a child with myelomeningocele.

Nephrolithiasis

Nephrolithiasis, or urinary calculi, may occur anywhere in the urinary tract (Fig. 21-4). Predisposing factors include stasis, obstruction, or infection. Children at greatest risk are those with abnormalities of the bladder or urinary tract, including neurogenic bladder, anatomic obstruction, and posterior urethral valves. Calcium oxalate accounts for the majority of urinary stones in children. These individuals often have gross or microscopic hematuria. Additional symptoms include abdominal pain and symptoms associated with UTI. UTI secondary to nephrolithiasis may be associated with loss of bladder control in a previously continent child.

Endocrine

Diabetes mellitus is the most common endocrine disorder of childhood. Most children have type I, or juvenile-onset, diabetes mellitus. This disorder is characterized by an insulin deficiency and dependence on exogenous insulin to prevent the complication of diabetic ketoacidosis. The insulin deficiency results in abnormal carbohydrate, protein, and fat metabolism. Common signs and symptoms include polydipsia and polyuria secondary to the associated osmotic diuresis. This physiologic condition frequently leads to enuresis in a previously continent child.

Diabetes insipidus (DI) is an endocrine disorder characterized by polyuria and polydipsia. The symptoms result from a lack of ADH (central DI) or from an abnormal renal re-

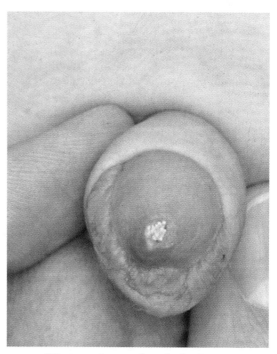

FIG. 21-4 Impacted urethral calculus.

TABLE 21-2

Polyuria

Differential diagnosis	Clinical clues
Water Diuresis	
Primary polydipsia	Abnormal parent-child interactions, normal physical examination and laboratory data
Dipsogenic DI	CNS infection and mass, head trauma, water deprivation test
Gestational DI	Pregnancy (return to normal 2 to 3 weeks after delivery)
Idiopathic DI (autoimmune)	MRI findings
Acquired DI	Mass lesions, CNS infection, trauma, medications
Nephrogenic DI	
Congenital	Family history
Autosomal recessive and X-linked	Drinking from toilets, sucking washcloths
Acquired	Medication history
Electrolyte disturbance	Check serum calcium, potassium; urinary calcium/creatinine ratio
Obstructive causes	Abdominal mass
Renal parenchymal disorders	Radiographic and laboratory findings
Solute Diuresis	
Organic solutes	
Glucose, urea, mannitol	Weight loss, polyphagia, laboratory results
Inorganic solutes	
Sodium chloride	Salt-wasting/renal disorders, (RTA)
Mineralocorticoid deficiency or excess	Key laboratory tests (hyperkalemia, hyponatremia, hypertension)
Alkali ingestion	History
Ammonium chloride, potassium chloride, sodium bicarbonate	Iatrogenic causes

CNS, Central nervous system; *DI,* diabetes insipidus; *RTA,* renal tubular acidosis.

sponse to ADH (nephrogenic DI). Children experience excess thirst to the point of distraction from play and disruption of sleep. In a child who has attained control of the bladder, enuresis may be the first symptom of this disease.

Abdominal/Pelvic Mass

Any mass leading to significant distortion and subsequent obstruction or extrinsic bladder compression may result in urinary incontinence. Neoplasia, such as childhood neuroblastoma or Wilms tumor, could present in this way. Neuroblastoma is a tumor arising from the neural crest cells, which normally form the adrenal medulla and sympathetic nervous system. Adrenal and retroperitoneal abdominal tumors are most common, although neuroblastoma may cause a pelvic mass in a small percentage of cases. Wilms tumor, or nephroblastoma, is a malignant tumor arising in the kidneys. As compared with neuroblastoma, Wilms tumor exhibits a greater incidence of distortion of the kidneys and urinary tract.

Encopresis refers to one condition leading to fecal incontinence after an age at which bowel control is expected. An organic cause is rarely identified. As with enuresis, fecal incontinence may be present since infancy. In this situation it is referred to as *primary encopresis.* The term *secondary encopresis* identifies those individuals in whom regression to fecal incontinence occurs after bowel control had been established. This condition often occurs after problems with constipation, fecal impaction, and stool withholding (see Chapter 17). Urinary incontinence may occur in this setting, secondary to extrinsic compression of the bladder by the fecal pelvic mass.

Polyuria

Water Diuresis

Primary Polydipsia

Primary polydipsia, also described as psychogenic polydipsia or compulsive drinking, is unusual in infants and children (Table 21-2). Initially it may be difficult to differentiate primary polydipsia from partial nephrogenic or central diabetes insipidus. In young infants, excessive drinking may be secondary to the infant's attachment to the bottle. This may have its origin in the caretaker offering a bottle at the first sign of an infant's distress. Excessive drinking is also a marker for problems in parenting. There are no reports on the frequency of psychogenic polydipsia in children, but in adolescents it can be a manifestation of a significant psychiatric disorder, such as schizophrenia. This disorder can also occur in the manic phase of bipolar disorders but is usually transitory. The diagnosis can be made by paying particular attention to the history and the presence of a normal physical examination. Laboratory studies are usually unnecessary, and a water deprivation test can be used in making the diagnosis. This is discussed further in the section on approach to the patient.

Dipsogenic Diabetes Insipidus

Dipsogenic refers to a primary thirst defect. This can be due to a number of disorders but can also be a consequence of chronic water intoxication. There can be a blunting of the maximal concentrating capacity in the medulla of the kidney secondary to a chronic water diuresis. In dipsogenic DI the excessive intake of fluid seems to be caused by a reduction in the osmotic threshold for thirst. Acquired defects, which may result in a thirst center defect, include granulomatous diseases, such as neurosarcoidosis; infection, such as tuberculous meningitis; multiple sclerosis; and certain drugs, such as

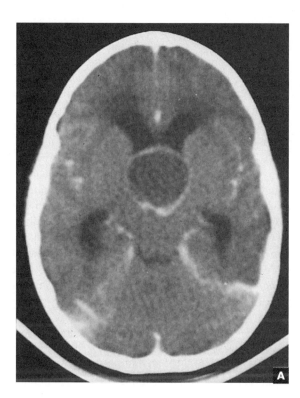

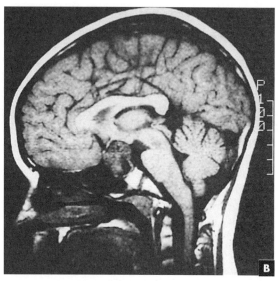

FIG. 21-5 Craniopharyngioma. *A,* CT scan shows a large spherical suprasellar mass, obliteration of the third ventricle, and associated hydrocephalus. *B,* MRI provides superior visualization of the anatomic relationship of this tumor to the optic chiasm and hypothalamus. (Courtesy Department of Neuroradiology, University Health Center of Pittsburgh.)

lithium and carbamazepine. Head trauma has also been associated with a thirst center defect. In these disorders, thirst and water intake continue to be regulated by osmotic factors, but they cannot be completely suppressed unless plasma osmolality and sodium concentration are reduced below the threshold for ADH release. However, there is a suppression of ADH, which results in the development of a maximal water diuresis. Subsequently the patient is left in a state of chronic thirst, polydipsia, and polyuria.

Gestational Diabetes Insipidus

During pregnancy there can be an increase in the degradation of ADH, which can result in polyuria and polydipsia. Delivery of the placenta usually results in a return to the normal ADH metabolism and urinary volume over a 2- to 3-week period.

Primary Diabetes Insipidus

FAMILIAL. To date there is only one clearly defined genetic form of central or neurohypophyseal DI. It is transmitted in an autosomal dominant mode and seems to result from postnatal degeneration of ADH-producing neurons. A number of mutations are responsible. These mutations result in the replacement or deletion of one or more amino acids in the protein precursor of ADH.

IDIOPATHIC. The idiopathic form of central DI occurs in the absence of any known cause, usually begins much later in life, and is not associated with a family history of DI. In one study by Imura and others, 17 patients with idiopathic DI were studied. They had duration of symptoms ranging from 2 months to 20 years. Biopsies of the neurohypophysis revealed lymphocytic infundibuloneurohypophysitis. Nine of the patients lacked the hyperintense signal in T-1 weighted

images seen in normal subjects. In addition, two patients had mild hyperprolactinemia and nine had impaired secretory responses of growth hormone to insulin-induced hypoglycemia. The natural course of the disorder was self-limited but could explain some of the patients diagnosed with DI without a known cause.

Secondary Diabetes Insipidus

The acquired forms of neurohypophyseal DI result from many different types of injury or disease. Traumatic causes include head injury or neurosurgical procedures, resulting in injury to the pituitary hypothalamic area. Infectious causes include meningitis, encephalitis, and central nervous system abscess. Granulomatous disease also can damage the anterior and posterior pituitary. Disorders such as neurosarcoidosis, histiocytosis X, and tuberculosis can result in injury to the neurohypophysis, with presentations of polyuria and polydipsia. Central nervous system tumors, such as craniopharyngioma (Fig. 21-5), hypothalamic or chiasmatic glioma, germinomas, and rarely metastases from other primary sites, can result in neurohypophyseal injury. There are also a number of medications that can result in DI. The central-acting medications, such as phenytoin, clonidine, and ethyl alcohol, can result in selective polyuria and polydipsia. Rarely, chemical toxins, such as snake venom and tetrodotoxin, can cause DI. Congenital malformations of the brain, aneurysms, and acquired coagulation disorders, such as a thrombus or embolus, can result in injury to the neurohypophysis.

Nephrogenic Diabetes Insipidus

CONGENITAL. There are two known modes of inheritance in the genetic etiology of nephrogenic DI—X-linked and autosomal recessive. The X-linked disorder is the more common of the genetic causes of DI and recently has been shown to be due to molecular defects in the vasopressin V_2 receptor gene. The severity of polyuria varies, probably because of the heterogeneity of the mutations that cause this disorder. Rarely the inheritance pattern is autosomal recessive. Recently, Kanno and others demonstrated that the autosomal recessive form is due to mutations in the gene encoding the water-channel protein, aquaporin-2. Aquaporin-2 is the vasopressin-regulated water channel in the collecting duct of the renal tubule. It has the primary role in concentrating the urine. It is now evident that mutations in the gene encoding aquaporin-2 can result in nephrogenic DI with an autosomal recessive inheritance pattern.

ACQUIRED. Reduced renal sensitivity to the antidiuretic action of ADH results in an imbalance of water homeostasis. Clinical manifestations include a decreased urinary concentration, a slight increase in urinary flow, and hypertonic dehydration. Occasionally the defect in this renal sensitivity is mild, and a rise in plasma ADH levels may be sufficient to overcome this insensitivity and restore urine concentration to normal. There are a number of inciting agents that can cause this renal insensitivity to ADH. A number of medications are associated with acquired nephrogenic DI. The most frequent offending agent is lithium. This medication can occasionally cause a permanent defect in renal response to ADH. Other medications that have been associated with nephrogenic DI include methoxyflurane, demeclocycline, amphotericin B, aminoglycosides, cisplatin, rifampin, and foscarnet.

Electrolyte disturbances should also be considered because hypercalcemia, hypercalciuria, or hypokalemia can result in a defect in the urinary concentrating ability of the kidney. This is caused by an interference with postreceptor biochemical mechanisms that mediate the effect of ADH on the permeability of the epithelium of the collecting tubules in the kidney.

OBSTRUCTIVE CAUSES. Obstructive uropathies and renal parenchymal disorders may result in nephrogenic DI and cause polyuria and polydipsia. There are a large number of obstructive lesions that may present with polyuria. In urethral obstruction, such as posterior urethral valves, the concentrating ability and the ability of the tubules to excrete hydrogen ions are decreased. Because of the defect in concentrating ability, polyuria and diluted urine may be early manifestations. One of the early presentations of familial nephronophthisis is characterized by polyuria, polydipsia, growth failure, and progressive renal insufficiency. In this uncommon disorder, renal medullary cysts are present and the patient usually is diagnosed in adolescence. Other medical renal disorders, such as medullary infarction secondary to sickle-cell disease, chronic pyelonephritis with reflux nephropathy, and other diseases that cause injury to the medullary and cortical concentrating ability, may result in nephrogenic DI. It is essential then that laboratory procedures to determine blood urea nitrogen and creatinine and a renal ultrasound be included in the evaluation of a child with polyuria and polydipsia.

Solute Diuresis

Organic Solutes. A solute diuresis may be the result of accumulated organic or inorganic solutes in the urine. The most common organic solutes that may cause a diuresis with symptoms of polyuria include glucose and urea. One other organic solute that causes a diuresis is mannitol, which is prescribed in the management of selected patients. This agent is an effective osmotic medication used in settings where rapid diuresis is necessary (e.g., suspected cerebral edema with increased ICP). The polyuria of diabetes mellitus and mannitol administration is related to osmotic diuresis, in which the osmolality of the urine approaches that of plasma. This is due to the presence of solutes that cannot be reabsorbed by the tubules or are present in amounts that exceed the tubular capacity for reabsorption. The greater the solute load to the tubules, the greater the urine flow. Glycosuria also can be caused by intravenous fluid administration of high concentrations of dextrose, which is seen in patients receiving hyperalimentation.

Inorganic Solutes. A number of inorganic solutes may contribute to an osmotic diuresis, resulting in polyuria. This includes the administration of excessive intravenous sodium chloride and the use of diuretic agents. A number of salt-wasting nephropathies can present with polyuria and impaired urinary concentrating ability. These conditions include Fanconi syndrome, which is associated with proximal and distal renal tubular acidosis, and chronic renal failure. Sodium-wasting is also seen in juvenile nephronophthisis. Renal disease is usually easily diagnosed by appropriate laboratory and radiographic tests. Mineralocorticoid deficiency may also present as a solute or osmotic diuresis. Children with mineralocorticoid deficiency may have polyuria and polydipsia caused by urinary sodium-wasting. This condition is seen in the context of a renal tubular acidosis and can result from either inadequate production of or reduced distal tubular responsiveness to aldosterone. This lack of aldosterone impairs the establishment of an electrochemical gradient favorable to hydrogen ion secretion. In the absence of aldosterone-mediated sodium resorption, hyperkalemia develops and urinary sodium-wasting is one of the findings. This may result in a solute-mediated diuresis. These children usually have a normal anion gap systemic metabolic acidosis. They also may have growth failure toward the end of the first year of life. Mineralocorticoid deficiency may also be found as an underlying feature of a primary kidney disease. Mineralocorticoid deficiency states can result from diseases of the adrenal gland, such as Addison disease (Fig. 21-6), congenital adrenal hyperplasia, and primary hypoaldosteronism. In these states, renal function is normal and the plasma renin level is elevated. Hypoaldosteronism, which may result from kidney disease, also can be associated with interstitial damage and destruction of the juxtaglomerular apparatus. In these conditions, plasma levels of renin are reduced. Renal function may also be compromised. Rarely, type IV renal tubular acidosis may be the result of a distal tubular unresponsiveness to aldosterone (pseudohypoaldosteronism);

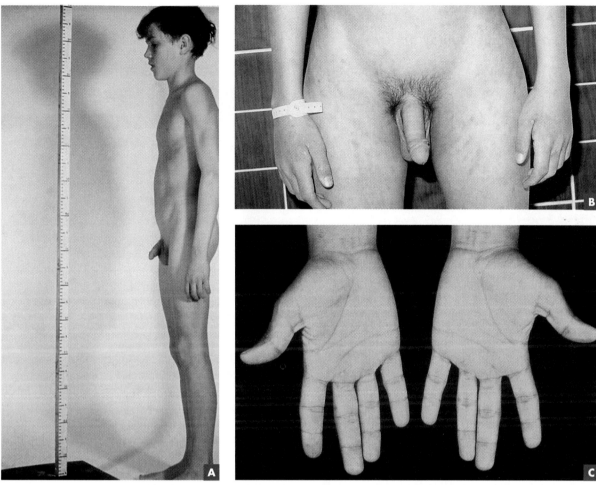

FIG. 21-6 *A,* This patient shows the thin habitus and ill appearance characteristic of Addison disease. *B* and *C,* Hyperpigmentation may be marked.

plasma renin and aldosterone levels are elevated; renal function is normal, and salt-wasting is the rule.

Mineralocorticoid Excess. In primary aldosteronism there are elevated levels of aldosterone. Primary states are independent of the renin-angiotensin system and are rare in children. They are characterized by hypertension and hypokalemia. Aldosterone-secreting adenomas, bilateral adrenocortical hyperplasia, and rare glucocorticoid-suppressible aldosteronism (an adrenocorticotropic hormone–dependent autosomal dominant form of hyperaldosteronism) may all present with hypokalemia, polyuria, nocturia enuresis, and polydipsia. Associated findings include hypertension, suppressed plasma renin activity, and occasionally elevated sodium and decreased serum chloride concentrations. The resulting hypokalemia, with its effect on renal tubular permeability, may result in decreased responsiveness to ADH, with resultant polyuria and polydipsia.

Rarely, ammonium chloride, potassium chloride, and alkali ingestion may result in a solute-mediated osmotic diuresis, causing polyuria and polydipsia. These states may be dif-

ferentiated by the history of ingestion or administration of these agents.

Functional Voiding Disorders

The functional voiding disorders of childhood represent a complex constellation of symptoms, leading to a pattern of bladder control that may be very disruptive to the patient and family (Table 21-3). Although rarely organic, such disorders may present with a pattern of symptoms that allows for a specific diagnosis and therefore approach to treatment of the functional voiding disorder. Urodynamic abnormalities have been documented in these children. Symptoms include changes in frequency, urgency, enuresis, dysuria, and abdominal or perineal pain. The discussion to follow summarizes some of the more common functional voiding disorders of childhood. It is critical for the physician to realize that throughout treatment of these disorders, he or she must continue to carefully monitor for development of a neurologic or urologic disorder contributing to the patient's symptoms.

TABLE 21-3

Functional Voiding Disorders

Differential diagnosis	Clinical clues
Daytime urinary frequency syndrome	Marked increase in urinary frequency during daytime, absence of increase frequency during nighttime
Unstable bladder syndrome	Frequency, urgency, daytime incontinence, nocturnal enuresis, recurrent UTI
Hinman syndrome	Urgency, infrequent voiding, intermittent stream, straining to void
Lazy bladder syndrome	Void only 2 to 3 times per day, overflow urinary incontenence, urgency with urge incontinence at bladder capacity, recurrent UTI
Stress incontinence	Release of small amount of urine with increased abdominal pressure (cough, exercise)
Giggle incontinence	Release of large amount of urine with laughter
Functional small bladder capacity	Frequency, urgency, urge incontinence, nocturia, recurrent UTI

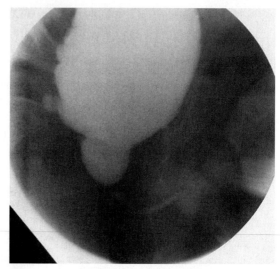

FIG. 21-7   Voiding cystourethrogram of a boy with Hinman syndrome shows severe dilation of the prostatic urethra. Severe bilateral hydronephrosis resulted from vesicoureteral reflux.

Daytime Urinary Frequency Syndrome

Daytime urinary frequency is one of the more common functional voiding disorders of childhood. In this case a previously toilet-trained child develops markedly increased frequency and urgency, progressing to up to 10 to 15 episodes per hour. This disorder is slightly more common in boys. Nocturnal enuresis may occur in approximately 20% of cases. Although the increase in urinary frequency does not occur at night, studies suggest that nocturnal enuresis indicates higher risk for relapse to daytime urinary frequency. Age ranges for this syndrome include children ages 2 to 14 years, although it most commonly occurs at approximately 5 years of age. This pattern of symptoms is also referred to as *pollakiuria,* from the Greek root *pollakis,* which means "often." Previous studies involving extensive evaluation of the urinary tract in these children have failed to identify an organic cause; therefore emotional factors must also be considered.

Unstable Bladder of Childhood

Unstable bladder is also referred to as *instability of the detrusor muscle* or *persistence of the infant bladder.* It is a common cause of voiding dysfunction in children with no evidence of a neurologic lesion. Symptoms include increased frequency, urgency, daytime incontinence, and nocturnal

enuresis. It is more common in girls, most often in the 6- to 12-year-old age range. Continued careful follow-up for the development of urologic disease is critical because involuntary detrusor muscle contraction in a child who would be expected to have obtained voluntary control of micturition can result in abnormally high intravesicular pressures. It has also been associated with the development of vesicoureteral reflux and UTI.

Hinman Syndrome (Nonneuropathic Dyssynergia)

Children with Hinman syndrome exhibit symptoms of upper and lower urinary tract dysfunction, similar to that observed with neuropathic bladder (Fig. 21-7). Further evaluation, however, reveals a neurologically intact child. Affected children experience a dyssynergia of detrusor and sphincter muscles. Symptoms include urgency, infrequent voiding, and an intermittent urinary stream with associated straining to void. The characteristic pattern is the absence of external sphincter relaxation during voiding, leading to increased intravesicular pressure and a weak or intermittent urinary stream. The result is a heavy, trabeculated, large, poorly compliant bladder associated with postvoid residual urine and subsequent development of hydroureteronephrosis and possible vesicoureteric reflux. There is no detectable obstructive or neurologic abnormality.

Lazy Bladder Syndrome or Infrequent Voiding

This relatively uncommon syndrome occurs almost exclusively in girls between 7 and 15 years of age. Affected children typically void 1 to 2 hours after awakening in the morning, and then void up to two additional times during the remainder of the day. The pattern of infrequent voiding leads to increased bladder capacity and decreased sensation of bladder fullness. These children begin to experience incontinence as the bladder fills beyond its capacity, leading to overflow incontinence. Affected individuals may experience urgency with urge incontinence at the time the bladder reaches capacity. Many also have symptoms of chronic constipation and associated encopresis. The pattern of micturition predisposes to development of UTI because of urinary stasis.

Stress Incontinence

Most commonly observed in women, stress incontinence is rare in childhood. Children with this disorder are predominantly girls between 9 and 15 years of age. They tend to have normal or infrequent voiding and experience incontinence of a small amount of urinary loss with increased abdominal pressure, such as coughing or exercise. Functional stress incontinence is a diagnosis of exclusion once organic causes have been eliminated. Children appear to respond well to a planned voiding schedule, and the condition tends to be benign and self-limited.

Giggle Incontinence

Giggle incontinence is another uncommon functional voiding disorder. It occurs predominantly in girls between 7 and 15 years of age. Typical symptoms include a normal voiding pattern except for spontaneous release of a large quantity of urine with laughing. Urologic or neurologic abnormalities are absent. Giggle incontinence is a benign condition of preadolescence, tends to be self-limited, and resolves with age.

Functional Small Bladder Capacity

Children with small bladder capacity may experience symptoms of frequency, urgency, urge incontinence, nocturia, and/or enuresis. Urodynamic studies document increased detrusor pressure during bladder filling. Unstable bladder contractions occur as the bladder reaches capacity, leading to markedly elevated intravesicular pressure. Incomplete relaxation of the ureteric sphincter during voiding leads to incomplete bladder emptying. Vesicoureteric reflux may be present, and recurrent UTIs are not uncommon.

History

The careful clinician directs the initial evaluation of urinary complaints by obtaining a thorough history. Voiding disorders are characterized by frequency of urination. This is the single most common symptom exhibited by children. It is crucial that the examiner differentiate between polyuria and frequency of urination. Polyuria is almost always associated with increased frequency of urination, whereas increased urinary frequency is not always associated with polyuria. True polyuria is associated with polydipsia, whereas urinary frequency is not. In the infant this distinction may be difficult to make, but a careful history may reveal a poor urinary stream or a persistent dribbling of urine. Poor or excessive fluid intake may be a manifestation of a neurogenic disorder. Occult

spinal dysraphism may not be clinically apparent initially. Clues to the diagnosis include recurrent UTI associated with gait disturbances when the infant becomes ambulatory. Other historic clues include a history of lumbar puncture with resultant spinal cord injury.

An infant's feeding schedule is important because rare causes of primary polydipsia in infants may include parental overfeeding resulting from a misunderstanding of the infant's needs. It is important that growth patterns and absence of dehydration and fever are noted. The nature of the parent-infant relationship should be explored, and the parents' response to infant crying may be a clue to the excessive fluid intake. In contrast to infants with psychogenic polydipsia, infants with nephrogenic DI tend to have polydipsia, polyuria, and frequent difficulties with dehydration, fever, vomiting, refusal of milk, and constipation. These infants are always thirsty for water and may have bizarre drinking habits, such as drinking from puddles or sucking washcloths. There may be a family history significant for early infant deaths, family members with polydipsia and polyuria, and infants with poor growth and chronic dehydration.

In the older toddler who has mastered toilet training, other voiding disorders may become more prominent. Symptoms of functional voiding disorders include changes in the urinary frequency, either increased or decreased. Urgency is a common finding, as is daytime and nighttime enuresis. Occasionally, dysuria and recurrent UTI may be notable in children with voiding disorders. Other symptoms include intermittent episodes of mild abdominal and perineal pain, constipation, and encopresis. It is important that the clinician note when the initial change in the urinary symptoms occurred. Does the child hold the urine for long periods of time? It is important that the physician inquire about family history of genitourinary disorders, the age of toilet training, and evidence of past urinary complaints, including UTIs and daytime incontinence.

It is important that the clinician quantitate the frequency of enuretic episodes at night. How often the child may have urinary incontinence during the day is also important. Questions regarding voiding habits may be revealing. For example, straining to urinate may be a clue to neurogenic bladder dysfunction. A complete voiding and stool history or diary may add much to the evaluation. If, for example, a youngster wets at night, it is helpful to know how often this occurs. Constant daytime thirst or chronic waking at night to drink could suggest renal insufficiency. Some children may refuse to void or defecate at school or in other settings and may consciously contract the external sphincter to prevent elimination.

In functional urinary disorders, children may have either increased daytime urinary frequency or excessive intervals between voiding. They may actually void just enough to relieve discomfort but may still have residual urine after voiding. Symptoms characteristic of neurogenic dysfunction include severe pain on urination; rectal, penile, or vaginal pain; straining to urinate; slow urinary stream; lower extremity weakness; or back and leg pain. If these findings are present, it is best to move rapidly to further evaluation.

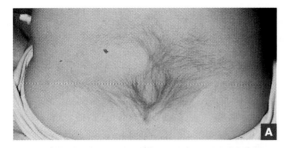

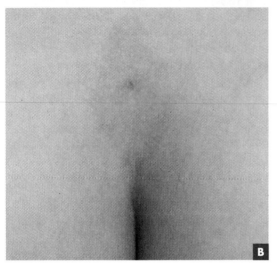

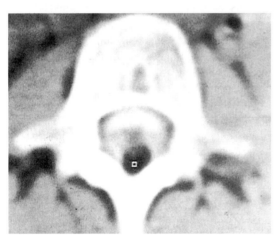

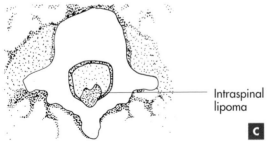

FIG. 21-8 *A,* Occult spinal dysraphism. Note hairy patch over lumbar region, here associated with diastematomyelia. *B,* Occult spinal dysraphism. Sacral sinus tract associated with intraspinal dermoid tumor. *C,* Occult spinal dysraphism. CT scan demonstrates an intraspinal lipoma in a child with a subcutaneous lipoma over the lumbar spine. (*A* and *B* courtesy Dr. Michael J. Painter, Pittsburgh.)

Intraspinal lipoma

It is important that the examiner ask about irritants, such as bubble baths, history of foreign body, or sexual abuse. Unstable bladder contractions may result in suppression of micturition, in which a child adopts characteristic posture, such as squatting, sitting on the heels, or holding the perineum. Attitudes shown during toilet training may be helpful because the child may have been encouraged to develop bladder or bowel control before he or she was emotionally ready or interested. This may result in functional disorders, such as problems with defecation, which may also complicate urinary voiding patterns. A proper history helps differentiate between neurogenic and nonneurogenic causes of urinary complaints and also differentiate between polyuria and urinary frequency.

Physical Examination

Physical examination is an essential feature in the evaluation of a child with urinary complaints. Children with functional voiding complaints, such as urinary frequency, unstable bladder, or bladder dyssynergia, generally have a normal physical examination. However, the examination should be detailed and should specifically emphasize the neurologic examination. A general overview of growth is essential because children with chronic illness may have evidence of growth failure when growth points are plotted. The abdominal examination may reveal an abdominal mass, such as a palpable distended bladder. The perineum may reveal excoriation caused by the presence of urine, which results from dribbling of urine in a child with a neurogenic bladder. It is essential to inspect the back, especially the lower lumbosacral area, for evidence of occult spinal dysraphism. The clinician may find a midline defect, such as a hairy patch, hyperpigmentation, dimple, sinus tract, hemangioma, or asymmetric gluteal cleft or lipoma (Fig. 21-8). These are all indications for further radiographic evaluation.

Flattened buttocks and asymmetry of the gluteal cleft may point to the diagnosis of sacral dysgenesis. A rectal examination may demonstrate laxity in the rectal sphincter tone, indicative of a neurogenic cause. It is essential that a complete neurologic examination, including deep tendon reflexes and demonstration of normal muscle strength in the leg and foot, be pursued. Abnormalities in these areas also may indicate a neurologic cause of the urinary complaints. Perineal sensation and an anal wink should be elicited because they indicate normal sacral nerve function. The child's gait should be observed and the lower back should again be inspected for sacral dimpling or cutaneous anomalies.

In the proper setting, it may be informative to observe a child's voiding pattern. The urinary stream can be a clue to ureteral obstruction, as in posterior urethral valves in boys. Constant dribbling of urine may indicate a neurogenic cause or the rare instance of an ectopic ureter, which is more common in girls. This results in continual leakage of urine and findings of perineal excoriation or a chronically damp diaper.

Finally the clinician should always inspect the external genitalia for evidence of trauma, which could be due to sexual abuse, resulting in the child's urinary symptoms. In summary a complete physical examination, concentrating on the neurologic component, helps to differentiate between the functional disorders and serious underlying neurologic anomalies.

Approach to the Patient

The approach to the patient with a urinary complaint requires a detailed history and physical examination, as noted in the previous sections. Again, a history of dysuria, intermittent daytime wetness, polydipsia, polyuria, central nervous system trauma, constipation, or encopresis may indicate medically treatable conditions. However, constant wetness or dampness, an abnormal urine stream, a change in gait, a past history of lumbar puncture, or snoring with obstructive sleep apnea may indicate surgically treatable conditions.

The history and physical examination should allow the clinician to obtain the critical information necessary to differentiate between urinary frequency, dysuria, and polyuria with polydipsia. A lack of urinary concentration and the presence of significant hypertonic dehydration excludes primary polydipsia as a cause of the polyuria. Therefore the first step after the examination is obtaining a urine specimen. The urine should be examined for infection, using an enhanced urinalysis and Gram stain. A 1993 study showed that greater than 10 white blood cells per cubic millimeter via an enhanced urinalysis, with bacteriuria noted on Gram stain, indicates a high likelihood of a UTI (see Hoberman reference). The urine specific gravity should be obtained to elicit defects in concentrating ability. The urine should also be screened for glycosuria to rule out the possibility of diabetes mellitus.

Because it is often difficult to differentiate the different causes of DI based on one urine sample or the history and physical examination, the 7-hour water deprivation test has been used effectively. The 7-hour water deprivation test requires hospitalization. This provocative test allows the clinician to assess the maximal concentrating power of the kidney in a patient with polyuria. Before the test, it is important that screening chemistries, including sodium, potassium, blood urea nitrogen, creatinine, calcium, and glucose, are performed to exclude other causes of polyuria and polydipsia. This test can be risky for the young patient, so it requires close monitoring. Free access to fluids and food is allowed until the morning of the test. All urine passed during the test is timed, the volume is recorded, and hourly measurements of urine volume and specific gravity are recorded. The patient is weighed, and urine and serum osmolality are measured at the beginning of the test and after completion of the 7-hour period. The test is terminated before the 7-hour time period if weight loss exceeds 5% or if the patient develops intolerable thirst. If the urine specific gravity rises to greater than 1.014, the test is terminated early and demonstrates normal concentrating ability of the kidney. At the completion of the 7-hour water deprivation period, the ADH analogue 1-deamino-8-D-arginine vasopressin (DDAVP) is administered intranasally. The patient is then monitored for another 4 hours, and serum and urine osmolality are determined. Oral fluids are permitted after the administration of the vasopressin at volumes equal to the urine output of the previous hour. Ways in which the results can be quantified have been determined. If the ratio of urine to serum osmolality is less than 1.5, the patient has abnormal urinary concentrating ability; a ratio greater than 1.5 indicates normal renal function. A positive response to DDAVP is defined as the ratio of urine to serum osmolality greater than 1.5, with the final urine osmolality greater than 450 mOsm, indicating sensitivity to ADH, and a diagnosis of central DI. Children with nephrogenic DI do not respond to the administration of DDAVP. Partial defects, both central and nephrogenic, can also be diagnosed with this procedure. It requires extensive monitoring and should be performed only in special settings. Appropriate treatment can then be initiated once the proper diagnosis has been made.

If the patient's signs and symptoms reflect a functional voiding disorder, urinary frequency, or dysuria, the approach should be directed accordingly. Again, it is crucial that the clinician obtain a urine sample and check for pyuria and bacteriuria. If present, UTI should be diagnosed with a urine culture. If hematuria is present, the evaluation should be directed toward a different differential diagnosis. It is critical that the physician determine the child's bladder capacity. This is an often overlooked step. One approach requires that the family take at least three measurements of the child's functional bladder capacity at the time of the initial evaluation. The normal bladder capacity in children is estimated to be the child's age plus 2 oz. Because urinary frequency and dysuria may be manifestations of hypercalciuria, a spot urine calcium-creatinine ratio can make this diagnosis. (A ratio greater than 0.21 is abnormal.) Again, close inspection of the meatus may reveal evidence of a foreign body or trauma.

In the evaluation for bladder instability or functional voiding disorders, postvoid residual urine volume should be measured. A child with detrusor instability voids to completion; a patient with obstructive anomalies of the lower tract (Hinman syndrome) or a neurogenic bladder may have a significant emptying disorder and a high volume of residual urine. Flowmetry is a noninvasive test performed in an urologist's office in which the child is asked to void in a commode containing a straining device that measures peak and average flows. The tracing reflects the interaction of detrusor contraction and bladder outlet resistance. If the flow rates and patterns are normal, it is unlikely that any significant disorder of emptying exists. Flowmetry is a good screening test, and the results should be normal for children with bladder instability.

Because UTI and vesicoureteral reflux may be associated with the functional voiding disorders, the voiding cystourethrogram (VCUG) is useful in looking for vesicoureteral reflux (Fig. 21-9). Ultrasonography of the kidneys and blad-

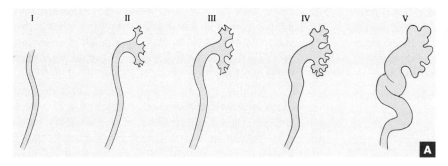

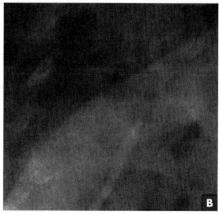

FIG. 21-9 *A,* Grades of vesicoureteral reflux, schematically presented. *B,* Grade I reflux—cystourethrogram shows reflux only into the ureter.

der is helpful in screening for congenital anomalies. The only ultrasonographic finding associated with detrusor instability is an occasional thick bladder wall, defined as greater than 3 mm when full and 5 mm when empty.

Rarely a cystometrogram may be indicated in a child with bladder instability. Involuntary detrusor contractions are present when the water pressure is greater than 15 cm. Small bladder capacity is also a common finding. Usually, cystometry is reserved for patients with an unclear diagnosis or for those who do not respond to subsequent treatment. If the history in a girl indicates continuous leaking of urine with no symptoms of urgency or frequency, the evaluation for ectopic ureters is indicated. Again, a VCUG would be diagnostic.

If the history and physical examination point toward the daytime urinary frequency of childhood, further evaluation is usually not indicated. This is a self-limited condition that resolves spontaneously, occasionally with the use of counseling if a psychosocial stressor has been elicited.

The child with constipation occasionally has associated urinary complaints, including incontinence, infrequent voiding, and recurrent UTI. When the constipation is treated appropriately, it is often found that the urinary symptoms improve as well.

When nocturnal enuresis is the most likely diagnosis, imaging studies are seldom indicated. Urinalysis and culture are the indicated diagnostic tests to rule out associated UTI or other urinary tract disorder. The approach to the patient with enuresis is multifaceted and can include behavioral modification treatment, including the use of enuresis alarms. Recently, medical management of enuresis has included the use of DDAVP, which may help a select group of children with enuresis but is primarily for short-term use. It can be effective when a child plans to attend an overnight camp or stay overnight with a friend.

The treatment for functional voiding disorders includes bladder retraining and the use of pharmacotherapy. This chapter does not detail the treatment for these disorders, but the use of comprehensive retraining programs and anticholinergic agents can be effective in helping children with these complaints.

SUMMARY

The busy clinician frequently sees patients with complaints related to the urinary tract. Functional disorders are common, whereas the incidence of polyuria is low. It is crucial for the practitioner to distinguish between these two symptoms. A thorough history, detailed physical examination, and organized approach allow for an effective diagnostic and interventional strategy. The use of limited laboratory and radiographic studies helps the clinician narrow the spectrum of urinary disorders that may present in childhood.

ILLUSTRATIVE CASES

Case 1. *A.B., a 3-year-old white boy, was brought to the doctor's office by his mother with a 4-week history of urinary frequency. A.B. would ask to void every 5 to 10 minutes during the day, but showed no change in the occasional episodes of nocturnal enuresis (1 to 2 episodes per week). There was no accompanying dysuria, fever, hematuria, or change in appetite or activity. The physical examination was normal. Of note, the family had moved to a new city in the previous month.*

This is a typical presentation for pollakiuria, or daytime urinary frequency. There was the abrupt onset of urinary frequency without other accompanying signs or symptoms. The recent move appeared to be a significant stressor, and with reassurance the frequency resolved over the following 3 weeks.

Case 2. *V.S., a 3-month-old white boy, was first evaluated in the emergency department. He was severely dehydrated, thin, and only 8 ounces above birth weight. The history revealed intermittent fever and refusal of milk, but he was always thirsty for water. The family history was notable for a male cousin who died at 2 months of age because of dehydration and presumed sepsis.*

This case is an example of a severe presentation of an infant with congenital nephrogenic DI. The family history was a clue, and after resuscitation and stabilization it was noteworthy that the urine remained dilute. A cautious water deprivation test and lack of response to DDAVP confirmed the diagnosis. Medical and dietary management have allowed the infant to be followed closely as an outpatient.

Case 3. B.T., a 6-year-old girl, was first seen for complaints of daytime and nighttime incontinence, a history of two previous UTIs, and constipation. Her mother observed that B.T. would attempt to stop the urge to void by frequently crossing her legs. The physical examination, a complete neurologic examination, radiographic studies (VCUG, renal ultrasound), and urinalysis were normal. The urine culture was negative.

This case represents a common problem seen more frequently in girls. This child was referred to a urologist, and urinary studies were consistent with the unstable bladder syndrome. The findings showed uninhibited detrusor muscle spasms with voluntary sphincter contractions, which resulted in high bladder-filling pressures. With intensive bladder retraining and pharmacologic treatment (anticholinergics), B.T. gradually improved and her enuresis and constipation resolved.

ANNOTATED BIBLIOGRAPHY

Fernandes E, Vernier R, Gonzalez R: The unstable bladder in children, *J Pediatr* 118:831-836, 1991.
This article is an excellent review of the functional voiding disorders.

Forsythe W, Redmond A: Enuresis and spontaneous cure rate: study of 1129 enuretics, *Arch Dis Child* 49:259-263, 1974.
This prospective study helps illustrate the incidence and natural history of childhood enuresis.

Leung A, Robson L, Helperin M: Polyuria in childhood, *Clin Pediatr* 30:634-640, 1991.
This article provides a review and discussion of causes of polyuria in childhood.

BIBLIOGRAPHY

Bass L: Pollakiuria, extraordinary daytime urinary frequency: experience in a pediatric practice, *Pediatrics* 87:735-737, 1991.

Bloom D, Faerber G, Bomalaski MD: Urinary incontinence in girls: evaluation, treatment, and its place in the standard model of voiding dysfunctions in children, *Urol Clin North Am* 22:521-538, 1995.

Cantani A, Bamonte G, Ceccoli D, et al: Familial juvenile nephronophthisis: a review and differential diagnosis, *Clin Pediatr* 25:90-95, 1986.

Casale J: Functional voiding disorders of childhood, *J Ky Med Assoc* 91:184-191, 1993.

Fernandes E, Reinberg Y, Vernier R, et al: Neurogenic bladder dysfunction in children: review of pathophysiology and current management, *J Pediatr* 124:1-7, 1994.

Hendricks SA, Lippe B, Kaplan S, et al: Differential diagnosis of diabetes insipidus: use of DDAVP to terminate the 7-hour water deprivation test, *J Pediatr* 98:244-246, 1981.

Hoberman A, Wald ER, Penchansky L, et al: Enhanced urinalysis as a screening test for urinary tract infection, *Pediatrics* 91:1196-1199, 1993.

Holtzman E, Harris HW, Kolakowski L, et al: Brief report: a molecular defect in the vasopressin V_2-receptor gene causing nephrogenic diabetes insipidus, *N Engl J Med* 328:1534-1541, 1993.

Imura H, Nakao K, Shimatsu A, et al: Lymphocytic infundibuloneurohypophysitis as a cause of central diabetes insipidus, *N Engl J Med* 392:683-689, 1993.

Kanno K, Sasaki S, Hirata Y, et al: Urinary excretion of aquaporin-2 in patients with diabetes insipidus, *N Engl J Med* 332:1540-1545, 1995.

Mikkelsen E, Rapoport J: Enuresis: psychopathology, sleep stage, and drug response, *Urol Clin North Am* 7:361-377, 1980.

Mundy A: Detrusor instability, *Br J Urol* 62:393-397, 1988.

Norgaard JP, Pedersen EB, Djurhuus JC: Diurnal antidiuretic-hormone levels in enuretics, *J Urol* 134:1029-1031, 1985.

Novello A, Novello J: Enuresis, *Pediatr Clin North Am* 34:719-733, 1987.

Robertson G: Diabetes insipidus, *Endocrinol Metab Clin North Am* 24:549-573, 1995.

Rushton HG: Wetting and functional voiding disorders, *Urol Clin North Am* 22:75-93, 1995.

Schmitt B: Special report on enuresis, *Contemp Pediatr* (special edition) 7:3-15, 1990.

VanGool J, Hjalmas K, Tamminen-Mobius T, Olbing H: Historical clues to the complex of dysfunctional voiding, urinary tract infection, and vesicourethral reflux, *J Urol* 148:1703-1705, 1992.

Yared A, Foose J, Ichikawa I: Disorders of osmoregulation. In Ichikawa I, editor: *Pediatric textbook of fluids and electrolytes*, Baltimore, 1990, Williams and Wilkins.

VIII

Skin

22

Swelling and Edema

ANDREW H. URBACH

Key Points

- The differential diagnosis of edema is broad and includes many significant organic causes that require prompt attention.

- Generalized edema often results from hypoalbuminemic states (e.g., nephrotic syndrome, malnutrition, protein-losing enteropathy, and liver disease), cardiac disease, renal vasculitis, and lymphatic abnormalities.

- Localized edema requires a more focused approach and may include life-threatening entities, such as superior vena cava syndrome caused by a tumor and orbital cellulitis, but may also include minor trauma, allergic reaction, and other relatively benign processes.

A previously healthy child who develops swelling presents a challenging diagnostic dilemma for the clinician. The differential diagnosis is broad and includes many significant organic causes that require prompt attention. Swelling generally results from edema, and therefore this chapter focuses on an approach to this particular finding. Edema represents an accumulation of excessive salt and water in the extravascular (also known as interstitial) component of the extracellular fluid space (Fig. 22-1). This extravascular space has the potential to sequester large volumes of water before clinical detection. A rapid weight increase of as much as several kilograms may predate overt symptoms or physical findings. Edema may or may not indent with prolonged application of pressure by the examiner. If indentation is visible, the term *pitting edema* is applied. Often edematous skin provides a doughy sensation to the affected subcutaneous tissues. From time to time the terms *dropsy* and *hydrops* are used synonymously with edema.

Edema may be generalized or localized, but in response to gravity it is typically confined to the dependent portions of the body, specifically the distal extremities or the lower back.

The tissues of the eyelids (Fig. 22-2), scrotum (Fig. 22-3), and labia majora by nature of their distensibility are also selectively affected. Edema involving the eyelids tends to remain confined to this area because tissues of the surrounding forehead, nose, and cheek are tightly adherent to the underlying tissues. Generalized edema often represents the body's response to a systemic disorder. Should this edema be "massive," the term *anasarca* is used. *Hydrops fetalis* refers to this condition in the fetus or newborn. Localized edema, on the other hand, may result from causes such as regional trauma or infection and rarely reflects systemic disease. Each type of localized edema (e.g., periorbital, scrotal, ascites, neck, and extremities) represents specialized circumstances, each of which is unique. The various aspects of these different presentations are addressed in this chapter. Hydrothorax (pleural fluid) and hydropericardium (pericardial fluid) do not cause swelling and are not discussed.

Pathophysiology

Four major pathogenic mechanisms result in the accumulation of fluid in the interstitial space. These include (1) increased intravascular hydrostatic pressure, (2) increased capillary permeability, (3) decreased plasma oncotic pressure (hypoalbuminemia), and (4) abnormal lymphatic drainage. In some instances, several mechanisms can participate in this abnormal process, making diagnosis more challenging.

Total body water and the relative amounts of water in the various body compartments change with age. Body water in the neonate accounts for about 75% of body weight, with the extracellular fluid comprising 45% and the intracellular fluid comprising 35%. By 1 year of age, extracellular fluid is 30% and intracellular fluid is 40%. With time, the total body water decreases to 60% to 65% of body weight, with extracellular fluid accounting for 20% to 25%. Plasma volume generally accounts for 25% of extracellular space and the rest is interstitial fluid. The physical laws that dictate the exchange of fluid between these two components are known as *Starling*

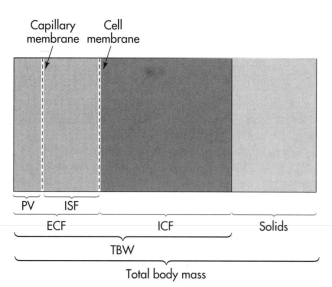

FIG. 22-1 Major subdivisions of the total body mass. *PV,* Plasma volume; *ISF,* interstitial fluid; *ECF,* extracellular fluid; *ICF,* intracellular fluid; *TBW,* total body water. (Modified from Winters RW: *The body fluids in pediatrics,* Boston, 1973, Little Brown.)

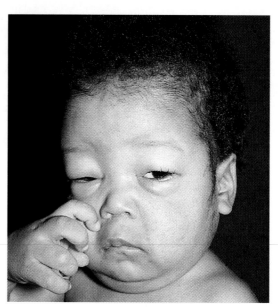

FIG. 22-2 Marked edema of the eyelids in a child with nephrotic syndrome.

forces. These forces are central to the understanding of the dynamic process that maintains fluid balance in this system.

Intravascular hydrostatic pressure and interstitial fluid oncotic pressure work in concert to encourage movement of fluid from intravascular space to extravascular space. The opposing forces of hydrostatic pressure within interstitial fluid ("tissue tension") and intravascular oncotic pressure promote movement of fluid into blood vessels. These dynamics result in a loss of vascular fluid at the arteriolar capillary end of this system and a movement of fluid into vessels at the venous capillary end of this system. Lymphatics are responsible for reclaiming any net loss of fluid from the vascular system and redepositing this fluid into blood vessels. Any disruption of this fine balance, if uncompensated, results in a pathologic process that may eventually lead to edema.

Increased intravascular hydrostatic pressure and the subsequent loss of vascular volume may result from local obstruction of venous drainage (i.e., venous thrombosis or tumor), cardiac failure, or inappropriate antidiuretic hormone (ADH) secretion. A decrease in plasma oncotic pressure and vascular fluid leak as a result of a low serum albumin level may occur because of poor protein intake (kwashiorkor) (see Fig. 18-1), decreased protein synthesis (liver disease), protein loss (nephrotic syndrome), or a significant catabolic state. When the level of albumin in the blood reaches a critical level of approximately 2.5 g/dl, this extravascular process is seen. Edema also may result from vascular injury and the loss of vascular proteins into the interstitial space. The oncotic pressure that these proteins exert shifts fluids in favor of nonvascular spaces. Examples of this type of vascular insult include bacterial infections, viral infections, allergic reac-

tions, and vasculitis. Impaired lymphatic drainage is another mechanism that can result in abnormal fluid dynamics. This can result from recurrent lymphatic inflammation, trauma, and tumors, to name just a few.

The hallmark of generalized edema is the retention of salt and water. Sodium balance is a result of sodium intake, renal sodium excretion, and extrarenal sodium loss, with the kidney playing a major regulatory role. Approximately two thirds of the glomerular filtrate is reabsorbed by the kidney's proximal tubule. ADH and aldosterone, by their actions on the distal tubule, regulate the remainder of fluid reabsorption or excretion. Alteration in the function of these hormones by the presence of disease states may result in the development of edema.

Differential Diagnosis

The differential diagnosis of edema is best approached by first determining whether the process is generalized or localized. Localized edema is considerably more common than generalized edema and is caused by conditions, such as insect bites, leading to changes in capillary permeability. It is, however, possible to focus on a localized process when the "local" edema may be only the first sign of a generalized process. For instance, bilateral periorbital edema may be the first sign of nephrotic syndrome, but without a careful search for other clues to this generalized process the correct diagnosis may be delayed. Several entities can mimic edema and mislead the clinician. These include myxedema, eosinophilic fasciitis, dermatomyositis, scleroderma, and scleredema.

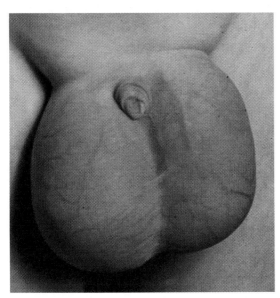

FIG. 22-3 Severe scrotal edema in a 6-year-old boy with nephrotic syndrome.

Generalized Edema in the Newborn: Hydrops

The earliest form of generalized edema is fetal hydrops, a condition affecting the fetus or neonate and associated with the accumulation of fluid in serous cavities and edema in the soft tissues. At birth the affected infant displays anasarca, with ascites, pleural effusion, and often pulmonary hypoplasia. With increasing frequency the diagnosis of hydrops is being made in utero, thus allowing earlier diagnosis and at times improving outlook.

The causes of hydrops in the newborn are varied, but a thoughtful approach often yields an underlying explanation. A very brief discussion is in order before an organized approach to edema in the older child is presented. The natural division between immune and nonimmune hydrops is a good place to begin. Before the use of anti-D globulin (RhoGAM), Rh isoimmunization was the most common cause of immune hydrops. Fetal red blood cell (RBC) destruction by maternal antibody results in anemia and eventually hypoxia, hypoalbuminemia, portal hypertension, and perhaps congestive heart failure (CHF). Currently the majority of cases of hydrops are nonimmune, with an estimated incidence of between 1 in 2500 to 3500 infants. Although mechanisms for the development of hydrops follow the same pathophysiologic rules as previously described (see the section on pathophysiology), a more functional approach to diagnosis in the neonate uses a number of other major diagnostic categories. These categories include hematologic, cardiovascular, respiratory, gastrointestinal, urinary or renal, chromosomal, placental abnormality, infection, metabolic, and miscellaneous (Table 22-1) causes. Anything leading to fetal anemia can result in hydrops. It is suggested that when fetal hemoglobin

drops to less than 6 to 7 g/dl, hydrops will occur. Immune processes, such as isoimmune disease, thalassemia, twin-twin transfusion, and fetomaternal transfusion, can result in a depression of normal fetal hemoglobin levels. In the instance of twin-twin transfusion, the simultaneous elevation of hemoglobin in the nonanemic "host" infant may lead to CHF and hydrops on the basis of polycythemia. In situations of RBC destruction or loss, increased marrow activity generally attempts to compensate for this lower hemoglobin level. In other circumstances, such as drug exposure or infections (e.g., parvovirus), marrow suppression may occur and lead to anemia of a different sort.

A variety of conditions may lead to cardiac dysfunction and result in hydrops. Severe structural disease, cardiac dysrhythmias, volume overload, arteriovenous malformation (AVM), myocarditis, premature closure of the foramen ovale, intracardiac tumors (i.e., rhabdomyoma in tuberous sclerosis), and, as already alluded to, anemia can result in fetal hydrops. Respiratory conditions, such as diaphragmatic hernia, cystic adenomatoid malformation, and pulmonary lymphangiectasia, may lead to lymphatic or vascular obstruction and excess fluid collection as a result.

Gastrointestinal conditions, such as volvulus, atresia, and duplication, may lead to protein loss into the developing bowel or lymphatic obstruction, and eventual hydrops may result. Renal conditions, either on the basis of obstruction or congenital nephrosis, are also well-described causes (Table 22-1). A wide range of genetic syndromes have also been noted to cause hydrops. Perhaps best known of these is Turner syndrome, in which it is postulated that an abnormally formed lymphatic system results in abnormal fluid collections. Table 22-1 provides a more complete list of chromosomal abnormalities and other syndromes associated with hydrops.

Intrauterine infections, such as cytomegalovirus (CMV) and toxoplasmosis, may lead to liver injury (hypoalbuminemia and portal hypertension) or anemia (marrow suppression) and eventual CHF. Also seen are placental anomalies, metabolic disease (especially resulting in hepatic injury), maternal diabetes, and toxemia.

Generalized Edema in the Older Child

Once it has been concluded that generalized edema is present, an excellent place to begin is the cardiac evaluation. Particular attention to CHF and pericarditis is essential. CHF may result from intracardiac pathology or from lesions outside of the heart, such as arteriovenous fistula and the high-output failure that results. The child with cardiac disease severe enough to cause edema has many other clues. CHF results in tachypnea, tachycardia, hepatomegaly, jugular venous distension, gallop rhythm, rales, rhonchi, wheezes, poor growth, and feeding difficulties. Pericarditis results in tachypnea, pulsus paradoxus of more than 10 to 20 mmHg, distant heart sounds, friction rub, chest pain, and evidence of poor venous return to the heart (i.e., neck vein distension, hepatomegaly, and perhaps protein loss in urine and stool).

TABLE 22-1

Differential Diagnosis and Frequency of Nonimmune Hydrops

Category	Frequency (%)	Category	Frequency (%)
Cardiovascular	20	Genetic/Chromosomal	5-30
Complex congenital heart disease		Noonan syndrome	
Atrioventricular septal defect		Turner syndrome	
Premature closure of the foramen ovale		Trisomy 13, 18, or 21 syndrome	
Hypoplastic left or right heart		Dwarfing syndromes	
Dysrhythmias, heart block		Thanatophoric	
Myocardial disease		Jeune syndrome	
Endocardial disease		Hypophosphatasia	
Cardiac tumors		Achondrogenesis	
Arteriovenous malformation		Multiple pterygium syndromes	
		Meckel syndrome	
Respiratory	5	Arthrogryposis	
Diaphragmatic hernia			
Intrathoracic mass		Metabolic	5-10
Cystic adenomatoid malformation		Gaucher disease	
Pulmonary lymphangiectasia		Lysosomal storage disease	
Pulmonary sequestration		Gangliosidosis	
Tracheoesophageal fistula		Sialidosis	
Tracheal stenosis			
		Infection	8
Hematologic	10	Cytomegalovirus	
Twin-twin transfusion		Toxoplasmosis	
Fetomaternal transfusion (chronic)		Syphilis	
Homozygous alpha-thalassemia		Parvovirus	
Hemorrhage		Parasitic disease	
Thrombosis			
Drugs (e.g., chloramphenicol)		Placental Abnormality	
		Umbilical vein thrombosis	
Gastrointestinal	5	Torsion on cord	
Gut atresia		Chorioangioma	
Gut duplication			
Volvulus		Miscellaneous	
Peritonitis		Amniotic band syndrome	
Hepatitis		Fetal tumors	
Cirrhosis and portal hypertension		Teratoma	
		Neuroblastoma	
Genitourinary	5	Wilms tumor	
Posterior urethral valves		Angiomas	
Cloacal malformation			
Ureteral and urethral atresia			
Bladder neck obstruction			
Nephrotic syndrome			
Bifid uterus			
Hydrocolpos			

Modified from McGillivray BC, Hall JG: Nonimmune hydrops fetalis, *Pediatr Rev* 9:197-202, 1987.

Causes of Generalized Edema in the Older Child

Increased Hydrostatic Pressure
Congestive heart failure
Pericarditis
Superior vena cava syndrome
Arteriovenous fistula
Venous thrombosis
Obstruction by tumors
Syndrome of inappropriate ADH secretion
Steroids
Iatrogenic fluid administration

Decreased Oncotic Pressure (Hypoproteinemia)
Nephrotic syndrome
Liver disease (e.g., alpha$_1$-antitrypsin deficiency,
    infectious hepatitis)
Cirrhosis (many causes)
Galactosemia
Kwashiorkor
Marasmus
Cystic fibrosis
Inflammatory bowel disease
Protein-losing enteropathy (e.g., cow's milk allergy)
Intestinal lymphangiectasia
Celiac disease
Bezoar
Infection (e.g., *Giardia* sp.)
Pancreatic pseudocyst
Severe anemia
Zinc deficiency

Increased Capillary Permeability
Rocky Mountain spotted fever
Stevens-Johnson syndrome

Modified from Tunnessen WW: Periorbital edema. In *Signs and symptoms in pediatrics*, Philadelphia, 1988, JB Lippincott.

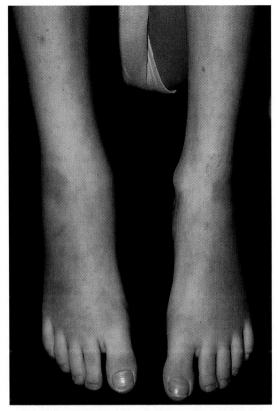

FIG. 22-4 The arthritis of Henoch-Schönlein purpura. Note the swelling of the right ankle in addition to the purpuric rash.

Additional data to support these diagnoses may come from electrocardiogram (ECG), chest x-ray films, and echocardiogram. The mechanism of generalized edema is increased hydrostatic pressure. Other causes are listed in Box 22-1.

If cardiac disease is eliminated as a diagnostic possibility, a full urinalysis provides valuable information about the possibility of a renal cause. Protein in the urine suggests nephrotic syndrome as an explanation for anasarca or less severe forms of generalized edema. Minimal change disease (nil disease) is a common cause of nephrotic syndrome and without renal biopsy is a diagnosis of exclusion. Hypoproteinemia, hypercholesterolemia, and an abnormal 24-hour urinary protein collection (> 150 mg protein/24 hours) are to be expected in any patient with nephrotic syndrome. Hypertension, hematuria, and an elevated creatinine or blood urea nitrogen level

increase the likelihood of an underlying glomerulonephritis (GN). Focal glomerulosclerosis, mesangial proliferative disease, membranoproliferative GN, and membranous GN are all examples of primary causes of nephrotic syndrome. A wide range of secondary causes should also be considered. These include Henoch-Schönlein purpura (HSP), polyarteritis nodosa, systemic lupus erythematosus, subacute bacterial endocarditis, syphilis, and human immunodeficiency virus (HIV) infection, to name a few. Clinical features and laboratory evaluation of these secondary causes of nephrotic syndrome are provided by Oliver and Kelsch. HSP presents an unusual situation. Although nephrotic syndrome is a possible mode of presentation, localized edema is more frequently a result of increased capillary permeability secondary to vasculitis. Typically a previously well child develops a distinctive purpuric rash in a waist-down distribution with arthritis (Fig. 22-4), microscopic hematuria, heme-positive stools, and abdominal pain. The edema of HSP is nonpitting and evanescent, usually affecting the hands and feet; children younger than 2 years of age are most likely to be affected in this fashion.

In the absence of cardiac disease and proteinuria and in the presence of a low serum albumin level, the clinician should search for evidence of gastrointestinal protein loss or malabsorption, poor nutrition, or impaired hepatic synthetic function. Hepatic function can be assessed by jaundice, hepatomegaly, splenomegaly, varices, and other stigmata of severe liver injury. Electrolytes, liver function tests, and studies that assess liver synthetic function may be abnormal and serve as clues. Transaminases are good markers for liver injury, as is bilirubin. When liver function is assessed, ammonia, cholesterol synthesis, and prothrombin time (PT) are of value. Vitamin K malabsorption may also result in abnormal clotting function. A parenteral dose of vitamin K should correct a deficiency state but not prolonged PT secondary to liver failure. Specific entities include infectious hepatitis, biliary atresia, portal hypertension, Budd-Chiari syndrome, and alpha₁-antitrypsin deficiency, to name several. If there is no clinical evidence of liver disease, the possibility of gastrointestinal disease must be considered. Protein malabsorption as a result of cystic fibrosis and its associated pancreatic dysfunction may cause edema. This occurs more often in soy- or breast-fed infants. Failure to thrive is a common finding despite what appears to be adequate caloric intake. Anemia is often associated with this form of generalized edema. When hypoproteinemia is secondary to gastrointestinal loss rather than malabsorption, protein-losing enteropathy (PLE) is implicated. Loss of protein can occur in the esophagus, stomach, and bowel as a result of a variety of mechanisms. Mucosal ulcers or erosions may occur; lymphatic obstruction leads to loss of fluid, protein, and lymphocytes, and cellular injury with impairment of mucosal barrier function may also occur. Clinical features include diarrhea, abdominal pain, and evidence of allergy. By far the most useful test for PLE is measurement of the stool alpha₁-antitrypsin level, which is increased in these abnormal states.

The range of disease entities causing abnormal PLE is broad. Although viral and bacterial pathogens, such as rotavirus and *Salmonella* organisms, cause PLE, they are less likely to cause edema than are parasites, such as *Giardia* and *Strongyloides* organisms. Noninfectious inflammatory disorders, such as allergy to cow's milk, may cause edema, poor growth, a severely depressed albumin level, eosinophilia, and anemia. Allergic phenomena, such as eczema, rhinitis, and wheezing, may also accompany this presentation. In children with previous bowel resection, the anastomosis itself may erode, leading to the subsequent development of anemia and hypoproteinemia. Intestinal ischemia, graft-versus-host disease, and drug hypersensitivity can produce a similar pattern.

Patients with inflammatory bowel disease, particularly Crohn disease, develop hypoalbuminemia, but often the degree of protein loss does not correlate with the severity of disease. Because very low albumin levels are seen in 50% to 60% of children with Crohn disease, albumin measurement should always be included when screening for this entity. Systemic lupus erythematosus, neuroblastoma, trypsinogen deficiency (diarrhea, anemia), bezoar, gastroesophageal reflux, and polyp syndromes rarely produce edema from stool protein loss. Intestinal lymphangiectasia, an entity with lacteal dilation and eventual rupture, leads to steatorrhea, diarrhea, and loss of lymph into the intestinal lumen. Serum studies confirm this process by the presence of lymphopenia, hypogammaglobulinemia, and depressed albumin level. This condition may be familial or secondary to Noonan syndrome or arsenic poisoning. Entities that increase right atrial pressure, such as pericarditis or cardiac surgical repair (i.e., Fontan procedure), also result in anasarca. Another unusual entity, known as *hypertrophic gastropathy* (Ménétrier disease), can result in vomiting, abdominal pain, and anasarca. Lastly, celiac disease can cause PLE, though malabsorption is perhaps a more prominent part of this edema-producing process. Weight loss, diarrhea, distended abdomen, and buttocks wasting are cardinal features.

In addition to loss of protein in the intestine and malabsorption of protein, poor dietary intake of protein, though rare in this country, is occasionally reported and is at times iatrogenically induced. The main features are pigmentary skin changes, skin peeling, monilia, hypotonia, apathy, pallor cheilitis, angular stomatitis, and edema. Psychosocial issues or vegetarian diets figure prominently in families of affected children. Marasmus with severely restricted caloric intake also has edema as a feature.

The patient with generalized edema may have cardiac failure, renal disease, liver or gastrointestinal disease, or hypoalbuminemia. Vasculitis, SIADH, excessive salt intake, and drug toxicity must also be considered. In the absence of these disorders, vasculitis and premenstrual syndrome may be associated with generalized edema with a normal serum albumin level.

An exhaustive discussion of each entity responsible for edema is beyond the scope of this text. Box 22-1 provides a list of examples of generalized edema.

Localized Edema

Periorbital

As suggested earlier, at times a systemic process can cause generalized or localized edema. The periorbital region has a particularly low threshold for the development of puffiness because of its low tissue tension. Nephrotic syndrome, GN, Rocky Mountain spotted fever, angioedema, CHF, serum sickness, and hypothyroidism all may begin with periorbital edema and never progress to more generalized swelling. On the other hand, many patients with periorbital disease may be suffering from a localized process. In the newborn the use of silver nitrate may lead to a chemical conjunctivitis; hypothyroidism may also give the eyelids a puffy appearance. In healthy infants, crying itself may lead to edematous eyelids. Tunnessen conveniently divides periorbital edema by cause as follows: (1) inflammatory, (2) noninflammatory, (3) systemic, (4) traumatic, (5) tumors, and (6) miscellaneous (Box 22-2). Inflammatory edema generally results from infection, spread of inflammation from nearby structures, allergy, or immunologic diseases. On the other hand, noninflammatory edema can occur as a result of trauma, fluid retention (on a systemic basis), impaired lymphatic drainage, or venous obstruction.

Evaluation of the child with periorbital edema should include the surrounding skin. A careful check for evidence of cellulitis and associated redness and pain may reveal group A streptococcal-induced erysipelas with a characteristic sharply demarcated, raised, indurated border and a hot, edematous, brawny, plaquelike lesion. Other forms of periorbital cellulitis may be associated with pain and redness (see Fig. 15-15). Orbital cellulitis involves the orbital space itself and is likely to be associated with proptosis, decreased extraocular muscle movement, and sinus pathology. Dacryocystitis is an inflammation of the lacrimal sac and is associated with a tender lesion lateral to the nose and below the medial aspect of the palpebral fissure. Gentle compression of the nasolacrimal sac may result in expression of exudate from the puncta. A hordeolum, or stye, is a very localized swelling of one or more of the sebaceous (meibomian) glands of the eyelid. Staphylococcal infection is usually the culprit. Redness, swelling, pain, photophobia, and lacrimation are the presenting complaints. Resolution is spontaneous and may be heralded by the release of purulent material. A chalazion is a chronic granulomatous reaction to released fat in the meibomian glands. Spontaneous resolution may not occur with this entity, and surgical drainage may be necessary.

Swollen eyes may also result from chemical or infectious conjunctivitis. Chemical conjunctivitis results from the prophylactic instillation of silver nitrate into the eyes of neonates to prevent *ophthalmia neonatorum*. This must be distinguished from bacterial gonococcal (usually days 2 to 4 of life) and chlamydial (days 8 to 14 of life) infection. History, scrapings, and cultures assist with diagnosis. Children with conjunctivitis display copious purulent discharge if gonococcal infection is present and typically watery discharge with chlamydial infection. In the older child, conjunctivitis is diagnosed by the presence of swelling, hyperemia, mucopurulent discharge (Fig. 22-5), mottling, and occasionally corneal ulcerations. Viral conjunctivitis caused by adenovirus often results in palpable preauricular lymph nodes. Allergic conjunctivitis results from exposures to animal dander, dust, pollens, and a variety of other allergens. Itching, tearing, and photophobia are often present. Chronic forms of allergic conjunctivitis lead to boggy and pale conjunctiva. Allergic rhinitis is often an associated feature. Scrapings of the conjunctiva may reveal eosinophils and their granules, and tears may have increased IgE levels. Insect bites also affect the periorbital tissues frequently, partly because the face is generally exposed. A punctum is often the clue to this lesion. A careful historic search for cat exposure and eye inoculation may explain a swollen eye and a preauricular node caused by cat-scratch disease. Epstein-Barr virus, which causes pharyngitis, posterior auricular lymph node enlargement, fever, and exhaustion, may have periorbital edema as a feature (Hoagland sign). A careful examination for dental abscess may reveal the cause of a swollen face and eye (Fig. 22-6). Tooth pain need not be a feature. In a patient with a past history of chickenpox; impetigo, with characteristic honey-colored

---

BOX 22-2

Selected Causes of Periorbital Edema

Inflammatory
Dacryocystitis
Chalazion or stye
Erysipelas
Orbital and periorbital cellulitis
Herpes zoster
Conjunctivitis
Cat-scratch fever
Iridocyclitis
Dental abscess
Sinusitis
Contact dermatitis
Epstein-Barr virus

Noninflammatory
Angioneurotic edema
Serum sickness
Foreign proteins from parasite
Acute glaucoma

Systemic
Renal disease (e.g., GN)
Thyroid disorder (e.g., hypothyroidism)
Cardiac disease (e.g., CHF)
Collagen vascular disease (e.g., SLE, dermatomyositis, scleroderma)
Infectious disease (e.g., EBV, roseola, diphtheria, scarlet fever)

Traumatic
Trauma
Insect stings/bites
Foreign bodies

Malignancies
Neuroblastoma
Leukemia
Neurofibroma
Hemangioma
Lymphangioma

Miscellaneous
Melkersson-Rosenthal syndrome
Cutis laxa
Subcutaneous emphysema
Superior vena cava syndrome
Rifampin toxicity

Modified from Tunnessen WW: Periorbital edema. In *Signs and symptoms in pediatrics,* Philadelphia, 1988, JB Lippincott.
CHF, Congestive heart failure, *EBV,* Epstein-Barr virus; *GN,* glomerulonephritis; *SLE,* systemic lupus erythematosus.

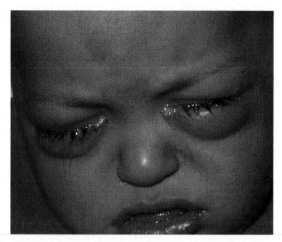

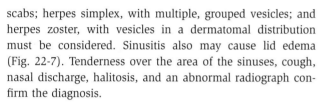

FIG. 22-5   Acute bacterial conjunctivitis. Copious amounts of mucopurulent discharge have made the upper and lower eyelids adherent to each other. Chemosis of the upper and lower eyelids may also make opening the eyes difficult.

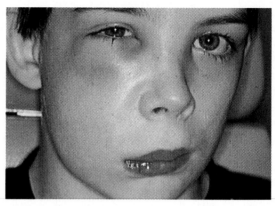

FIG. 22-6   Facial cellulitis associated with an abscessed maxillary tooth. Hospital admission for intravenous antibiotics, incision and drainage, and extraction of the abscessed tooth was necessary.

scabs; herpes simplex, with multiple, grouped vesicles; and herpes zoster, with vesicles in a dermatomal distribution must be considered. Sinusitis also may cause lid edema (Fig. 22-7). Tenderness over the area of the sinuses, cough, nasal discharge, halitosis, and an abnormal radiograph confirm the diagnosis.

Dermatitis, atopic and contact, can cause eyelid swelling. When atopic dermatitis is the cause of allergic shiners, Dennie-Morgan lines (see Fig. 15-6) and dry, scaly skin (with lichenification secondary to rubbing) may be seen. An eczematoid rash elsewhere on the body may serve as a confirmatory clue. Contact dermatitis can result from an allergic or irritant reaction secondary to substances that contact the skin. Redness, swelling, and a papular or vesicular lesion are present.

Hives (urticaria) and angioedema are well-described causes of eyelid swelling. Hives are a transient vascular reaction of the skin, with edema secondary to increased dilation and permeability of vessels. The rash is extremely itchy and raised, with an irregular red border. Deeper versions of the same lesions are termed *angioedema*. Because of the abundant number of mast cells in the eyelids, this rapidly developing lesion has a predilection for and may recur at this particular site (Fig. 22-8). Drugs, airborne agents, and ingested allergens may be the culprits. Hereditary angioedema is an autosomal dominant condition with either absence or dysfunction of C1 esterase inhibitor. In half of the instances the nonpitting, nonpruritic swelling results from trauma. Half of the lesions occur spontaneously, and most notably the absence of itching and gradual onset distinguish this condition from hives. Although visceral involvement, abdominal pain, and airway edema can occur, the eyelids alone can be involved.

Dermatomyositis and its associated proximal muscle weakness, distinctive extensor surface rash, facial rash, and purplish lid involvement is part of the differential diagnosis. Lid edema may result from primary ocular pathology, such as uveitis, glaucoma, endophthalmitis, and corneal infection. Cardinal features of ocular disease include photophobia, corneal clouding, blurry vision, and perilimbal conjunctivitis. Blepharochalasis is an uncommon cause of recurrent, nonpitting, painless lid swelling. Swelling persists for 3 to 4 days and causes injury to the upper lid and surrounding structures, resulting in a wrinkled, drooping appearance. Onset in the first two decades of life is typical. Cutis laxa of the upper lid (dermatochalasis) may mimic this entity. Other very unusual inflammatory causes of periorbital swelling include vaccinia, tularemia, anthrax, and cavernous sinus thrombosis.

Noninflammatory causes for lid swelling may include drug-induced swelling (e.g., barbiturates, antibiotics, and aspirin). Systemic disorders, such as renal disease, cardiac disease, and collagen vascular disease, have already been discussed. A wide range of infectious diseases remain considerations. These include malaria, Rocky Mountain spotted fever, trichinosis, roseola, diphtheria, and streptococcal infections. Other features of these entities provide the clues to diagnosis.

Trauma is a relatively common cause of lid edema, though the associated bruising almost always gives this diagnosis away. Occasionally, in dark-skinned individuals the signs of bruising may be obscure and delayed onset of swelling may confuse the clinician. Injury to the cornea itself may result from a foreign body and cause prominent symptoms of lacrimation and pain.

Tumors, such as leukemia and neuroblastoma, are known to metastasize to the orbit. Leukemia causes swelling, eye discoloration from hemorrhage, and perhaps proptosis. Neuroblastoma may cause periorbital ecchymosis ("raccoon eyes"), swelling, proptosis, and hemorrhage of the subconjunctiva. The benign masses of neurofibromatosis should also be included in this differential diagnosis, with skin findings of six 1.5-cm café au lait spots assuring a correct diagnosis. Any tumor that compresses lymphatics may sec-

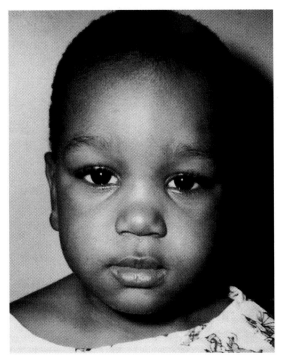

FIG. 22-7 Sympathetic periorbital swelling with sinusitis. This 2-year-old boy was seen late in the afternoon with high fever, wet cough, decreased activity, and mild infraorbital puffiness. The puffiness was neither red, indurated, nor tender and reportedly had been more marked upon awakening in the morning. He also had a scant cloudy nasal discharge. His chest x-ray film was normal, but sinus films showed opacification of the maxillary sinuses.

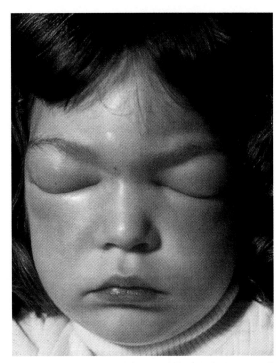

FIG. 22-8 Eyelid angioedema in a child with venom allergy. Onset was explosive after a bee sting. (From Fireman P, Slavin RG: *Atlas of allergies*, New York, 1990, Gower.)

ondarily lead to puffy eyelids. Primary abnormalities of the lymphatic system may also do the same. On occasion a tumor or a lymphangiomatous lesion precipitates superior vena cava syndrome. Edema of the face, neck, upper torso, and superficial chest veins; stridor; cough; cyanosis or plethora; and headache are cardinal features. Other lesions, such as abscess or vascular occlusion as a result of a central venous catheter, are other potential causes. Melkersson-Rosenthal syndrome is associated with recurrent facial nerve palsy, edema, and furrowed tongue; sickle-cell disease, subcutaneous emphysema (crepitation makes the diagnosis), and hypothyroidism and hyperthyroidism round out the differential diagnosis of periorbital edema.

Neck

Edema of the neck can occur as part of generalized edema, but when this region is the only affected area the clinician should carefully search the oral cavity for evidence of infections, such as herpetic stomatitis and diphtheria. Superior vena cava syndrome, although rare, is an important cause of neck swelling. Because of its association with a malignancy (i.e., lymphoma or Hodgkin disease), the importance of searching for an underlying cause is heightened. The most common cause of superior vena cava syndrome is obstruction after surgery for congenital heart disease. Children

who have a central venous catheter in place should be considered at risk. Though the neck may be a striking feature of the presentation, swelling may involve the face and upper chest as well. Periorbital puffiness may be the earliest sign and not surprisingly may be most visible in the morning. Prominence of neck and chest veins can be another clue to the diagnosis. In addition the patient may appear cyanotic or plethoric and may show signs of respiratory distress. Chest pain and headache may accompany these other physical signs. When superior vena cava syndrome is suspected, it should be approached as a medical emergency.

Various conditions may mimic edema, including enlarged lymph nodes (see Chapter 25), tumors of the neck (neuroblastoma or rhabdomyosarcoma), subcutaneous air, and lymph abnormalities (cystic hygroma). Children with Noonan or Turner syndrome often have a webbed neck (pterygium colli) (see Fig. 29-14) as a result of lymphedema. Especially early in life, this lymph fluid may be a prominent feature of the neck examination. Lymphedema in Turner syndrome may recur later in life, especially during periods of estrogen replacement during adolescence.

Ascites

Fullness of the abdomen has many causes, including obesity, megacolon, mesenteric cysts, hepatomegaly, spleno-

Categories in the Differential Diagnosis of Ascites

Portal Hypertension
Prehepatic
   Portal vein thrombosis
     or occlusion
Hepatic
   Fibrosis
   Cirrhosis
   Tumors
   Cysts
Posthepatic
   Budd-Chiari syndrome
   Constrictive peri-
     carditis
   Congestive heart
     failure

Hypoalbuminemia
Nephrotic syndrome
Protein-losing en-
   teropathy
Malnutrition
Hydrops fetalis

Infectious Causes
Bacterial peritonitis
Fungal peritonitis
Tuberculous peritonitis
Cytomegalovirus
Toxoplasmosis
Syphilis

Chylous
Traumatic
Lymphatic obstruction
Lymphatic abnormalities

Urinary Causes
Posterior urethral valves
Bladder perforation
Ureteral stenosis
Urethral stenosis
Neurogenic bladder

Gastrointestinal Causes
Pancreatic causes
Intestinal atresia
Meconium peritonitis
Bile peritonitis

Miscellaneous Causes
Gynecologic disorders
Ventriculoperitoneal
   shunts
Eosinophilic peritonitis
Hypothyroidism

Pseudoascites
Omental cysts
Mesenteric cysts
Enteric duplication

Modified from Cochran WJ: Ascites. In Oski FA, et al, editors: *Principles and practice of pediatrics*, Philadelphia, 1994, JB Lippincott.

megaly, hydronephrosis, and a wide range of intraabdominal tumors. The diagnosis of these entities is often made by radiographic imaging procedures, but they are not the focus of this chapter. Ascites, or the collection of fluid in the peritoneal cavity, is a diagnostic challenge in its own right, and its detection and differential diagnosis are important. As with other areas of the body, ascites occurs when there is an alteration of Starling forces and the extravasation of fluid overloads the lymphatic system's ability to return that fluid to the vascular compartment. As a rule there are three major pathophysiologic mechanisms for its occurrence (1) decreased plasma oncotic pressure (hypoalbuminemia), (2) peritoneal irritation (infection, neoplasm, and trauma), and (3) venous or lymphatic obstruction (thrombosis or mass effect).

Ascites has its root in the Greek word for *bladder* or *bag*. An apparently fluid-filled abdominal cavity with a fullness or prominent appearance generally calls clinical attention to ascites. This observation can be reinforced by a variety of tech-

niques, including fluid wave, shifting dullness, and ballottement (see section on physical examination). The development of ascites can be either rapid or insidious. As a result of increased intraabdominal pressure and in some cases decreased muscle mass, several types of hernias may be associated (umbilical, femoral, or inguinal). Additional features may include scrotal edema (Fig. 22-3). Both portal hypertension and obstruction of the inferior vena cava may cause prominent veins over the abdomen (see Fig. 19-2). In the case of the patient with cirrhosis there is a sallow and dehydrated appearance and significant muscle wasting. Ascites resulting from hepatic disease is generally gradual in its appearance. Various imaging modalities help confirm the presence of fluid and rule out other processes that might be confused with ascites (omental and mesenteric cysts or tumors). Whereas the plain film can be used to screen, the abdominal sonogram and computed tomography are most effective at identifying fluid and its volume and location. Sonographic imaging is particularly effective for this purpose because it can detect as little as 150 ml of fluid, and the dynamic nature of the study allows for easy distinction between free fluid and loculated fluid. Its sensitivity, specificity, cost, and noninvasive nature make it the procedure of choice.

The differential diagnosis of ascites is varied and includes a wide range of fluid types as its cause (Box 22-3). Portal hypertension is a broad category and can be caused by intrinsic liver disease or obstruction of the portal vein (prehepatic) or hepatic veins (posthepatic). Portal vein obstruction generally results in splenomegaly and esophageal varices, but ascites is uncommon. Any number of liver diseases can cause cirrhosis or fibrosis and subsequent portal hypertension. Included are Alagille syndrome, biliary atresia, congenital hepatic fibrosis, alpha$_1$-antitrypsin deficiency, cystic fibrosis, and congenital hepatic fibrosis. Posthepatic causes include any pathophysiologic process that obstructs the outflow of blood from the liver and increases pressure in the vessels on the venous side of the liver, such as Budd-Chiari syndrome, CHF, and constrictive pericarditis. Careful cardiac history and physical examination can assist in the diagnosis of these latter two entities.

As discussed earlier, decreased oncotic pressure secondary to hypoalbuminemia has several causes, including albumin loss in the urine (nephrotic syndrome), protein loss in the gut (PLE), malnutrition, and severe liver disease (decrease in protein production). Chylous ascites results from abnormalities of lymphatic channels or obstruction of previously normal lymph vessels. Chyle also may collect in the peritoneal cavity as a result of traumatic injury to lymph structures (e.g., child abuse or surgery). Infections with bacteria, including *Mycobacterium* organisms, viruses, and fungi, cause peritoneal fluid. Perforation of organs can result in extrusion of a variety of fluids. These fluids include urine (e.g., secondary to posterior urethral valves or neurogenic bladder), bile (e.g., secondary to posterior perforated biliary tree), and meconium. Other causes of ascites include pancreatitis and gynecologic disorders (pelvic inflammatory disease).

For accurate diagnosis of many of these causes, ascitic fluid must be obtained by paracentesis. This is a relatively safe procedure that provides detailed information about the cause of the ascites. Transudate and exudate are two common ways to differentiate between various causes. Transudates generally result from processes, such as portal hypertension, that increase hydrostatic pressure or hypoalbuminemia that decreases serum oncotic pressure. Transudates generally have low protein, lactic dehydrogenase, and white blood counts, whereas exudates, which result from inflammation (infection, pancreatitis, and neoplasia), have high levels of these three parameters. Specific characteristics can assist in the diagnosis of free bile, urine, or chyle. Gram stains and cultures also provide critical information.

Scrotum

Swelling of the scrotal sac is alarming and should be viewed as an emergency. The danger of irreversible testicular injury should prompt an immediate emergency room visit, a urologic consult, and a detailed evaluation. Because surgical exploration is a possibility, the child should refrain from eating or drinking until a surgical problem has been eliminated. The presence of pain is helpful in approaching the differential diagnosis of the swollen scrotum. Torsion of the appendix testis or the testicle itself, trauma, epididymitis, and incarcerated hernia are all associated with scrotal pain.

Several embryologic remnants of testicular development, such as the appendix of the testis, are located on the testes and epididymis. These can twist on themselves, causing venous engorgement, pain, and, if blood supply is compromised enough, infarction. Typically this occurs even in the prepubertal child. The symptoms of acute pain, swelling, diaphoresis, nausea, and vomiting can mimic torsion of the testis itself. If the child is seen early in the course of this process, the testis itself is not painful, but rather the pain is localized to the area of the torsed appendage. If the pain is localized to the upper portion of the testicular structures, a diagnosis of testicular torsion is unlikely. "Blue dots" in the area of the affected structure may be present and can further support the clinician's impressions. Over the course of several days the pain should lessen, confirming the diagnosis of torsion of testicular appendicial structures.

Torsion of the testis itself presents acutely and dramatically, often after minor trauma or activity. It is the most common cause of acute painful swelling of the scrotum in children. Because the testis is not well attached to the scrotum, it is able to twist on itself, resulting in impaired venous and lymphatic drainage, eventual compromise of arterial blood supply, and resultant testicular injury (Fig. 22-9). As opposed to a twisted appendage, torsion of the testis in this case is very tender, with pain often radiating to the abdomen. The scrotal skin may be discolored, and fever may be a clinical feature. Nausea and vomiting may also accompany these findings. On examination the involved testis is located higher than the normal testis. Further elevation of the testis exacerbates the child's discomfort. The leg on the affected side may

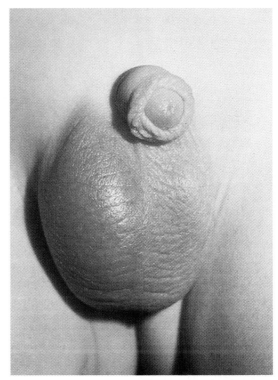

FIG. 22-9 A red, tender hemiscrotum may be due to torsion of the testis with gangrene, a surgical emergency.

be held in flexion. The emergent nature of this process cannot be overemphasized. Ideally, surgery should be performed within 6 hours of onset of symptoms for the testis to have the best chance of being saved. Surgery involves untwisting the affected testicular structures and bilateral exploration and orchiopexy.

Because of the minor trauma frequently associated with testicular torsion, the diagnosis may be delayed. Trauma as the sole cause of testicular swelling and pain can cause mild symptoms on one end of the spectrum to outright rupture with a hemiscrotum and tenseness at the other end. As with testicular torsion, timely surgical exploration is indicated.

Epididymoorchitis generally occurs in pubertal boys and is not associated with underlying urogenital anomalies. Typically, onset of symptoms is gradual, and often the epididymis is the first structure to show swelling and tenderness. Epididymitis is associated with inguinal pain as well. With time the testis and scrotum itself become symptomatic. In adults, elevation and support of the scrotum for an hour may relieve the painful sensation. The scrotum may be erythematous and have a parchmentlike appearance but typically is not edematous. Chills, fever, urethral discharge, and pain on urination occur. White blood cells may be present in the urine, and on occasion urine culture may be positive. *Chlamydia trachomatis,* gonorrhea, and the bacteria responsible for urinary tract infections may be the culprit.

In the postpubertal boy who has not been immunized for mumps, orchitis may be either unilateral or bilateral. Typi-

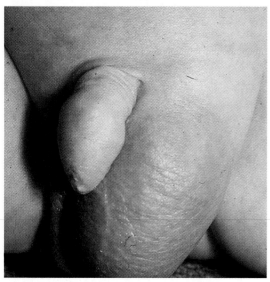

FIG. 22-10   A complete inguinal hernia extends into the scrotum, obscuring the testis.

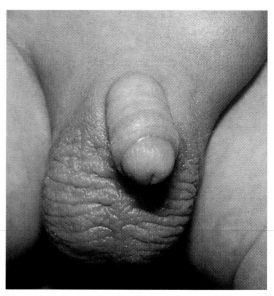

FIG. 22-11   Incomplete inguinal hernia produces a bulge in the left groin but does not extend into the scrotum.

cally, orchitis occurs 4 to 6 days after parotitis. Other agents include echovirus and coxsackievirus. In addition to pain and swelling of the testicular and scrotal areas, fever, chills, and rectal pain may accompany orchitis.

Inguinal hernia may be another cause of scrotal pain and swelling (Fig. 22-10). At times, however, the hernia may sit above the scrotum itself (Fig. 22-11). Often the testis is felt and no abnormality is found. The process of straining and coughing (increased intraabdominal pressure) may exacerbate the degree of swelling. Lastly, cellulitis of the scrotum and surrounding tissues can also result in swelling and pain.

Painless scrotal swelling is not as urgent as testicular torsion or incarcerated inguinal herniation but nonetheless can indicate significant pathology. One of the more common causes of scrotal swelling is a hydrocele (a collection of fluid within the tunica vaginalis, which surrounds each testis). In the infant this may represent residual fluid that remains after the processus vaginalis has already closed. If the size of the hydrocele does not change with time, the fluid is generally reabsorbed by $1\frac{1}{2}$ years of age. A hydrocele also may be secondary to torsion of the testis, a testicular appendage, trauma, epididymitis, or a tumor. If the size of the hydrocele waxes and wanes, the processus vaginalis is surely open and the hydrocele communicates. The likelihood of closure is small, and a true hernia may develop. Because of the fluid-filled nature of a hydrocele, it transilluminates easily. A noncommunicating hydrocele is not reducible. On the other hand, parents often describe a relative increase in volume as the day progresses and the effects of gravity bring fluid into the patent processus vaginalis. In the supine or prone position (during sleep), fluid is reabsorbed, lessening its volume. This indicates that an indirect inguinal hernia exists. Further examination using the thumb and index finger in the area above the testes but below the internal ring reveals a thickening that represents the processus vaginalis.

"Silk sign" can be elicited by palpating the region of the inguinal canal and sensing the anterior and posterior portions of the processus rolling over each other (the feeling of rubbing two pieces of silk together). These physical examination maneuvers can allow for accurate diagnosis even when an obvious inguinal or scrotal bulge is not present. Although inguinal hernia is less common in girls, it does occur, and it is usually detected by the observation of this bulge or the presence of a palpable processus vaginalis. As already suggested, inguinal hernia can occur with or without pain.

Another common cause of painless swelling is a varicocoele, which is found in 10% of pubertal boys. A varicocoele is palpated in the scrotum while the patient is standing. It represents varicosities of the pampiniform venous plexus and has a soft, irregular feel described as a "bag of worms." It almost always occurs on the left side; rarely it is bilateral.

Testicular tumors typically present as indurated, firm, painless, unilateral testicular masses. A hydrocele often is seen along with testicular tumors. In children with known leukemia the testes are common sites of relapse.

Idiopathic scrotal edema accounts for approximately 2% to 5% of all normal patients with acute scrotal swelling. The scrotum may be swollen bilaterally, and the abdominal wall also may be affected. The testes, however, are normal and nontender on examination. Some authors suggest that this condition may be a form of angioneurotic edema. The swelling and erythema typically resolves in about 48 hours. A variety of other entities can cause scrotal swelling or scrotal masses, including Henoch-Schönlein purpura, healed meconium peritonitis, fat necrosis, sarcoidosis, and elephantiasis. As alluded to earlier, the scrotum may be affected in isolation or as part of a generalized process in many entities causing edema. These entities include nephrotic syndrome and liver disease.

Extremities

A child with a swollen extremity poses a challenging diagnostic dilemma. As with other forms of localized edema, focal areas of altered capillary permeability, such as insect bites, should be sought. A central punctum, pruritus, firmness of the affected area, and excoriation all may be clues to diagnosis. Lesions can be multiple or solitary. Evidence of trauma or surgery should be sought historically and by physical examination. Local allergic reactions should be considered as well, and a search for inciting agents should be pursued. Cellulitis of the extremities can also cause swelling. The pain, tender skin, erythema, and induration that accompany this diagnosis often solidify clinical suspicion. A break in the skin may be found, and rapid response to an antibiotic confirms the diagnosis. Osteomyelitis is a common cause of focal swelling in childhood. Fever may or may not be present, but focal tenderness over bone, pseudoparalysis or limp, local warmth, and soft tissue swelling often are part of the clinical picture. A positive blood culture and radiologic imaging assist in diagnosis.

Kawasaki syndrome causes swollen, red, and at times tender distal extremities (see Fig. 7-5). Diagnosis is clinical and is made when the Centers for Disease Control criteria are met. These criteria include prolonged high fever, oropharyngeal infection, rash, cervical lymphadenopathy, and bilateral nonexudative conjunctivitis. As already alluded to, Henoch-Schönlein purpura can cause extremity swelling. Often a purpuric rash, hematuria, heme-positive stools, abdominal pain, and joint pain accompany the swelling (Fig. 22-4). In the patient with sickle-cell disease, a "log-jam" phenomenon of the distal extremities can lead to swelling and pain. This form of tissue infarction is known as *dactylitis* or *hand-foot syndrome* (see Fig. 4-1). Many causes of arthritis can play into the differential diagnosis of limb swelling, and these are discussed in detail in Chapter 6. In addition, some patients with paralysis from the thoracic level down display lower extremity-dependent edema.

Venous obstruction of a major vessel caused by mass effect (tumor), vessel injury, or a clotting disorder (thrombosis) can also cause limb swelling. Deep venous thrombosis, although uncommon in children, must be considered in the evaluation of limb swelling. A deep venous line is often the culprit.

Lymphatic abnormalities comprise a major group of disorders that result in limb swelling. These entities can be divided into primary and secondary disorders. Secondary lymphedema can be caused by recurrent lymphangitis, filariasis, tuberculosis, neoplasm, surgery, or radiation therapy. Lymphatic injury, obstruction, inflammation, and scarring may play a role in these entities. Primary lymphedema can occur as a result of an underlying syndrome, such as Turner syndrome or Noonan syndrome. In Turner syndrome, it is postulated that hypoplasia and delayed maturation of the lymphatic system cause the distinctive findings of lymphedema (see Fig. 29-9). The yellow nail syndrome is an aptly named entity characterized by dystrophic yellow nails, pleural effusion, bronchiectasis, and sinusitis. Inheritance is autosomal dominant. Edema with districhiasis is another unusual syndrome presenting with impaired lymphatic drainage and an extra set of eyelashes. Other forms of primary lymphedema include congenital lymphedema, which evolves early in life; lymphedema praecox, which develops with puberty; and lymphedema tarda, which begins at approximately age 35. Several hereditary forms of primary lymphedema exist, congenital lymphedema (Milroy disease) and lymphedema in the older child (lymphedema praecox). Additional details of this classification system are available in several excellent reviews.

History

Edema may present in dramatic fashion with generalized swelling or a more localized distribution. In either case, information about the intermittent or persistent nature of the swelling should be sought. The date of original onset should be established, as should changes in the amount and location of swelling throughout the day. As a result of gravity, periorbital edema may dominate the clinical picture upon arising in the morning and ankle edema may predominate during the evening. The temptation to rapidly focus on a particular region of the body without accounting for the changes that occur during the day may lead the clinician in the direction of localized edema instead of a generalized process. At times the presence of edema may not be immediately obvious. As suggested earlier, adults can harbor 5 to 10 pounds of extra fluid before pitting edema is detected. Careful questioning about the tightness of shoes, pants, rings, or belts may lead to the suspicion of edema. Dependent areas, such as the feet, may be particularly affected after the day's activities. Shoes that fit in the morning may be uncomfortable at day's end. It is important to emphasize that a particular region of swelling, such as the scrotum, may simply be the first affected or detected area in a systemic process. Accurate weights are extremely helpful in assessing fluid status, though the distinction between a true increase in tissue mass and an increase in body fluid can be historically difficult to confirm even when weights are available.

When more than one body region is affected by edema, the historic approach should focus on systemic processes. Any family history of systemic disorders (e.g., lupus erythematosus or cystic fibrosis) or renal disease (e.g., Alport syndrome) should be sought. Questions about hereditary angioedema should also be asked. Changes in stooling pattern (frequency or consistency) or evidence of malabsorption may suggest an underlying gastrointestinal cause for a child's edema. Cardiac disease (CHF) may be the underlying cause of edema when a history of poor exercise tolerance, fatigue, or inability to keep up with other children is elicited. Questions about shortness of breath and increased heart and respiratory rates may add further evidence for heart failure. The infant may have less specific features, such as poor feeding, fussiness, and a sense of restlessness. Renal causes may surface when evidence of changes in urine volume and character are discovered. Blood in the urine (e.g., smoky or colored) or decreased urine output may be a valuable clue to a renal cause for edema. Historic evidence for liver disease, including pruritus, spider angiomata, gastrointestinal bleeding, and jaundice, should be sought.

Allergic reactions to foods (cow's milk) and poor protein intake (kwashiorkor) cause edema, necessitating a careful dietary history. Exposure to a variety of toxins, drugs, and chemicals (e.g., antihypertensives, estrogen, lithium, or alcohol) should be explored.

Careful attention should be paid to use of over-the-counter drugs, illicit drugs, and physician-prescribed medications. Edema may result from an allergic reaction, toxic reaction, idiosyncratic reaction, or even an infectious agent transmitted by a "dirty" needle. Environmental factors should be addressed. An entity called *tropical edema* occurs when normal adults leave a temperate climate and travel to hot regions of the world. Edema rapidly develops in the ankles (within 2 days) and disappears without therapy in several days. Edema is also known to occur in high altitudes. A history of the menstrual cycle and sexual activity should be explored. Premenstrual "bloating" is a common finding, as is oral contraceptive–induced edema. During the later 6 months of pregnancy, gravity-dependent regions may become puffy. Rash should suggest an infectious cause, collagen vascular disease, or possibly an allergic process.

Localized edema is generally a marker for minor trauma, allergic reactions, or subcutaneous tissue infection. Evidence of burns, bites, and contact with various agents (e.g., poison ivy) should be included in the history-taking process. History gathering should focus on causes of these regional processes.

Physical Examination

As with the history, a prime focus of the physical examination should be the distinction between generalized and localized edema. Generalized edema often is recognized in a localized region of the body first. The absence of additional local clues, such as rash, insect bite puncta, or skin irritation, should increase suspicion of a generalized process. If bilateral edema of the extremities is noted, a generalized process is more likely. Whereas children with mild edema may escape detection without the use of sequential weight measurements, others have swelling so obvious that easy recognition is assured. Lean, muscular individuals are more likely to hide their edema. Direct pressure over a bony prominence of the tibia, fibula, or sacrum may elicit pitting and can be visualized as a depression or indentation of the subcutaneous tissue. It is incumbent upon the examiner to have the supine patient turn over and to examine the sacral area and the tissue of the posterior aspect of the calf. Because of gravity, edema collects in the most dependent areas. The same caveat holds true for the ambulatory patient. If socks are not removed during an examination, a key physical sign may be overlooked. The obliteration of the normal anatomic landmarks of a struc-

ture can be another helpful clue. The formation of lymphedema as a result of lymph obstruction mimics edema produced by other mechanisms.

Many processes that result in generalized edema also affect vital signs. Tachycardia (e.g., CHF) and tachypnea (e.g., pulmonary edema) can both be seen, as can hypotension and hypertension. If intravascular volume depletion is severe enough, orthostatic changes or baseline hypotension may exist. Hypertension can be seen in states such as acute glomerulonephritis and iatrogenically induced volume overload (intravenous gammaglobulin). Elevated temperature should suggest infection or perhaps collagen vascular disease. Height and head circumference should be measured and used as general markers of nutritional state and endocrine, renal, and gastrointestinal well-being. Children with cystic fibrosis, hepatic failure, and HIV infection may not grow well, making these parameters invaluable clues.

In the search for causes of generalized edema, findings of specific disease processes should be sought. If cystic fibrosis is suspected, nasal polyps, clubbing, and rectal prolapse are additional clues. If liver disease is a consideration, xanthomata, spider angiomata, caput medusa, scleral icterus, and palmar erythema may be visible. In the child with high-output cardiac failure as a result of an arteriovenous fistula, cranial or abdominal bruits may be present. The list of potential physical findings is obviously extensive, necessitating a meticulous general examination.

When the focus of the examination is localized edema, detailed observation again serves the clinician well. In a child with unilateral periorbital swelling, a careful search for evidence of an abrasion, cut, or puncta is critical. The conjunctiva and sinuses require equal attention. Although bilateral periorbital edema may be a sign of Epstein-Barr virus infection, the presence of pharyngitis and splenomegaly confirm the diagnosis. Clearly the physical examination holds many valuable clues to the differential diagnosis of the child with edema.

Approach to the Patient

Laboratory Tests and Radiologic Procedures

The laboratory provides useful tools to the clinician for the management of edema. Evaluations should be focused and used to assist with clinical "branch points" (Fig. 22-12) or to confirm diagnoses that are suspected on the basis of the history and physical examination. Localized edema rarely warrants extensive laboratory evaluation. Often, trauma or infection dictates the type of radiographs or cultures obtained. Allergic causes should be sought when possible with the assistance of a pediatric allergist. Ascites requires its own detailed laboratory evaluation with specific attention to liver function (liver enzymes and functional parameters) and sonography. Other conditions that result in ascites can be diagnosed with sonogram as well (tumors or pancreatitis). More specific laboratory examinations, (e.g., a voiding cystoure-throgram) may be indicated in specific circumstances, such as suspected urinary tract obstruction with perforation. When generalized edema is present and cardiac disease is suspected, a chest radiograph may show pulmonary edema, pleural effusion, an enlarged heart (CHF or pericardial effusion), or even calcifications (constrictive pericarditis). Echocardiogram can differentiate pericardial fluid from an enlarged heart. Information about cardiac anatomy and function also can be obtained. Electrocardiogram may show evidence of dysrhythmia, low-voltage QRS complexes, and myocardial ischemia. Blood gases can be used to assess tissue hypoperfusion and hypoxia. Lastly, electrolytes, glucose, calcium, and creatine phosphokinase values may be abnormal.

The most common cause of generalized edema in children is renal disease. Fortunately, the diagnosis of proteinuria is easily made by urine dipstick. A value of 1+ (or 30 mg/dl) is suspicious and warrants a formal 24-hour collection for protein. Values greater than 150 mg per 24 hours are considered abnormal, though double this amount may be considered normal in select circumstances. Other markers for significant proteinuria are a urine protein/urine creatinine ratio greater than 0.2 (in nephrotic syndrome the ratio usually is greater than 3.5). Another rule of thumb for nephrotic syndrome is protein spillage of greater than 50 mg/kg/day. A 24-hour creatinine clearance can easily be obtained simultaneously with urine collection for protein. This assists in the assessment of renal function, which may be impaired by the same pathologic process or may be secondarily affected by the hemodynamic changes of nephrotic syndrome. Urinalysis should include microscopic examination for hematuria, white blood cells and casts, and a specific gravity should be measured. Additional assessment of the patient with renal disease might include serum urea nitrogen, creatinine level, electrolytes, cholesterol value, triglycerides, total protein and albumin levels, complete blood count, and sedimentation rate. Complement levels (C3 and C4) can help diagnose postinfectious GN and membranoproliferative GN. If post-streptococcal GN is a concern, serology for streptococcal antibody titers and a throat or skin culture may be indicated.

If cardiac disease and renal disease seem unlikely, further laboratory testing might include an antinuclear antibody test, liver function tests, a detailed gastrointestinal workup, and C1 esterase inhibitor.

Consultation

The initial workup of edema is certainly within the generalist's purview, but often there is need for consultation as a specific diagnosis becomes clearer. The pediatric cardiologist, gastroenterologist, and nephrologist often play a major role in the later phases of diagnosis and are invaluable in management of patients with specific disease processes. Severe allergic entities, such as anaphylaxis with laryngeal edema or abdominal visceral edema, suggest the need for consultation with a pediatric allergist. As with most diagnostic entities, however, the generalist is central in identifying the affected organ system(s) and embarking on a direction at that point. It is vital that the generalist remain involved to coordinate care and provide ongoing direction and support.

Management

The focus of proper management of edema should be on the underlying condition. In the case of localized edema, therapies such as topical steroids, heat, ice, or elevation may prove effective. In the case of infection (e.g., periorbital cellulitis), antibiotics are indicated. Other settings may require the use of antihistamines or nonsteroidal antiinflammatory drugs.

Generalized edema is best managed by addressing the underlying cause (e.g., CHF or nephrotic syndrome), but some basic principles may help to augment this therapy. Activities can continue if the child is able to participate. Fluid restriction is difficult to accomplish and generally is not critical. At times, however, restriction is needed (e.g., renal failure), and only daily insensible plus urinary losses should be replaced. Salt restriction is important and should be maintained to a degree that provides adequate palatability. Ideally, 2 gm/m^2 of sodium (4 gm/m^2 of sodium chloride) should be used as a starting point. Attempts to further restrict salt may lead to poor caloric intake. Diuretics should be used very judiciously, especially when low protein states are being treated. Close attention to intravascular volume is essential to avoid hypoperfusion. Infection is also a significant risk to the patient with edema, and fever should prompt a rapid and detailed assessment. In situations, such as nephrotic syndrome where immunoglobulins are lost (along with albumin), the risk of infection is heightened.

Algorithm

As stated several times earlier, the first branch point in the algorithmic approach to edema is whether there is localized or generalized edema (Fig. 22-12). If the edema is localized, a historic search for trauma can provide an explanation. Should this history be negative, a search for redness or fever may lead to evidence of infection, such as cellulitis or osteomyelitis. If this aspect of the examination is negative and there is no history to suggest allergy, lymphatic abnormalities become likely possibilities.

In the event that the edema is generalized, cardiac examination then urinary evaluation for protein may reveal the primary cause. The loss of protein in the urine may be secondary to GN, nephrotic syndrome, renal failure, or collagen vascular disease. If protein is not found in the urine, other sources of loss or poor production or intake may be the cause. These include PLE, hepatic disease, and malnutrition. If serum protein is also normal, vasculitis and premenstrual syndrome should be considered.

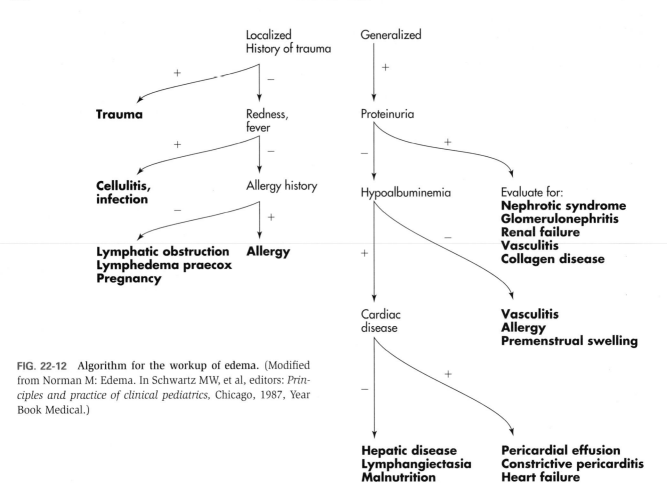

FIG. 22-12 Algorithm for the workup of edema. (Modified from Norman M: Edema. In Schwartz MW, et al, editors: *Principles and practice of clinical pediatrics*, Chicago, 1987, Year Book Medical.)

SUMMARY

In summary, edema is the abnormal swelling of tissues as a result of fluid accumulation in the interstitial compartment. The body has the capacity to accumulate large amounts of fluid that are not clinically detectable until substantial amounts are present. At other times, with focal processes, small amounts of fluid are rapidly detectable and parents respond with alarm. Fluid may be generalized or localized, acute or chronic, and a result of systemic disease or very focal processes. The four major pathogenic mechanisms include low oncotic pressure, increased capillary permeability, abnormal lymphatic function, and elevated hydrostatic pressure.

A detailed history, searching for familial incidence, preceding events, and other systemic symptoms is essential. In addition, a meticulous and complete physical examination may provide essential clues to diagnosis. After it is determined whether the process is generalized or localized, a thoughtful and pointed workup generally leads to an explanation. Therapy can then be tailored to the underlying disease process. Although many causes of edema are benign and of little consequence to a child's health, other processes are life-threatening, heightening the need for rapid and accurate diagnosis.

ILLUSTRATIVE CASES

Case 1. A 2½ year-old boy has puffy eyelids upon awakening. He is seen in his pediatrician's office in the late afternoon. By this point the edema in his eyelids has lessened, and he is noted to have scrotal and ankle edema. There is no significant preceding medical history, and the child is on no medications. Physical examination reveals normal vital signs and no other evidence of abnormality.

Because of the presence of edema in three distinct areas of the body, a diagnosis of generalized edema is considered. Because of the absence of cardiac findings and normal liver size, cardiac disease is considered unlikely. A urine dipstick done in the office reveals 4+ protein. Further laboratory evaluation reveals hypoalbuminemia and hypercholesterolemia. A tentative diagnosis of nephrotic syndrome is made, and the patient is referred to a pediatric nephrologist.

This case illustrates a generalized process beginning with focal edema of the eyelids and provides a typical scenario for the presentation of nephrotic syndrome.

Case 2. A 4-year-old girl has unilateral eyelid swelling that was first noticed in the early afternoon. An upper respiratory tract infection had been present for approximately 2 weeks, with minimal systemic signs. Five days before being seen in her pediatrician's office, she developed thick green nasal discharge, exacerbation of her cough, and halitosis. Careful physical examination of her eyelid reveals erythema, swelling, and enough puffiness to partially occlude the visual access. On palpation the lesion feels somewhat boggy and is surprisingly nontender. Further physical examination reveals that the child is afebrile and shows no other abnormalities. Sinus x-ray films are obtained and show sinusitis of the ethmoid and maxillary sinuses on the ipsilateral side. A diagnosis of sinusitis-induced inflammatory edema is made, and antibiotic therapy is initiated. The patient is sent home and improves slowly over a period of 3 to 4 days.

This case illustrates sinusitis as a local cause of edema affecting the periorbital space. The absence of tenderness distinguishes this lesion from an infectious periorbital or orbital cellulitis.

Case 3. A 9-year-old boy comes to his pediatrician with abdominal swelling. His past medical history is significant for neonatal jaundice that was considered physiologic but persisted for approximately 4 to 6 weeks. After the resolution of his jaundice, he was well and developing and growing normally. On careful examination, he is noted to have shifting dullness of his abdomen, and the possibility of ascites is raised. The presence of ascites is confirmed by sonogram, and in addition an enlarged spleen and a possibly cirrhotic liver are noted. Liver enzymes are markedly elevated, and serum albumin level is well below the normal range. Referral to a pediatric gastroenterologist is initiated. After further evaluation, a liver biopsy is performed and reveals alpha$_1$-antitrypsin deficiency. Over the next 3 to 6 months, there is a deterioration of synthetic liver function, and a liver transplantation is performed.

This case provides an example of a hepatic disorder leading to ascites and eventually end-stage liver disease. Rapid diagnosis and appropriate referral led to swift initiation of the transplantation process and improved this child's chance for survival.

ANNOTATED BIBLIOGRAPHY

Fleisher GR: Edema. In Fleisher GR, Ludwig S, editors: *Textbook of pediatric emergency medicine*, Baltimore, 1993, Williams and Wilkins.

This text provides an excellent overview of edema with pathophysiology, differential diagnosis, and an excellent (but brief) algorithm.

Norman M: Edema. In Schwartz MW, Chaney EB, Curry TA, et al, editors: *Principles and practice of clinical pediatrics*, Chicago, 1987, Year Book Medical.

This is a brief, but helpful review of edema with a focus on history, physical examination, laboratory evaluation, and an algorithm.

Tunnessen WW: Edema. In *Signs and symptoms in pediatrics*, Philadelphia, 1988, JB Lippincott.

This is the most comprehensive chapter available on the differential diagnosis of edema with all the major categories outlined in a very clinically functional fashion.

BIBLIOGRAPHY

Baliga R, Lewy JE: Pathogenesis and treatment of edema, *Pediatr Clin North Am* 34:639-648, 1987.

Berman S: Scrotal swelling. In *Pediatric decision making*, Philadelphia, 1991, BC Decker.

Chase HP, Kumar V, Caldwell RT, et al: Kwashiorkor in the United States, *Pediatrics* 66:972-976, 1980.

Cochran WJ: Ascites. In Oski FA, et al, editors: *Principles and practice of pediatrics*, Philadelphia, 1994, JB Lippincott.

Etches PC, Lemons JA: Nonimmune hydrops fetalis: report of 22 cases including three siblings, *Pediatrics* 64:326-332, 1979.

Fitzgerald JF: Ascites. In Wyllie R, Hyams JS, editors: *Pediatric gastrointestinal disease: pathophysiology, diagnosis, management*, Philadelphia, 1993, WB Saunders.

Gleason WA: Protein-losing enteropathy. In Wyllie R, Hyams JS, editors: *Pediatric gastrointestinal disease: pathophysiology, diagnosis, management*, Philadelphia, 1993, WB Saunders.

Goldbloom RB: *Pediatric clinical skills*, New York, 1992, Churchill-Livingstone.

Green M: *Pediatric diagnosis: interpretation of symptoms and signs in infants, children, and adolescents*, Philadelphia, 1992, WB Saunders.

Hilliard RI, McKendry JBJ, Phillips MJ: Congenital abnormalities of the lymphatic system: a new clinical classification, *Pediatrics* 86:988-994, 1990.

Hutchison AA, Drew JH, Yu VYH, et al: Nonimmune hydrops fetalis: a review of 61 cases, *Obstet Gynecol* 59:347-352, 1982.

Issa PY, Brihi ER, Janin Y, et al: Superior vena cava system in childhood: report of ten cases and review of the literature, *Pediatrics* 71:337-341, 1983.

Lee PA, Dietrich WR, Howatt WF: Hypoproteinemia and anemia in infants with cystic fibrosis: a presenting symptom complex often misdiagnosed, *JAMA* 228(5):585-588, 1974.

Lewis JM, Wald ER: Lymphedema praecox, *J Pediatr* 104:641-648, 1984.

McGillivray BC, Hall JG: Nonimmune hydrops fetalis, *Pediatr Rev* 9:197-202, 1987.

Murph JR, Woodhead JC: Edema. In Dershewitz RA, editor: *Ambulatory pediatric care*, Philadelphia, 1993, JB Lippincott.

Oliver WJ, Kelsch RC: Nephrotic syndrome due to primary nephropathies, *Pediatr Rev* 2:311-317, 1981.

Smeltzer DM, Stickler GB, Schirger A: Primary lymphedema in children and adolescents: a follow-up study and review, *Pediatrics* 76:206-218, 1985.

Tunnessen WW: Periorbital edema. In *Signs and symptoms in pediatrics*, Philadelphia, 1988, JB Lippincott.

Weiss AH: The swollen and droopy eyelid: signs of systemic disease, *Pediatr Clin North Am* 40:789-804, 1993.

Winters RW: *The body fluids in pediatrics*, Boston, 1973, Little Brown.

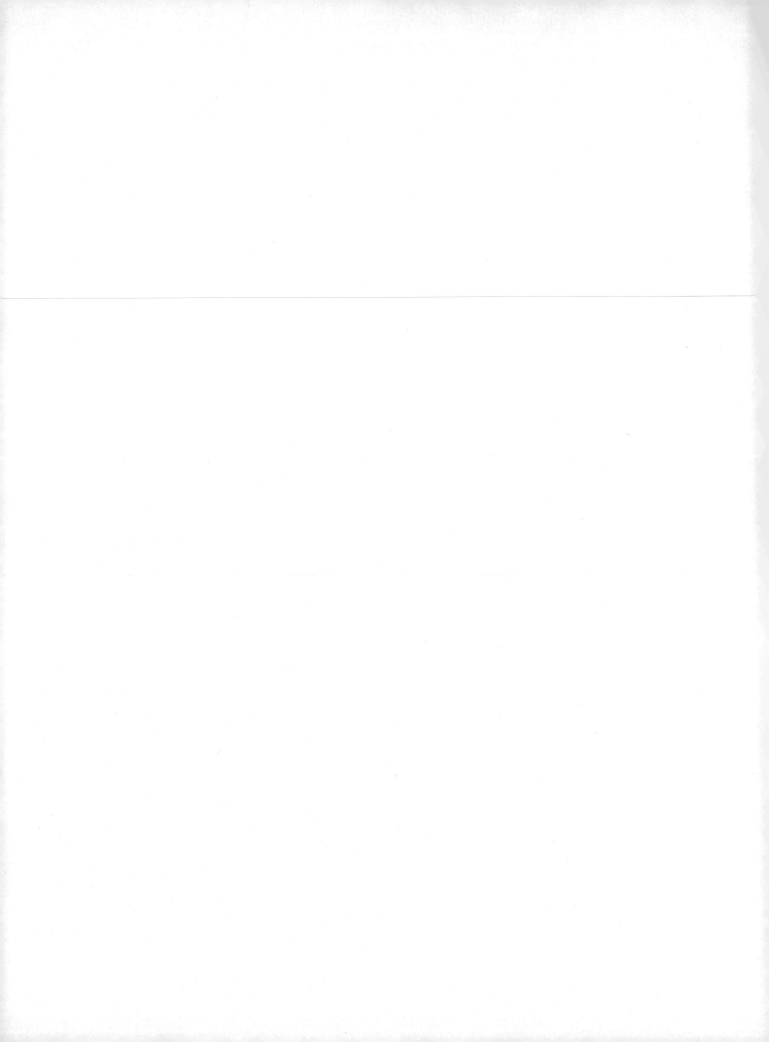

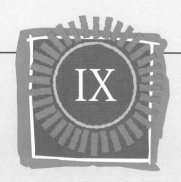

Hematology and
Immunology

23

Bruising and Bleeding

J. JEFFREY MALATACK ❧ MARY M. MORAN
BETH MOUGHAN

 Key Points

- Failure of platelet action because of decreased platelet number or decreased platelet function leads to symmetric petechiae and bruising with mild trauma.

- Historic clues to a clotting-factor defect include delayed umbilical cord separation, oozing from the umbilical stump, poor wound healing, and bleeding at intramuscular injection sites.

- Inflammation of the blood vessel wall (vasculitis) is commonly manifested by palpable purpuric lesions, often involving the lower extremities.

Cardinal features of disease may be divided into those that infer pathology by their presence and those that infer disease when present beyond some acceptable norm. Additionally, features of a disease must be interpreted, as must all signs and symptoms in the pediatric patient, with reference to the patient's age. Jaundice may be "physiologic" in the newborn but always is abnormal beyond the neonatal age. Bruising and bleeding in the neonate or the older child suggest disease only if present in excess. Everyday activities can cause bruising in children who have no defects in hemostasis (Fig. 23-1). Because of their unsteady gait, toddlers often have bruises on the extensor surfaces, particularly the shins. They may have head bruises from an occasional head bump incurred during a fall. Bruises also may occur in patients with defects in hemostasis. However, in these cases the bruise is often large, has a central nodule, and is disproportionate to the degree of trauma (Fig. 23-2).

Bruises on the thorax, abdomen, and back are less common in normal children but are a frequent result of everyday activity in children who have a bleeding disorder. Nosek-Cenkowska and colleagues attempted to differentiate normal children from children with bleeding disorders on the basis of a questionnaire. No combination of historic questions was both sensitive and specific in separating the two groups com-pletely, but children who report large bruises, frequent hematoma formation, bruising in many different body locations (not always the shins), or nosebleeds that either occur at least once a year or last longer than 10 minutes should be suspected of having a bleeding problem.

Pathophysiology

A complex interaction of vascular changes, platelet activity, and soluble clotting factors maintains normal hemostasis. These aspects of normal control of bleeding are integrated to trigger coagulation at the moment of tissue injury and avoid spontaneous coagulation at all other times. The system should work only when needed, but the response must be controlled and appropriate to the need.

The blood vessels play an important role in the coagulation scheme. Injury to the vessel exposes subendothelial structures, including collagen fibers, which become the site for platelet adhesion and also initiate platelet aggregation. The injured surface of the vessel interacts with certain circulating procoagulants to initiate the intrinsic coagulation path. Additionally, vessel injury is the source of tissue thromboplastin, which is needed to initiate the extrinsic coagulation pathway. Finally, stimulated endothelial cells release intermediates, triggering fibrinolysis and activating anticoagulant activity. Vascular tone, which is controlled by nitric oxide, plays a role in overall hemostasis.

Once tissue injury has occurred, providing a site for platelet aggregation, a thrombin-dependent and thrombin-driven process prompts a series of steps, leading to a fibrin-enmeshed platelet plug. The process is influenced by blood flow characteristics in the injured vessel (shear stress), viscosity of blood (hematocrit level), humoral factors, interaction with the endothelial cell, and the number of platelets per cubic millimeter.

The platelet plug (primary clot) is stabilized by the plasma coagulants, which provide a fibrin meshwork to hold the plug together and form the so-called secondary clot. The mecha-

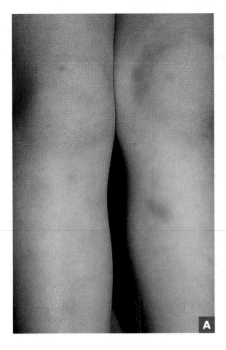
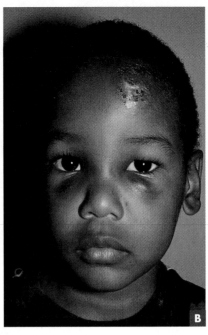

FIG. 23-1   Normal bruises. *A,* A number of small, nonspecific bruises are present over the knees and shins of this active youngster. *B,* Black eyes after a forehead contusion. This boy fell from a slide 3 days earlier. Blood from his forehead hematoma tracked down through the facial soft tissues, creating these shiners.

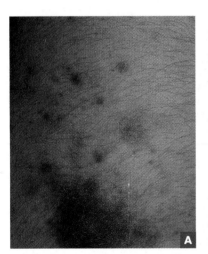
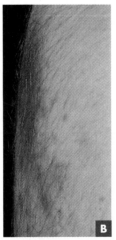

FIG. 23-2   *A,* Dramatic bruises with thick, round centers can be seen in children with clotting factor deficiencies. *B,* This view from the side demonstrates the elevation of the central portion of the ecchymosis.

nisms that create this meshwork are juxtaposed to mechanisms that dissolve it. Promoters of further fibrin clot formation are offset by inhibitors of such formation in an intricate pattern of control and countercontrol that allows for a very finely tuned system.

Literature Survey

There is a massive amount of literature dealing with specific defects in hemostasis that may lead to excessive bruising or bleeding, but little literature focuses on the child who has bruising and bleeding and guides the reader toward a diagnosis.

A Medline search for articles on bruising and bleeding written during the last 30 years lists 114 citations. Few are reviews, rather most are case reports of unusual entities presenting as bruising and bleeding. Only one in every five published articles focuses on children. Though four pediatric reviews are available, prospective studies are lacking.

Prospective studies are unlikely to be forthcoming because inclusion criteria for such a study are difficult if not impossible to develop. How much bruising is enough to warrant inclusion of a patient in such a study? How are the substantial differences in children's activity levels and aggressive behaviors corrected for?

An interesting attempt has been made to distinguish children who have prominent bruising and bleeding secondary to a bleeding diathesis from those who are normal. The attempt used a questionnaire and carefully selected normals and controls (bleeders). The authors noted that, although a pattern of response to certain questions provided some ability to differentiate normals from bleeders, overlap persisted. When responses to a series of questions included more than 90% of bleeders, 40% of nonbleeders were also included. Alternatively, when responses to a series of questions captured more than 85% of normals, 35% of bleeders were also included.

An additional diagnostic difficulty in the child with excessive bruising and bleeding was described by O'Hare and Eden. Their study of 50 children with suspected nonaccidental injury (child abuse) noted that a small but significant number of children had evidence of a bleeding disorder, though several features supported the diagnosis of abuse (Figs. 23-3 and 23-4). They concluded that laboratory evidence of altered hemostasis and child abuse should not be

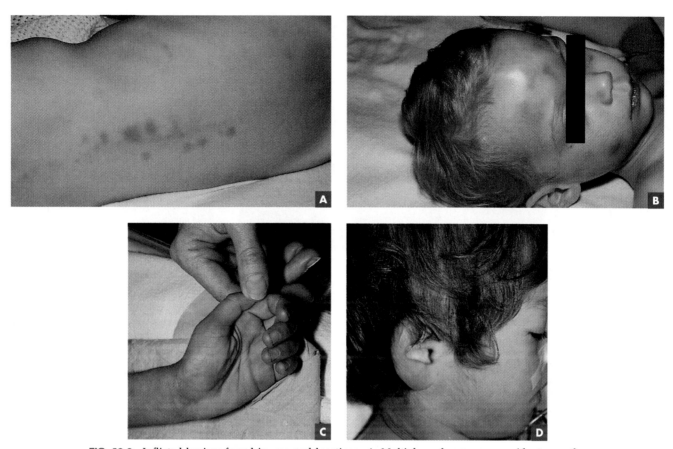

FIG. 23-3   Inflicted bruises found in unusual locations. *A*, Multiple ecchymoses are evident over the back and upper chest of this child who is poorly nourished but has normal coagulation studies. *B*, The same patient has multiple bruises of the face and forehead. *C*, This child has severe contusions that were inflicted with a ruler over the hands. *D*, The same child has a markedly swollen and contused ear as well.

considered mutually exclusive. Eden and O'Hare argued that it is as significant an error to accuse a family of nonaccidental injury when a bleeding disorder exists as it is to dismiss the possibility of child abuse in the child with laboratory evidence of abnormal hemostasis. The child with a bleeding disorder is at particular risk of serious injury from abuse.

Differential Diagnosis

When excessive, bruising and bleeding represent either a disturbance in normal hemostasis or significant trauma. Trauma may be incurred accidentally or inflicted (child abuse). When excessive bruising and bleeding are the result of hemostatic dysfunction, the differential diagnosis may be divided into three broad categories as follows: (1) pathology that alters normal platelet function, (2) pathology of normal fibrin clot formation, or (3) pathology affecting normal vascular integrity. Although all three of these phases are intricately related, discussion deals with each broad category separately.

Platelet Disorders

Platelet disorders may be further divided into quantitative and qualitative defects. Inadequate platelet number or function leads to the hallmark clinical findings listed in Box 23-1. Purpura (defined as either petechiae or ecchymoses) occurs when blood escapes from its vascular compartment and leaks into the skin. If the escape is contained within a small distribution, petechiae are seen. Petechiae are flat, red or reddish-purple, 1 to 3 mm in diameter, nonpulsatile, nonblanching lesions. In the setting of decreased platelet number or function, petechiae are generally found in a symmetric pattern throughout the torso and extremities (Fig. 23-5). (This pattern is in dramatic contrast to petechiae found in dependent areas, which are indicative of altered vascular integrity.) Typically in quantitative or qualitative platelet defects, patients exhibit symmetric petechiae and small ecchymoses (Fig. 23-6). If excessive bleeding complicates an injury, the bleeding occurs immediately after the injury (in contrast to the delayed onset of bleeding seen in defects of the plasma coagulant system). Bleeding from mucous membranes (nose, mouth, and gastrointestinal and genitourinary tracts) is characteristic. Large hematomas and

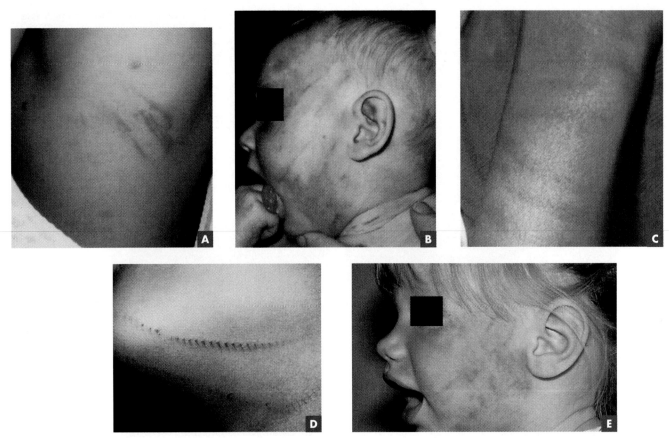

FIG. 23-4 Imprint marks reflecting the weapons used to inflict them. *A,* Fresh looped cord marks. *B,* Characteristic parallel lines as a result of being beaten with a leather belt. *C,* Multiple linear contusions inflicted with a switch. *D,* Chain imprints on the neck and chin. *E,* Handprint contusion of the face.

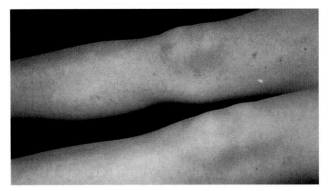

FIG. 23-5 This school-age child had a chief complaint of a rash after a viral upper respiratory tract infection. Examination revealed diffuse petechiae and scattered purpuric lesions. Her hemoglobin level and white blood cell count and differential were normal, but her platelet count was markedly reduced.

hemarthroses are not typical, unless they are induced by trauma.

Quantitative Disorders

Normal platelet count as determined on a standard Coulter counter is between 150,000 and 400,000/mm³. Generally,

> ### BOX 23-1
>
> ## *Clinical Findings of Platelet Defects*
>
> Petechiae (usually symmetric)
> Ecchymoses
> Mild to moderate mucousal membrane bleeding
>   Gastrointestinal
>   Genitourinary
>   Pulmonary
>   Epistaxis
> History of easy bruising
> History of spontaneous bruising
> Frequent gingival bleeding with tooth eruption

Modified from Bick RL: Pathophysiology of hemostasis and thrombosis. In Sodeman WA, Sodeman TA, editors: *Pathologic physiology: mechanisms of disease,* Philadelphia, 1985, WB Saunders.

platelet counts must decrease to less than 50,000/mm³ for trauma to result in excessive bleeding or bruising. Consequently, every instance of apparent excessive bleeding and/or bruising requires a standard platelet count determination. Counts less than 20,000/mm³ are associated with the spontaneous appearance of petechiae.

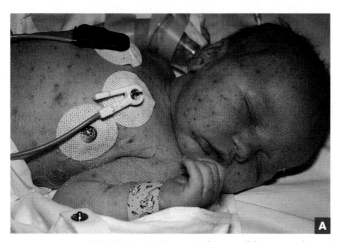
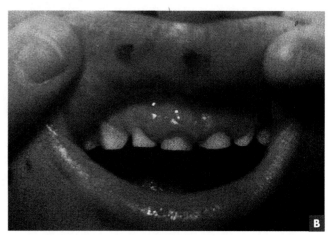

FIG. 23-6 *A,* Tiny petechiae and larger ecchymosis in an infant with severe immunologic thrombocytopenia. *B,* Purpura occurring on the oral mucosa or retina is called *wet purpura* and may suggest an increased tendency for major bleeding in the thrombopenic patient.

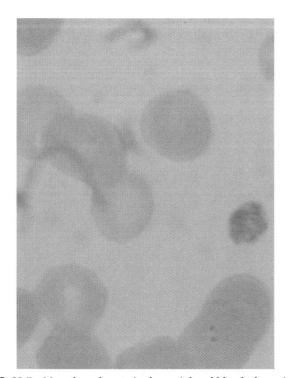

FIG. 23-7 Megathrombocyte in the peripheral blood of a patient with idiopathic thrombocytopenic purpura.

Thrombocytopenia may be the result of inadequate platelet production (approximately 10% of circulating platelets must be replaced daily to compensate for platelet senescence), excessive platelet destruction, or both. When thrombocytopenia is discovered, the process of diagnosing its cause begins with evaluation of the standard Wright-stained blood smear.

The smear confirms the presence of thrombocytopenia. Each platelet observed per high-power field corresponds to a platelet count of 10,000 to 15,000/mm³. (Consequently a normal platelet count corresponds to a smear with a minimum of 10 to 15 platelets per high-power field.) Clumped platelets in adequate number may inappropriately be counted by the Coulter counter as white blood cells (WBC), providing a falsely low platelet count. Pseudothrombocytopenia (the term applied to falsely reported low platelet counts because of platelet clumping) is most often noted when a platelet count is obtained as part of a routine complete blood count (CBC) and not as a part of purpura evaluation. The absence of purpura, despite a reported platelet count less than 20,000/mm³, is the usual clinical setting of pseudothrombocytopenia.

Other important clues to the cause of thrombocytopenia may be gained from evaluation of platelet morphology (Fig. 23-7). The presence of young platelets, indicated by their large size, generally indicates rapid platelet turnover and destruction. Features of red and white cell morphology may also be helpful. Red blood cell (RBC) fragments, suggesting disseminated intravascular coagulation (DIC), may explain thrombocytopenia. Immature WBCs may suggest that a marrow-based malignancy led to failure of platelet production.

When caused by thrombocytopenia, bruising and bleeding, regardless of the age of the patient, are acquired or inherited and may be primarily the result of destruction of platelets or impaired platelet production. Neonatal thrombocytopenia with purpura is best discussed separately because of the unique role of maternal influence on the differential diagnostic considerations. Maternal factors may cause (1) immunologic thrombocytopenia from maternal autoantibodies or alloantibodies and (2) congenital infection.

Neonatal Thrombocytopenia

Clinical recognition of purpura in the newborn is complicated by the wide range of normal bruising seen because of

TABLE 23-1

Comparison of Neonatal Immune Thrombocytopenia and Neonatal Alloimmune Thrombocytopenia

Feature	NITP	NAIT
Antiplatelet antibody	Yes	Yes
Affected neonates per year in US	50-100	800-2000
Incidence of severe thrombocytopenia	15%	>50%
Complication of thrombocytopenia	ICH (1.5%)	ICH (20%)
Postnatal ICH	All of ICH	50% of ICH
Prenatal ICH	Rare	50% of ICH
Subsequent effect on sibling	Equal to index case	Worse than index case
Fetal treatment recommendation	None	IVIG/steroids
Neonatal treatment	IVIG and steroids	IVIG, steroids, and matched (maternal) platelet transfusion

ICH, Intracranial hemorrhage; *IVIG,* intravenous gamma globulin; *NAIT,* neonatal alloimmune thrombocytopenia; *NITP,* neonatal immune thrombocytopenia.

TABLE 23-2

Other Causes of Neonatal Thrombocytopenia Without Hepatosplenomegaly

Condition	Mechanism	Comment
Bacterial sepsis	Platelet destruction with or without DIC	May be seen with hepatosplenomegaly
Congenital malformation		
Thrombocytopenia-absent radius syndrome	Absence of normal platelet production	Most severe in first year of life then improves
Chromosomal defects	Absence of normal platelet production	Trisomies 13 and 18
Kasabach-Merritt syndrome	Platelet destruction in large hemangioma	Hemangioma may be apparent on physical examination
Renal vein thrombosis	Platelet use on clot surface	Inability to compensate for rapid platelet use leads to thrombocytopenia
Asphyxia	May be related to hypoxic-related tissue injury with DIC and/or megakaryocyte injury secondary to hypoxia	Frequent cause of thrombocytopenia in the asphyxiated newborn
Miscellaneous		
Respiratory distress syndrome	Similar to asphyxia	Mild thrombocytopenia
Maternal drug use	Tolbutamide, thiazide, heparin	Other drugs reported as single cases
Polycythemia	Mechanism unknown	

DIC, Disseminated intravascular coagulation.

childbirth trauma. Diffuse, symmetric petechiae are never an accompaniment of a difficult delivery. Excessive bruising occasionally may occur if the birth was unusually traumatic. Petechiae or bruising warrants a platelet count and screen of plasma coagulation.

A helpful clinical algorithm divides neonatal thrombocytopenia into those infants without hepatosplenomegaly (usually of immunologic origin) and those infants with hepatosplenomegaly (usually of infectious origin).

THROMBOCYTOPENIA WITHOUT HEPATOSPLENOMEGALY

NEONATAL ALLOIMMUNE THROMBOCYTOPENIA. Neonatal alloimmune thrombocytopenia (NAIT) is the platelet analog of Rh disease of the red cell. Platelet membrane antigen derived from a paternally contributed gene crosses the placenta as part of whole platelets. Maternal antibody (IgG) produced to this antigen crosses the placenta, causing platelet destruction in the fetus. Because there is no routine screen for NAIT, siblings of an index case must be anticipated. The index case usually presents to the clinician with bruising and bleeding, and a subsequently determined platelet count is significantly depressed. Alternatively the clinician may recognize thrombocytopenia when a CBC and platelet count are obtained for reasons other than bruising or bleeding (usually a sepsis workup). NAIT is responsible for significant morbidity. Of

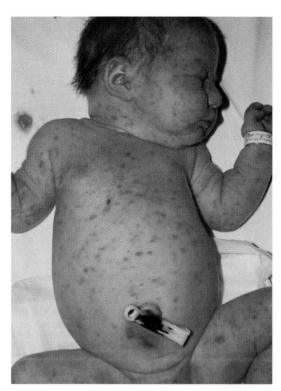

FIG. 23-8 Congenital rubella. This newborn had the full-blown picture of expanded rubella syndrome, including a generalized blueberry muffin rash, diffuse petechiae, hepatosplenomegaly, early onset of jaundice, and neurologic depression. (Courtesy Dr. Michael Sherlock, Baltimore.)

recognized cases, 20% suffer intracranial hemorrhage (ICH), with half of these occurring prenatally. The first clue to NAIT in the infant with thrombocytopenia is the severity of the decrease in platelets. Platelet count is often less than 20,000/mm³. When the clinical setting allows for conjecture as to the cause of thrombocytopenia, it is prudent to investigate NAIT as the primary cause or an additional cause of thrombocytopenia. The implication for subsequent pregnancies is profound, and prenatal treatment of NAIT is effective in most instances.

Postnatal treatment is directed by knowledge of central nervous system (CNS) imaging. A posttreatment platelet count goal of greater than 100,000/mm³ is sought if an ICH or life-threatening bleeding is present. In the absence of ICH or serious bleeding, a platelet level of 30,000 to 50,000/mm³ is the goal. Treatment consists of intravenous gamma globulin (IVIG), with or without corticosteroids, and random donor platelet transfusion until maternally donated platelets can be obtained. The diagnosis of NAIT rests on testing the parents for platelet incompatibility within a short time of the infant's birth.

NEONATAL IMMUNE THROMBOCYTOPENIA. Neonatal immune thrombocytopenia (NITP) occurs when the mother suffers from immune thrombocytopenia (ITP) and her circulating an-

tiplatelet antibodies pass through the placenta to the fetus. Unlike NAIT, prenatal ICH does not occur and postnatal ICH is much less frequent (1.5%) in NITP. Postnatal management is more conservative than with NAIT and includes daily IVIG until the target platelet count (30,000 to 50,000/mm³) is achieved. Corticosteroids also may be used, but platelet transfusions should be considered only in the setting of ICH or other life-threatening bleeding. Although NITP most often occurs in an infant born to a mother known to have ITP, occasionally the mother may have compensated ITP, in which her marrow is able to increase platelet production sufficiently to allow for a normal platelet count. The antibody-mediated platelet destruction may not be compensated for by the less competent neonatal marrow. Table 23-1 compares the features of NAIT and NITP.

OTHER CAUSES OF BRUISING AND BLEEDING WITHOUT HEPATOSPLENOMEGALY. In addition to NAIT and NITP, a heterogenous group of disorders may lead to thrombocytopenia that results in bruising and bleeding in the neonate. It has been pointed out that "almost anything that makes the newborn sick makes the newborn thrombocytopenic." Table 23-2 lists the other causes of neonatal thrombocytopenia without hepatosplenomegaly. Most of the causes listed are associated with a mild degree of thrombocytopenia in which bruising and bleeding are minimal if apparent at all.

THROMBOCYTOPENIA WITH HEPATOSPLENOMEGALY

Congenital infection accounts for most neonates with thrombocytopenia and hepatosplenomegaly. Although the constellation of findings in these infants often suggests the diagnosis, on occasion purpura is the only manifestation. The so-called blueberry muffin baby of congenital rubella is an example (Fig. 23-8). These infants have purpura out of proportion to the degree of thrombocytopenia. This apparent inconsistency is explained by the fact that only a minority of the purpura is due to bruising. Most purpura is due to extramedullary (cutaneous) hematopoiesis. The mechanism of thrombocytopenia in rubella and other congenital infections is poorly understood and may represent both decreased platelet production and increased platelet destruction.

Other congenital infections, including cytomegalovirus, toxoplasmosis, syphilis, and human immunodeficiency virus (HIV), may cause bruising as a result of thrombocytopenia. Herpesvirus, which is perinatally rather than congenitally acquired, also may cause thrombocytopenia and bruising. Finally, bacterial infection often is associated with thrombocytopenia.

Infectious causes of thrombocytopenia generally are associated with a self-limited low platelet count and rarely cause significant bleeding. Platelet transfusions are occasionally necessary, though often no direct management of the thrombocytopenia is necessary. Steroids are contraindicated in light of the infectious nature of this process.

Table 23-3 lists the remaining causes of neonatal thrombocytopenia with hepatosplenomegaly and includes some causes in older infants and children.

TABLE 23-3

Other Causes of Thrombocytopenia With Hepatosplenomegaly

Condition	Mechanism	Comment
Congenital leukemia	Decreased platelet production	Thrombocytopenia's consequences overshadowed by direct evidence of leukemia
Alloimmune hemolytic disease	Probably related to reactive reticuloendothelial cells in enlarged liver or spleen	Present with severe alloimmune hemolysis Rh- rather than ABO-mediated
Liver disease	Destruction of platelets in liver and spleen	Includes congenital osteopetrosis, congenital thyrotoxicosis, and congestive heart failure
Hypersplenism and portal vein obstruction	Destruction of platelets in spleen	May coexist with liver disease

TABLE 23-4

Drugs Reported to Induce Immune Thrombocytopenia

Drug	Comment
Anticonvulsants	
Phenytoin	
Valproic acid	Has two mechanisms causing thrombocytopenia; one is immune mediated
Antidysrythmics	
Quinidine	Infrequently used in pediatrics
Phenytoin	
Anticoagulants	
Heparin	Most frequent drug associated with immune thrombocytopenia worldwide, but rare in children
Other	
Quinine	Used primarily in treatment of autoimmune disease

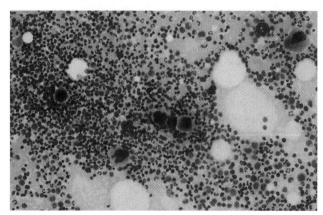

FIG. 23-9 Bone marrow aspirate in ITP, with prominent megakaryocytes. In children with thrombocytopenia—on the basis of decreased platelet production—megakaryocytes are decreased in number.

Thrombocytopenia Beyond the Neonatal Period

IMMUNE THROMBOCYTOPENIC PURPURA

ITP is the most frequent condition causing thrombocytopenia. It is the leading diagnosis in a child who has bruising and bleeding, excluding nonaccidental trauma. Its exact cause remains unknown, but it occurs when IgG antibody attaches to the platelet, resulting in immune sensitization of platelets, which are then destroyed by the monocyte-macrophage system. The condition is seen most often in the aftermath of a viral infection, and it is presumed that the immune response to the virus somehow triggers the sensitizing IgG antiplatelet antibody. ITP is most common in children and young adults, with more than half of all cases occurring in children under 15 years of age.

Typically the child develops petechiae and bruising (often at sites of incidental trauma) over a brief time period measured in hours or days. The platelet count is often less than 30,000/mm^3. The diagnosis is likely when purpura is found in a well-appearing child with an otherwise normal physical examination. Specifically, absence of significant adenopathy, hepatosplenomegaly, bone tenderness, pallor, jaundice, or a focus of infection reassures the physician, though rarely the parent.

A standard blood count and peripheral blood smear that reveal normal RBC and WBC lines and large young platelets

---

TABLE 23-5

Differences Between Hemolytic Uremic Syndrome and Thrombotic Thrombocytopenic Purpura

Feature	HUS	TTP
Peak age incidence	1–4 years	20–25 years
Male/female ratio	1:1	1:2
Prodromal illness	Usual	Variable
Shiga-like toxin	Frequent	Unusual
Neurologic abnormalities	Variable	Usual
Renal disease	Usual	Usual
Renal failure	Common	Rare
Hypertension	Common	Rare
Major organs affected	Kidneys	Kidneys, brain, heart, pancreas, and adrenals
Prognosis	Relatively good	Relatively poor

Modified from Berman N, Finkelstein JB: Thrombotic thrombocytopenic purpura in childhood: results of a survey and reexamination of the literature, *Scand J Haematol* 14:286-294, 1975.

HUS, Hemolytic uremic syndrome; *TTP,* thrombotic thrombocytopenic purpura.

---

further define the process as probable ITP. However, because diagnoses such as leukemia and aplastic anemia also may cause bruising and bleeding, controversy exists about the need for bone marrow evaluation in these children (Fig. 23-9). Consensus opinion among pediatric hematologists has moved steadily in the direction of eliminating routine bone marrow aspiration. A children's cancer group study, which included thousands of children with leukemia, demonstrated that it is unlikely for acute leukemia to cause isolated thrombocytopenia, an otherwise normal blood count, and a normal physical examination except for petechiae and bruising.

This lingering controversy has almost disappeared since IVIG was found to be efficacious in the treatment of ITP. IVIG's more rapid onset of action in increasing the platelet count and the relative absence of side effects resulted in displacement of corticosteroids as the primary treatment. The use of corticosteroids in ITP has the potential for inducing at least a partial remission in 60% of children with acute lymphocytic leukemia, thus supporting the need for a marrow aspiration before treatment. IVIG, which works by decreasing platelet destruction rather than impacting marrow platelet production, obviates the need for a marrow evaluation before treatment. Marrow aspiration in the child with thrombocytopenia is required in the following cases: (1) when the condition is refractory to IVIG treatment; (2) when physical examination, blood count, or blood smear is abnormal (other than thrombocytopenia); and (3) when the initial treatment is corticosteroids.

A few further points are worth noting. The child with significant bruising and bleeding whose platelet count is greater than 50,000/mm³ should be suspected of having a disorder that reduces platelet number and function; platelet counts greater than 50,000/mm³ usually are associated with minimal symptoms.

Even when the diagnosis of ITP is made correctly, the issue of whether the diagnosis is primary ITP or secondary ITP must be considered, for example, as a manifestation of a wider immunologic process, such as systemic lupus or HIV. Finally, because many processes may mimic ITP, at least initially the clinician must continue to follow the patient's course, including response to therapy.

DRUG-INDUCED IMMUNE THROMBOCYTOPENIA

A short list of drugs has been reported to trigger immune-mediated thrombocytopenia (Table 23-4). This condition is rare, and when a child taking one of the offending drugs has bruising and bleeding, classic ITP is as likely a diagnosis as drug-induced ITP. Fortunately, management of ITP and drug-induced thrombocytopenia is identical. Only after recovery can the clinician decide whether the possible offending drug should be used again. As a rule, if alternative effective treatment is available, prudence argues for its use.

MICROANGIOPATHIC PLATELET DESTRUCTION

Hemolytic uremic syndrome (HUS) and thrombotic thrombocytopenia purpura (TTP) are listed together because they generally are regarded as widely varying expressions of a unitary pathologic process involving small blood vessels. Berman and Finkelstein compared these two entities. Table 23-5 is an extension of that comparison.

Petechiae, bruising, and bleeding may be seen in either of these conditions; however, the degree of thrombocytopenia is usually moderate, and the other nonhemostatic disease features dominate the clinical concerns. A child with a prodromal illness—either gastrointestinal with diarrhea (often bloody) or respiratory—who then develops pallor, evidence of acute renal failure, petechiae, jaundice, hepatosplenomegaly, hypertension, a peripheral blood smear revealing normocytic anemia, platelet reduction to less than 100,000/mm³ but usually greater than 20,000/mm³, and typical red cell fragments (schistocytes) clearly has microangiopathic disease.

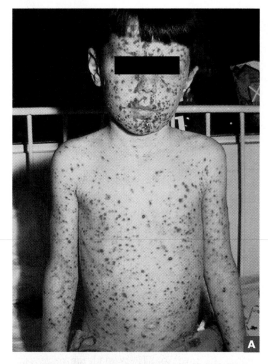

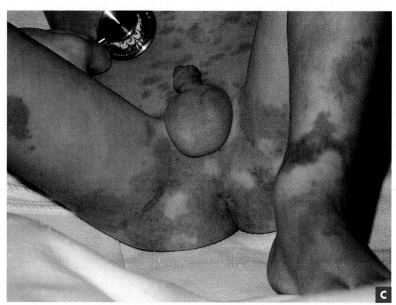

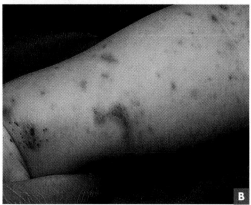

FIG. 23-10 Meningococcemia. *A,* This youngster manifests the generalized purpuric and petechial rash characteristic of acute meningococcemia. *B,* Petechiae are more apparent in this close-up of an infant. Gram stain of petechial scrapings may reveal organisms. *C,* Purpura may progress to form areas of frank cutaneous necrosis, especially in cases with DIC.

Management requires overall support, particularly support of renal failure. Some suggest that early dialysis, before it is biochemically necessary, may shorten the course of the renal failure. High-dose corticosteroids with plasma infusion and plasma exchange have been used in some TTP series with excellent response rates. Specific treatment of the purpura is not usually necessary, and there is evidence that platelet transfusions may exacerbate TTP. TTP's far greater CNS involvement and more guarded prognosis differentiate it from HUS.

A number of other diseases may be associated with microangiopathic hemolytic disease in children. These disorders include vasculitis, DIC, and giant hemangiomas (Kasabach-Merritt syndrome). Bruising and bleeding may complicate these conditions, but rarely if ever are they the presenting complaint.

INFECTION

Although infection may trigger ITP during convalescence, a number of acute infections may be associated with thrombocytopenia. Bacterial septicemia and certain viral infections commonly are associated with thrombocytopenia (Figs. 23-10

and 23-11). The degree of thrombocytopenia is mild, and bruising and bleeding are rarely significant.

Infection also may trigger hemophagocytic syndrome, which has associated thrombocytopenia. This condition has features identical to familial erythrophagocytic lymphohistiocytosis, often manifesting bleeding when the patient requires venipuncture. Fever, pancytopenia, lymphadenopathy, coagulopathy, and erythrophagocytosis by histiocytes characterize these two conditions. Bruising and bleeding rarely are responsible for the child's presentation.

*Thrombocytopenia Caused by Ineffective
Platelet Production*

The child who has excessive bruising and bleeding and recognized thrombocytopenia raises the concern that failure of platelet production is the basis for the decrease. Concern exists because most patients with platelet production failure suffer from serious disease.

When suspicious historic information or provocative physical findings are present or a presumed destructive platelet

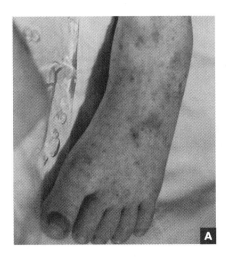
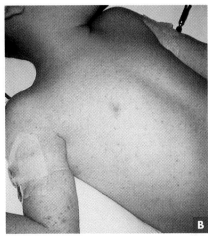

FIG. 23-11 Rocky Mountain spotted fever. *A,* The exanthem characteristic of this disease first appears distally on the wrists, ankles, palms, and soles. It may be petechial from the outset, or it may start as an erythematous, blanching, macular or maculopapular eruption, which then becomes petechial as it spreads centripetally. *B,* In this child the rash has become generalized. Both petechial and blanching erythematous lesions are present. (*A* Courtesy Dr. Ellen Wald, Children's Hospital of Pittsburgh; *B* courtesy Dr. T.F. Sellers, Jr.)

process fails to respond to therapy, a bone marrow evaluation is necessary to determine the cause of the platelet production failure. The child with a history of recurring infections, malaise, fatigue, and subjective complaints of diffuse bone and joint pain requires a marrow evaluation, as does a child with adenopathy, pallor, hepatosplenomegaly, bone tenderness, or abdominal mass(es).

ACQUIRED APLASTIC ANEMIA

Bruising and bleeding are the most common manifestations of acquired aplastic anemia. Findings associated with anemia, including pallor, fatigue, and dyspnea, are the second most common presenting feature of acquired aplastic anemia. Occasionally, infectious presentations occur. Physical examination rarely reveals findings beyond the presenting symptoms. CBC reveals pancytopenia with a low reticulocyte count for the degree of anemia, and a peripheral smear demonstrates normochromic, normocytic, or macrocytic RBCs; normal-sized rare platelets; and normal morphology of all WBC lines. Bone marrow biopsy is diagnostic.

LEUKEMIA AND METASTATIC TUMORS OF THE MARROW

Leukemia and other tumors that replace normal bone marrow often cause excessive bruising or bleeding. A history of malaise, fatigue, dyspnea, and/or bone and joint pain is common. Examination may reveal bone tenderness, adenopathy, hepatosplenomegaly, and/or an abdominal mass (particularly in neuroblastoma and marrow replacement) in addition to the purpura. Marrow aspirate is usually diagnostic; though in the setting of completely replaced marrow, a marrow biopsy may be necessary.

HYPOPLASTIC THROMBOCYTOPENIA

Acquired hypoplastic thrombocytopenia is a rare condition in which platelet marrow precursors are depressed but RBC and WBC lines are normal. Occasionally this condition actually represents a plateau, halting temporarily the downhill course of marrow failure caused by acquired aplastic anemia. It is occasionally a preleukemia presentation. A minority of affected children have decreased thrombopoiesis as an isolated finding that recovers spontaneously. Androgenic steroids have been useful in treatment.

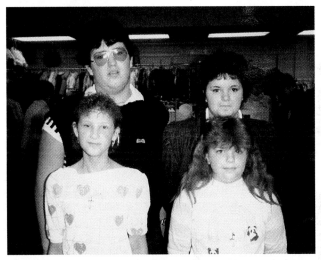

FIG. 23-12 A patient with Fanconi anemia (shortly after bone marrow transplantation) and her three siblings. The patient *(front left)* had a hemoglobin of 3.5 g/dl, short stature, and increased skin pigmentation. Note the patient's diminutive size with respect to her more robust siblings.

PAROXYSMAL NOCTURNAL HEMOGLOBINURIA

Paroxysmal nocturnal hemoglobinuria (PNH) is a rare acquired disorder in which an altered clone of bone marrow stem cells fails to endow its mature effector cell progeny with membrane factor(s) that protect against complement-mediated cell destruction. Clinical presentation is usually due to pallor and malaise resulting from anemia. Occasionally, venous thrombosis leads to clinical presentation. Bruising and particularly bleeding may complicate the course of PNH because thrombocytopenia evolves as part of pancytopenia, but bruising and bleeding are not usually part of the initial presentation.

FANCONI ANEMIA

Fanconi anemia is an inherited disorder in which the phenotype includes short stature, café au lait spots, variable musculoskeletal and genitourinary anomalies, and evolving pancytopenia (Fig. 23-12). Presentation is most often due to

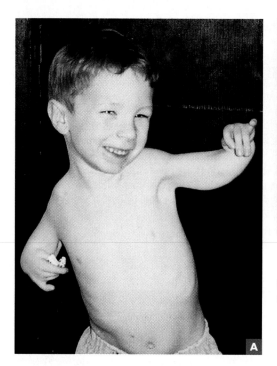

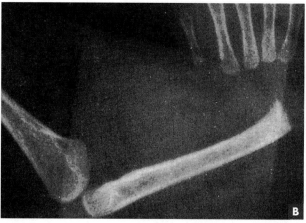

FIG. 23-13   *A*, A child with TAR syndrome. *B*, Radiograph of the same patient. Note the absence of radii.

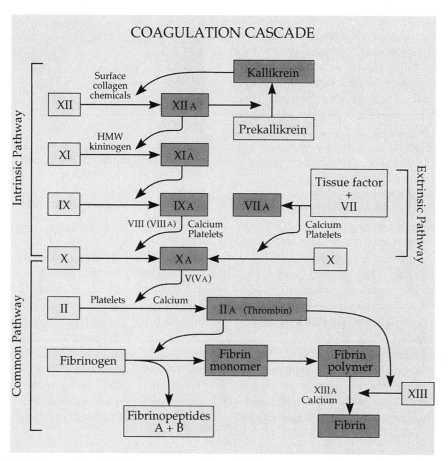

FIG. 23-14   The prothrombin time measures the extrinsic-common pathway, whereas the partial thromboplastin time measures the intrinsic-common pathway.

TABLE 23-6

Acquired Platelet Dysfunction Secondary to a Primary Disease Process

Condition	Disease state
Uremia	Renal failure
Paraproteinemia	Multiple myelomas
	Waldenström macroglobulinemia
	Monoclonal gammopathy
Myelodysplastic	Essential thrombocytopenia
syndrome	Agnogenic myeloid metaplasia
	Paroxsymal nocturnal hemoglobinuria
	Polycythemia vera
	Chronic myelogenous leukemia
	Sideroblastic anemias

anemia, but frequently bruising or bleeding brings the patient to attention.

THROMBOCYTOPENIA-ABSENT RADIUS SYNDROME

Thrombocytopenia-absent radius (TAR) syndrome is an inherited syndrome causing isolated thrombocytopenia associated with bilateral absent radii (Fig. 23-13). The thrombocytopenia is caused by failure of platelet production, a process that ameliorates with the increasing age of the patient. The dramatic dysmorphic feature of shortened forearms generally brings the patient to attention before bruising and bleeding occur, although bruising resulting from the birthing process itself may be the initial presentation. Because intrauterine ultrasound is becoming the standard of obstetric care, it is anticipated that TAR will become an intrauterine diagnosis.

Qualitative Disorders

Qualitative platelet disorders most often are characterized by defective platelet function but normal platelet number. A few of these disorders may cause recognizable platelet morphologic abnormalities, some of which may result in a mildly decreased platelet count because of shortened platelet survival. The common clinical findings of symmetric petechiae and mucous membrane bleeding with a normal or near-normal platelet number should raise suspicions that a functional platelet defect is operative.

A review of the peripheral smear may help make the diagnosis. The Bernard-Soulier syndrome, in which platelet adhesion is decreased, is characterized by giant platelets and borderline thrombocytopenia. May-Hegglin anomaly (also characterized by giant defective platelets) has the additional finding of leukocyte inclusions. One third of the patients with May-Hegglin anomaly also have thrombocytopenia.

Platelet function defects more often are associated with a normal peripheral blood smear and platelet number.

Glanzmann thrombasthenia is caused by failure of primary platelet aggregation. Essential athrombia, a different defect than Glanzmann thrombasthenia, has the same functional platelet defect—failure of primary aggregation. Hereditary platelet storage pool defects cause failure of secondary platelet aggregation. Conditions that cause failure of secondary platelet aggregation are more likely to present with mucocutaneous hemorrhage, hematuria, and epistaxis. Petechiae are less common. Hereditary aspirin-like defect is yet another rare disease of secondary platelet aggregation that causes bruising and bleeding.

Acquired platelet dysfunction is seen as an epiphenomenon in a number of diseases. Table 23-6 lists the disease entity and the associated platelet dysfunction.

Drug-induced platelet dysfunction also may lead to clinically significant hemorrhage. The following three mechanisms of drug-induced platelet dysfunction exist: (1) interference with the platelet membrane or membrane receptor sites, (2) interference with prostaglandin biosynthesis, and (3) interference with phosphodiesterase activity. A list of drugs causing platelet function defects and their mechanisms is available. Most of these drugs impact coagulation studies but have minimal clinical effect.

Miscellaneous

Wiskott-Aldrich syndrome is a rare, X-linked recessive disorder characterized by chronic thrombocytopenia, eczema, and immunodeficiency resulting in frequent infections. It generally presents with petechiae and increased bruising in affected infant boys and is seen in association with atopic dermatitis and frequent trivial and serious infections.

Diagnosis depends on finding the clinical triad in association with small platelets, relative lymphopenia, and variable degrees of a normochromic, normocytic anemia without reticulocytosis. Thorough immunologic workup usually confirms the diagnosis.

Disorders of the Coagulation Cascade

Once the platelet plug or primary clot is formed on damaged subendothelium, a complex series of steps, called the *coagulation cascade*, results in stabilization of the fibrin network and formation of the secondary clot (Fig. 23-14). Disorders of secondary clot formation include congenital deficiencies of one or more of the coagulation factors (Box 23-2) and acquired disorders that interfere with coagulation factor functions, as with vitamin K deficiency (Box 23-3). The intrinsic part of the clotting cascade includes factors VIII, IX, XI, and XII; defects here result in prolongation of the partial thromboplastin time (PTT). The extrinsic pathway includes factor VII; deficiency of this factor results in a prolonged prothrombin time (PT). Deficiency of the factors in the common part of the cascade results in prolongation of both the PT and the PTT. Factor XIII helps galvanize the loosely associated fibrin polymers. Although von Willebrand factor (vWF) is vital to the primary part of clot formation, deficiency of

Congenital Disorders of the Coagulation Factors

Afibrinogenemia/dysfibrinogenemia
Factor V deficiency
Factor VII deficiency
Factor VIII deficiency (hemophilia A)
Factor IX deficiency (hemophilia B or Christmas disease)
Factor X deficiency
Factor XI deficiency
Factor XIII deficiency
von Willebrand disease

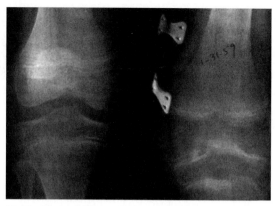

FIG. 23-15 Hemophiliac arthritis after recurrent hemarthroses. Note the widened joint space on the left knee as compared with that of the normal right knee.

Acquired Disorders of the Coagulation Cascade

Vitamin K deficiency
  Hemorrhagic disease of the newborn
  Malnutrition
  Broad-spectrum antibiotic use
  Malabsorption
  Warfarin or "superwarfarin" ingestion
Nonspecific inhibitors of coagulation factors
Specific inhibitors (IgG) of coagulation factors
Liver failure
Snake envenomation
Consumption of coagulation factors
  Kasabach-Merritt syndrome
  Disseminated intravascular coagulation
  Congenital heart disease (polycythemia)

this factor is addressed here along with the rest of the coagulation cascade. Table 23-7 summarizes the clinical clues and laboratory features of specific clotting factor deficiencies.

Congenital Deficiencies

Factor VIII and Factor IX

Factor VIII and factor IX deficiencies, hemophilia A and B respectively, are clinically indistinguishable. Inheritance for both disorders is X-linked recessive. Spontaneous mutations occur frequently; family history is negative in 20% to 30% of cases. The severity of the disease corresponds to the level of factor activity. In 20% of the most severely affected boys (less than 0.5% factor VIII activity), presentation may occur at the time of circumcision. Most boys with hemophilia, however, come to medical attention when they become more mobile and begin walking.

Unlike children with other disorders resulting in bruising and bleeding, children with hemophilia have a tendency for deep rather than superficial hemorrhage. Bleeding events most often are oral (frenulum tears in youngsters or tooth extraction in the older child), occur within a joint, or involve a muscle, and the frequency tends to decrease with age (Fig. 23-15). CNS hemorrhage occurs in 1% to 2% of neonates and can occur in the older child. Because factors VIII and IX are involved in secondary clot formation, bleeding after trauma is not usually immediate.

Because factors VIII and IX are crucial in the intrinsic pathway of the clotting cascade, screening laboratory evaluation is marked by prolongation of only the PTT. Bleeding time, PT, and platelet counts are normal. These clinical and laboratory findings necessitate measurement of specific factor levels.

von Willebrand Factor

vWF is crucial for adherence of platelets to the damaged endothelium. It accomplishes this by interacting with the glycoprotein Ib receptor of the platelet, thereby activating it and inducing aggregation of more platelets targeted to the damaged area. This results in formation of the primary clot. vWF also functions as a carrier protein for factor VIII.

von Willebrand disease (vWD) is a heterogeneous disorder caused by congenital quantitative vWF deficiency or structural abnormality resulting in functional vWF deficiency. The disease prevalence is approximately 1%. It is usually transmitted in an autosomal dominant manner. Men and women are equally affected. The clinical course is variable; 80% of patients experience only a mild bleeding diathesis. Patients with certain subtypes of the disease, however, tend to have clinical courses similar to those of patients with hemophilia. Frequent symptoms are mucous membrane bleeding, menorrhagia, and recurrent nosebleeds. Because it is a disorder of primary clot formation, bleeding tends to begin shortly after trauma.

Laboratory evaluation is remarkable for prolongation of the bleeding time and perhaps an increase in the PTT. In the

TABLE 23-7

Clinical and Laboratory Features of Congenital Clotting Factor Deficiencies

Factor	Inheritance (chromosome)	Usual sites of bleeding	Severity	Distinguishing features	Screening laboratories
Intrinsic					
Factor XII	Autosomal recessive? (5)	No clinical bleeding	0	Identified preoperatively, occasionally associated with vWD	Markedly increased PTT
Factor XI (hemophilia C)	Autosomal recessive (4)	Skin, with or without surgical bleeding	+ to ++	Ashkenazi Jews	Increased PTT
Factor IX (hemophilia B)	X-linked recessive	Mouth, joints, muscles, circumcision (about 30% overall)	++ to +++	Males, positive family history in about 65% of cases	Increased PTT
Factor VIII (hemophilia A)	X-linked recessive	Mouth, joints, muscles, circumcision	++ to +++	Males, positive family history in about 70% cases	Increased PTT
Extrinsic					
Factor VII	Autosomal recessive (13)	Skin, tooth extraction, uterus, surgical bleeding possible	+ to +++	—	Increased PT; normal PTT
Common					
Factor X	Autosomal recessive (13)	Umbilical stump, skin, nose, uterus	++	Prenatal CNS bleeding	Increased PT, PTT
Factor V	Autosomal recessive (1)	Skin, nose uterus	++	Prenatal CNS bleeding	Increased PT, PTT
Factor II	Autosomal recessive (11)	Skin, nose, uterus	+ to ++	—	Increased PT; slightly increased PTT; normal TT
Fibrinogen	Autosomal dominant (4)	Umbilical stump, gastrointestinal, skin	0 to +++	Bleeding in only 50%, poor wound healing, rare thrombotic episode	Increased PT, PTT, BT, TT
Other					
Factor XIII	Autosomal recessive	Umbilical stump >90%, skin	++	Delayed cord separation, bruising 24 hours after trauma	Normal PT, PTT, BT, TT; clot solubility test abnormal
vWF	Autosomal dominant (12)	Mucous membranes, nose, uterus	+ to +++	Males and females equally	Increased BT, with or without increased PTT, decreased factor VIII-vWF complex activity

0, None; +, mild; ++, moderate; +++, profound; BT, bleeding time; PT, prothrombin time; PTT, partial thromboplastin time; TT, thrombin time; vWD, von Willebrand disease.

patient with a history suggestive of vWD the activity of each component of the factor VIII–vWF complex should be measured (factor VIIIc:vWF, and ristocetin cofactor [vWF:RcoF]) and each will have decreased activity. Because many physiologic factors (e.g., pregnancy, hormones, and stress) can affect the measured level of vWF and because results in affected individuals can vary within the normal range, the patient with a history suggestive of vWF should be evaluated repeatedly.

Acquired Disorders

Vitamin K Deficiency

Synthesis of clotting factors II, VII, IX, and X is dependent on vitamin K. Sources of this vitamin are dietary, and synthesis is performed by bacteria that normally inhabit the small intestine. Coagulopathy resulting from vitamin K deficiency is encountered in children in several instances.

Hemorrhagic disease of the newborn (HDN) may occur within 24 hours of birth (the "early" form), usually in the infant whose mother is taking anticonvulsants, warfarin, or antituberculins. The "classic" form of HDN affects the breast-fed infant between the first and seventh days postpartum and presents with gastrointestinal, cutaneous, and nasal bleeding and perhaps bleeding after circumcision. HDN also occurs between 3 and 8 weeks of age (the "late" form) and presents with ICH 50% of the time. Pathophysiology of HDN is multifactorial as follows: (1) neonates have only 25% of vitamin K stores when compared with adults, (2) human milk has low concentrations of vitamin K, and (3) in the classic form the intestinal flora of a 1-week-old infant is not yet effective in producing vitamin K. Parenteral vitamin K is effective in preventing the classic and late forms of HDN, and its routine administration has made HDN a rare occurrence.

Broad-spectrum antibiotic use may alter the intestinal flora of the critically ill and perhaps somewhat malnourished patient, leading to coagulopathy from vitamin K deficiency. Children with inadequate excretion and absorption of bile salts (e.g., those with cystic fibrosis and biliary atresia) have difficulty absorbing fat-soluble vitamins and may have decreased vitamin K stores.

Accidental ingestion of rodenticides containing superwarfarins may result in severe coagulopathy. These compounds interfere with vitamin K metabolism, resulting in a functional vitamin K deficiency. The coagulopathy may be quite resistant to vitamin K administration, and abnormalities in the coagulation profile may persist for months.

Children with coagulopathy secondary to deficiency of vitamin K generally have increased bruising and epistaxis. Because the vitamin K–dependent coagulation factors represent all three arms of the cascade (intrinsic, extrinsic, and common), prolongation of the PT and the PTT occurs. Platelet count and bleeding time are normal.

Inhibitors of Clotting Factors

Acquired inhibitors of coagulation are common in patients with severe, congenital factor deficiencies (14% of patients with hemophilia A) who have received factor replacement. They also may develop in patients with autoimmune disease, drug sensitivity, allergy, or malignancy. Healthy children may develop coagulation inhibitors after a viral illness. Such children generally come to medical attention because of moderate bruising, or more frequently they are asymptomatic with a prolonged PTT identified on routine preoperative screening.

Acquired inhibitors may impair coagulation in a nonspecific way or may be directed at a specific clotting factor. When the latter is the case, the inhibitor is usually an antibody (IgG). Inhibitors can be identified by mixing the patient's plasma with normal plasma. If a true factor deficiency is present, the PTT shortens. Continued prolongation of the PTT is diagnostic of an inhibitor.

Acquired inhibitors are generally transient in children and do not require therapy. Their presence should be considered in the child with an appropriate history and prolongation of the PTT.

Other Disorders

Consumption of clotting factors (and platelets) may occur in DIC, resulting in prolongation of the PT and PTT and a decrease in fibrinogen. DIC is generally secondary to a severe illness (sepsis or hypoxia) resulting in widespread endothelial damage. Although bruising and bleeding may be identified, they are rarely hallmark features of the primary illness, and often the diagnosis of DIC is made before bleeding is clinically apparent.

The coagulopathy of liver failure has multiple causes, including a decrease in clotting factor synthesis, vitamin K deficiency secondary to decreased absorption of vitamin K, and thrombocytopenia from hypersplenism. Again, bleeding accompanies this disorder but generally occurs after the diagnosis of liver failure is made.

Blood Vessel Disorders

Bruising or bleeding may result from increased transmural pressure across the blood vessel wall, an abnormality of the vessel wall or supporting tissue, or direct damage to the vessel wall (Box 23-4). The blood vessel disorders can be differentiated according to the nature of the purpuric lesions (petechiae, bruises, and palpable purpura), the distribution of the lesions, and associated clinical features.

Increased Transmural Pressure

Appearance of petechiae at the site of tourniquet placement is common and occurs as a result of increased vascular pressure and capillary leakage of blood into the skin. More frequently, petechiae arising from this mechanism are located on the upper body, face, neck, and subconjunctival area as the result of forceful crying, coughing, or vomiting. This is rarely a matter of concern unless there is accompanying fever or toxicity, which may be indicative of a more serious infectious process.

Abnormal Vessel or Supporting Tissue

Several inherited diseases are associated with decreased integrity of the blood vessel wall and supporting perivas-

Blood Vessel Disorders

Increased Transmural Pressure
Tourniquet placement
Forceful coughing, vomiting, crying

Abnormal Vessel or Supporting Tissue
Ehlers-Danlos syndrome
Marfan syndrome
Osteogenesis imperfecta
Hereditary telangiectasia
Corticosteroid excess
Vitamin C deficiency
Pseudoxanthoma elasticum

Damage to the Vessel
Trauma
  Accidental
  Inflicted
Vasculitis
  Primary
  Secondary
Miscellaneous
  Pigmented

cular tissues. These diseases include Ehlers-Danlos syndrome, Marfan syndrome, osteogenesis imperfecta, and pseudoxanthoma elasticum. Each of these disorders has some abnormality of collagen or other connective tissue element and is identified by distinctive clinical features. Easy bruising as a clinical manifestation is most prominent in Ehlers-Danlos syndrome. Ten subtypes of Ehlers-Danlos syndrome have been classified based on genetic, biochemical, and clinical characteristics. The majority are inherited in an autosomal dominant fashion. These patients are identified by their soft, hyperextensible skin; joint hypermobility; and poor wound healing. A generalized bruising tendency of varying severity, especially prominent in areas subject to trauma (i.e., the shins), is seen in many of the subtypes. Type IV may be associated with severe bruising and life-threatening arterial rupture. Although platelet abnormalities and coagulation factor deficiencies have been reported in patients with Ehlers-Danlos syndrome, the majority of patients studied have had normal hemostasis, supporting the belief that abnormal structure of the blood vessel wall and supporting skin causes the vascular fragility, easy bruising, and bleeding.

Hereditary hemorrhagic telangiectasia (Rendu-Osler-Weber syndrome) is an autosomal dominant inherited disorder of mucocutaneous and visceral vascular dysplasia. Bleeding is associated with rupture of malformed vessels. Recurrent epistaxis is the most common bleeding manifestation (80%) and is usually the initial symptom. This epistaxis is followed in decreasing frequency by gastrointestinal, genitourinary, pulmonary, and intracerebral bleeding. Severity of bleeding is variable. Typically, 1- to 3-mm, reddish-purple, blanching, macular lesions representing telangiectactic vessels occur on the face, lips, nasal mucosa, tongue, ears, chest, hands, feet, and nailbeds. The size and number of lesions increase with age, and lesions usually are not detected in the young child. Vascular ectasias of the viscera, with bleeding and resultant iron deficiency anemia, occur. In this setting, cutaneous lesions provide an important diagnostic clue to the cause of visceral bleeding.

Corticosteroid excess (exogenous or endogenous) leads to breakdown of collagen and thinning of the epidermis, making cutaneous vessels more fragile. Reddish-purple lesions precipitated by minor trauma typically involve extensor surfaces. The lesions' appearance remains unchanged for a prolonged time because of delayed resorption of extravasated blood, presumably resulting from inhibition of the cellular response by the corticosteroid. The diagnosis should be considered in a child who has a compatible medication history or stigmata of Cushing syndrome (moon facies, truncal obesity, and hypertension). However, easy bruising is unlikely to be the presenting complaint of a child with Cushing syndrome.

Vitamin C deficiency (scurvy) is uncommon in the United States. Bleeding manifestations include perifollicular petechiae; ecchymoses, particularly of the lower extremities; gum bleeding; and in infants, subperiosteal hemorrhages manifesting as very painful, tender leg muscles and pseudoparalysis. Associated features include hyperkeratosis of the skin, corkscrew hairs, and arthralgias. A diet particularly devoid of fresh fruits and vegetables is the major risk factor for this disease.

Damage to the Vessel

Direct damage to the blood vessel occurs as a result of trauma to (accidental or inflicted) or inflammation of (vasculitis) the blood vessel wall. Palpable purpura is common with vasculitis and most frequently involves the lower extremities. Bruises result from traumatic injury to the blood vessel. Palpable lesions caused by trauma occur in the setting of severe injury or an underlying abnormality of hemostasis.

Bruising as a result of trauma may be the presenting complaint or may be noted incidentally during evaluation for another problem. The physician must differentiate accidental from inflicted injury. Although bruising from accidental injury is common in childhood, bruises are also the most common manifestation of physical abuse in childhood. Accidental bruises typically are found in ambulatory children on the shins, forearms, elbows, and forehead. The following "red flags" should heighten the physician's suspicions of physical abuse: (1) a history incompatible with either the physical findings or the developmental stage of the child; (2) bruises in areas rarely injured accidentally (buttocks, face, back, etc.); (3) bruises in multiple stages of healing, implying repeated trauma; (4) bruises in unusual patterns (circumferential) or geometric shapes, reflecting an object used to strike the child (belt, cord, kitchen utensil, etc.); (5) imprints of a

BOX 23-5

Vasculitides

Primary	Secondary
Large vessel	*Collagen vascular disease*
Giant cell (temporal) arteritis	Systemic lupus erythematosus
Takayasu arteritis	Juvenile rheumatoid arthritis
Medium vessel	Mixed connective tissue disease
Classic polyarteritis nodosa	Dermatomyositis
Cutaneous polyarteritis nodosa	Scleroderma
Kawasaki syndrome	*Infection*
	Bacteria
Small vessel	Viruses
Henoch-Schönlein purpura	Fungi
Leukocytoclastic ("hypersensitivity") vasculitis	Spirochetes
	Rickettsia sp.
Wegener granulomatosis	*Medications*
Churg-Strauss syndrome	
Essential cryoglobulinemia	*Malignancy*

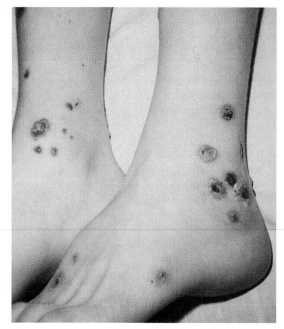

FIG. 23-16   Cutaneous vasculitis in systemic lupus erythematosus. Purpuric, ulcerative, and necrotic skin lesions of active disease.

hand or finger on the skin; and (6) bruises in a nonambulatory child (Figs. 23-3 and 23-4). Signs of neglect further raise suspicion. Evidence of additional injuries (e.g., fractures) should be sought in the very young infant or child. Because bleeding disorders are also associated with unusual bruising patterns, it is prudent to screen children who are suspected victims of physical abuse for a defect in coagulation or platelets. The presence of a bleeding disorder does not exclude the possibility of physical abuse.

Folk remedies, such as coin rubbing *(cao gio)* and cupping *(ventosas),* produce bruising over the trunk in a linear or circular configuration. Coin rubbing involves massaging the trunk with oil and then firmly rubbing the skin with the edge of a coin until petechiae or bruises appear. Cupping involves applying a heated cup to the skin until a lesion appears. The history is usually readily obtained from the caretaker, who is often of Asian or Mexican descent.

Psychogenic purpura (autoerythrocyte sensitization) is a poorly understood entity of spontaneous, recurrent bruising of the extremities seen primarily in young women and occasionally in adolescents. The onset of bruising is usually preceded by painful sensations of burning or stinging of the skin and systemic complaints of malaise, headache, and gastrointestinal distress. These patients usually suffer from emotional and psychologic problems that predate the onset of bruising episodes. In these cases bruising cannot be explained by a bleeding disorder or systemic illness, and at least some evidence to exclude the possibility of self-induced bruising has been documented in a few patients. Autosensitivity to blood

components is postulated to be part of the pathogenesis of this disorder.

Factitious or self-induced bruising is reported mostly in teenage and young adult women and may be difficult to distinguish from psychogenic purpura. Blunt trauma, biting, and sucking on the skin are some of the methods used to induce bruising. Like patients with psychogenic purpura, these patients suffer from emotional and psychologic disturbances.

Inflammation of the blood vessel wall occurs in a primary vasculitic syndrome or secondary to an association with infection, collagen vascular disease, medication exposure, and malignancy (Box 23-5). Skin is a frequent target of involvement when there is inflammation of small blood vessels (arterioles, capillaries, and venules) (Fig. 23-16). Inflammation of the capillary and postcapillary venules in the superficial layers of the dermis results in extravasation of erythrocytes and inflammatory cells, producing palpable purpura. Inflammation of arterioles in the deeper dermis and subcutaneous fat produces tender nodules rather than purpuric lesions. Associated features of the primary vasculitic syndrome or features of the underlying disorder causing secondary vasculitis usually allow the correct diagnosis.

All classes of infectious pathogens are capable of causing vascular inflammation by direct invasion of the blood vessel wall (e.g., meningococci or *Rickettsia rickettsii*), septic embolization (e.g., subacute bacterial endocarditis), immune-mediated mechanisms (e.g., meningococci or hepatitis B virus), or the effects of microbial toxins on the vasculature (e.g., *Staphylococcus aureus*). Rarely in these instances is the

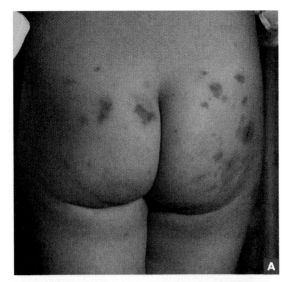

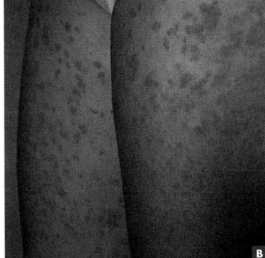

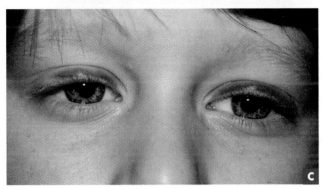

FIG. 23-17 The distinctive rash of HSP. *A* and *B,* It characteristically involves the buttocks and lower extremities, with purpuric coalescent lesions. Note the striking waist-down distribution. *C,* Eyelid involvement has been reported.

primary complaint bruising or bleeding alone. Generally, other signs and symptoms of an infection predominate.

Similarly, cutaneous vasculitic lesions of collagen vascular diseases are usually accompanied by other systemic complaints. Clues to these diseases include insidious onset of malaise, fever, weight loss, and joint complaints. Classic features of particular diseases may be present, such as the malar rash of systemic lupus erethematosus, the "gelling" phenomenon of juvenile rheumatoid arthritis, and the proximal muscle weakness of dermatomyositis.

Drugs have been implicated in causing a small vessel ("hypersensitivity") vasculitis presumably resulting from immune complex deposition. Numerous reports have implicated antibiotics, anticonvulsants, and diuretics, to name a few. Vasculitic lesions (usually on the lower extremities) erupt within 8 to 10 days of drug exposure. Fever and eosinophilia may accompany the lesions. Discontinuation of the drug is curative.

The most common vasculitis of childhood by far is Henoch-Schönlein purpura (HSP), which is a necrotizing vasculitis of small blood vessels primarily affecting children ages 2 to 10 (Figs. 23-17 to 23-21). Palpable purpura, arthritis, ab-

dominal pain, and nephritis are the classic clinical features of HSP, but several other organs may be involved as well. The onset is acute, and the child is previously well, although frequently there is a history of a preceding upper respiratory tract infection. The usual presenting feature is palpable purpura on the lower extremities and buttocks ("dependent"), but lesions can involve any area of the body, particularly if the child is not yet ambulatory. The lesions may start as blanching wheals and maculopapules but evolve into red, palpable, nonblanching lesions. Frequently, angioedema of the scalp and extremities is an associated skin finding. Arthritis, abdominal pain, and nephritis can occur in any combination before the onset of purpura, sometimes making the diagnosis difficult. Although infections and allergens have been implicated, the cause of the vasculitis is unknown. Vessel damage appears to be IgA mediated because IgA levels are elevated and IgA is deposited in the vessels. Patients usually recover fully, although recurrences may occur weeks to years after the initial onset. Nephropathy and end-stage renal disease are the most serious, though infrequent, sequelae of HSP. Children less than 2 years of age tend to have a milder course with less frequent renal and gastrointestinal manifes-

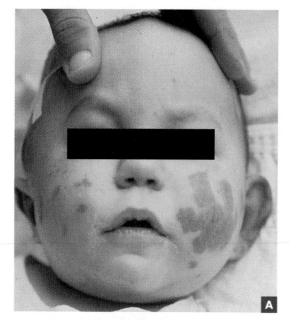

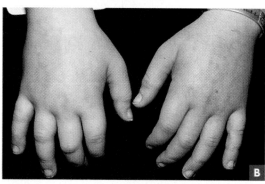

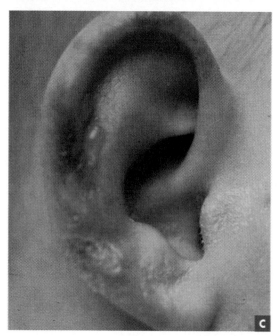

FIG. 23-18   An infant with HSP. *A,* The rash may occur on the face, along with edema. *B,* Rash and edema may be present in the extremities. *C,* Ulceration and vesicles are unusual manifestations of HSP.

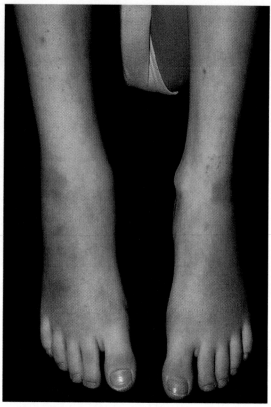

FIG. 23-19   The arthritis of HSP. Note the swelling of the right ankle in addition to the purpuric rash.

tations. It is worth noting that Wegener granulomatosis, although uncommon in children, presents similarly to HSP. Evidence of chronic upper or lower respiratory tract disease differentiates Wegener granulomatosis from HSP.

Progressive pigmentary dermatosis (Schamberg disease) is one of the dermatologic entities known as *pigmented purpuras.* Although more common in adults, there are reports of this disorder occurring in children. The lesions occur predominantly on the lower extremities and appear as reddish-brown, nonblanching macules (Cayenne pepper spots) that may eventually coalesce to form larger patches. As the lesions age, they become darker brown. Skin biopsy shows lymphocytic perivascular infiltration, extravasated erythrocytes in dermal capillaries, hemosiderin-laden macrophages, and dilated capillaries. Distinction from HSP is made by the more insidious onset of the lesions, the macular nature and brownish color of the lesions, and the lack of systemic involvement. The course is benign but may be prolonged, with chronic pigmentation persisting for months or even years.

History

Children with excessive bruising based only on history can be divided into those with trauma-induced ecchymoses and those with a bleeding diathesis. Initial questions should be di-

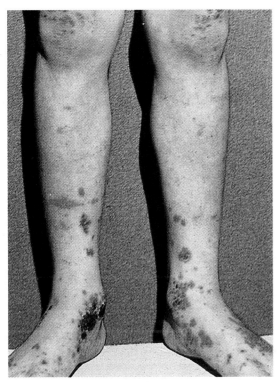

FIG. 23-20   An older child with severe HSP vasculitis resulting in cutaneous necrosis just below and anterior to the right malleolus.

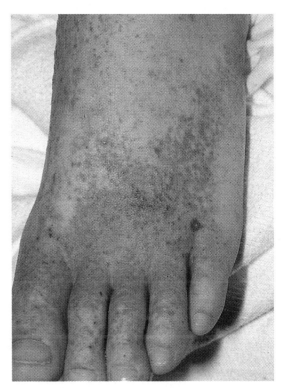

FIG. 23-21   The typical vasculitic rash of HSP is evident in the dorsum of the foot of this 15-year-old youngster. He went on to develop rapidly progressive glomerulonephritis and pulmonary hemorrhage, which were managed by pulse methylprednisolone.

rected at the cause of bruising, the time of onset, and the time course of appearance. The child with platelet dysfunction (either quantitative or qualitative) who has developed spontaneous ecchymoses has petechiae in a diffuse symmetric pattern predating the ecchymoses. The internal consistency of the story provided must be assessed. Is the reported mechanism of injury consistent with the physical findings and the developmental level of the child? In cases of child abuse the interviewer should not expect even the most verbal children to be forthcoming about the injuries because they may have been coerced into silence or a contrived story by the perpetrator.

Further history should attempt to separate those patients with self-limited disease from those with life-threatening disease. Constitutional symptoms should be sought; weight loss, recurring fever, pallor, jaundice, exercise intolerance, and recurring infection suggest severe systemic illness, such as malignancy or collagen vascular disease. Bone pain, joint pain, and abdominal discomfort all may be important. A complete review of systems is necessary to look for clues suggesting that the bleeding diathesis is secondary to a systemic illness.

The past medical history may be helpful. Delayed umbilical cord separation, oozing from the umbilical stump, poor wound healing, and bleeding at intramuscular injection sites

may be clues to defective clotting factor function. Is this episode of purpura a repeat of prior episodes, or is this the first event? Has the patient tolerated prior injury with less ecchymoses? Has minor surgery been tolerated (e.g., circumcision or loss of primary teeth)? Family history of a bleeding diathesis or syndrome associated with increased vascular fragility may be very important and must be obtained. Does any family member take anticoagulants that the patient may have ingested? Are other anticoagulant (e.g., rodenticides) or antiplatelet drugs (e.g., aspirin or other nonsteroidals) present in the home? A thorough social history may uncover risk factors for child abuse.

Physical Examination

The physical examination provides important clues to the cause of bruising and bleeding. It is first directed at identifying immediate life-threatening illness. The child with ITP, aside from purpura, is perfectly well and behaves normally. In the ill-appearing child with purpura, documentation of fever and assessment of blood pressure with orthostatic changes may implicate infection with vascular involvement.

Evidence of malignancy or collagen vascular disease includes cachexia, lymphadenopathy, organomegaly, bone tenderness, and arthritis. Signs of bone marrow failure with resultant anemia may include pallor (best evaluated by looking at the palms and conjunctivae), tachypnea, and tachycardia. Neutropenia may manifest itself with gingivitis, folliculitis, or local soft tissue infection.

Physical stigmata of a syndrome associated with bruising or bleeding should be sought. Examples include the hyperextensible skin and joint hypermobility of Ehlers-Danlos syndrome, the partial albinism of Hermansky-Pudlak syndrome, and the radial anomalies of TAR syndrome.

The appearance and distribution of the lesions give direction to the diagnosis. Petechiae distributed diffusely and symmetrically suggest platelet pathology, whereas ecchymotic lesions may arise in all disorders of hemostasis. Ecchymoses from an inflicted injury may have a peculiar configuration (e.g., belt buckle or doubled-over phone cord) or unusual location (e.g., trunk, buttocks, or perineum). Localized petechiae on only the face or neck suggest increased venous pressure (e.g., coughing). Palpable lesions in dependent locations are typical of vasculitis (HSP). Nodular ecchymoses suggest an infiltrating hematoma typical of either severe trauma or a coagulation factor defect. Finally, bleeding at a number of sites, including muscles or joints, also suggests a coagulation factor defect.

Approach to the Patient

A complete history and physical examination should be complemented by coagulation screening tests. Choice of laboratory screening tests should be individualized and based on clinical suspicion of a specific disease entity when possible. In the patient with bleeding that is deemed excessive but without history or physical examination findings suggestive of any of the specific disorders mentioned, it is reasonable to begin with a CBC, differential, platelet count, peripheral blood smear, PT, and PTT. However, in the adolescent girl with menorrhagia and a positive family history of easy bruising, screening tests should also include measurement of factor VIII:vWF activity.

To rule out pseudothrombocytopenia, thrombocytopenia must be confirmed by visual evaluation of the peripheral smear. When thrombocytopenia is severe enough to account for the presenting signs, the history and physical examination dictate whether an evaluation of the bone marrow is necessary to differentiate a defect in platelet production from a destructive platelet process.

If performed, the marrow evaluation dictates further approaches to the thrombocytopenic patient. For those patients without compelling evidence favoring marrow aspiration, a search for the primary cause of platelet destruction should precede the institution of IVIG. The search should include evaluation of autoimmune markers, including an antinuclear antibody (ANA) test, antineutrophil cytoplasmic antibody (ANCA) test, serum complement levels, Coombs test, and HIV screen. Platelet antibodies currently are not useful outside of a research setting.

A good response to IVIG in the patient with suspected ITP supports the diagnosis and leads to expectant management, perhaps with subsequent doses of IVIG if the platelet count falls to less than 30,000 mm³. A failed response to IVIG warrants a bone marrow evaluation; the results of this examination dictate further care.

If the platelet count is normal or inadequately depressed (greater than or equal to 60,000/mm³) to explain the failure of platelet function (diffuse symmetric petechiae and mucous membrane bleeding), then specific, thorough platelet function studies are indicated.

The child with excessive bruising or bleeding and a normal platelet count but prolonged PT or PTT suffers from a primary or secondary defect in a serum clotting factor. The majority of hereditary factor deficiency states demonstrate a normal PT and a prolonged PTT. Isolated prolongation of the PT implicates warfarin ingestion or factor VII deficiency. When combined with prolonged PTT, vitamin K deficiency, liver disease, or some of the other rare clotting factor deficiencies should be considered.

Although controversy exists over use of the bleeding time in children, it is the best available in vivo measure of a patient's platelet function and ability to form a primary clot. Bleeding time norms have been established for different age groups. If bleeding time is to be performed, the Ivy method (forearm puncture) is preferred because the Duke method (earlobe puncture) is more likely to lead to hemorrhagic complications in children. Measurement of bleeding time may be considered in the patient with suspected platelet dysfunction or unexplained bleeding with normal PT and PTT. Results must be interpreted with the recently delineated limitations in mind.

Normal screening studies can support a vascular defect as the cause of bruising, as well as the need for evaluation of possible vascular-related diseases.

SUMMARY

Bruising and bleeding are normal features in the growing, active child. When bruising and bleeding are considered excessive, the astute clinician must first decide that the trauma inducing the signs is not at issue (question abuse) and then categorize the cause as either platelet-, procoagulant-, or vascular-related pathology. In most instances the generalist is able to pursue the diagnosis to a conclusion. Sophisticated coagulation laboratory studies are necessary to characterize a defect of either the clotting cascade or platelet function.

ILLUSTRATIVE CASES

Case 1. A previously well 3-year-old boy awoke with petechiae and extensive bruising of his legs. A large ecchymotic area of the left buccal mucosa was noted by his mother. He had been ill approximately 2 weeks earlier with an upper respiratory tract infection.

Examination revealed a well-appearing, white boy with diffuse symmetric petechiae. Notably there was no adenopathy, organomegaly, or bone tenderness. A CBC with platelet count revealed a hemoglobin of 12.5 g, WBC count of 10,000/mm³, a normal differential count, and a platelet count of 9000/mm³. Intravenous immunoglobulin was given at a dose of 1 g/kg. Within 48 hours the platelet count had risen to 58,000 mm³ with a normal differential count, and the patient was discharged on mildly restricted activities until follow-up in 1 week. The parent was instructed to contact the physician if an accidental head injury occurred. This is a typical history and course for ITP.

Case 2. A 15-month-old African-American boy was brought to the office because of concern regarding multiple large bruises over his shins, left thigh, and left buttock. He had been completely well and walking for the past 2 months, and the parents denied any history of significant trauma. The family history was negative for bleeding disorders.

Physical examination revealed a pleasant, interactive toddler with multiple ecchymoses over the pretibial areas bilaterally; the ecchymoses ranged in size from 2 to 5 cm in diameter and were in various stages of resolution. Some were quite recent and intensely purple, with a central nodule. Ecchymoses on the left lateral thigh and buttock were ovoid and measured 12 × 9 cm and 18 × 10 cm respectively. No petechiae or mucosal bleeding was noted.

Given the severity of bruising disproportionate to history of trauma, evidence of bruises at varying stages, and central nodules of hematoma formation, a defect in clotting factor function was suspected. PTT was 81 seconds. PT and platelet count were normal. Factor VIII activity was approximately 2%, making the diagnosis of hemophilia A clear.

Case 3. A 5-year-old healthy boy recently recovered from an upper respiratory tract infection. Two days before presenting he complained of diffuse mild to moderate abdominal pain. On the day of presentation, his mother noted what appeared to be hives on the lower legs. The hives evolved into red, raised lesions over several hours and progressed up to the buttocks and lower back.

On physical examination, the boy was cooperative but in mild discomfort. Abdominal examination was remarkable for diffuse mild tenderness but no peritoneal signs. Skin examination revealed scattered petechiae and reddish, nonblanching, palpable lesions of various sizes over the lower back, buttocks, and legs.

New lesions erupted over several days, but 3 weeks after onset all lesions had faded. Initial urinalysis had microhematuria.

The classic features of HSP evolved in this patient, but the initial abdominal pain without skin lesions could have

been misleading. The boy recovered fully and had normal follow-up urinalyses.

ANNOTATED BIBLIOGRAPHY

Bussel JB, Corrigan JJ: Platelet and vascular disorders. In Miller DR, Baehner RL, editors: *Blood disease of infancy and childhood,* ed 7, St Louis, 1995, Mosby.

This is an excellent chapter from a highly regarded pediatric text with thorough and well-referenced information on all quantitative and qualitative platelet disorders written by two authors expert in pediatric coagulation.

Johnson CF: Inflicted injury versus accidental injury, *Pediatr Clin North Am* 37:791-814, 1990.

The definition, epidemiology, and differential diagnosis of physical abuse are given in this review article. An excellent medical approach is detailed, emphasizing historic and physical examination clues that distinguish accidental from intentional injury.

von Kries R, Shearer MJ, Gobel U: Vitamin K in infancy, *Eur J Pediatr* 147:106-112, 1988.

This is an informative review, addressing pathophysiology, risk factors, and diagnosis of hemorrhagic disease of the newborn. It nicely organizes data regarding controversy surrounding enteral versus parenteral vitamin K prophylaxis.

BIBLIOGRAPHY

Anstey A, Mayne K, van de Pette J, et al: Platelet and coagulation studies in Ehlers-Danlos syndrome, *Br J Dermatol* 125:155-163, 1991.

Austin HA III, Balow JE: Henoch-Schönlein nephritis: prognostic features and the challenge of therapy, *Am J Kidney Dis* 2:512-520, 1983.

Aversa LA, Vazquez A, Penalver JA, et al: Bleeding time in normal children, *J Pediatr Hematol Oncol* 17:25-28, 1995.

Baehner RL, Strauss HS: Hemophilia in the first year of life, *N Engl J Med* 275:524-528, 1966.

Barrai I, Conn HM, et al: The effect of parental age on rates of mutation for hemophilia and evidence for differing mutation rates for hemophilia A and B, *Am J Hum Genet* 20:175, 1968.

Berman N, Finkelstein JB: Thrombocytopenic purpura in childhood: results of a survey and reexamination of the literature, *Scand J Haematol* 14:286-294, 1975.

Bick RL: Pathophysiology of hemostasis and thrombosis. In Sodeman WA, Sodeman TA, editors: *Pathologic physiology: mechanisms of disease,* Philadelphia, 1985, WB Saunders.

Brodeur GM, O'Neill PJ, Willimas JA: Acquired inhibitors of coagulation in nonhemophiliac children, *J Pediatr* 96:439-441, 1980.

Bussel JB: Thrombocytopenia in newborns, infants, and children, *Pediatr Ann* 19:181-193, 1990.

Bussel JB, Kaplan C, MacFarland JG: Working party in neonatal immune thrombocytopenia of the neonatal hemostasis subcommittee of the scientific and standardization committee of the ISTH: recommendation for the evaluation and treatment of neonatal autoimmune and alloimmune thrombocytopenia, *Thromb Haemost* 65:631-634, 1991.

Dubost JJ, Souteyrand P, Sauvezie B: Drug-induced vasculitides, *Ballier Clin Rheum* 5:119-138, 1991.

Montgomery RR, Scott JP: Hemostasis: diseases of the fluid phase. In Nathan DG, Oski FA, editors: *Hematology of infancy and childhood,* Philadelphia, 1993, WB Saunders.

Morse EE: The fibrinogenopathies, *Ann Clin Lab Med* 8:234-238, 1978.

Nosek-Cenkowska B, Cheang MS, Bizzi NJ, et al: Bleeding/bruising symptomatology in children with and without bleeding disorders, *Thromb Haemost* 65(3):237-241, 1991.

O'Hare AE, Eden OB: Bleeding disorders and nonaccidental injury, *Arch Dis Child* 59:860-864, 1984.

Ratnoff OD: The psychogenic purpuras: a review of autoerythrocyte sensitization, autosensitization to DNA, "hysterical" and factitial bleeding, and the religious stigmata, *Semin Hematol* 17:192-213, 1980.

Rodeghiero F, Castaman G, Dini E: Epidemiological investigation of the prevalence of von Willebrand disease, *Blood* 69:454-459, 1987.

Rogers RP, et al: A critical reappraisal of the bleeding time, *Semin Thromb Hemost* 16:1-20, 1990.

Sherertz EF: Pigmented purpuric eruptions, *Semin Thromb Hemost* 10:190-194, 1984.

Travis SF, Warfield W, Greenbaum BH, et al: Spontaneous hemorrhage associated with accidental brodifacoum poisoning in a child, *J Pediatr* 122:982-984, 1993.

24

Hepatosplenomegaly

J. CARLTON GARTNER, Jr.

Key Points

- Careful physical examination should allow distinction between a normal and an abnormal size of the liver (span) or spleen.

- History must be inclusive (perinatal, family, etc.), and physical examination should seek findings of chronic disease.

- Treatable disorders, such as metabolic disease in infancy and Wilson disease in older children, must be recognized quickly.

The finding of enlargement of either the spleen or liver on physical examination may help confirm a suspected diagnosis. On the other hand, this finding in a well patient may lead to anxiety, multiple laboratory procedures, and an inconclusive or frustrating evaluation. In this chapter we discuss the evaluation of patients with enlargement of the liver, spleen, or both for weeks (subacute) or months (chronic). Although the differential diagnosis of *all* possible causes is not discussed, an organized, stepwise approach to the patient based on categories of disease is presented. By obtaining key pieces of information from the history and examination, along with some screening laboratory tests, the physician may then plan further evaluation, if necessary.

Pathophysiology

The discussion of enlargement of organs must start with what is normal. Conclusions from several investigators suggest that about 30% of newborns and 10% of healthy 1-year-old infants have palpable spleens, generally just below the costal margin. Only 1% of children at 12 years of age have spleens 1 cm below the rib margin. McNicholl found that overall 11% of healthy children had a palpable spleen, which usually becomes less prominent with increasing age. With the advent of

newer imaging techniques, standards for spleen and liver size have developed, especially using ultrasound. Although not routine, the use of such techniques may eliminate the need for even more costly procedures in certain cases. Liver size in both adults and children has been systematically studied. The distance below the costal margin is inconsistent, even among careful observers. Span is more useful. In a study of 105 healthy school children (5 to 12 years of age), only 1 had a span beyond 11 cm. Size correlated with age and weight (Fig. 24-1). Unfortunately, there are no good standards for liver size or span in infants and toddlers, but a clinician could extrapolate them from Fig. 24-1. A span of less than 12 or 13 cm in adults is generally normal, with the upper border percussed gently and the span measured in the midclavicular line. Apparent enlargement is then the first consideration; in this case an unusual position of the liver or mobility of the spleen (visceroptosis) is a distinct possibility, especially in the well-appearing child. Even in an ill child, palpable liver or splenic "enlargement" may not represent a true increase in size. Because of the mechanics of diaphragm function, over-inflation of the chest (as in asthma) may lower the liver and spleen into the abdominal cavity.

True enlargement of the spleen in the newborn period, but rarely later in infancy, may be caused by hematopoiesis. After infancy the spleen generally acts as a filter to remove old or damaged formed elements and pathogens from the blood. Immune reaction, both humoral and cellular, is a second major function of the spleen. Macrophages can ingest material and lead to "storage" enlargement. Finally, the blood returning from the spleen enters the portal circuit and is susceptible to obstruction.

The liver, the largest reticuloendothelial organ in the body, is the center of metabolism. It is arranged in a series of plates with a dual blood supply from the hepatic artery and the portal vein. Sinusoids lined by Kupffer cells extend from the portal area (arteriole, venule, and bile canaliculus) to a central vein, all of which then combine to form the hepatic veins. Many factors may lead to hepatic enlargement, including congestion (usually from right-sided heart failure

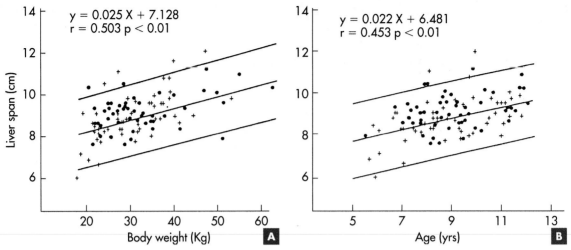

FIG. 24-1 Liver span (estimates of height in the right midclavicular line) in normal boys and girls was obtained by palpating the lower border and percussing the upper border. The closed circles (•) represent values for girls, and the crosses (+) represent values for boys. Each mark is a *mean* of the measurements obtained by two investigators. In *A*, liver span is plotted against body weight, and in *B*, it is plotted against age. The middle lines are the regression lines, and the outer lines represent the 95% confidence limits. The slopes of the lines were significantly different from zero ($p < 0.01$). (From Younoszai MK, Mueller S: Clinical assessment of liver size in normal children, *Clin Pediatr* 14:378-380, 1975.)

or hepatic venous obstruction), storage of material in hepatocytes or Kupffer cells, inflammation or immune stimulation, infiltration of neoplastic cells, and overgrowth of cells intrinsic to the liver (neoplasia or hyperplasia). Some of these mechanisms are similar to those affecting the spleen. Congestion, infiltration, and storage of abnormal material affect both organs, whereas metabolic and inflammatory disorders more frequently affect the liver.

Literature Survey

Few reviews, if any, deal with hepatosplenomegaly in children. In textbooks the differential diagnosis is covered extensively but *separately* under sections on hepatomegaly and splenomegaly. These meticulous listings are useful in difficult or unusual cases. The broad categories of conditions that produce hepatomegaly are well defined in an older review, and perhaps the best mnemonic for the causes of splenic enlargement is contained in the first volume of *The Whole Pediatrician Catalogue*. The remainder of the literature generally deals with enlargement of the liver or spleen as a part of an individual disease process or as a feature of a group of disorders, such as the mucopolysaccharidoses.

Differential Diagnosis

Although somewhat artificial, it is clinically useful to divide the approach to differential diagnosis into the disorders in which splenomegaly is the predominant feature, those in

which hepatomegaly is primary, and finally, those in which both are equally prominent. Although there is obviously extensive overlap, the distinction between the conditions may be quite helpful when patients are seen early in the course of a disease. An example might be congenital hepatic fibrosis in which hepatomegaly is prominent early but tremendous enlargement of the spleen occurs later. Although not discussed in the medical literature, it is probably true that enlargement of the spleen is more frequently noted by examiners than enlargement of the liver. Liver span is often difficult to percuss precisely, and subtle enlargement may be more difficult to discern by examination alone. An example might be infectious mononucleosis in which splenomegaly is a prominent feature. However, almost all patients have hepatitis, as manifested by elevation of transaminase levels, and mild hepatomegaly in the course of the illness.

Predominant Splenomegaly

Infection represents the most common cause of splenomegaly. Perhaps the most frequent office scenario for this condition is the healthy child found to have an enlarged spleen during a visit for a febrile illness. Nonspecific viral illness predominates and may include Epstein-Barr virus, cytomegalovirus (which has been reported as a chronic disorder in the immunologically normal host), and more recently parvovirus B19. Bacterial causes include subacute bacterial endocarditis and chronic infections by low-grade pathogens (such as from a coagulase-negative staphylococcal shunt or central line infection). Protozoal infections include malaria (rare in the United States but common worldwide) and a disorder of increasing frequency, babesiosis.

Hematologic disorders that commonly produce spleno-megaly can be grouped as follows: immune mediated (isoimmune [such as ABO incompatibility] and autoimmune), membrane defects (hereditary spherocytosis, elliptocytosis, and stomatocytosis), hemoglobinopathies (sickle-cell disease and variants and the thalassemias), and enzyme deficiencies (glucose-6-phosphate dehydrogenase deficiency, pyruvate kinase deficiency, etc.). The porphyrias may also be associated with splenomegaly. Disorders of the bone marrow, such as myelofibrosis and osteopetrosis may lead to splenomegaly because of extramedullary hematopoiesis.

Vascular disorders increase splenic size usually because of portal hypertension resulting from liver disease. However, the liver may seem normal on initial examination until further studies demonstrate signs of chronic liver disease. Primary involvement of the splenic or extrahepatic portion of the portal vein may produce splenomegaly with normal liver function, as in cavernous transformation of the portal vein.

Tumors and infiltrations are the final causes of spleno-megaly. Splenic cysts, hemangiomas, hamartomas, and primary lymphoreticular malignancies, such as Hodgkin disease, may be found. Metastatic involvement is rare, the most common being neuroblastoma.

Predominant Hepatomegaly

It is useful to categorize the disorders responsible for predominant liver enlargement. In addition, the clinician should be aware of the age at presentation. With each etiology, infancy, childhood, and adolescence are discussed in a sequential fashion but the discussion also allows for significant overlap.

Infection and inflammation again represent the most frequent cause of hepatomegaly. Nonspecific viral infection is usual. Primary viral hepatitis is next in incidence, beginning in the newborn period with neonatal hepatitis that encompasses many specific diagnoses but may be idiopathic as well. Infection with the multiple hepatitis viruses (A, B, C, D, and E) must be considered and appropriate serologic tests performed. In early infancy the possibility of congenital infection must be considered. Although many congenital infections are associated with hepatosplenomegaly, several conditions, such as congenital syphilis or cytomegalovirus, may produce hepatomegaly only. Granulomatous disorders (tuberculosis and sarcoidosis) may occur at any age because of the current rise in the incidence of tuberculosis. Another uncommon disorder is chronic granulomatous disease, a white-cell killing defect usually inherited as an X-linked disorder. Drug reactions may be associated with prominent hepatomegaly but usually include lymphadenopathy and even cutaneous involvement (e.g., with phenytoin toxicity). Cholangitis may be caused by structural disorders of the hepatobiliary system (e.g., after a portoenterostomy procedure) and is also associated with disorders such as inflammatory bowel disease. Hepatic abscess may be a primary disorder or follow intraabdominal infection, as occurs after appendicitis

> ### BOX 24-1
>
> ## Obstructive Jaundice in the Neonate: Major Causes
>
> ### Anatomic
> Biliary atresia, extrahepatic
> Biliary atresia, intrahepatic (hypoplasia)
>   Syndromic (Alagille syndrome)
>   Nonsyndromic
> Choledochal cyst
> Spontaneous perforation of bile duct
>
> ### Hepatitis
> Idiopathic neonatal
> Other—cytomegalovirus, hepatitis B, etc.
> Toxic—sepsis, urinary tract infection, parenteral nutrition
>
> ### Metabolic
> Alpha$_1$-antitrypsin deficiency
> Cystic fibrosis
> Tyrosinemia
> Galactosemia
> Storage diseases—Niemann-Pick, etc.
> Other
>
> ### Genetic and Familial
> Familial cholestasis (Byler disease)
> Chromosomal disorders (trisomy E)

with rupture. Patients with inflammatory bowel disease may develop hepatic inflammation, cholangitis, or both. Sclerosing cholangitis may be seen in children.

Finally, chronic active hepatitis may follow infection from one of the hepatitis viruses, especially B and C, but may have an immunologic etiology. Antibodies against nuclear, mitochondrial, and smooth muscle antigens may be present with hyperglobulinemia.

Vascular disorders leading to hepatomegaly should be considered, especially in early infancy, when enlargement of the liver may be a sign of congestive heart failure. A more subtle and rarer disorder is pericardial disease with venous obstruction, which may present with hepatomegaly. Obstruction of the hepatic veins (Budd-Chiari syndrome) may be subacute or chronic. A rare disorder that may lead to obstruction of small and large hepatic veins is paroxysmal nocturnal hemoglobinuria, which is associated with thrombophlebitis, hemolysis, and bone marrow hypoplasia.

It is important for the clinician to recognize structural and intrinsic disorders of the liver. In early infancy, hepatomegaly may be a presenting sign of extrahepatic biliary atresia or intrahepatic biliary hypoplasia (see Fig. 19-1). Jaundice is common but initially may be mild and may be mistaken for physiologic hyperbilirubinemia if the conjugated bilirubin is not measured (Box 24-1). Similarly a choledochal cyst may be associated with true or apparent liver enlargement. In late infancy or early childhood congenital hepatic fibrosis, part of the spectrum of infantile polycystic disease, may present with a large, firm liver on routine examination. Recently, several authors have called attention to the finding of hepatomegaly (and elevation of transaminase levels) as findings in child abuse with abdominal trauma. This is a very important disorder to recognize because the episodes may be recurrent and life-threatening.

Storage and metabolic disorders may be grouped together because they have similar features. In early infancy, disorders of carbohydrate metabolism (glycogen storage disease, galactosemia, and hereditary fructose intolerance) and amino acid metabolism (especially tyrosinemia and urea cycle disorders) may present with hepatomegaly, usually with other signs and symptoms. Cystic fibrosis may be associated with early liver enlargement without other signs. A well-appearing infant with hepatomegaly may have alpha$_1$-antitrypsin deficiency. These patients may improve over time or may progress to cirrhosis. It is important to note that the major glycogenoses, such as type I (glucose-6-phosphate dehydrogenase deficiency), present in early infancy with multiple metabolicderangements, hepatomegaly, and increased transaminase levels. Other glucogenoses such as type VI (hepatic phosphorylase deficiency), may be associated only with hepatomegaly in a well-appearing child evaluated for other reasons. Type IV (branching enzyme deficiency) is associated with early cirrhosis.

Important metabolic disorders occurring in older children are Wilson disease and hemochromatosis. Presentations for the former may be multiple and include an enlarged liver, "hepatitis," neuropsychiatric symptoms, portal hypertension, and hemolytic anemia. Early recognition is critical because treatment is lifesaving. Hemochromatosis is more frequent than generally recognized. An enlarged liver with increased transaminase values should suggest hemochromatosis as a possible diagnosis; iron studies are confirmatory.

Fatty change of the liver is a cause of hepatomegaly. The most frequent causes are undernutrition or overnutrition and drug effects from agents such as corticosteroids and alcohol. Poorly controlled diabetes mellitus (Mauriac syndrome) may be a factor.

Tumors and infiltrations of the liver may be primary or secondary and benign or malignant. Hemangioma or hemangioendothelioma may be large enough to lead to congestive heart failure. Hepatoblastoma is more common in infancy, whereas hepatoma is seen in older children. The latter may occasionally be a late effect of congenital metabolic disorders, such as tyrosinemia. Common metastatic tumors in infancy are neuroblastoma, Wilms tumor, leukemia and lymphoma, and histiocytosis syndromes.

Miscellaneous disorders that do not fit neatly into any category are perhaps best listed as syndromes. Examples most frequently occur in the neonatal period. Zellweger syndrome (a peroxisomal disorder; Fig. 11-1) and Beckwith-Wiedeman syndrome are recognized by features that characterize each of them.

Hepatosplenomegaly

Finding enlargement of both the liver and spleen may be a helpful clue to a disease entity or the stage of a disease process. The spleen may enlarge secondarily from portal hypertension in conditions with progressive scarring or fibrosis of the hepatic architecture. Enlargement early in the course of an illness suggests inflammation or storage, which is similar in both organs.

Infection and inflammation are likely the most common causes of hepatosplenomegaly; they are usually associated with generalized adenopathy secondary to a viral infection. Congenital infection must be considered, especially with cytomegalovirus and herpes simplex. Epstein-Barr virus may occur at any time in childhood, but older children have a more typical illness with generalized reticuloendothelial stimulation. Congenital or acquired infection with the human immunodeficiency virus also falls into this category. Bacterial infection is less frequent and includes congenital syphilis, tuberculosis, brucellosis, and cat-scratch disease (often with prominent findings on imaging procedures but mild organomegaly). Protozoal infections, such as toxoplasmosis, malaria, and babesiosis, or helminthic infections, such as visceral larva migrans, are unusual in this country. Fungal infection (histoplasmosis or coccidiomycosis) is uncommon. Sarcoidosis may produce generalized enlargement. Once again, chronic granulomatous disease may be associated with generalized involvement of both the liver and spleen. The connective tissue diseases, most commonly juvenile rheumatoid arthritis and systemic lupus erythematosus, may present with organomegaly. Usually these presentations are associated with fever and other systemic complaints.

Vascular disorders involving the liver may lead to portal obstruction or decreased venous return. Cirrhosis is usually associated with a smaller-than-normal liver. Pericarditis, congestive heart failure, and Budd-Chiari syndrome may be associated with engorgement of hepatic and splenic vessels.

A classic structural disorder is congenital hepatic fibrosis, usually involving greater enlargement of the left lobe of the liver and splenic enlargement. Splenic enlargement may be massive and may result from the obstruction caused by the broad bands of fibrous tissue in the liver (Fig. 24-2).

Special attention should be given to the storage and metabolic disorders. Most of the generalized disorders, with the exception of glycogen storage disease, lead to storage of abnormal material in both the liver and spleen (although type IV glycogen storage disease may produce enlargement of both the liver and spleen secondary to cirrhosis). Examples are mucopolysaccharidoses, gangliosidoses, Niemann-Pick disease, Gaucher disease, Wolman disease, sea-blue histiocyte syndrome, and others. One feature of most of these disorders is enlargement of both the liver and spleen from the onset, rather than later in the course. Other associated features of these disorders assist the clinician in making the diagnosis; they include neurologic signs, developmental delay, bone changes, unusual appearance, etc. Amyloidosis, rare in childhood, may also produce hepatosplenomegaly.

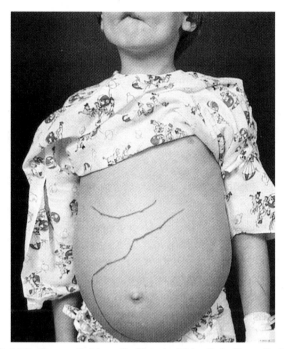

FIG. 24-2 Congenital hepatic fibrosis. This clinically well child had hematemesis and hypersplenism with normal liver function studies. Note the massive splenic size and large left lobe of the liver. Portosystemic shunting was an effective therapy.

Generalized involvement of the reticuloendothelial system by tumors or infiltrations may cause hepatosplenomegaly. Leukemia, lymphoma, histiocytosis X, and histiocyte proliferation syndromes are the most common causes.

The differential diagnoses of splenomegaly and hepatomegaly are presented in Box 24-2.

History

As with most pediatric disorders, a carefully performed history leads to the correct diagnosis or, in the case of organomegaly, helps define the most likely category of disease. A child with an acute illness may simply need followup to ensure that the organ's size has decreased before an extensive investigation is undertaken. Persistent enlargement of the liver, spleen, or both requires a more thorough history and physical and laboratory examination. A family history of illness is important because many conditions, such as storage diseases, metabolic disorders, hepatic fibrosis, and alpha$_1$-antitrypsin deficiency, may be hereditary. A history of neonatal death may be especially important. In neonates the prenatal history may be crucial; infections, drug use, and exposures are important clues to congenital infection. General health, nutritional history, and growth and development are key data. Neurodevelopmental information may be especially important in children with suspected storage and metabolic diseases in which a delay or loss of milestones may occur.

Previous episodes associated with organomegaly, especially if associated with neurologic symptoms, are very suggestive of metabolic disorder, such as urea cycle defects, or disorders of fatty acid oxidation. Current and past drug and medication use should be reviewed. In addition to damage resulting from hepatic injury from medications, such as anticonvulsants, the liver may be damaged by alcohol or other toxins used by the adolescent population.

A careful review of systems may produce data. Prolonged neonatal jaundice, especially in an infant who is not breastfed, suggests cystic fibrosis or alpha$_1$-antitrypsin deficiency. Symptoms of systemic illness or chronic liver disease should be sought; a few of these symptoms are fever, pallor, bruising, weight loss, jaundice, fatigue, respiratory distress, abdominal fullness, and joint complaints. At some point the examiner must decide whether the patient is generally well or whether he or she has a disorder affecting general health. Inflammatory, infectious, and neoplastic disorders are usually associated with constitutional symptoms; an exception is the young infant with neuroblastoma and hepatic involvement. Many storage disorders—especially "milder" variants of glycogen storage disease, nonneurologic storage disorders, and congenital hepatic fibrosis—are discovered during routine examinations in well children. Patients with developing cirrhosis may initially appear well, but their condition deteriorates under observation.

Physical Examination

Clues to a systemic illness should be sought on examination (Box 24-3). Documentation of growth on a growth curve is important. Vital signs, especially in young infants, may suggest cardiorespiratory compromise. The general appearance should be noted. Is there a prominent abdomen? Wasting? Subtle coarsening of facial features may be the only symptom of mucopolysaccharidoses. Skin examination may reveal signs of pruritus; icterus; spider angiomas (chronic liver disease, obstruction of the biliary tract, or both; Fig. 24-3); pallor, petechiae, and bruising (malignancy or chronic liver disease); erythema nodosum (inflammatory bowel disease or sarcoidosis); and prominent superficial abdominal veins (portal hypertension; see Fig. 19-2). Head size and shape should be noted in infants in relation to congenital infection (see Chapter 8). Eye examination may reveal cataracts (galactosemia) and Kayser-Fleischer rings (Wilson disease; see Fig. 19-3). The location and size of lymphadenopathy should be noted. Chest and cardiac examinations are most important in infancy because there may be clues that the hepatosplenomegaly is secondary to heart failure. Cystic fibrosis may be associated with adventitious pulmonary sounds. Abdominal examination should be methodical, starting with inspection. Distension, prominent superficial veins, fullness, and umbilical hernia should be noted. Auscultation may reveal bruits. Percussion of the flanks for shifting dullness and then the chest and right upper quadrant for liver span should be done

BOX 24-2

Differential Diagnosis of Hepatosplenomegaly

Predominant Splenomegaly
Infection
Viral—usual, EBV, CMV, parvovirus B19
Bacterial—endocarditis, shunt or central line
Protozoal—malaria, babesiosis

Hematologic
Hemolytic anemias
Porphyrias
Marrow reduction—osteopetrosis, myelofibrosis

Vascular
Portal vein anomalies
Hepatic scarring or fibrosis

Tumor and infiltration
Cysts, hemangiomas, hamartomas
Lymphoreticular malignancies—with or without
   hepatomegaly
Metastatic disease—neuroblastoma

Predominant Hepatomegaly
Infection and inflammation
Neonatal—CMV, syphilis, neonatal hepatitis
Hepatitis—A, B, C, D, E, etc.
Granulomatous disease—tuberculosis, sarcoidosis, CGD
Drugs—alcohol, phenytoin, etc.
Cholangitis—sclerosing, infectious
Abscess
Chronic active hepatitis—immune mediated

Vascular
Cardiac—failure, pericarditis
Budd-Chiari syndrome
PNH

Structural and intrinsic
Biliary atresia or hypoplasia
Choledochal cyst—multiple locations
Congenital hepatic fibrosis—with or without splenomegaly
Child abuse—trauma

Storage and metabolic
Carbohydrate metabolism—galactosemia, glycogen
   storage disease, fructose intolerance
Amino acid metabolism—tyrosinemia, urea cycle disorders
Cystic fibrosis
Alpha$_1$-antitrypsin deficiency
Older child—Wilson disease, hemochromatosis

Predominant Hepatomegaly—cont'd
Fatty change
Nutritional—malnutrition, obesity
Drug—alcohol, corticosteroids
Diabetes—poor control (Mauriac syndrome)

Tumors and infiltrations
Primary—benign or malignant: hemangioma, hemangioendothelioma, hepatoblastoma, hepatoma
Secondary or metastatic—neuroblastoma, Wilms tumor,
   leukemia or lymphoma, histiocytosis syndromes

Miscellaneous
Syndromes—Zellweger, Beckwith-Wiedemann

Hepatosplenomegaly
Infection and inflammation
Viral—congenital, acquired (especially EBV)
Bacterial—congenital syphilis, tuberculosis, brucellosis, cat-
   scratch disease
Protozoal—malaria, babesiosis, toxoplasmosis
Helminthic—visceral larva migrans
Fungal—histoplasmosis, coccidiodomycosis
Granulomatous—sarcoidosis, CGD
Connective tissue—juvenile rheumatoid arthritis, systemic
   lupus erythematosus

Vascular
Cirrhosis—scarring and portal obstruction
Cardiac—failure, pericarditis
Hepatic veins—Budd-Chiari syndrome, PNH

Structural
Congenital hepatic fibrosis (later in course)

Storage and metabolic
Mucopolysaccharidoses
Gangliosidoses
Lipidoses (e.g., Niemann-Pick and Gaucher diseases)
Glycogen storage disease (type IV only)
Other—Wolman disease, sea-blue histiocyte syndrome, etc.
Amyloidosis

Tumors and infiltrations
Leukemia and lymphoma
Histiocytosis X
Histiocyte proliferation syndromes

EBV, Epstein-Barr virus; *CMV,* cytomegalovirus; *CGD,* chronic granulomatous disease; *PNH,* paroxysmal nocturnal hemoglobinuria.

Diagnostic Clues in Hepatosplenomegaly

History

Age of onset—early suggests congenital infection, metabolic disorders

General health—illness suggests infection or inflammation, tumor, major metabolic disorder; good health suggests structural defect, more benign storage disease (e.g., nonneurologic Gaucher disease)

Growth—poor with severe liver dysfunction, CF

Family history—metabolic disorders, CF, storage disease, hepatic fibrosis

Jaundice—hemolysis, inflammation (hepatitis), bile duct abnormalities (congenital or acquired)

Development—delay in many patients; regression suggests neuronal storage disease

Physical examination

Growth—curve mandatory; poor in CF, hepatic dysfunction

Skin—icterus in hemolysis, hepatic inflammation, bile duct injury
  pallor—anemia
  edema—increased venous pressure, hypoalbuminemia
  pruritus—cholestasis
  spider nevi—chronic liver disease
  petechiae and bruises—bone marrow process, hypersplenism (decreased platelet level), child abuse
  rashes—juvenile rheumatoid arthritis, systemic lupus erythematosus, inflammatory bowel disease

Head—microcephaly or macrocephaly in congenital infection

Eyes—cataract (galactosemia); Kayser-Fleischer rings (Wilson disease)

Nodes—generalized with infection or inflammation, neoplasia

Chest—adventitious sounds in CF, infection

Heart—gallop, tachycardia in failure; signs of pericarditis (rub, pulsus paradoxus)

Abdomen—ascites with cirrhosis, portal hypertension
  large kidneys—hepatic fibrosis
  prominent veins—portal or hepatic vein obstruction
  size of liver or spleen—related to differential diagnosis

Rectal—hemorrhoids with increased venous pressure; fissures, fistulas, and skin tags with inflammatory bowel disease

Neurologic—delay in development
  dystonia, tremor—Wilson disease
  absent reflexes, ataxia—decreased levels of vitamin E (cholestasis)

CF, Cystic fibrosis.

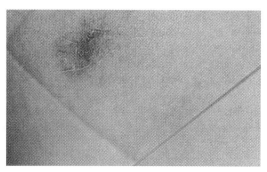

FIG. 24-3 Spider nevus. The vascular lesion blanches on compression with a glass slide, but it reappears when pressure is released.

carefully. Palpation is the final step. The consistency, texture, and symmetry of the liver should be noted. Irregularity is seen with cirrhosis, and the left lobe tends to enlarge with end-stage liver disease and congenital hepatic fibrosis. Occasionally, what appears to be the liver edge may actually be a choledochal cyst. Spleen size and texture are important because careful measurements allow more accurate subsequent examination. In addition, the relative enlargement of both organs should be noted. Are they similar in size or is there disproportionate enlargement? Next, the perianal area should be inspected for hemorrhoids (possible portal hypertension) or fissures, skin tags, and fistulas (inflammatory bowel disease). Edema of the extremities may be a symptom of liver or other disorders (see Chapter 22). Bone and joint evaluation may reveal subtle clues of arthropathy or stiffness (juvenile rheumatoid arthritis or mucopolysaccharidoses). Clubbing of the digits is seen with a variety of disorders, including chronic oxyhemoglobin desaturation and intestinal and hepatic disorders (see Fig. 1-3).

Approach to the Patient

After completing a thorough history and physical examination, the physician should be able to categorize the possible diagnoses. Answers to several questions may provide guidance. What was the age of onset of the problem? Is there evidence that the current findings may be long-standing? Key information about the perinatal period, especially maternal illness, neonatal problems, umbilical catheterization, and persistent icterus, should be obtained. How have the patient's general health and nutrition been since birth? What are the patient's developmental milestones? Is there a clue to the diagnosis in the family history if the problem seems chronic? Have other family members undergone investigation for disorders of the liver or spleen? Is the patient's problem less chronic and of more recent onset? These data begin to limit the possible diagnoses; a shorter duration of symptoms increases the chances of an inflammatory, infectious, or neoplastic disorder.

Physical examination should be done looking for signs of a systemic illness or subtle clues to chronic liver disease. A very important sign is enlargement of the liver, spleen, or both. Splenic enlargement alone with a normal liver may be "postinfectious" but suggests extrahepatic portal obstruction if there is progressive enlargement. At times the examiner may be frustrated by the inability to decide whether there is involvement of the liver. The liver's lower edge may not be palpable and its span difficult to percuss. Such an evaluation may require further assessment of liver size or involvement using laboratory or imaging procedures. Purely hepatic enlargement is a clue to several diagnoses, such as glycogen storage disease, but may be an early finding (i.e., occurring before portal hypertension develops) in many more chronic liver disorders. Hepatosplenomegaly suggests a more generalized process, especially inflammatory, infectious, or neoplastic disease if the process is subacute or storage disease or cirrhosis if it is chronic.

Selective laboratory tests should then be done. Key tests evaluate inflammation of the liver (alanine aminotransferase [ALT] or serum glutamate pyruvate transaminase; aspartate aminotransferase [AST] or serum glutamic-oxaloacetic transaminase), obstruction of the biliary tract (fractionated bilirubin, gamma-glutamyl transferase [GGT] levels), and ability to synthesize major products (prothrombin time, partial thromboplastin time, albumin and cholesterol levels). Serologic testing for hepatitis is important in subacute disorders. In older patients with prolonged symptoms, tests for the etiology of chronic disorders are important; these tests include ceruloplasmin levels (which may be normal in Wilson disease); 24-hour copper levels; ferritin levels; and antinuclear, antimitochondrial, and antimicrosomal antibody values ("liver, kidney, microsomal antibody" levels, a marker for autoimmune hepatitis). In younger children it is important to look for metabolic disorders, such as tyrosinemia, with quantitative amino and organic acids (for disorders of fatty acid metabolism). It is also reasonable to obtain a complete blood count (CBC), differential count, and platelet count when considering a malignant process or hypersplenism. At this point it may be useful to obtain a limited imaging procedure, such as ultrasound, to confirm the enlargement and assess the architecture. In selected cases this procedure may be diagnostic (e.g., when a localized hepatic tumor or a splenic cyst is present). An additional finding on ultrasound may be the flow in the portal circuit; a reversal of flow (hepatofugal) suggests portal hypertension.

At this point decisions about further investigation should be made. Patients with normal findings on all tests and with enlargement of the liver and spleen likely have a process not intrinsic to those organs; these may include metastatic tumor, leukemia or lymphoma, storage disorders (except glycogen storage disease, which is associated with an increase in transaminase levels), and congenital hepatic fibrosis. A bone marrow examination or skin fibroblast enzyme assay may be considered first in some cases in which metabolic or storage disease is suspected, or a liver biopsy may be performed to confirm congenital hepatic fibrosis unless typical cysts are seen on abdominal imaging.

Patients with inflammation of the liver should have further study for a cause. In subacute cases, viral titers (Epstein-Barr virus, cytomegalovirus, human immunodeficiency virus, etc.) should be done. Patients with chronic signs should eventually undergo liver biopsy. An ophthalmologic examination for Kayser-Fleischer rings is sometimes helpful and may allow treatment without a biopsy. In addition, if glycogen storage disease remains a possibility in a well-appearing child with hepatomegaly, a leukocyte assay of many of the enzymes may be possible, eliminating the need for liver biopsy.

If the clinician can eliminate serious, potentially life-threatening disorders such as metabolic disease in infants and Wilson disease in older children, a course of close outpatient follow-up without liver biopsy may be undertaken. As with most pediatric conditions, time usually allows recovery from common disorders, such as mild inflammation. There is no substitute for knowing the patient and the course of the illness over time.

SUMMARY

Although relatively uncommon, persistent enlargement of the liver, spleen, or both suggests a myriad of possible diagnoses ranging from mild and transient to potentially life-threatening. By taking a stepwise approach and collecting key information from the history and examination, the physician can limit the differential diagnosis to several major categories and then collect several tests of function (e.g., laboratory tests and imaging studies). A decision can then be made to pursue more invasive investigation, such as liver biopsy, or simply follow the patient over time. An organized approach allows the correct diagnosis to be made promptly and spares patients with benign conditions a needlessly aggressive approach.

ILLUSTRATIVE CASES

Case 1. B.R. *was first seen at 1 year of age when enlargement of the liver was found by his family pediatrician on two examinations that were several months apart. He was healthy, was growing well, and had never been hospitalized. His perinatal history was unremarkable, as was the family history. The pediatrician had delayed referral because the child was so healthy. On initial examination the child appeared well; growth was at the 75% percentile, but the infant had a somewhat prominent abdomen. The liver was firm in consistency and 5 cm below the costal margin with a span of 10 cm, and the spleen was palpable 4 cm below the left costal margin. The remainder of the examination was normal. Laboratory data, including transaminase levels, prothrombin time, CBC, and hepatitis serologic tests, were completely normal. An abdominal sonogram confirmed organomegaly and also indicated that the kidneys were mildly hyperechoic.*

Because of the chronicity of the process and normal liver function, storage disease, cirrhosis, and congenital hepatic fibrosis were considered the most likely diagnoses. The alpha₁-antitrypsin level was normal. Bone marrow examination and skin fibroblast enzyme assay were considered, but liver biopsy was done because of the abnormal renal ultrasound. A diagnosis of congenital hepatic fibrosis was confirmed. The patient has remained asymptomatic, but the spleen has slowly enlarged.

This case demonstrates the importance of normal enzyme levels in categorizing the disease process, the relative enlargement of both organs, and the value of ultrasound. If the spleen had been enlarged as much as the liver and the sonogram basically normal, a disorder such as Gaucher disease would have been more likely, and the order of testing may have been changed.

Case 2. A 10-month-old boy was referred for further evaluation because of poor growth and elevated liver enzyme levels. Growth had fallen off after 6 months, from the 50th to the 10th percentile, without a change in appetite or bowel movements. The pediatrician found the liver to be enlarged and ordered liver function tests, which included an ALT level of 450 IU and an AST level of 500 IU; normal levels of bilirubin and gamma-GTP and negative hepatitis A and B serologic tests led to the referral. A more-detailed history revealed an uneventful perinatal period, negative family history, and general good health. Examination revealed a generally healthy child with good nutrition. The liver was 4 cm below the costal margin with a smooth soft margin and a span of 9 cm. The spleen was not palpable. The child was well except for the inability to get to a sitting position or stand with support. Reflexes and the remainder of the examination were normal.

This child has isolated prominence of the liver with elevated enzyme levels. Initial impressions centered on a type of chronic hepatitis, but two features were peculiar. First, the transaminase values showed that the AST level, a feature more consistent with muscle disease, was higher than the ALT level. The ALT level is usually significantly higher with hepatic disorders. Second, the child had a mild delay in motor development. A test to determine creatine phosphokinase levels was ordered before other tests, and the level was strikingly elevated at 15,000 IU. Neurologic evaluation and a later muscle biopsy confirmed muscular dystrophy.

This case illustrates that liver enlargement must be taken in context as only one feature of a disease process. The span of this child's liver is likely at the upper limit of normal, since there are no standards on physical examination for a 1-year-old. In addition, the edge of the liver was soft and smooth, another unusual finding in disease.

Case 3. A 12-year-old boy (J.W.) was referred for further evaluation of abdominal swelling and peripheral edema. The past history was unremarkable. The parents had noted a prominent abdomen for several weeks and brought the child to the family physician. A routine chemistry profile demonstrated mild transaminase elevation (ALT, 200 IU; AST, 150 IU) and a bilirubin level at 2.0 mg/dl with conjugated bilirubin of 1.5 mg/dl. The family history and past medical history were unremarkable. Examination revealed a boy with numerous spider nevi, mild icterus, mild peripheral edema, and ascites. The liver was palpable 3 cm below the costal margin with a span of 10 cm and an irregular, firm margin. The spleen was palpable 4 cm below the costal margin. Neurologic examination was normal. Further laboratory testing revealed an albumin level of 2.8 g/dl, a prothrombin time of 18 seconds (control, 12 seconds), mild anemia with a hemoglobin level of 11 g/dl, and mild reductions in both the leukocyte and platelet counts.

This boy had not appeared ill until a few weeks before evaluation but had signs of chronic liver disease. Hepatitis and cirrhosis were considered, so serologic and antinuclear antibody tests were done. An ophthalmology consultation revealed Kayser-Fleischer rings. Both 24-hour urinary copper and serum ceruloplasmin levels were abnormal. D-Penicillamine therapy was started immediately, and the patient is well some 15 years later.

Every physician needs to be aware of Wilson disease because the presentations are multiple and the treatment is usually effective if started early enough. Even when significant liver scarring has taken place, the course may be reversed. Occasionally the course is fulminant, and liver transplantation is the only option.

ANNOTATED BIBLIOGRAPHY

Coant PN, Kornberg AE, Brody AS, Edwards-Holmes K: Markers for occult liver injury in cases of physical abuse in children, *Pediatrics* 89:274-278, 1992.

> *The spectrum of child abuse extends to occult liver injury. This may be the only clue and, if missed, may allow further injury or even death for the child.*

Dobyns WB, Goldstein NP, Gordon H: Clinical spectrum of Wilson's disease (hepatolenticular degeneration), *Mayo Clin Proc* 54:35-42, 1979.

> *This disorder is treatable if considered early. Presentations may include hepatitis, neurologic disorder, and even hemolytic anemia.*

Tunnessen WW: *Signs and symptoms in pediatrics,* Philadelphia, 1988, JB Lippincott.

> *This book includes useful lists for the differential diagnoses of hepatomegaly and splenomegaly. In difficult cases, a list may alert the physician to a possibility that had not been considered previously.*

BIBLIOGRAPHY

Alvarez F, Bernard O, Brunelle F, et al: Congenital hepatic fibrosis in children, *J Pediatr* 99:370-375, 1981.

Alvarez F, Bernard O, Brunelle F, et al: Portal obstruction in children. I and II. *J Pediatr* 103:696-702, 703-707, 1983.

Balistreri WF: Neonatal cholestasis, *J Pediatr* 106:171-184, 1985.

Boles ET, Baster CF, Newton WA: Evaluation of splenomegaly in childhood, *Clin Pediatr* 2:161-168, 1963.

Crystal RG: α_1-Antitrypsin deficiency: pathogenesis and treatment, *Hosp Pract* 26:81-94, 1991.

Currie JM, Adamson DJ, Brown T, et al: The fifth cause of splenomegaly? Parvovirus B_{19}, *Clin Lab Haematol* 14:327-330, 1992.

Gentil-Kocher S, Bernard O, Brunelle F, et al: Budd-Chiari syndrome in children: report of 22 cases, *J Pediatr* 113:30-38, 1988.

Green M: *Pediatric diagnosis,* Philadelphia, 1980, WB Saunders.

Maggiore G, Bernard O, Homberg J, et al: Liver disease associated with anti–liver-kidney microsome antibody in children, *J Pediatr* 108:399-404, 1986.

McMillan JA, Nieberg PI, Oski FA: *The whole pediatrician catalog,* vol I, Philadelphia, 1977, WB Saunders.

McNicholl B: Palpability of the liver and spleen in infants and children, *Arch Dis Child* 32:438-440, 1957.

Morse RP, Rosman NP: Diagnosis of occult muscular dystrophy: importance of the "chance" finding of elevated serum aminotransferase activities, *J Pediatr* 122:254-256, 1993.

Nowicki MJ, Balistreri WF: Hepatitis A to E: building up the alphabet. I. *Contemp Pediatr* 9(11):118-128, 1992.

Nowicki MJ, Balistreri WF: Hepatitis A to E: building up the alphabet. II. *Contemp Pediatr* 9(12):23-42, 1992.

Scriver CR, Beaudet AL, Shy WS, et al: *The metabolic and molecular basis of inherited disease,* New York, 1995, McGraw-Hill.

Walker WA, Mathis RK: Hepatomegaly: an approach to differential diagnosis, *Pediatr Clin North Am* 22:929-942, 1975.

Ware RE, Hall SE, Rosse WF: Paroxysmal nocturnal hemoglobinuria with onset in childhood and adolescence, *N Engl J Med* 325:991-996, 1991.

Younoszai MK, Mueller S: Clinical assessment of liver size in normal children, *Clin Pediatr* 14:378-380, 1975.

Lymphadenopathy

BASIL J. ZITELLI

 ## Key Points

- Normally, lymph nodes can be palpated in children and even neonates. Lymphoid tissue increases in mass as children grow older, reaching maximum mass during puberty.

- The most common cause of lymph node enlargement in children is viral infection. With frequent infections, nodes may not fully regress in size over time. Generalized lymph node enlargement usually is associated with systemic disorders, whereas regional adenopathy suggests a more localized process.

- Lesions of the head and neck include congenital anomalies, adenopathy secondary to a variety of infections, and malignancies. Careful history, physical examination, and selected laboratory tests aid the physician in sorting out the potential causes of adenopathy.

*L*umps under a child's skin raise fears and concerns among the parents and physicians. Although superficial lumps are rarely malignant, the differential diagnosis is difficult and requires a systematic approach to the patient. Enlarged lymph nodes that cause superficial lumps are common in children and may tax even the most astute physician. This chapter summarizes normal lymphoid development and related physical findings in children, discusses a general approach to generalized and regional adenopathy (with special emphasis on cervical adenopathy), reviews mechanisms of lymph node enlargement, presents common differential diagnoses of generalized and regional adenopathy, and finally offers an approach to the patient via history, physical examination, and simple laboratory tests.

Pathophysiology

Enlargement of lymph nodes can occur because of proliferation of elements intrinsic to the node or infiltration of the node by cells extrinsic to node tissue. Intrinsic proliferation of lymphocytes occurs after antigenic and cytokine stimulation. Normal histiocytes within the node may proliferate and ingest material or expand by storing products of abnormal metabolic processes, such as those found in storage disorders (e.g., Gaucher disease). Nonantigenic stimulation of lymphocyte proliferation also occurs, with hyperthyroidism and lymphomas.

Invasion of cells extrinsic to the lymph node is most commonly caused by polymorphonuclear leukocytes resulting from viral or bacterial infections. Abscess formation may occur, especially as a result of bacterial infection. Metastatic tumors and leukemic infiltration also cause lymph node enlargement.

Literature Survey

Palpable lymph nodes commonly are found in children of all ages, ranging from birth to adulthood (Table 25-1). Lymphoid tissue steadily increases during infancy, childhood, and adolescence to achieve approximately twice the adult lymphoid volume and then undergoes a relative reduction. More than one third of neonates have palpable lymph nodes, primarily in inguinal, cervical, and axillary areas. As the child ages, 57% of children up to 1 year of age have palpable lymph nodes, with cervical nodes palpated most frequently, followed by inguinal and axillary nodes. Normally no supraclavicular nodes are detected before 1 year of age. Occipital lymph nodes often can be palpated in young infants, especially in the presence of scalp lesions, such as seborrhea. Generally, lymph nodes 3 mm or smaller in size are considered normal. Nodes larger than 5 mm in the epitrochlear area, larger than 10 mm in the cervical area, and larger than 15 mm in the inguinal area are considered abnormal. The spleen can be palpated normally in 14% of newborns, but the frequency decreases to about 7% of children under 10 years of age (see Chapter 24). A thymic shadow usually is visible on routine chest radiographs up to 1 year of age and most often disappears by age 3.

The increasing ability to palpate lymph nodes with increasing age most likely reflects the developmental aspects of

TABLE 25-1

Frequency of Palpable Lymph Nodes in Children (Percentage of Children Examined)

Age	Axillary	Occipital	Postauricular	Submandibular	Cervical	Inguinal	None palpated
0-6 mo	6	32	13	2	2	22.7*	62
7-12 mo	14	26	13	3	26	36.7†	52
13-23 mo	—	10	7	18	28	—	52
2-3 yr	—	7	0	26	33	—	41
4-5 yr	—	0	5	21	63	—	26

Modified from Bamji M, Stone RK, Kaul A, et al: Palpable lymph nodes in healthy newborns and infants, *Pediatrics* 78:573-575, 1986; and Herzog LW: Prevalence of lymphadenopathy of the head and neck in infants and children, *Clin Pediatr* 22:485-487, 1983.
*1 to 6 months.
†6 to 12 months.

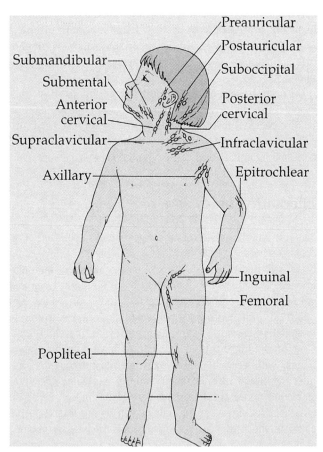

FIG. 25-1 Lymph node regions that may be involved in generalized adenopathy.

lymphoid growth, as well as chronic and recurrent stimulation. It is not uncommon to find lymph node enlargement after acute infection, with only partial return to normal size after resolution of the infection. Healing of the node is often accompanied by fibrosis; palpable nodes sometimes persist for months or years.

Adenopathy commonly is divided into generalized and regional involvement. The initial approach to the patient should be directed toward determining the extent of involvement. Generalized lymph node enlargement implies a systemic disease (benign or malignant). Regional lymph node enlargement more frequently but not exclusively indicates a pathologic process localized to the regional drainage area of the involved nodes. Despite the distinction between generalized and regional disease, many pathologic processes have overlapping features. Epstein-Barr virus (EBV) infection is only one example of such a process, presenting as regional cervical adenopathy with pharyngitis or generalized lymphadenopathy.

Differential Diagnosis

Generalized Lymphadenopathy

Generalized lymphadenopathy is defined as enlargement of two or more noncontiguous lymph node regions (Fig. 25-1 and Box 25-1). The liver and spleen—components of the lymphoreticular system—frequently are also enlarged. Infections account for the majority of generalized lymphadenopathy cases, and malignancies are found in less than 20% of biopsied peripheral lymph nodes. Pyogenic infections of virtually any cause may stimulate nodes or cause direct bacterial invasion. Chronic streptococcal infection in young children is associated with fever, mucopurulent rhinorrhea, weight loss, and generalized adenopathy. Viral exanthems of nearly any cause, especially rubella or rubeola, have noncontiguous lymph node enlargement; nodes usually are moderately enlarged and minimally tender. Infectious mononucleosis caused by cytomegalovirus (CMV) or EBV infection can cause both regional (cervical) and generalized palpable lymph nodes. Hepatitis, especially associated with papular acrodermatitis (Gianotti-Crosti syndrome), and mycoplasmal infections less commonly cause generalized adenopathy. Although

Differential Diagnosis of Generalized Lymphadenopathy

Systemic Infections

Pyogenic bacterial infections
Scarlet fever
Viral exanthematous diseases (e.g., rubella or rubeola)
Epstein-Barr virus
Cytomegalovirus
Infectious hepatitis
Cat-scratch disease
Mycoplasma organisms
Bacterial endocarditis
Tuberculosis
Syphilis
Toxoplasma organisms
Brucella organisms
Histoplasmosis
Coccidioidomycosis
Typhoid fever
Malaria
Chronic granulomatous disease
HIV infection

Immune-Mediated Inflammatory Disorders

Systemic lupus erythematosus
Juvenile rheumatoid arthritis
Serum sickness
Kawasaki syndrome
Hyper IgD syndrome
Hyper IgE syndrome

Storage Diseases

Gaucher disease
Niemann-Pick disease
Tangier disease

Malignancies

Leukemia
Lymphoma
Neuroblastoma
Histiocytosis X
X-linked lymphoproliferative syndrome
Kawasaki-like syndrome after therapy for acute monocytic leukemia

Metabolic Disorders

Hyperthyroidism
Adrenal insufficiency

Miscellaneous

Drug reactions (phenytoin, hydralazine, allopurinol, etc.)
Hemolytic anemias
Immunoblastic lymphadenopathy
Sarcoidosis
Sinus histiocytosis

cat-scratch disease usually is associated with regional lymph node involvement, multiple sites are involved in nearly 40% of cases as reported by Margileth. Other infectious causes of generalized adenopathy are listed in Box 25-1. Infection with the human immunodeficiency virus (HIV) may cause adenopathy as a feature of chronic infection or as a sign of lymphoma (less commonly in children). Acute HIV infection may have a similar presentation to infectious mononucleosis; persistent adenopathy also may occur.

Approximately two thirds of children with immune-mediated inflammatory disorders, such as systemic lupus erythematosus or juvenile rheumatoid arthritis, have generalized adenopathy during the acute stages of the illness. As activity of the disease subsides, lymph nodes tend to regress in size. Similarly, enlarged noncontiguous lymph nodes found in serum sickness subside as the exanthem disappears. The hyperimmunoglobulinemia D (hyper IgD) syndrome, a rare disorder resulting in periodic fevers in children, usually causes cyclic fevers, chills, headache, adenopathy, and occasional abdominal pain and diarrhea. Kawasaki syndrome usually causes unilateral cervical adenopathy, but rarely is generalized node enlargement seen.

A variety of storage diseases cause generalized adenopathy because the reticuloendothelial system sequesters products of metabolism. Hepatosplenomegaly is a prominent finding in both the rapidly progressive infantile form and the chronic forms of Gaucher disease, a disorder of lipid metabolism with accumulation of glucocerebrosides. In Niemann-Pick disease, sphingomyelin and nonesterified cholesterol are stored in the reticuloendothelial system. At least six major forms of the disease exist, and adenopathy and hepatosplenomegaly are common in most forms. Tangier disease is a rare familial disorder of apolipoprotein A-I metabolism, causing very low levels of high-density lipoproteins and high levels of serum triglycerides. Cholesterol esters are stored in the reticuloendothelial tissues, causing hepatosplenomegaly, adenopathy, and large yellowish-gray or orange tonsils.

Malignancies are associated with generalized adenopathy caused by lymphomatous changes of cells within lymph nodes or by invasion of metastatic cells. About 70% of patients with acute lymphocytic leukemia and 30% of patients with acute myelocytic leukemia have generalized adenopathy at presentation. These percentages may be decreasing, however, because the diagnosis is being made earlier. Neuroblas-

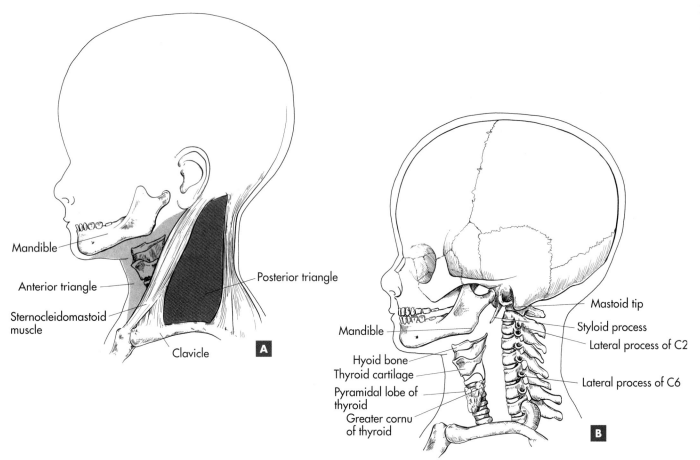

FIG. 25-2 Anatomy of the neck. *A,* The anterior triangle is bounded by the inferior border of the mandible, the SCM, and the midline of the neck. The posterior triangle is bounded by the SCM, the outer two thirds of the clavicle, and the posterior midline of the neck. *B,* Normal structures that can be palpated include the angle of the mandible, mastoid tip, styloid process, pyramidal lobe of the thyroid, greater cornu of the thyroid, and lateral processes of C2 and C6 vertebrae.

toma causes lymph node enlargement through metastasis, whereas malignant histiocytosis X results from generalized neoplastic proliferation of Langerhans cells. EBV infection in an immunocompromised male host is responsible for the X-linked lymphoproliferative syndrome. EBV also is associated with posttransplantation lymphoproliferative disease. Both lymphoproliferative disorders can cause generalized adenopathy simulating or leading to lymphoma. In addition, therapy for acute monocytic leukemia may cause a Kawasaki-like syndrome with generalized adenopathy.

Uncommon causes of generalized adenopathy include metabolic disorders, such as hyperthyroidism and adrenal insufficiency, although the exact mechanism is not well understood. Drugs, especially phenytoin, have been associated with enlarged nodes, rash, and eosinophilia. Hemolytic anemias have been linked with lymph node enlargement, especially when occurring with viral infections, such as CMV. Immunoblastic lymphadenopathy, rare in children, presents with fever, sweats, weight loss, hemolytic anemia, hyperglobulinemia, and generalized adenopathy. Sarcoidosis, uncommon in children and more common in African-Americans, is a granu-

lomatous disorder with frequent pulmonary involvement and hilar adenopathy. Peripheral adenopathy occurs in about 40% of patients. Sinus histiocytosis with massive lymphadenopathy is a rare disorder characterized by massive lymph node enlargement, which is usually cervical, although other lymph nodes and extranodal sites, such as the orbit, can be involved. Nodes often are bilateral and painless, but fever, leukocytosis, neutrophilia, and hypergammaglobulinemia are also components of the illness. Nodal architecture shows dilation of sinuses and numerous intrasinusoidal histiocytes. The disease course is protracted, with eventual spontaneous regression of nodes and recovery.

Regional Adenopathy

Head and Neck

Perhaps the most complicated region to evaluate for enlarged lymph nodes is the head and neck area. The differential diagnosis of a child with a neck mass may include adenopathy, congenital lesions, and malignancy. A brief review of surface anatomy can help in the evaluation of cervical

TABLE 25-2

Common Congenital Neck Masses

Mass	Distinguishing features
Thyroglossal duct cyst	Midline neck location, retracts with tongue protrusion
Second branchial cleft cyst	Located anterior to the middle third of the SCM, may have fistula opening at base of SCM, may retract with swallowing
Vascular malformations	
Hemangioma	Soft spongy mass, may increase in size with Valsalva maneuver, does not transilluminate, may have reddish-blue skin discoloration
Cystic hygroma	Soft spongy mass, may increase in size with Valsalva maneuver, transilluminates
Congenital muscular torticollis	Firm, noninflamed spherical or oval mass within the belly of the SCM, head tilted to affected side, chin pointed to contralateral side

SCM, Sternocleidomastoid muscle.

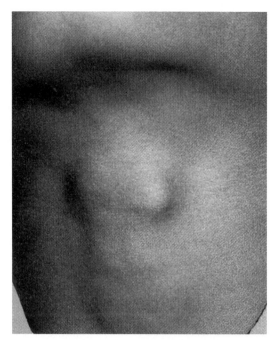

FIG. 25-3 A thyroglossal duct cyst located slightly to the left of the midline. Usually these cysts are midline in location.

masses. The neck is divided into two major anatomic triangles. The anterior triangle is bounded by the mandibular border, the sternocleidomastoid muscle (SCM), and the midline of the neck (Fig. 25-2, *A*). The posterior triangle is bounded by the SCM, the outer two thirds of the clavicle, and the midline neck posteriorly. Some normal structures that can be palpated and confused with abnormal neck masses include the angle of the mandible, mastoid tip, styloid process, pyramidal lobe of the thyroid, greater cornu of the thyroid, and lateral processes of C2 and C6 vertebrae (Fig. 25-2, *B*).

Generally, lesions that enlarge slowly over several months are benign, whereas those that grow rapidly (in the absence of inflammation) are more frequently neoplastic. Risk factors for malignancy include fixation to deep tissues; size greater than 3 cm; hard or firm consistency; matting of nodes into a single, large indistinct mass; and constitutional symptoms, such as fever, night sweats, and weight loss.

Location of the mass is an important detail. Most masses lying anterior to the SCM are benign. Thyroid nodules are the exception; at least 70% of thyroid nodules are malignant in children under 10 years of age. Therefore any thyroid nodule in a child should be considered malignant until proved otherwise. Malignancies can present as a single mass in the posterior triangle or as multiple matted masses crossing into the anterior and posterior triangles.

Cervical masses are grouped into three general categories—congenital lesions, lymphadenopathy, and malignant tumors.

Congenital Lesions

Three major lesions—thyroglossal duct cysts (72%), branchial cleft cysts (24%), and vascular malformations (4%)—account for most diagnoses of congenital defects (Table 25-2).

Thyroglossal duct cysts are the most common congenital neck mass. During the third week of gestation the thyroid anlage descends as a hollow-stalked structure from the base of the tongue. This stalk (thyroglossal duct) usually atrophies; however, failure to do so may lead to a fistula, sinus tract, or cyst along the path of descent. Usually a fluctuant cystic mass is palpated in the midline or slightly off center, below the level of the hyoid bone (Fig. 25-3). Infection of the cyst leads to acute swelling and tenderness. With the neck extended the cyst can be palpated easily. Although the cyst characteristically retracts with tongue protrusion, this clinical sign is not infallible because not all cysts are attached to the fistulous connection to the tongue. Lingual thyroid cysts, cysts of the thyroid pyramidal lobe, lipomas, dermoids, and sebaceous cysts easily can be confused with thyroglossal duct cysts.

Branchial cleft cysts occur because of incomplete fusion of the branchial grooves and pouches. Although branchial cleft anomalies may arise from any of the first four clefts, 95% arise from the second cleft, perhaps because of its greater

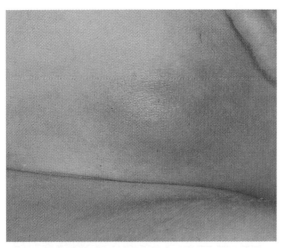

FIG. 25-4   An inflamed cyst from the second branchial cleft beneath the anterior border of the SCM.

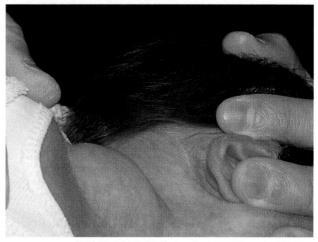

FIG. 25-6   Cystic hygroma arising from the posterior triangle.

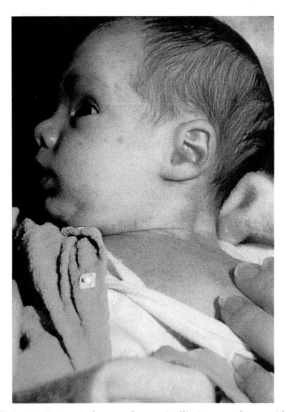

FIG. 25-5   Congenital muscular torticollis in a newborn with a fibrous mass in the belly of the SCM.

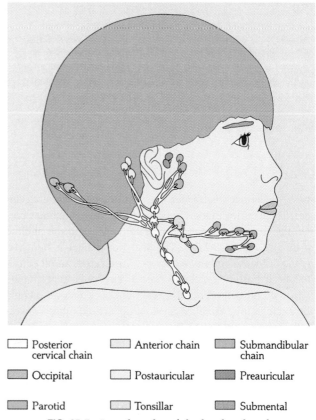

☐ Posterior cervical chain	☐ Anterior chain	☐ Submandibular chain
☐ Occipital	☐ Postauricular	☐ Preauricular
☐ Parotid	☐ Tonsillar	☐ Submental

FIG. 25-7   Lymph nodes of the head and neck.

depth and persistence. Cysts of the second branchial cleft usually are found in the carotid triangle, anterior but deep to the middle third of the SCM (Fig. 25-4). Sinus tracts, found in less than one third of patients, frequently are seen as small slits anterior to the lower third of the SCM. Skin appendages and fistulas accompany branchial cleft cysts in 63% of cases,

making diagnosis somewhat easier. The cysts may fluctuate in size or become acutely inflamed with infection, requiring antibiotic therapy and subsequent excision. These cysts can be confused with lymph nodes, congenital muscular torticollis (although affected children have an associated head tilt to the affected side, with the chin pointing away; Fig. 25-5), cys-

Some Common Causes of Cervical Lymphadenopathy

Disorder	Associated characteristics
Viral upper respiratory tract infection	Soft, discrete, mobile, minimally tender lymph nodes
EBV or CMV infection	Infectious mononucleosis presentation, pharyngitis
Suppurative infections (staphylococcal, streptococcal)	Fever, swelling, erythema, tenderness, sometimes fluctuant lymph nodes
Cold inflammation	
Cat-scratch disease	Exposure to a kitten, history of a pustule, regional adenopathy, minimal symptoms
Atypical mycobacterial adenitis	Thin, scaly, parchmentlike overlying skin; asymptomatic; reactive PPD test; normal chest radiographs
Toxoplasmosis	Asymptomatic, painless swelling in posterior triangle; high titers to *Toxoplasma* organisms
Miscellaneous	
Systemic disorders causing generalized adenopathy	Specific signs or symptoms of each disorder
Kawasaki syndrome	Prolonged fever, rash, conjunctivitis, oral and extremity changes
Kikuchi disease	Necrotizing lymphadenitis, usually affects young adults
Hyper IgD syndrome	Periodic fevers, adenopathy
Hyper IgE syndrome	Recurrent infections, immunodeficiency
Sinus histiocytosis	Massive, persistent cervical adenopathy; may cause minimal symptoms; extranodal involvement
Sarcoidosis	Scalene node enlargement, pulmonary disease, uveitis, mediastinal adenopathy
Drugs	Phenytoin, hydralazine, allopurinol

PPD, Purified protein derivative.

tic hygromas, dermoid cysts, fibromas, ectopic thyroid, lipomas, and hemangiomas.

Vascular malformations are relatively uncommon congenital neck lesions but usually are easy to recognize. Hemangiomas and cystic hygromas generally are more diffuse and more easily compressible than other lesions. Both lesions may enlarge with Valsalva maneuver, and cystic hygromas sometimes transilluminate. Overlying skin discoloration with a reddish or bluish hue may be a clue to the presence of a hemangioma. Frequently these lesions are not noted at birth but increase in size during infancy, plateauing at around 1 year of age and in about half of cases regressing by the time the child enters school. Cystic hygromas arise from lymphatic sacs near the jugular vein. Over 90% of these lesions are found in the posterior triangle behind the SCM in the supraclavicular fossa (Fig. 25-6). Compression of vital structures necessitates surgical excision.

Lymphadenopathy

Palpable lymph nodes in the neck are common at virtually any age and are stimulated constantly by recurrent upper respiratory tract infections in children. Fig. 25-7 shows common sites of regional lymph nodes in the head and neck and their drainage areas. Common causes of cervical lymphadenopathy are summarized in Table 25-3.

Viral infections are by far the most common cause of enlarged cervical nodes, producing bilateral, discrete, minimally tender, soft lymph nodes. Usually the history of recent infection and characteristic benign findings do not create much diagnostic confusion. Size of the lymph nodes usually parallels the acute infection. However, at times total regression to the previous size may not occur because of recurrent stimulation, fibrosis during healing, or both.

Adenovirus, enterovirus, EBV, and CMV have been shown to cause cervical adenopathy. EBV infection may produce fever, malaise, exudative pharyngitis, mild hepatitis, and rash. Whereas this presentation is typical in older children, younger children may have a more atypical course. In addition, younger children, especially those under 5 years of age, may not develop heterophile antibodies. Heterophile antibodies are found in 27% to 91% of EBV-infected patients between 2 and 5 years of age and 53% to 94% of patients between 6 and 10 years of age. CMV may produce a constellation of symptoms similar to those of EBV infection and accounts for a large proportion of "heterophile-negative" infectious mononucleosis.

Acute suppurative infection of a cervical lymph node often is accompanied by fever and a tender, swollen, erythematous neck mass. Bacterial lymphadenitis is most likely the result of an upper respiratory tract infection or an infection of the teeth or gums or is secondary to trauma. *Staphylococcus aureus* and *Streptococcus pyogenes* cause 40% to 80% of acute unilateral cervical adenitis in children. Lymph nodes may become fluctuant and require incision and drainage (Fig. 25-8). Infants up to 7 weeks of age may develop lymphadenitis associated with otitis media, poor feeding, and bacteremia. *S. aureus* and group B streptococci have been implicated. Anaerobic and mixed aerobic-anaerobic infections are increasingly recognized as causative agents in lymphadenitis, representing 18% and 20% of bacterial infections respectively. Less commonly, *Haemophilus influenzae* type B may present in a fashion similar to more common staphylococcal or streptococcal infections. Brucellosis and tularemia both have cervical adenopathy as part of the associated febrile illness and should be suspected if the patient had contact with potentially infected animals. Cervical adenopathy (Winterbottom sign) is a rare presenting sign of syphilis, which usually is diagnosed after careful history and appropriate serologic tests.

Lymphadenitis also may occur without substantial associated constitutional symptoms. Several disorders may produce this "cold inflammation." Perhaps the most common agent producing this inflammatory process is cat-scratch disease, a zoonotic infection (usually contracted from a kitten) occurring after a bite, scratch, or salivary contamination of an open wound. In one series, only 9% of patients had temperature greater than or equal to 102° F. Generally a patient develops a primary pustule 3 to 10 days after contact with the kitten; this pustule may last up to 8 weeks (Fig. 25-9). If the eye is the site of inoculum, conjunctivitis or an ocular granuloma with preauricular adenopathy occurs. Impressive regional adenopathy develops approximately 2 weeks after inoculation but may be delayed up to 7 weeks. Nodes are tender and usually drain the area of the pustule. Over 25% of involved nodes are in the head and neck, although isolated mesenteric adenitis and systemic cat-scratch disease without adenopathy have been described. Lymph node biopsy typically demonstrates stellate granulomas with suppurative or caseous centers. A gram-negative pleomorphic rod seen with Warthin-Starry silver impregnation stains has been identified as *Bartonella henselae* (previously *Rochalimaea henselae*). Lymphadenopathy may persist for months.

Atypical mycobacterial adenitis causes between 1% and 6% of all cases of serious cervical lymphadenitis. It typically presents as a relatively asymptomatic, progressive swelling of submandibular or anterior cervical nodes. With time, nodes become matted, and overlying skin becomes thin, scaly, and parchmentlike with diffuse erythema. Despite these changes the area is minimally tender and not warm to the touch (Fig. 25-10). Children between 1 and 5 years of age are affected most commonly with *Mycobacterium scrofulaceum* and *M. avium-intracellulare.* Nodes are usually unilateral, in contrast to *M. tuberculosis* infection, which frequently causes bilateral adenopathy. Generalized adenopathy does not occur, and chest radiographs are normal. These findings and a lack of exposure to tuberculosis help distinguish atypical mycobacterial infection from *M. tuberculosis* infection. Diagnosis is based on the presentation and intradermal reaction of 5 to 10 mm of induration to an intermediatestrength tuberculin (5-TU) dose of purified protein derivative (PPD). Specific skin tests for atypical mycobacterial infection are not generally available at this time but have shown promise in helping to distinguish these infections.

Acquired toxoplasmosis most frequently presents as a painless, solitary, asymptomatic lymph node enlargement in the posterior triangle. It easily may be confused with a malignancy. Nearly two thirds of patients have posterior triangle disease, and three fourths of patients are asymptomatic. Some patients may exhibit minimal symptoms, such as low-grade fever, malaise, sore throat, cough, or anorexia. Diagno-

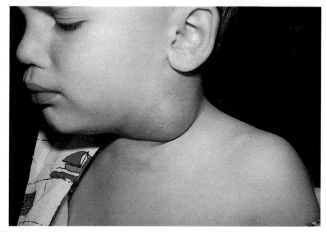

FIG. 25-8 Acute suppurative cervical adenitis secondary to *S. pyogenes.*

sis is made by demonstrating high or rising titers to *Toxoplasma* organisms. No specific therapy is indicated, and the course is benign.

Although systemic disorders with associated generalized adenopathy as described previously may have cervical lymph node enlargement as well, some miscellaneous disorders deserve special mention. Kawasaki syndrome has cervical adenopathy as part of its diagnostic criteria, although only 50% of white children demonstrate this finding. A particular presentation of Kawasaki syndrome, however, has lymphadenitis as the dominant manifestation. Children tend to be older (mean age, 5 years) and were initially treated for bacterial adenitis before the diagnosis of Kawasaki syndrome was made. Necrotizing lymphadenitis (Kikuchi disease) is a benign, self-limited disorder that pathologically resembles a malignant lymphoma. Cervical nodes are affected in three fourths of children, although young adults are affected most frequently. Minimal constitutional symptoms of low-grade fever, vomiting, and weight loss may accompany mild node tenderness, leukopenia, and a mildly elevated sedimentation rate. Lymph nodes are characterized by loss of architecture with necrosis, histiocytes, and lack of neutrophils. Hyper IgD and hyper IgE syndromes may have cervical adenopathy as part of their presentation. The former disorder has cervical adenopathy and periodic fevers, whereas the latter is associated with immunodeficiency and recurrent infections. Sinus histiocytosis usually has cervical adenopathy associated with other, minimal symptoms, and sarcoidosis may have enlarged cervical glands, especially scalene nodes, as part of its presentation. Uveitis, pulmonary disease, and mediastinal adenopathy are commonly seen with sarcoidosis as well. Drugs, including phenytoin, hydralazine, and allopurinol, may produce enlarged nodes without infection.

Malignancies

More than 25% of malignant tumors in children occur in the head and neck, and one of every seven children admitted with a neck mass has a malignant tumor. For every six chil-

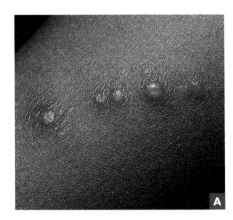

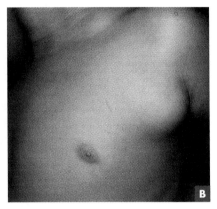

FIG. 25-9 Cat-scratch disease. Note a series of papules at the inoculum site in this patient *(A)*, who subsequently developed axillary adenopathy *(B)*.

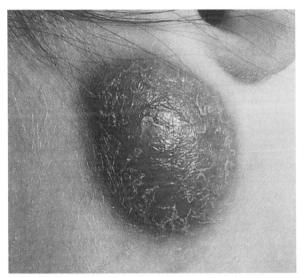

FIG. 25-10 Mycobacterial adenitis. Despite erythema and thin, parchmentlike changes of overlying skin, the node is minimally tender and not warm.

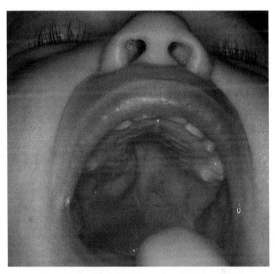

FIG. 25-11 Intraoral extension of a rhabdomyosarcoma.

dren with a malignant tumor of the head and neck, one has an associated tumor of the nasopharynx. This underscores the importance of a thorough examination and evaluation of the head and neck of any child who has a neck mass (Fig. 25-11). Warning signs suggestive of malignancy include the following: (1) onset of an enlarging mass in the neonatal period, (2) a history of rapid or progressive growth, (3) skin ulceration, (4) fixation to or location deep to fascia, and (5) a firm mass greater than 3 cm in diameter. When these signs are present, malignancies are identified in 80% of cases. Similarly, in the absence of these risk factors, 99.7% of lumps in children are benign.

Tumors of the head and neck in children usually are mesenchymal in origin, with lymphoid tumors predominating (e.g., Hodgkin disease, lymphosarcoma, rhabdomyosarcoma, fibrosarcoma, thyroid malignancies, and epidermoid carcinoma).

Age may be a helpful clue in determining which type of tumor is most likely. Children younger than 6 years of age generally have neuroblastoma, which is followed in frequency by lymphosarcoma, rhabdomyosarcoma, and Hodgkin disease. In preadolescent children, Hodgkin disease and lymphosarcoma occur with almost equal frequency, whereas thyroid cancers and rhabdomyosarcoma are less common. In the adolescent, Hodgkin disease is the most common malignancy of the head and neck.

Hodgkin disease often presents as a painless or minimally tender, unilateral (80%) mass developing in the upper one third of the neck, posterior triangle, or supraclavicular area. If the last area is involved, a mediastinal tumor is usually present as well. About 6% of patients have preauricular adenopathy simulating parotid swelling or possibly cat-scratch disease. A child with a neck mass has an equal chance of having Hodgkin disease or lymphosarcoma. Although lymphosarcoma occurs approximately twice as frequently as Hodgkin disease, the latter disorder presents twice as frequently with a neck mass (80% versus 40% respectively). Lymphosarcoma is more common among younger patients, and extranodal sites, such as the tonsils, are involved up to 4 times more frequently in lymphosarcoma than in Hodgkin disease.

Rhabdomyosarcoma is the most common solid tumor of the head and neck, accounting for 10% of head and neck malignancies. It presents as a painless mass at virtually any site, although the nasopharynx, middle ear, mastoid, and orbit are common points of origin. Symptoms depend on the anatomic location of the tumor.

Fibrosarcoma and neurofibrosarcoma occur with half the frequency of rhabdomyosarcoma. These tumors present as a painless mass arising from the cheek, jaw, nose, or sinuses, and they have a low tendency to metastasize.

Thyroid nodules are rare in children but when present often are malignant. Tumors usually are of the medullary or mixed papillary and follicular types. A history of radiation to the neck may increase the likelihood of thyroid malignancy. Thyroid nodules are generally midline or slightly off center and in close proximity to the thyroid gland. Prognosis after lobectomy and node dissection generally is excellent.

Neuroblastoma in the neck most frequently is the result of metastasis from other sites. In metastatic disease of the lymph node, neurologic signs develop later than they do in primary neuroblastoma of the neck, which arises from a ganglion and causes early neurologic manifestations, such as Horner syndrome.

Other metastatic tumors of the cervical nodes must be considered and include leukemias, thyroid malignancies, nasopharyngeal carcinoma, and any tumor that metastasizes via lymphatic channels.

Other Regional Adenopathy

Although regional adenopathy most commonly is caused by localized infection or inflammation, any disorder causing generalized lymph node involvement can cause regional disease as well.

Occipital nodes drain the back of the scalp and neck and enlarge when inflammatory conditions affect those areas. Infants as young as 2 weeks of age may have palpable nodes in this area, especially if eczema or seborrhea affects the scalp. Systemic viral infections also cause enlargement of these nodes, with rubella classically causing occipital adenopathy.

Posterior cervical nodes can be involved in the same pathologic processes as nodes in any other lymphoid region. However, the presence of a single, enlarging, painless node raises the specter of malignancy. In a study examining lymph node biopsies from the upper posterior triangle, 41 of 53 nodes were reactive. Six patients had toxoplasmosis. However, three patients had Hodgkin disease, and another patient had metastatic neuroblastoma.

Preauricular adenopathy occurs when infections and inflammatory conditions drain the ipsilateral conjunctiva and preauricular area. Chlamydial conjunctivitis, adenovirus, tularemia, lymphogranuloma venereum, and cat-scratch disease have been associated with enlarged preauricular nodes. In a small number of patients, Hodgkin disease presents with preauricular lymph node enlargement. These nodes must be distinguished from branchial cleft cysts (particularly those involving the first branchial cleft) and parotid gland inflammation.

Submaxillary and submental nodes drain the mucous membranes of the lips and mouth and enlarge when infections involve those areas. Herpetic gingivostomatitis may produce high fever and impressive adenopathy. Notably, adenopathy may persist for several months after herpes infection.

Supraclavicular nodes normally are not palpable in infants and children. Significant progressive pathologic processes usually involve these lymph nodes when they are palpable. Of 23 patients with supraclavicular adenopathy undergoing biopsy, 14 had a malignancy, 5 had cat-scratch disease, 2 had nondiagnostic granulomatous disease, and 2 had reactive nodes. Supraclavicular adenopathy fixed to underlying tissue and associated with persistent fever and weight loss indicated significant risk of malignancy. Chest radiographs were abnormal in most children who had Hodgkin disease associated with enlarged supraclavicular nodes, and abnormal chest radiographs in general were associated with serious progressive disease in 21 of 27 children. In another study, all five children with supraclavicular adenopathy had mediastinal disease, and three of them had abnormal chest radiographs. The patients with abnormal chest radiographs were diagnosed with lymphoma (2) or tuberculosis (1). The other two patients had atypical mycobacterial infection and sarcoidosis.

Axillary node enlargement generally is caused by infections of the hand, arm, chest wall, breast, and upper lateral abdominal wall. Cat-scratch disease may have a predilection for axillary nodes because of the frequency of scratches on the hands and arms. Syphilis and HIV infection also may cause axillary adenopathy. These nodes may be involved in localized antigenic stimulation as a result of vaccines administered in the deltoid muscle, such as BCG, typhoid, and tetanus.

Epitrochlear nodes are rarely palpable and demonstrate reactive hyperplasia as does any other node group. Cat-scratch disease is a common cause of swollen nodes in this location, but other disorders include lymphoproliferative diseases, such as Hodgkin and nonHodgkin lymphoma, infectious mononucleosis, tularemia, sarcoidosis, rheumatoid arthritis, and HIV infection.

Inguinal adenopathy is most frequently caused by inflammatory conditions of the penis and scrotum, vulva and vaginal mucosa, lower abdomen, perineum and gluteal region, and lower extremities. Of neonates, only 25% have palpable inguinal nodes, compared with 36% of 1 year olds. This increase may reflect recurrent superficial skin infection and inflammation in infancy. Lesions of the lower extremities, lymphogranuloma venereum, chancroid, rickettsial infections resulting from tick bites to lower extremities, and malignancies also cause enlarged inguinal nodes. Swelling in this area must be differentiated from inguinal hernia, ectopic testes, aneurysms, and lipomas.

Iliac nodes are palpated over the inguinal ligament and may be infected by staphylococci or streptococci. Acute inflammation may cause limp and hip pain but no limitation of hip motion, except possibly in extension. Malignancy, particularly lymphoma, also may affect these nodes.

Popliteal nodes, located behind the knee, generally are not palpable, except with severe local infections of the knee and the lateral aspect of the lower leg and foot.

Mesenteric lymph nodes are not palpable but can be involved in any of the pathologic processes of other regional lymph nodes. Viral upper respiratory tract infections or any disorder causing generalized adenopathy may affect these nodes, causing abdominal pain, back ache, constipation, and possible intestinal obstruction as a result of intussusception. Involvement of the nodes surrounding the ileocecal valve may cause symptoms mimicking acute appendicitis. Rarely, cat-scratch disease may cause mesenteric adenitis.

History

Because the differential diagnosis of adenopathy is so extensive, a detailed history and physical examination are most important in narrowing the diagnostic possibilities (Table 25-4). Early in the course of evaluation the examiner must determine whether the patient has generalized or regional adenopathy. Key differential diagnosis for adenopathy is listed in Box 25-1. Systemic infections may be associated with fever, and at times the pattern of fever may be helpful in directing the diagnostic workup (see Chapter 7). High, spiking fevers occurring several times a day may suggest abscess formation, whereas relapsing fever or persistent fever may indicate brucellosis. An exanthem and its character might point to scarlet fever, viral infection, EBV, endocarditis, secondary syphilis, or even chronic granulomatous disease. Exposure to infectious persons might suggest hepatitis, EBV, or other viruses, and a travel history might point to illnesses, such as histoplasmosis, coccidioidomycosis, or even malaria, contracted in endemic areas. Animal exposure suggests possibilities such as cat-scratch disease, brucellosis, and tularemia. A history of blood product use may point to hepatitis A, B, or C; CMV; or HIV. An adolescent or a parent of a younger child with a history of blood product exposure, intravenous drug abuse, or high-risk sexual behavior may have HIV infection.

Arthralgia, arthritis, or both and characteristic rashes may indicate immune-mediated inflammatory disorders. Systemic lupus erythematosus may cause a malar rash (see Fig. 7-12), Raynaud phenomenon, alopecia, and cardiopulmonary disease; typical laboratory findings include autoantibodies and hematologic and renal abnormalities. Juvenile rheumatoid arthritis, especially Still disease, may feature constitutional symptoms of fever, rash, and joint involvement accompanying adenopathy (see Fig. 7-11). Serum sickness usually pre-

TABLE 25-4

Some Key Historic Questions for Lymphadenopathy

History	Possible indication
Generalized adenopathy	Systemic illness
Regional adenopathy	Localized infection, congenital lesion, neoplasm
Fever	Infection, inflammation, neoplasm
Rash	Viral infection, EBV, SBE, syphilis, SLE, JRA
Exposure to infection	Contagious infectious illness
Travel	Endemic disease, hepatitis, coccidioidomycosis, histoplasmosis, malaria
Animal exposure	Cat-scratch disease, brucellosis, tularemia, toxoplasmosis
Blood product use	Hepatitis, CMV, HIV
Arthralgia/arthritis	Collagen disorder, SLE, JRA
Delayed growth/development	Storage disease, chronic illness
Weight loss, night sweats	Malignancy, tuberculosis
Lesion present at birth	Congenital cyst, vascular anomaly
Torticollis	Congenital muscular torticollis
Neck fistula	Branchial cleft cyst

CMV, Cytomegalovirus; *EBV,* Epstein-Barr virus; *HIV,* human immunodeficiency virus; *JRA,* juvenile rheumatoid arthritis; *SBE,* subacute bacterial endocarditis; *SLE,* systemic lupus erythematosus.

sents after drug exposure and causes rash, hepatosplenomegaly, and joint pain or swelling with adenopathy. Kawasaki syndrome is characterized by prolonged fever, rash, conjunctivitis, oral and extremity changes, and adenopathy. Patients with hyper IgD syndrome often have periodic relapsing fevers beginning early in childhood. Hyper IgE syndrome is associated with recurrent infections.

Storage diseases frequently involve other organ systems, so abdominal distension caused by hepatosplenomegaly, alterations in developmental progress, and growth failure without other constitutional symptoms may point to a storage disease.

Warning signs of malignancy include fever, weight loss, night sweats, and joint and bone pain accompanying enlargement of a noninflammatory mass. Location in the supraclavicular area or posterior cervical triangle raises suspicions of malignancy. Pallor and easy bruising are other signs that raise concerns of malignancy.

Evaluation of regional adenopathy demands knowledge of regional drainage areas and usually entails asking many of the same questions asked for generalized adenopathy and localized trauma or infection. Regional cold inflammatory masses may be due to cat-scratch disease or toxoplasmosis, and therefore questions about animal exposure, particularly kittens, are important. Atypical mycobacterial infections may not have many historic clues other than those that distinguish them from tuberculosis; hence the examiner must inquire about exposure to tuberculosis.

Questions regarding head and neck masses help differentiate congenital lesions from adenopathy and malignancies. Neck masses found at birth or in early infancy and recurrent inflammatory masses in the same location suggest congenital cysts or anomalies. A head tilt and a neck mass in a young infant most commonly suggest congenital muscular torticollis. A midline neck mass that retracts with tongue protrusion is characteristic of a thyroglossal duct cyst. Draining fistulas lower in the neck might indicate a branchial cleft cyst. Lesions that are soft and spongy and grow slowly after birth or enlarge as infants cry are indicative of a vascular lesion.

Questions pertaining to lymph node enlargement are similar to those pertaining to other regional disorders; upper respiratory tract infections are the most common cause of enlargement. Hence questions regarding the 3 Ts—tonsils, teeth, and trauma—frequently lead to the cause of bacterial cervical adenitis. Exposure to kittens or other animals and other systemic signs may be clues to a particular cause.

Physical Examination

The physical examination must confirm whether adenopathy is generalized or regional and then determine whether other signs are present before a specific diagnosis can be made (Table 25-5). First, measuring growth parameters and plotting growth percentiles help indicate whether a chronic illness exists. Vital signs, particularly temperature, may indicate the presence of infection or inflammation. Tachycardia or wide pulse pressure may signal hyperthyroidism. Particular attention should be given to lymph node characteristics, such as location, size, number, discreteness, mobility, consistency, and presence of tenderness or fluctuation. Rashes may be specific for different disorders (e.g., the rash of scarlet fever, splinter hemorrhages of endocarditis, usual viral exanthems or exanthems, systemic lupus erythematosus, and juvenile rheumatoid arthritis). Hepatosplenomegaly frequently accompanies systemic infections, EBV infection, and especially storage diseases. A noninflamed, fixed, matted, hard confluence of nodes suggests a malignancy, especially if located in the supraclavicular or posterior triangle area.

A meticulous examination of regional drainage areas may point to the cause of localized adenopathy. An acute punctum or pustule or a recently healed extremity lesion might indicate the inoculum site of cat-scratch disease. Examination of the conjunctivae may indicate another inoculum site, conjunctivi-

TABLE 25-5

Clues on Physical Examination

Physical finding	Possible indication
Generalized adenopathy	Systemic illness
Regional adenopathy	Localized infection, inflammation, neoplasm
Growth failure	Chronic illness
Fever	Infection, inflammation, neoplasm
Tachycardia, wide pulse pressure, brisk reflexes	Hyperthyroidism
Rash/exanthem	Viral illness, scarlet fever, SBE, SLE, JRA
Hepatosplenomegaly	Systemic infection, EBV, storage diseases
Fixed, noninflamed, matted, hard confluence of nodes	Malignancy, mycobacterial infection
Skin pustule/punctum	Cat-scratch disease
Conjunctivitis/uveitis	Viral infection, Kawasaki syndrome, autoimmune disease, sarcoidosis
Midline neck mass that retracts with tongue protrusion	Thyroglossal duct cyst
Soft, spongy mass	Vascular malformation (hemangioma, cystic hygroma)
Location of mass in posterior triangle or crossing anterior and posterior triangles	Malignancy, *Toxoplasma* sp. infection
Supraclavicular mass	Malignancy, granulomatous disease

EBV; Epstein-Barr virus; *JRA,* juvenile rheumatoid arthritis; *SBE,* subacute bacterial endocarditis; *SLE,* systemic lupus erythematosus.

tis with viral illness or uveitis accompanying Kawasaki syndrome, autoimmune disease, or sarcoidosis. One fourth of children with malignancies have a tumor of the head or neck, and more than 15% of these children have a tumor in the nasopharynx. It is imperative therefore that any child with a suspected malignancy undergo a thorough examination of the head and neck, including the nasopharynx.

Approach to the Patient

Often a good history and physical examination are sufficient to determine the cause of adenopathy, and no other laboratory tests are required. For example, viral illness associated with mild, minimally tender cervical nodes may require only supportive care. An acutely swollen, erythematous, warm lymph node in a patient with fever may require only antibiotics for a presumed bacterial adenitis. However, if the cause of enlarged nodes is not apparent, selected and directed laboratory tests may be indicated.

Because generalized adenopathy usually indicates a systemic disorder, some simple screening tests can begin the evaluation. A complete blood count (CBC) looking for anemia, thrombocytopenia or thrombocytosis, and alterations in white blood cell number and morphology is important. Atypical lymphocytes on a peripheral smear should be reviewed by a pathologist to ensure they do not represent malignant cells. An elevated erythrocyte sedimentation rate (ESR) often accompanies systemic inflammatory disorders. Any drug that the patient is taking that could cause adenopathy should be discontinued if possible. A PPD with control skin tests and chest radiographs are helpful in determining the presence of tuberculosis, and mononucleosis serology is especially helpful in the older patient to confirm EBV infection. Cultures of materials from regional lesions and suppurative nodes or blood cultures may reveal a cause. If these tests are unrevealing and adenopathy persists, further testing for hyperthyroidism, CMV, toxoplasmosis, cat-scratch disease (if indicated), syphilis, and HIV can be carried out. Serologic tests for other, less common disorders such as coccidioidomycosis, brucellosis, histoplasmosis, and systemic lupus erethematosus also can be obtained. Follow-up serologic tests may reveal diagnostic rises in titers to specific agents. If after 3 to 4 weeks the nodes are not regressing in size and the evaluation has not revealed the cause of the adenopathy, a lymph node biopsy should be considered.

Regional adenopathy in an area other than the head and neck may demand a similar approach. A CBC and differential count, ESR, and local cultures, including lymph node aspiration, may be diagnostic. In one study, fine-needle aspirations of lymph nodes in children were 98% accurate and caused no significant complications in 110 cases. Culture of aspirated material was positive in 14% of cases, and no examples of false-negative aspirates for malignancy were noted. Approximately 10% of cases had insufficient material for adequate pathologic examination. Excisional biopsy should be entertained if fine-needle aspiration is inadequate or histopathologic examination is necessary.

Masses of the head and neck may be more complicated because of the consideration of congenital lesions. If the patient has an acutely inflamed neck mass, careful examination for pharyngitis or auro-facial-dental infection may be all that is necessary. A throat culture or a rapid test for streptococci may be done in the face of pharyngitis. A CBC, differential count, and serology tests for EBV infection, CMV, or toxoplasmosis might be considered. If the lesion has no characteristics of a congenital lesion as noted in Table 25-2, the lesion should be considered an enlarged lymph node. If the node is fluctuant, fine-needle aspiration can obtain culture material. However, aspiration or incomplete excision in mycobacterial disease may lead to chronic fistula formation, and aspirated material frequently is nondiagnostic in cat-scratch disease, although it may be therapeutic. Ultrasound of the neck may be helpful in determining location, extent, and internal characteristics of the neck mass (i.e., solid or cystic). Various lesions, such as thyroglossal duct cyst, neonatal torticollis, cystic hygroma, and adenopathy, have characteristic sonographic appearances. Nuclear medicine studies are helpful in determining the presence and location of thyroid tissue. A computed tomography (CT) scan with contrast may be helpful in determining the location, extent, and sometimes characteristics of the mass. Magnetic resonance imaging is especially useful in delineating soft tissue structures but requires sedation in small children, as does the CT scan. If bacterial infection is most likely, antibiotic therapy should be given, using a first-generation cephalosporin or semisynthetic penicillin to cover staphylococci and streptococci. If no resolution occurs, repeat evaluation and examination for uncommon organisms, including fungi, should be considered.

If the node has persisted for 2 to 3 weeks without resolution, application of a PPD with control skin tests and *Toxoplasma* organism and *B. henselae* titers should be considered (Fig. 25-12). The presence of fever with weight loss, progressive adenopathy, and malaise should lead to excisional biopsy. Noninflammatory nodes in the supraclavicular triangle should be considered for biopsy without an extensive observation period, especially if the chest radiograph shows mediastinal adenopathy or other abnormalities. If the patient is on medications that may cause adenopathy, these drugs should be discontinued if possible. Thyroid function tests and tests for systemic lupus erythematosus or juvenile rheumatoid arthritis should be pursued if the clinical history and physical examination warrant evaluation. If no regression occurs after 4 weeks, excisional biopsy should be entertained.

The decision to proceed to biopsy can be challenging. Malignancy or granulomatous disease is found in a high percentage of patients with supraclavicular adenopathy. Torsiglieri and others found 12 lymphomas and 3 granulomatous disorders in 34 supraclavicular node biopsies. Knight and others diagnosed 14 malignancies and 7 granulomatous disorders from biopsies in this area, and Lake and Oski found that all 5 patients with supraclavicular adenopathy had significant mediastinal disease. Over three fourths of children with abnormal chest radiographs had serious progressive disease, and granulomatous disease or malignancy was frequently present when abnormal chest radiographs, nodes larger than 2 cm, night sweats, and weight loss were noted in any patient.

The overall diagnostic yield of lymph node biopsies has been 20%. Malignancies have been diagnosed in 11% to 17% of children undergoing lymph node biopsy, but 37% to 55% of biopsies yield nondiagnostic results. When children with initial nondiagnostic biopsies are followed, however, specific diagnoses may be made on subsequent biopsies in 17% to 24% of cases. Kissane and Gephardt followed 34 patients for up to 20 years, and 6 ultimately died (4 with Wiskott-Aldrich syndrome and 2 with malignancies). Lake and Oski found that 7 of 41 patients with initial nondiag-

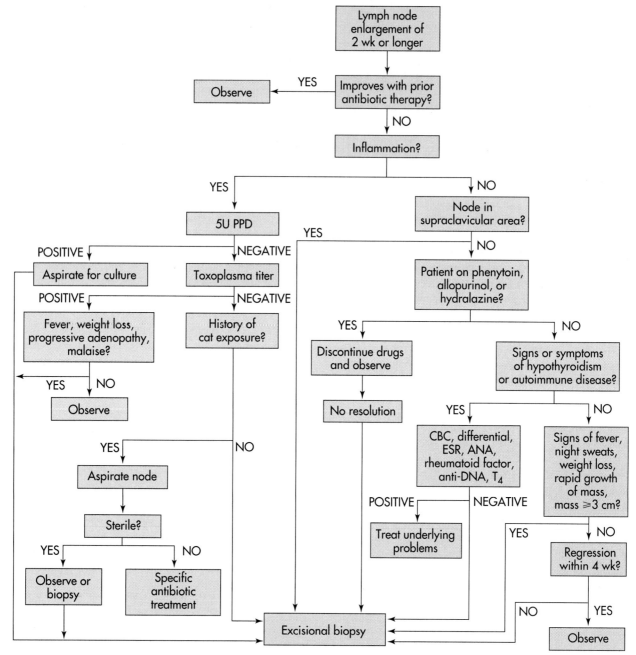

FIG. 25-12   Evaluating the child with a neck mass. (From Zitelli BJ: Evaluating the child with a neck mass, *Contemp Pediatr* 7:90-112, 1990.)

nostic biopsies ultimately proved to have specific pathologic processes (4 lymphomas, 2 tuberculosis, and 1 mycoplasmal infection. In patients for whom a diagnosis was subsequently made, the diagnosis was established in the majority within 8 months of the first biopsy. Hence close follow-up of patients with nondiagnostic biopsies is essential, especially if symptoms do not resolve.

SUMMARY

Lymphadenopathy in the child can be vexing to even the most experienced clinician. Generalized lymph node enlargement encompasses many systemic disorders, and regional adenopathy expands the differential diagnosis even more. Congenital disorders and malignancies must be considered when lesions of the head and neck are present. Evaluation begins with a detailed history and physical examination, and selected and specific laboratory tests frequently confirm the clinical diagnosis. Lymph node biopsy may not always be diagnostic, but continued careful follow-up is essential.

ILLUSTRATIVE CASES

Case 1. A 3-month-old infant boy was seen for the acute onset of fever to 103.4° F, poor feeding, and a warm, tender erythematous mass underlying the left SCM. Bacterial adenitis was suspected, and a first-generation cephalosporin was given, with rapid resolution of signs and symptoms within 3 to 4 days. The patient remained well until 6 weeks later when the same signs and symptoms recurred. Antibiotics were readministered, with rapid resolution. An ultrasound of the neck revealed a cystic structure underlying the SCM. After resolution of the infection, the patient underwent surgical exploration of the neck with excision of a branchial cleft cyst and a fistula tract that ended blindly. This patient demonstrates the typical presentation of a branchial cleft cyst with recurrent inflammation and infection at the same location. Ultrasound was helpful in distinguishing this cyst from a solid mass.

Case 2. A 4-year-old girl had a painless swelling under the left mandible for over 2 weeks. No constitutional symptoms were present, and examination was normal except for a firm, nontender 2 × 2 cm mass with matted nodes in the left submandibular region. A CBC, differential count, ESR, and throat culture were normal. A 10-day course of antibiotics had no effect, and the child returned with progressive swelling, diffuse erythema, and parchmentlike thinning of the overlying skin. A 5-TU PPD was placed, and a chest radiograph was obtained. The radiograph was normal, but the skin test showed 9-mm induration at 48 hours. Surgical excision was recommended. The lymph node demonstrated caseous necrosis but no acid-fast bacilli on staining. However, 6 weeks later cultures grew M. avium-intracellulare.

Atypical mycobacterial infections initially may simulate a malignancy before overlying skin changes occur. Absence of constitutional symptoms, location, ultimate progressive skin changes, and a reactive tuberculin skin test help confirm the diagnosis. Therapy can be excision or observation.

Case 3. A 14-year-old boy was seen for routine physical examination and was found to have a 2 × 3 cm painless right posterior triangle mass. He denied having fever, night sweats, or weight loss. The mass was firm, fixed to underlying tissue, and matted. CBC showed a mild normochromic, normocytic anemia; chest x-ray film was normal, and Toxoplasma sp. titers were negative. A brief course of antibiotics was given, but no change in the nodes occurred.

The patient was referred for lymph node biopsy, which demonstrated Hodgkin disease.

Posterior triangle lesions have a greater incidence of malignancy. Toxoplasmal adenopathy frequently occurs in the posterior triangle and has few other symptoms. The lack of constitutional symptoms suggested a nonmalignant process; however, the physical examination had features consistent with lymphoma. A biopsy was done earlier in the evaluation rather than after a prolonged period of observation.

ANNOTATED BIBLIOGRAPHY

Jaffe BF, Jaffe N: Head and neck tumors in children, *Pediatrics* 51:731-740, 1973.
This is an excellent, still timely review of tumors of the head and neck in children.

Lake AM, Oski FA: Peripheral lymphadenopathy in childhood, *Am J Dis Child* 132:357-359, 1978.
This is an excellent review of adenopathy and especially biopsy results, with follow-up of pediatric patients.

Zuelzer WW, Kaplan J: The child with lymphadenopathy, *Semin Hematol* 12:323-334, 1975.
This classic paper discusses regional and generalized adenopathy in children.

BIBLIOGRAPHY

Bamji M, Stone RK, Kaul A, et al: Palpable lymph nodes in healthy newborns and infants, *Pediatrics* 78:573-575, 1986.
Carithers HA: Cat-scratch disease, *Am J Dis Child* 139:1124-1133, 1985.
Fleisher G, Lenette ET, Henle G, et al: Incidence of heterophile antibody responses in children with infectious mononucleosis, *J Pediatr* 94:723-728, 1979.
Herzog LW: Prevalence of lymphadenopathy of the head and neck in infants and children, *Clin Pediatr* 22:485-487, 1983.
Jaffe BF: Pediatric head and neck tumors: a study of 178 cases, *Laryngoscope* 83:1644-1651, 1973.
Kissane JM, Gephardt GN: Lymphadenopathy in childhood, *Hum Pathol* 5:431-439, 1974.
Knight PJ, Mulne AF, Vassy LE: When is lymph node biopsy indicated in children with enlarged peripheral nodes? *Pediatrics* 69:391-396, 1982.
Kraus R, Han BK, Babcock DS, et al: Sonography of neck masses in children, *Am J Roentgenol* 146:609-613, 1986.
Marcy SM: Infections of lymph nodes of the head and neck, *Pediatr Infect Dis J* 2:397-405, 1983.
Margileth A, Hadfield TL: Could the infection be cat-scratch disease? *Contemp Pediatr* 2:62-72, 1985.
May M: Neck masses in children: diagnosis and treatment, *Ear Nose Throat J* 57:12-54, 1978.
Pounds LA: Neck masses of congenital origin, *Pediatr Clin North Am* 28:841-844, 1981.

Schuit KE, Powell DA: Mycobacterial lymphadenitis in childhood, *Am J Dis Child* 132:675-677, 1978.

Slap GB, Brooks JSJ, Schwartz JS: When to perform biopsies of enlarged peripheral lymph nodes in young patients, *JAMA* 252:1321-1326, 1984.

Torsiglieri AJ, Tom LWC, Ross AJ III, et al: Pediatric neck masses: guidelines for evaluation, *Int J Pediatr Otorhinolaryngol* 16:199-210, 1988.

Ward PH, Strahan RW, Acquarelli M, et al: The many faces of cysts of the thyroglossal duct, *Trans Am Acad Ophthalmol Otolaryngol* 74:310-318, 1970.

26

Recurrent Infections

BASIL J. ZITELLI

Key Points

- Recurrent infections are common in children, especially in the first several years of life, and generally do not indicate immunodeficiency.

- A primary immunodeficiency should be suspected if a child has recurrent, severe infections; unusual infections with opportunistic organisms; chronic infections; or unusually severe infections that are normally mild in childhood.

- The screening evaluation for cellular and humoral deficiencies and major defects in complement and phagocytic functions frequently can be accomplished by careful history, physical examination, and selected skin and blood tests and radiographs.

*I*nfections account for nearly one third of pediatric office visits in the United States, and respiratory tract infections account for the majority of them. Recurrent infections present a frustrating problem for patients and families and are a challenge for the pediatrician. Frequent infections disrupt the family lifestyle and create significant financial stress because of costs of medications, office visits, and loss of income. The role of the pediatrician is to care for each illness as expeditiously as possible and be wary of possible alterations in host defense mechanisms that predispose to increased morbidity.

Literature Survey

Normal healthy children often experience their first respiratory tract infection before 6 months of age and may develop three to five additional respiratory illnesses, an episode of gastroenteritis, and two additional infectious illnesses all before the first birthday. The number of respiratory illnesses rises from three to seven during the first year to up to eight per year until 6 years of age, and then it drops slightly to six

respiratory illnesses per year after 6 years of age. Children who were not in daycare during the first year of life experienced nearly five infections and averaged nearly 6 weeks of illness during that time. Normal healthy children may experience 100 different infections by the time they are 10 years of age. Because most infections occur during fall, winter, and spring and the ordinary respiratory tract infection takes nearly 2 weeks to resolve, the time consumed every year by illnesses can approximate nearly half the time at risk. It is no wonder then that parents can perceive that their child is "always sick." It is challenging for the physician to discern whether the pattern of illness is within the normal range so that the family may be reassured.

Frequently, when confronted with the child who has recurrent infections, the physician turns the diagnostic evaluation toward immunodeficiency states. Except for isolated IgA deficiency, which affects as many as 1 in 500 live births, primary immunodeficiency disorders are rare, with the incidence approaching 1 in 10,000 live births. It is estimated that 400 children with immunodeficiency (excluding selective IgA deficiency) are born every year in the United States, and up to 10,000 children with immunodeficiency are cared for. Thus other mechanisms account for the frequency of infections in the majority of children.

Disorders other than primary immunodeficiency that lead to increased susceptibility to infection are listed in Box 26-1. Obstruction and stasis of urine, respiratory tract mucus, or decreased clearance of pathogens may lead to infections of the urinary tract, lung, sinuses, or middle ear. Closely allied to obstruction are mucociliary disorders, such as cystic fibrosis with thick, tenacious mucus; ciliary dyskinesia disorders, such as Kartagener syndrome (dextrocardia, situs inversus, sinusitis, and bronchiectasis associated with a ciliary defect [see Chapter 14]); and disorders secondary to pollutants, such as tobacco smoke, which interfere with ciliary function. Recurrent or chronic disruption of the integrity of the skin or mucous membranes allows pathogens easy entry into the circulation and lymphatic systems. Foreign bodies, whether a festering splinter or an iatrogenic indwelling catheter, allow

Disorders Leading to Increased Susceptibility to Infection

Obstructive disorders—genitourinary tract stenosis, asthma, eustachian tube dysfunction, allergic rhinitis, bronchial stenosis

Mucociliary disorders—active or passive smoking, cystic fibrosis, ciliary dyskinesia disorders

Integumentary disorders—eczema, burns, repeated trauma, sinus tracts, epidermal defects

Mechanical disorders—foreign bodies, indwelling catheters, aspirated foreign body, artificial heart valves

Environmental factors—prolonged systemic or cutaneous steroid use; broad-spectrum antibiotics; repeated exposure to contaminated water, food, or equipment; daycare and school exposure

Circulatory disorders—sickle-cell disease, diabetes mellitus, nephrosis, varicose veins, congenital cardiac disease

Secondary immunodeficiencies—malnutrition, prematurity, malignancy, splenectomy, uremia, immunosuppressive therapy, protein-losing enteropathy

Primary immunodeficiencies

bacteria to colonize on their surfaces, and foreign body aspiration can lead to chronic or recurrent pneumonia. Chronic use of steroids can lead to increased infection; even prolonged use of topical steroids can interfere with normal adrenal function. Use of chronic or broad-spectrum antibiotics permits bacterial overgrowth, opportunistic infections, or the development of antibiotic-resistant pathogens. Exposure to contaminated water or food and use of contaminated equipment (e.g., respiratory equipment) can cause chronic or recurrent infections. Stasis of blood flow leads to tissue injury and increased infection. Common examples include sickle-cell disease and diabetes mellitus. Several disorders may have associated defects of the immune system and frequent infections as a consequence. For example, prematurity, malnutrition, malignancies, and splenectomy are relatively common. Nearly every serious illness alters immune function to some degree and creates secondary immune defects.

Daycare and school exposures greatly increase the number of infections in children. Wald and others reported that children in daycare during the first year of life suffered more than 7 illnesses per year, whereas children cared for at home had an average of 4.7 illnesses per year. Over 3 times as many children in daycare experienced at least 4 severe illnesses with high fever and prolonged illness or requiring a physician visit when compared with children cared for in the home (67% versus 21% respectively). Also, children in daycare were ill a total of 96 days per year compared with 41 days for children cared for at home. Respiratory tract infections are by far the

most common illnesses in daycare settings, although gastrointestinal pathogens (e.g., *Shigella* sp., *Giardia* sp., rotavirus, hepatitis A virus, and *Cryptosporidium* sp.) have been identified. Invasive organisms (e.g., *Haemophilus influenzae,* streptococci, staphylococci, scabies, and lice) and herpesviruses (e.g., varicella-zoster virus and cytomegalovirus [CMV]) cause disease among children and staff members. Hence a wide variety of disorders and circumstances other than primary immunodeficiencies can lead to frequent infections.

Primary immune defects often are hereditary and congenital, with 80% of cases having their onset in childhood. Because many of the disorders are X-linked, 70% occur in boys. Children who may be at risk for a primary immunodeficiency are those who have suffered (1) chronic infections (osteomyelitis, pneumonia, or encephalitis), (2) unusual infections caused by opportunistic organisms (*Pneumocystis carinii* or *Pseudomonas* species), (3) recurrent infections (pneumonia or mucosal or cutaneous abscesses), and (4) severe infections caused by organisms that normally cause mild or no illness (varicella or live vaccines). Normal children with frequent infections often are able to handle the infection with little or no intervention and have periods of wellness between infections. Also, children who have recurrent infections limited to one site (e.g., otitis media) are unlikely to have a systemic immunodeficiency. Allergic respiratory disease, asthma, allergic rhinitis, and associated otitis media may easily be confused with recurrent pulmonary and sinus infections. Hence manifestations of an allergy frequently are confused with immunodeficiency. However, if a child has two systemic bacterial (e.g., sepsis, meningitis, and osteomyelitis) infections or three serious respiratory (e.g., pneumonia or sinusitis) or bacterial (e.g., cellulitis or lymphadenitis) infections per year, an evaluation may be warranted.

Stiehm classifies children who have recurrent infections into four categories. The first category is the child who is probably well. Approximately half of evaluated children fall into this category. Children may have a relatively brief history of recurrent infections or a single, prolonged illness and delayed recovery. The onset of illness may coincide with enrollment in daycare, preschool, or kindergarten. Physical examination generally is normal, and little or no evaluation is needed, although much reassurance is indicated. The second group accounts for about 30% of children with recurrent lower respiratory tract symptoms. These children have allergies causing most symptoms. Fever is usually absent, and antibiotics have little effect on the illness. Chronic cough, poor exercise tolerance, nighttime cough, wheezing, food intolerance, a history of colic, eczema, and a family history of atopy may be clues to the allergic nature of symptoms. Chronic nonimmunologic disease accounts for only 10% of presenting children and comprises the third category. Symptoms might include failure to thrive, recurrent pneumonia, chronic diarrhea, or recurrent fever. Disorders that should be considered include pulmonary anomalies, such as bronchial stenosis and pulmonary sequestration; bronchopulmonary dysplasia; cystic fibrosis; ciliary dyskinesia syndromes; gastroesophageal reflux; and foreign body aspiration. The fourth category represents the truly immunodeficient child. Approximately 10% of children evaluated for recurrent infections fall into this category. Infections often begin early in childhood and vary according to the causative organism, location, and severity. Often, infections may respond to antibiotics initially, but illness recurs shortly after medications are stopped.

Differential Diagnosis

Well over 70 different primary immune disorders are recognized, encompassing each major component of the immune system, including lymphocytes (B and T cells are involved most frequently), phagocytic cells, and complement. Although it is impossible to discuss all of these disorders, some relatively common and important examples of defects in each area are presented as examples. Table 26-1 lists some primary immunodeficiency diseases.

Human Immunodeficiency Virus Infection

Any current discussion of differential diagnosis of immunodeficiency must include human immunodeficiency virus (HIV) infection, which would not have been included 20 years ago. Well over 3000 children in the United States have acquired immunodeficiency syndrome (AIDS), a state of symptomatic HIV infection meeting specific criteria established by the Centers for Disease Control. AIDS is highly lethal; the majority of affected patients are predicted to die as a result of the infection. AIDS is caused by HIV-1 (most common in the United States) or HIV-2. Both serotypes have an affinity for the CD4 antigen on T lymphocytes, macrophages, and other cells. The virus enters the cell and ultimately causes cell death, rendering the immune system incompetent.

Of children with HIV infection, approximately 15% acquired HIV infection from contaminated blood products, largely before mass screening became effective in March 1985. Another 5% contracted the virus from blood products used in the treatment of hemophilia or other coagulation disorders. The majority of infants, nearly 80%, contracted HIV from an infected mother. Approximately 30% to 40% of infants born to HIV-infected mothers contract the infection. Transmission of the virus through breast-milk has been reported. Less frequently, children and adolescents are infected by routes more commonly associated with adult risk factors, such as needle sharing among intravenous drug abusers or sexual activity. Casual contact or nonsexual household contact is not a risk for contracting HIV infection.

With destruction of $CD4^+$ lymphocytes, the $CD4^+:CD8^+$ (helper/suppressor ratio) decreases from a normal of 2 to less than 1. This may also reflect a rise in $CD8^+$ lymphocytes. Functional lymphocyte abnormalities, cutaneous anergy, polyclonal B-cell proliferation, and immunoglobulin secretion with markedly elevated serum immunoglobulin levels (IgG, IgM, IgA, and IgD) are the hallmarks of HIV infection. The elevated immunoglobulins can be determined before other laboratory features, such as lymphopenia or low $CD4^+$ lymphocytes. Despite elevated immunoglobulin levels, children have impaired antibody production.

The majority of children who acquire perinatal HIV infection become symptomatic between 4 and 6 months of age, often experiencing failure to thrive, lymphadenopathy (especially axillary adenopathy), hepatosplenomegaly, and opportunistic infection. Median age at diagnosis is 9 months. Most children are diagnosed within the first year of life, and 82% are usually diagnosed by age 3 years. In children infected by HIV-contaminated blood products, the median interval between transfusion and diagnosis is 17 months, although the onset of AIDS may be delayed for over 7 years in some children.

Clinical manifestations of AIDS are protean and include an enlarged liver, spleen, and lymph nodes; oral candidiasis; failure to thrive; chronic diarrhea; rash; and fevers. Bacterial infections with common pathogens and gram-negative organisms, such as *Pseudomonas* organisms and Enterobacteriaceae, can cause serious systemic infection. Opportunistic infections with *P. carinii*, atypical mycobacteria, *Candida* organisms, CMV, *Cryptosporidium* organisms, and herpesviruses occur with increased frequency. Viral infections with varicella-zoster, rubeola, and Epstein-Barr virus (EBV) may be life-threatening. Although some complications (e.g., lymphocytic interstitial pneumonitis) are more common in children, others (Kaposi sarcoma) are much more common in adults.

Primary Antibody Deficiencies

Antibody deficiency, accounting for about 50% of primary immunodeficiencies, is associated with recurrent infections often caused by encapsulated organisms. The development of serum immunoglobulins is age dependent (Fig. 26-1 on p. 386), and most children with gross deficiencies of IgG are protected from serious infection until maternally derived IgG wanes at 6 to 9 months of age. Selective IgA deficiency is by far the most common immunoglobulin deficiency, and although most patients have recurrent infectious complications, allergies, and autoimmune diseases, some may have minimal or no symptoms.

X-Linked Agammaglobulinemia

X-linked agammaglobulinemia (Bruton disease) is the prototype for antibody deficiency diseases and was first described in 1952. Boys with this disease generally remain well for the initial 6 to 9 months of life before developing infections with pneumococci, streptococci, and *Haemophilus* species in a variety of locations. Fungal infections are generally handled without difficulty, as are most viral infections, with the exception of hepatitis and enteroviruses. Hepatitis may be particularly severe, and central nervous system infections with enteroviruses, including live attentuated poliovirus, may lead to a chronic, progressive, potentially lethal encephalitis. Lymphoid hypoplasia of the tonsils, adenoids, and lymph nodes is found

TABLE 26-1

Summary of Some Primary Immunodeficiencies

Name	Inheritance	Incidence	Organisms	Sites	Carrier detection	Prenatal diagnosis
Primary Antibody Defects						
X-linked agammaglobulinemia	XL	1:103,000	Pneumococci, streptococci, *Haemophilus* sp., hepatitis virus, enterovirus	Middle ear, sinus, lung, bone, skin, blood, meninges	Yes	Yes
Common variable immunodeficiency	AR, AD	1:83,000	*Haemophilus* sp., pneumococci, streptococci, staphylococci, *Giardia* sp., echovirus	Sinus, lung, middle ear, liver, intestine	—	—
IgG subclass deficiency	—	—	*Haemophilus* sp., pneumococci	Sinus, middle ear	—	—
Transient hypogammaglobulinemia of infancy	—	—	Pneumococci, staphylococci, streptococci	Middle ear, skin, lung	—	—
Selective IgA deficiency	AR, AD	1:500	Pyogenic bacteria, *Giardia* sp., viruses	Middle ear, sinus, lung, GI, GU	—	—
Elevated IgM with immunodeficiency	XL, AR	—	Pyogenic infections	Middle ear, sinus, lung (pneumonia, pneumocystis)	—	—
X-linked lymphoproliferative disease	XL	—	Epstein-Barr virus	—	—	—
Primary Cellular Defects						
DiGeorge syndrome	AD	1:66,000	Fungi, viruses, *Pneumocystis* sp.	Sinus, ear, lung	—	—
Nezelof syndrome	AR	—	Fungi, viruses, *Pneumocystis* sp.	Lung, blood (sepsis) GI, GU	—	—
PNP deficiency	AR	—	Viruses	Lung	Yes	Yes
Mucocutaneous candidiasis	AR, AD	—	*Candida* sp.	Skin, nails, mucous membranes	—	—

AD, Autosomal dominant; *AR*, autosomal recessive; *CNS*, central nervous system; *GI*, gastrointestinal tract; *GU*, genitourinary tract; *PNP*, purine nucleoside phosphorylase; *SCID*, severe combined immunodeficiency; *XL*, X-linked.

on physical examination (Fig. 26-2). A maturational block in the pre-B cell is postulated, leading to low serum immunoglobulins, with IgG, IgA, and IgM levels far below the 95% confidence limits for age. The patient does not make protective antibodies to protein or polysaccharide antigenic challenge. Occasional patients may have neutropenia. Therapy generally consists of aggressive antibiotics for infections, prophylactic antibiotics, and intravenous immunoglobulin replacement.

Common Variable Immunodeficiency

Common variable immunodeficiency (CVID), also known as *late-onset hypogammaglobulinemia*, is clinically similar to congenital (Bruton) agammaglobulinemia, with profoundly depressed immunoglobulin levels. Children of both genders are equally affected, although onset of infections may occur later in childhood or adolescence. Chronic sinopulmonary infections predominate the clinical presentation, and slowly progressive bronchiectasis is common. Organisms causing infection are similar to those causing infection in congenital agammaglobulinemia. Physical examination, however, may differ, with an affected patient having normal or enlarged lymph nodes, tonsils, and spleen. Splenomegaly is found in 25% of patients. CVID has been associated with numerous autoimmune phenomena and the development of autoanti-

TABLE 26-1

Summary of Some Primary Immunodeficiencies—*cont'd*

Name	Inheritance	Incidence	Organisms	Carrier Sites	Prenatal detection	diagnosis
Primary Cellular Defects—cont'd						
Short-limbed dwarfism	AR	—	Varicella-zoster virus, poliovirus	Skin, CNS	?	Yes
Primary Combined T- and B-Cell Defects						
SCID	AR, XL	1:66,000	Viruses, fungi, *Pneumocystis* sp.	Sinus, lung skin, GI, blood (sepsis)	Yes (XL)	Yes (XL)
SCID with adenosine deaminase deficiency	AR	—	Viruses, fungi, *Pneumocystis* sp.	Sinus, lung	—	—
Partial T- and B-Cell Defects						
Ataxia telangiectasia	AR	—	Viruses, pyogenic bacteria	Sinus, lung	—	—
Wiskott-Aldrich syndrome	XL	—	Bacteria, viruses, herpesvirus	Middle ear, lung, sinus	Yes	Yes
Hyperimmunoglobulinemia E	Possible AD	—	Staphylococci	Skin, lung, joints	—	—
Leukocyte adhesion defect	AR	—	Bacteria, fungi	Skin, lung, mucous membrane	—	—
Phagocytic and Complement Defects						
Chronic granulomatous disease	XL, AR	1:181,000	Staphylococci, *Klebsiella, Proteus, Serratia, Candida, Nocardia,* and *Aspergillus* sp.	Lung, skin, bone, liver	Yes (XL)	Yes (XL)
Chédiak-Higashi syndrome	AR	—	Pyogenic bacteria	Lung, bone	—	—
Complement	AR	—	Pneumococci, meningococci	Bone, lung, blood, meninges	—	—

bodies. Hemolytic anemia, thrombocytopenia, neutropenia, pernicious anemia, and many syndromes resembling rheumatoid arthritis, dermatomyositis, systemic lupus erythematosus, and scleroderma have been described in conjunction with CVID. Nodular lymphoid hyperplasia of the intestine has been noted as well. Affected women in the fifth and sixth decades of life are at a 438-fold increased risk for developing lymphoma. Patients may have normal numbers of circulating B lymphocytes, but these cells do not differentiate into immunoglobulin-producing cells. T-cell function usually is normal, although some patients may have depressed T-cell function. Frequently, first-degree relatives of CVID patients

may have a variety of immune abnormalities, including autoimmune diseases, autoantibodies, and selective IgA deficiency. Therapy is similar to that for congenital agammaglobulinemia; careful observation for autoimmune phenomena or malignancy is especially important.

IgG Subclass Deficiency

Deficiencies of one or more of the IgG subclasses may cause patients to suffer recurrent episodes of otitis media, sinusitis, or pneumonia. Patients with more serious infections, such as meningitis or sepsis, may have a more profound immunodeficiency. Although significant depression of one or

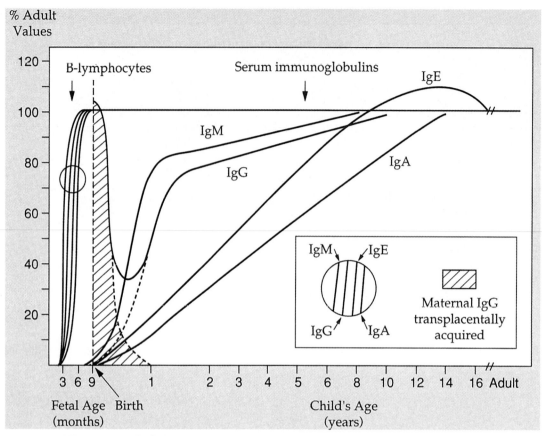

FIG. 26-1   Antibody levels according to age expressed as a percentage of adult values.

more IgG subclasses may occur, the total IgG level usually is normal or near normal. In addition, some patients have profound depression of several subclasses yet are virtually asymptomatic. Hence the clinical significance of IgG subclass deficiency is still questioned. All subclasses are passively transferred transplacentally, and IgG1 and IgG3 subsequently rise to adult levels within the first year, whereas IgG2 and IgG4 are slower to achieve adult levels. IgG1 accounts for two thirds of IgG serum levels, binds complement, adheres to phagocytic cells, and constitutes a strong response to protein and viral antigenic challenges. Antibodies to *H. influenzae* are found within the IgG1 fraction as well. IgG2 also constitutes a large fraction of the antibody response to polysaccharide antigens, particularly group A streptococci. IgG2 represents 23% of the serum IgG concentration. IgG3 reacts with protein antigens similar to IgG1 but reacts minimally to polysaccharides, and the exact clinical significance of IgG4 deficiency is unclear because levels may be near zero in asymptomatic individuals. Patients with selective IgA deficiency and IgG subclass deficiency are particularly vulnerable to recurrent infections. The physician must be cautious in making a diagnosis of IgG subclass deficiency based solely on serum subclass levels because little epidemiologic data exist concerning IgG subclass deficiencies, difficulty exists in inter-

preting low IgG subclass levels, and age-related standardization of levels is lacking. A better evaluation includes the patient's functional ability to respond to protein and polysaccharide antigens by measuring titers of diphtheria-tetanus and pneumococcal vaccines before and 4 weeks after immunization. Current conjugated *H. influenzae* type B immunizations probably should not be used to test the patient's response to polysaccharides because conjugation increases immunogenicity. Rather, response to a pneumococcal polysaccharide vaccine can be used as a test, although interpretation may be difficult because children under 2 years of age normally react poorly to polysaccharide antigens. Older children also may have varied responses to the pneumoccal subtypes. Generally, treatment of children with IgG subclass deficiency requires only aggressive antibiotic therapy, although intravenous immunoglobulin therapy may be indicated for children who demonstrate a defective response to a wide variety of antigens and are not IgA deficient.

Transient Hypogammaglobulinemia of Infancy

Transient hypogammaglobulinemia of infancy results from an abnormally prolonged recovery from the physiologic nadir of serum immunoglobulins that normally occurs between 3 and 6 months of age. Serum immunoglobulin levels are low,

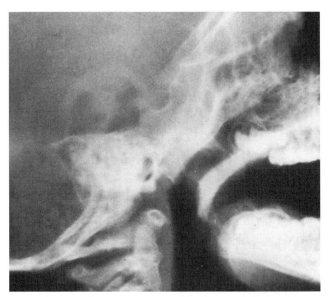

FIG. 26-2 A lateral neck radiograph shows absent adenoidal shadow in a patient with X-linked agammaglobulinemia.

but B cells are normal or near normal in number. Children may have gram-positive infections of the skin, lungs, and upper respiratory tract, although many children have mild or few infections. Children with this disorder can develop antibodies to red cell antigens and diphtheria-tetanus toxoids, often by 12 months of age (long before immunoglobulin levels normalize by 18 to 36 months of age). Some clinicians treat patients with intravenous gamma globulin until the clinical picture becomes clearer. However, because this is a benign, self-limited disorder, therapy with parenteral immunoglobulin generally is not indicated.

Selective IgA Deficiency

Virtual absence of secretory and serum IgA is the most common specific primary immunodeficiency, occurring in about 1 in every 500 individuals. Although some individuals with selective IgA deficiency are healthy, most have infections of the mucosal surfaces, primarily the respiratory, gastrointestinal, and urogenital tracts. Approximately 90% of patients have deficiencies of both the serum and secretory IgA, and 3% of patients have normal secretory IgA but low serum levels. Serum IgA levels are usually less than 5 mg/dl. Most patients suffer pyogenic bacteria infections of the middle ear, sinuses, and lower respiratory tract. Giardiasis and prolonged diarrhea resulting from viral infections can be troublesome. Serum IgA deficiency also has been associated with IgG subclass deficiency, causing frequent infections and significant morbidity greater than that of either deficiency alone. Autoantibodies and autoimmune disorders have been found in selective IgA-deficient patients, which is similar to patients with CVID. Antibodies to cow's milk, a spruelike syndrome in adults that is responsive to a gluten-free diet, and an in-

creased incidence of malignancies have been described as well. Therapy remains symptomatic, and immunoglobulin replacement may be dangerous. Antibodies to IgA, which may lead to severe and potentially fatal anaphylactic reactions to even trace amounts of IgA in standard immunoglobulin preparations (generally greater than 99% IgG), have been found in as many as 44% of patients with selective IgA deficiency. Packed red cells administered to these patients should be washed 5 times, or other products should be obtained from other IgA-deficient patients. Selective IgA deficiency has been noted in families of individuals afflicted with CVID, suggesting a common genetic basis. IgA deficiency has been observed in some patients taking medications, such as phenytoin, sulfasalazine, D-penicillamine, and gold, suggesting that the defect may be exposed by certain environmental factors.

Immunodeficiency With Elevated IgM Levels

Immunodeficiency with elevated IgM levels is characterized by low IgG and IgA levels but normal or elevated IgM. Onset of symptoms is within the first 2 years of life and is marked by an increase in pyogenic infections, particularly of the upper and lower respiratory tracts. Lymph node and tonsillar enlargement, occasional thrombocytopenia, hemolytic anemia, and neutropenia can be found. T-cell function usually is normal, although it is postulated that the defect lies in T-cell regulation of B-cell immunoglobulin synthesis. Inheritance appears to be X-linked.

X-Linked Lymphoproliferative Disease

An unusual disorder, X-linked lymphoproliferative disease, also known as *Duncan disease,* is caused by an aberrant immunologic response to infection with EBV. Patients are healthy with no evidence of immunodeficiency until infected with EBV. Most patients develop potentially fatal, overwhelming, EBV-induced B-cell proliferation during infection. Antibody response to EBV is variable, with no to markedly elevated antibodies to viral capsid antigen and no antibodies to nuclear antigen. Patients have symptoms suggestive of lymphoma. Those who survive may develop hypogammaglobulinemia, B-cell lymphoma, or both.

Primary T-Cell Defects

Patients who have defects in the T-cell system generally have an earlier onset of infections than patients who have only antibody deficiencies because no maternal protection exists. Infecting organisms usually are different, with yeasts, fungi, protozoa, viruses, and opportunistic bacteria predominating the clinical presentations. Treatment options are limited as well. Patients with cellular defects account for about 10% of individuals with primary immunodeficiencies.

DiGeorge Syndrome

DiGeorge syndrome, described in 1965, has a wide spectrum of clinical presentations, although most children have

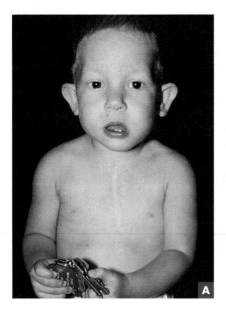
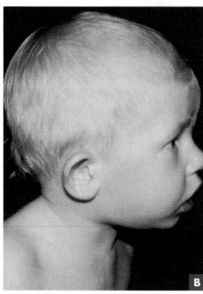

FIG. 26-3 Patient with DiGeorge syndrome. Note hypertelorism and low-set, malformed ears. The patient underwent repair of an aortic arch anomaly.

a constellation of congenital heart defects, dysmorphic facial features, and immune defects associated with thymic hypoplasia or aplasia. Not all features need be present, leading to the term *partial DiGeorge syndrome.* Dysmorphogenesis of the third and fourth pharyngeal pouches and resulting hypoplasia or aplasia of the thymus and parathyroid glands are responsible for most of the clinical features. Cardiovascular defects, particularly aortic arch anomalies, are frequent, as is hypocalcemia presenting after 1 week of age. Dysmorphic features of micrognathia; low-set, rotated ears; hypertelorism; and anteverted nostrils are observed in most patients (Fig. 26-3). Immune defects are limited mostly to poor lymphocyte mitogen stimulation and poor intradermal delayed hypersensitivity response, with normal immunoglobulins and a normal helper/suppressor ratio. Purulent rhinorrhea, maculopapular rashes, and failure to thrive begin the child's frequent infections, and severely affected patients may have infections with fungi, viruses, and *P. carinii.* In addition these patients are susceptible to graft-versus-host disease (GVHD) resulting from nonirradiated blood transfusions. In some children, immunodeficiency improves or resolves with time, although fetal thymic transplant may be considered if the diagnosis is made early in infancy and the child is profoundly affected.

Cellular Deficiency With Elevated Immunoglobulins

Cellular deficiency with elevated immunoglobulins, also known as *Nezelof syndrome,* frequently presents in infancy with chronic pulmonary, gastrointestinal, urogenital, and skin infections, as well as oral candidiasis. Lymphopenia, poorly developed lymphoid tissue, and an abnormal thymus coexist with normal to elevated immunoglobulins, causing this syndrome to be confused with AIDS in children. The helper/suppressor ratio usually is normal, despite a profound deficiency in total T-cell number.

Purine Nucleoside Phosphorylase Deficiency

The purine nucleoside phosphorylase (PNP) enzyme is involved in the purine salvage pathway, ultimately leading to the formation of uric acid. Deficiency of PNP leads to the accumulation of potentially toxic metabolites, thus affecting immune function. Two thirds of patients have had neurologic dysfunction with spasticity or mental retardation. Serum uric acid levels are low. T cells are markedly decreased, as is lymphocyte response to mitogens, but B-cell numbers and antibody formation appear to be normal. Patients often succumb to overwhelming viral infections, pneumonia, or GVHD. Some patients with Nezelof syndrome have PNP deficiency as well.

Chronic Mucocutaneous Candidiasis

Chronic mucocutaneous candidiasis, a specific defect in T-cell function toward candidal infection, leads to chronic candidiasis of the skin, nails, and mucous membranes. *Candida* organisms are the primary pathogen, although other organisms can be involved as well. Polyglandular endocrine dysfunction has been seen, with autoantibodies directed against thyroid, adrenal, pancreas, and gastric parietal cell antigens. Although some patients have defects in intradermal delayed hypersensitivity responses, generally no immunologic defect is found, and the diagnosis is based on clinical presentation. Systemic infection is rare. Ketoconazole and related antifungal drugs are the mainstays of therapy. Sporadic, autosomal recessive, and autosomal dominant modes of inheritance have been observed, depending on clinical presentation.

Short-Limbed Dwarfism

Short-limbed dwarfism with immunodeficiency is an autosomal recessive disorder associated with metaphyseal or spondyloepiphyseal dysplasia. The immunodeficiency may be T cell, B cell, or combined. The prototype of this syndrome

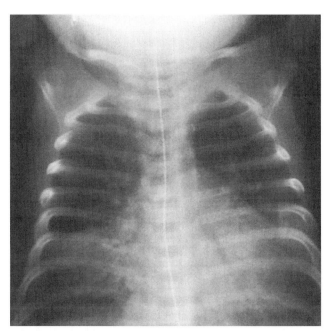

FIG. 26-4 A chest radiograph from a patient with SCID. Note the absent thymic shadow and bilateral pulmonary infiltrates.

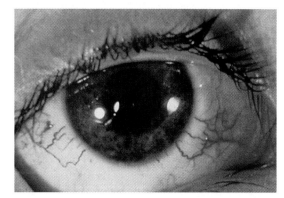

FIG. 26-5 Ataxia telangiectasia. Bulbar telangiectasia usually appears by 6 years of age.

is cartilage-hair hypoplasia (CHH) with T-cell deficits. Infections with viruses, particularly poliovirus and varicella-zoster virus, are potentially lethal. Bony defects; redundant skin; fine, sparse hair; and megaloblastic anemia are associated findings.

Combined T-Cell and B-Cell Deficiencies

Profound deficiencies in both T-cell and B-cell systems usually lead to early, overwhelming infection (caused by viruses, fungi, *Pneumocystis* organisms, and low-grade pathogens) and death before the first birthday unless immunologic reconstitution can be accomplished. Of primary immune defects, 20% are represented among these disorders.

Severe Combined Immunodeficiency

Although autosomal recessive and X-linked forms of severe combined immunodeficiency (SCID) have been described, 75% of affected patients are male. Children present early in infancy with persistent candidal infection, chronic diarrhea, failure to thrive, and potentially fatal viral or opportunistic infections, such as *P. carinii* pneumonia (Fig. 26-4). GVHD resulting from transplacentally acquired maternal lymphocytes or nonirradiated blood transfusions is also a threat. Profound lymphopenia, absent mitogen responses, absent cutaneous delayed hypersensitivity, profoundly depressed serum immunoglobulin levels, absent antibody formation, and variable B-cell numbers characterize the immune defects. Some patients with a subtype of reticular dysgenesis also have congenital aleukocytosis (absence of lymphocytes and granulocytes from marrow and peripheral blood). The disease is uniformly fatal unless immunologic

reconstitution can be accomplished, usually through bone marrow transplantation.

SCID With Adenosine Deaminase Deficiency

Approximately 50% of patients with autosomal recessive SCID are also deficient in adenosine deaminase (ADA), an enzyme involved in purine metabolism. Lack of this enzyme leads to toxic metabolite accumulation and lymphocyte dysfunction. Patients have a similar presentation to that of SCID but usually exhibit more profound lymphopenia and do not have elevated B cells. In addition, patients frequently have anomalies of the ribs and scapulae. Treatment has included enzyme replacement and bone marrow transplantation; with recent successful cloning of genes, ADA deficiency has become the first disorder treated successfully with gene-replacement therapy.

Partial Defects of T-Cell and B-Cell Function

Several syndromes are characterized by only partial immunodeficiencies and may be associated with other major defects. Ataxia telangiectasia is an autosomal recessive disorder delineated by progressive ataxia (usually beginning by age 3), telangiectasis (often appearing on the bulbar conjunctivae by age 5; Fig. 26-5), recurrent sinopulmonary infections caused by T-cell deficiency (commonly occurring with selective IgA deficiency and low IgG levels), elevated serum alpha-fetoprotein, malignant neoplasms, and frequent chromosomal aberrations, including breakage. Wiskott-Aldrich syndrome (thrombocytopenia, eczema, and immunodeficiency; Fig. 26-6) is an X-linked disorder characterized by thrombocytopenia; abnormally small platelet size and volume; atopic dermatitis; infections with organisms containing polysaccharide

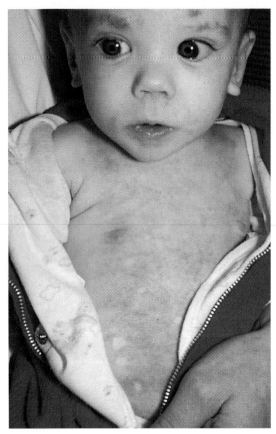

FIG. 26-6 Child with Wiskott-Aldrich syndrome. Note the eczematoid rash on the face and trunk. Petechiae resulting from thrombocytopenia cannot be visualized.

capsules, herpesviruses, and *Pneumocystis* species; excessive catabolism of immunoglobulins, with variable but usually low IgM, elevated IgA and IgE, and normal to slightly low IgG levels; cutaneous anergy; and poor lymphocyte mitogen response. Patients with hyperimmunoglobulinemia E (hyper IgE) syndrome have severe, recurrent staphylococcal abscesses of the skin, lungs, joints, and other areas along with a maculopapular dermatitis, markedly elevated IgE concentrations, elevated numbers of eosinophils in the blood and sputum, and poor antibody and cell-mediated responses to antigens. The leukocyte adhesion defect is the result of a mutation on chromosome 21, leading to poor cytotoxic lymphocyte function; interference with immune-cell interaction; and abnormal phagocytic-cell adherence, chemotaxis, and metabolic activity during phagocytosis. Patients often have a history of delayed umbilical cord separation, omphalitis, mucous membrane infections, sinopulmonary infections, and perianal abscesses. Bacterial and fungal infections can be severe, but viral infections or malignancies are not more prevalent.

Phagocytic and Complement Deficiencies

Phagocytic defects account for about 18% of primary immunodeficiencies, whereas complement disorders are much rarer, accounting for only 2%. The classic example of a phagocytic defect is chronic granulomatous disease. Nearly two thirds of cases are X-linked, and the remainder are autosomal recessive. Children are plagued by chronic suppurative infections, lymphadenitis, pneumonia, abscesses, osteomyelitis, and dermatitis. Elevated immunoglobulin levels frequently are noted, but the defect resides in the neutrophil's inability to kill catalase-positive organisms (*Staphylococcus aureus, Klebsiella* organisms, *Proteus* organisms, and *Serratia marcescens*) and fungi (*Candida* organisms and *Aspergillus* organisms). The phagocyte cannot convert oxygen to hydrogen peroxide, superoxide anion, and hydroxyl radicals necessary for killing because of any one of several possible enzyme defects. Diagnosis can be made by using the nitroblue tetrazolium (NBT) test, which uses oxidative products to reduce the dye to a blue color. Phagocytes from affected patients fail to reduce the dye, and no color change occurs. Specific enzyme analysis can delineate the defect. Aggressive antibiotic therapy, including trimethoprim sulfamethoxazole prophylaxis, is helpful. Interferon-gamma administration significantly reduces rates of infection as well.

Chédiak-Higashi syndrome is an autosomal recessive disorder that causes pyogenic infections as a result of defects in intracellular killing and chemotaxis. Patients may have oculocutaneous albinism, photophobia, and nystagmus. Granulocytes contain giant granules, which in turn contain lysosomal enzymes and peroxidase. Poor granule fusion leads to the defect in killing, and the chemotactic defect contributes to recurrent infections.

Deficiencies of complement proteins and their dysfunction lead to recurrent infections. Deficiencies in C2, C3, and C4 lead to recurrent pyogenic infections, often with pneumococci and meningococci causing bacteremia, pneumonia, and meningitis. Autoimmune disorders, especially systemic lupus erythematosus and glomerulonephritis, have also been associated with these deficiencies. Defects in any of the more terminal components of complement from C5 to C9 predispose to gram-negative infections, especially recurrent or chronic meningococcal infection. Diagnosis can be made by measuring CH_{50} assay. If the amount is low, specific complement protein assays can define the defect.

History

Initial evaluation of the patient searches for historic clues to nonimmunologic causes of recurrent infection and primary immunodeficiency (Table 26-2). The pregnancy history should examine issues of maternal illness, prematurity, birth weight, and perinatal illnesses. If the mother received blood transfusions between 1981 and 1985, she may be at risk for HIV infection, which can be transmitted to the infant. In addition, parents should be questioned about participation in behaviors that put them at high risk of HIV infection (e.g., sexual promiscuity, anal intercourse, homosexual behavior, and intravenous drug abuse). Prematurity and chronic lung disease resulting from respiratory distress syndrome may predispose to recurrent pulmonary complications and infections. Exposure to medication, such as chronic antibiotics or steroids, may induce secondary immune defects. Evidence of delayed cord separation might suggest a white-cell defect. Symptoms beginning after weaning from breast-feeding may suggest food allergy.

The frequency, location, severity, and complications of infections should be described. Respiratory symptoms account for the majority of infections that children develop. If infections tend to be self-limited with periods of good health between infections, immunodeficiency is unlikely. Similarly, if infections primarily involve a single site, local factors may be responsible. Allergy may be suspected on the basis of (1) absence of fever, (2) nonpurulent nasal discharge, (3) past history of eczema or atopic disease, (4) positive family history for allergy, (5) seasonal pattern of illness, and (6) poor response to antibiotics and good response to antihistamines or bronchodilators. Reactive airway disease is the most common cause of recurrent pulmonary infiltrates. A careful review of the immunization history may provide important clues. A child who has received live or BCG vaccines with no adverse reaction or has exhibited the rash of a viral exanthem or poison ivy most likely has an intact T-cell system. The age of onset of infection may provide information regarding the cause of the infection. Normal children have mostly respiratory infections, beginning before 6 months of age. Illnesses generally are mild and self-limited or respond quickly to usual therapy with periods of good health between illnesses. Children with T-cell defects have onset of chronic fungal infections or opportunistic infections early in life, before 6 months of age. Infants with B-cell defects, however, usually are protected by maternal antibodies until 6 months of age or after.

Past history should include the type of infection. Chronic candidal infection after 6 months of age suggests a T-cell defect, as does severe viral, fungal, or opportunistic infection. Pyogenic bacterial infections of multiple sites may indicate a humoral defect, and recurrent staphylococcal infections may point to chronic granulomatous disease. The past history also should be explored for prior surgeries, such as lymph node excision, tonsilloadenoidectomy, or splenectomy. Retrospective examination of these tissues may provide histopathologic evidence for an immunodeficiency. Prior illnesses requiring blood transfusions, chronic antibiotic therapy, steroid therapy, immunoglobulin replacement, chemotherapy, or radiation should be noted.

Family history should include information about atopy, recurrent infections, and autoimmune disorders. A history of consanguinity should be sought, and early deaths or a strong history of lymphoreticular malignancies may suggest immunologic disease. Family members who smoke tobacco or marijuana place household children at risk for recurrent infection and pulmonary symptoms.

TABLE 26-2

Clues from the History and Physical Examination

Finding	Characteristic
History	
Prenatal/Perinatal	
Maternal illness	Underlying illness
Parental high-risk behavior for HIV	HIV transmission
Prematurity	Poor immunity, chronic lung disease
Medication exposure	Increased infection with antibiotics, steroids
Delayed cord separation	White-cell defect
Feeding method	Protective effect of breast-feeding
Infancy/Childhood	
Chronic candidal infection after 6 months	T-cell defect
Immunization history	Adverse reaction to live virus vaccines
Frequency, location, severity, complications of infection	May distinguish normal child from one with immunodeficiency
Atopic disease	Allergy
History of splenectomy/ malignancy	Acquired immune defect
Exposures to tobacco smoke, contaminated water, farm animals, pollutants	Recurrent infections
Daycare/school attendance or siblings in school	Increased infections in preschool children
Physical Examination	
Poor growth, failure to thrive	Chronic illness
Allergic shiners, Dennie lines, conjunctivitis, eczema, wheezing	Allergy
Skin rash	Viral illness, chronic granulomatous disease, Wiskott-Aldrich syndrome
Telangiectasia	Ataxia telangiectasia
Absent lymphoid tissue	Agammaglobulinemia
Enlarged lymph nodes, hepatosplenomegaly	CVID
Thrush	T-cell defect
Arthritis, subcutaneous nodules	Autoimmune disease, CVID, Selective IgA deficiency

A history of exposures, including animals, chemicals, farm animals, or contaminated water sources, should be obtained. A history of travel may indicate exposure to unusual organisms. In addition, recent enrollment in daycare or school increases the incidence of infections.

Physical Examination

The physical examination may help determine whether the child with recurrent infections is among the 50% of children who are generally well or has some chronic disorder. Children with chronic illness may fail to thrive; hence careful, sequential monitoring of weight, length, and head circumference is essential. Because allergy is high among the disorders in the differential diagnosis, clues suggesting the presence of atopic disease should be sought. These clues include allergic shiners, Dennie Morgan lines, follicular conjunctivitis, pale and swollen nasal turbinates with a clear nasal discharge, a transverse nasal crease resulting from the "allergic salute," eczema, or wheezing.

Children with immunodeficiencies frequently appear chronically ill, with pallor and decreased subcutaneous fat. The skin may reveal rashes seen with chronic granulomatous disease, pyoderma (chronic granulomatous disease or white blood cell defect), eczema (Wiskott-Aldrich syndrome), petechiae (Wiskott-Aldrich syndrome), and telangiectasia (ataxia telangiectasia). Children with antibody deficiencies frequently have chronic otitis media, scarred tympanic membranes, sinusitis, and chronic conjunctivitis. Cervical lymph nodes may not be palpable despite recurrent infection in congenital X-linked agammaglobulinemia or may be normal or enlarged as in CVID. Oral mucosa may have placques of *Candida* organisms, which when persistent or resistant to therapy after 6 months of age, may be indicative of a T-cell defect. Tonsil and adenoid size may parallel that of the cervical lymph nodes, being virtually absent in congenital agammaglobulinemia. Chronic pulmonary disease with loose cough, wheezing, rales, and rhonchi may indicate an allergic diathesis, local pulmonary disease (right middle lobe syndrome), systemic disease (cystic fibrosis), or virtually any of the primary immunodeficiencies. The liver and spleen frequently are enlarged in systemic disorders causing frequent infections, including many immune defects. Generalized wasting and decreased subcutaneous tissue and muscle mass are seen in many chronic illnesses and are not specific but should alert the physician to a serious, long-term illness. Perianal excoriations may accompany chronic diarrhea. Physical signs of autoimmune disease, such as joint swelling, subcutaneous nodules, and rashes, may be associated with antibody deficiency, particularly CVID or selective IgA deficiency. Neurologic abnormalities, such as developmental delay or ataxia, can be found in patients with ataxia telangiectasia, although such findings may not be present early in the illness. Dysmorphic features, including short limbs, redundant skin, and fine or sparse hair, may suggest CHH.

BOX 26-2

Initial Evaluation of the Child with Recurrent Infections

Complete blood count, differential count, platelet count
Peripheral blood smear
Erythrocyte sedimentation rate
Chest x-ray*
Sinus x-ray*
Lateral neck x-ray*
Sweat test*
Urinalysis, urine culture*
Stool analysis, ova and parasites*
HIV testing*

*Performed only when indicated by the history and physical examination.

Approach to the Patient

Laboratory evaluation of the child should be focused, specific, and dependent on information obtained from the history and physical examination (Box 26-2). Because primary immunodeficiencies are uncommon compared with other nonimmune causes of infections, selected tests should concentrate on the factors listed in Box 26-1, depending on the organ system involved. In general a complete blood count can be helpful in many cases (e.g., looking for anemia; leukopenia; leukocytosis; lymphopenia; abnormal cell morphology, such as in sickle-cell disease and leukemia; large white-cell granules, such as in Chédiak-Higashi syndrome; and thrombocytopenia, such as in Wiskott-Aldrich syndrome). Review of the blood smear may show Howell-Jolly bodies, indicating anatomic or functional asplenia. In addition, small platelets associated with eczema and thrombocytopenia in a boy who has recurrent infections may point to Wiskott-Aldrich syndrome. An erythrocyte sedimentation rate is frequently elevated in patients who have systemic disorders, whereas most often it is normal in children with simple recurrent viral infections. If recurrent sinopulmonary disease is present, sinus x-ray films may show thickening of mucosa or air fluid levels, particularly if the child is older than 1 year of age. A lateral view may indicate whether adenoid tissue is present. Chest radiographs may show evidence of airtrapping, such as that seen in asthma and allergy, or chronic infiltrates in different areas of the lung suggestive of a systemic disorder. If chronic changes are noted on chest x-ray films, a sweat test also may be indicated. In children under 3 years of age, a thymic shadow sometimes can be noted if significant physiologic stress has not occurred. Urinalysis, urine culture, and stool analysis for lymphocytes, culture, and ova and parasites should be obtained if those organ systems are involved. HIV tests (ELISA and Western blot) should be performed for the child if high-risk factors are present and should be per-

TABLE 26-3

Laboratory Tests for Primary Immunodeficiency Disorders

Screening tests	Second level tests*	Advanced tests*
B-Cell Deficiency		
IgG, IgA, IgM levels	B-cell enumeration	Lymph node biopsy
Isohemagglutinin levels	IgE level	IgG catabolism
Antibody assay to previously administered vaccines	Antibody response to administered antigens	IgG synthetic rates
T-Cell Deficiency		
Lymphocyte count	T-cell enumeration	ADA
Chest x-rays	CD4$^+$:CD8$^+$	PNP
Intradermal skin tests for delayed hypersensitivity	Lymphocyte proliferation to mitogens, antigens, allogenic lymphocytes	Lymphokine assays, cytotoxicity assays, thymic hormone assays
Phagocytic Deficiency		
White blood cell count, morphology	Motility and chemotaxis assays	White blood cell enzymes
NBT test	Phagocytosis ability	Oxidative metabolism
IgE level	Bactericidal assays	Assays for adherence, aggregation
Complement Deficiency		
C3 level	Individual component assay	Alternative pathway activity
C4 level	Opsonic activity	Functional assay
CH$_{50}$ assay	—	In vivo component survival

Modified from Stiehm ER: Clinical and laboratory evaluation of the child with suspected immunodeficiency, *Pediatr Rev* 7:53-61, 1985.
*Tests in these categories may be performed after consultation with an immunologist.

formed for the mother if the child is under 18 months of age and there are strong clinical suspicions and abnormal laboratory tests.

Screening for immunodeficiencies can be done in stages, and most are simple and reliable and can be performed or ordered through a physician's office (Table 26-3). Because most primary immune defects involve the antibody system, the single best screening test is serum IgA level. A normal value essentially eliminates serious permanent antibody deficiency states. If the IgA level is low, IgG and IgM levels should be quantified and compared with age-related normal values. A total immunoglobulin level (IgG + IgA + IgM) greater than 600 mg/dl or an IgG level greater than 400 mg/dl excludes the diagnosis of antibody-deficiency states, providing that antibody function is normal. Total immunoglobulin levels less than 400 mg/dl and IgG levels less than 200 mg/dl usually indicate an antibody-deficiency state. Intermediate values are of concern and should be correlated with antibody function tests.

Antibody function can be tested simply. Children between 6 and 12 months of age with blood types other than AB develop IgM isohemagglutinin antibodies (anti-A, 1:8; anti-B, 1:4). Antibody response to protein antigens can be determined by measuring preimmunization and postimmunization titers to the pneumococcal vaccine.

H. influenzae type B vaccines may not be the best source of polysaccharide antigen because current vaccines are conjugated to make them more immunogenic. Children under 2 years of age normally mount poor antibody responses to polysaccharide antigens, and response to the various pneumococcal serotypes is variable among individual patients. Tests for specific antibody function (testing response to diphtheria-tetanus and pneumococcal vaccines) may be the best method for the evaluation of IgG subclass deficiency because age-related normal values vary from one laboratory to the next. The biologic significance of low levels is questioned, since asymptomatic individuals have been identified with total lack of IgG1, IgG2, and IgG4.

If immunoglobulin levels are low, B-cell enumeration should be performed. Normally 4% to 10% of circulating lymphocytes carry surface membrane immunoglobulin, and low levels may indicate disorders, such as X-linked agammaglobulinemia.

IgE levels should be measured also. Although low levels generally have no clinical significance, high levels are seen in some antibody-deficiency states, allergies, parasitic infections, chemotactic disorders (hyper IgE), and partial T-cell immunodeficiencies.

Specialized tests for B-cell function include lymph node biopsy to examine for architecture and malignancy, IgG catabolism studies, and IgG synthetic rates.

Tests examining for T-cell defects can be done easily in the office and include intradermal skin testing to *Trichophyton* organisms, *Candida* organisms, and tetanus toxoid. Skin testing is dependent on antigen exposure and may be unreliable for patients younger than 6 years of age. Chest radiographs may show a thymic shadow, and a complete blood count can estimate the total lymphocyte count and morphology. More specialized tests include T-cell enumeration with the helper/suppressor ratio ($CD4^+:CD8^+$) and lymphocyte proliferation response to mitogens, antigens, and allogenic lymphocytes. Enzymes involved in purine salvage (ADA and PNP) should be measured in specialized laboratories if a T-cell deficiency has been identified. Lymphokine, cytotoxicity, and thymic hormone assays also can further define a specific T-cell defect.

Phagocytic function can be screened for simply by examining the complete blood count for total white count and white blood cell morphology. The NBT test is an excellent screen for chronic granulomatous disease. The hyper IgE syndrome can be determined by an appropriate clinical presentation along with high levels of IgE (greater than or equal to 2000 IU/ml). More specialized tests examine for mobility, chemotaxis, phagocytic ability, and specific bactericidal assays. Further testing elucidates specific enzyme defects involved in intracellular killing of microorganisms. White blood cell turnover, adherence, and aggregation require specialized laboratories.

Complement deficiencies are extremely uncommon but can be screened for by measuring CH_{50} or CH_{100} and C3 and C4 levels. If the CH_{50} or CH_{100} assay is abnormal, specific components can be measured along with opsonic activity. The alternative pathway, in vitro survival, and functional assays should be assessed only after consultation and through a specialized laboratory.

Management

The approach to the patient with recurrent infections depends greatly on the underlying cause. Most frequently, children have no underlying illness, and frequent infections represent one end of the normal spectrum. The greatest difficulty may be trying to allay parental fears of serious disease. The same tenets used in other clinical situations apply here as well. A complete and thorough history should be obtained and all records reviewed, so parents are assured that all information is being obtained. The physical examination should be meticulous and is preferably performed with the parents in the room to verify the examiner's thoroughness. The history and physical examination should be done in a relaxed, professional manner and should not be rushed by other demands. Adequate time should be allowed for the evaluation. After arriving at a diagnosis, the physician should not present an air of ambiguity because this creates more tension and uncertainty. In addition the physician should not contribute to anxiety by ordering numerous laboratory tests without specific indication. Each test ordered and the anticipated result should be explained to the family. If abnormal tests return, a focused, staged evaluation can be pursued. If tests are normal and confirm clinical suspicion, the physician should carefully explain the pattern of normal infections in children, emphasizing that some children may normally experience up to 10 infections per year. Also, if possible, factors leading to frequent infections, such as daycare attendance or contact with older siblings who attend school, and clinical and laboratory features that eliminate serious illness from consideration can be explained. Emphasizing that most children improve with time and recommending a relaxed approach to this non–life-threatening problem may avert potential hypochondriac behavior.

Viral infections often can be treated symptomatically and with reassurance. Bacterial infections should be treated on the basis of culture and sensitivity data. Recurrent infections, such as otitis media and sinusitis, may require prophylactic antibiotic therapy, particularly during high-risk seasons such as fall and winter. The use of prophylactic antibiotics, however, must be weighed against the potential for developing antibiotic-resistant organisms. Controlling environmental situations that may lead to infections, such as exposure to cigarette smoke, also may help. Specific medical conditions that are associated with infections can be treated as indicated.

Treatment of various primary immunodeficiencies depends on the specific defect and available therapeutic options. Replacement immunoglobulin therapy is not recommended for all B-cell antibody-deficiency states. Generally, transient hypogammaglobulinemia, IgG subclass deficiencies, and selective IgA deficiency do not require replacement therapy. In other disorders, however, intravenous immunoglobulin (IVIG) may be lifesaving. Minimal standards for IVIG preparation have been set up by the World Health Organization. In addition to other preparation requirements, they recommend that IVIG contain 90% of IgG1, with all subclasses represented; have little IgA; and be free of aggregates. Normal individuals have an IgG serum half-life of 21 days, and hypogammaglobulinemia patients have a slightly prolonged half-life of about 28 days. The dose of IVIG given should be such that the serum level at 4 weeks ranges between 200 to 400 mg/dl. This may require doses of IVIG from 100 to 400 mg/kg/month. IgG level at the seventh day postinfusion is predictive of the level at day 28; the day-28 level is 50% of the day-7 level. Treatment with IVIG cannot transmit hepatitis B virus or HIV. Preparation methods essentially eliminate these agents, so that no proven cases of hepatitis B or HIV infection resulting from IVIG have been reported in the United States. Rare cases of hepatitis C resulting from IVIG have been reported, but preparation methods have been changed to include a viral inactivation step that should minimize the risk of hepatitis C infection.

Treatment of T-cell deficiency relies on immunologic reconstitution with fetal thymic tissue or bone marrow transplantation. Enzyme replacement in patients with ADA deficiency has beneficial effects, but more recently correction of the defect has been accomplished by gene therapy.

Chronic granulomatous disease, as a prototype of phagocytic dysfunction, requires aggressive antibiotic and antifungal therapy. Prophylactic trimethoprim sulfamethoxazole is particularly helpful in this disease. More recently these patients have benefited from regular subcutaneous injections of interferon-gamma. This therapy has also benefited patients with hyper IgE syndrome by enhancing neutrophil chemotactic responses.

Complement disorders currently are best managed by aggressive antibiotic therapy, prophylactic antibiotic therapy, and active immunization against *H. influenzae* type B, pneumococci, and meningococci.

SUMMARY

Recurrent infections in children are common and are rarely caused by serious underlying disease. Careful history and physical examination usually guide the evaluation through the maze of diagnostic possibilities. Environmental factors often account for many symptoms of recurrent infections. However, if a patient experiences numerous infections beyond the range for a normal child, unusual infections, chronic infections, or unusually severe infections, then an underlying immunodeficiency must be considered. Again, history and physical examination help tailor the laboratory investigation, which includes surveying humoral and cellular arms and phagocytic and complement abnormalities, leading to a diagnosis and possible therapy.

ILLUSTRATIVE CASES

Case 1. A 22-month-old boy comes to his pediatrician with a history of recurrent infections. He had an uncomplicated prenatal and perinatal course and was breast-fed until 8 months of age. He was well until 6 months of age, when he developed fever and rash consistent with roseola. He recovered without antibiotic therapy and was well until 9 months of age, when he developed fever and otitis media that improved after antibiotics were begun. At 13 months of age, he developed diarrhea that lasted for 2 weeks and resolved when lactose was omitted from the diet. At 15 months of age, fever, otitis media, and diarrhea occurred. The otitis media improved after medication, but the diarrhea persisted until antibiotic therapy was discontinued. At 17 months of age the patient developed fever, cough, and conjunctivitis associated with a lingular infiltrate. Otitis media occurred again at 20 months of age and resolved easily, but wheezing associated with clear rhinorrhea developed shortly after antibiotics were discontinued.

Physical examination shows a well-grown, healthy-appearing child with height and weight at the 25th percentile for age. Tympanic membranes are scarred. Lymph nodes and tonsils are normal size. The chest is clear to auscultation, and no hepatosplenomegaly is noted. The skin is normal.

This child falls into the category of a "well child" with recurrent infections. Infections vary as to site and cause and respond appropriately to treatment, and the patient has periods of good health between episodes. Growth data are normal, and no physical signs suggest a systemic disorder. Appropriate therapy is to treat each infection appropriately and provide reassurance to the family. Minimal laboratory tests are indicated.

Case 2. A 15-month-old girl has recurrent pneumonia. She had an uncomplicated prenatal and perinatal course and was fed proprietary formula. At 2 months of age, she was admitted to the hospital with cough and wheezing that slowly resolved. No pneumonia was noted. At 3½ months of age, cough and dyspnea recurred; a chest x-ray film showed hyperinflation and a right middle lobe infiltrate. Treatment with antibiotics and bronchodilators aided resolution. She remained well until 6 months of age, when fever, otitis media, cough, and wheezing were noted. Rales were heard in the left lung, and a chest x-ray film showed a lingular infiltrate with atelectasis. Antibiotics and bronchodilators were given. She improved, but nighttime cough occurred at 10 months of age and continued for 4 weeks. Bronchodilator therapy improved the cough, but she developed an eczematoid skin rash in the flexural creases of her knees and nape of her neck. This was treated with topical corticosteroid cream and emollients. At 13 months of age, recurrent cough without fever occurred and a chest x-ray film showed a right upper lobe atelectasis with compensatory hyperinflation of the right lower lobe. She slowly improved after admission to the hospital and treatment with systemic corticosteroids, bronchodilators, and sodium cromolyn.

Physical examination now reveals a thin but well-appearing child. Height and weight are at the 40th and 25th percentiles respectively. Eczema is noted in the areas previously described. No clubbing is seen. The chest has minimal end-expiratory wheezes.

Laboratory data show a normal complete blood count and white blood count, but the differential shows 13% eosinophils (780 absolute count). A chest x-ray film shows minimal hyperinflation and no infiltrates. Serum IgE level is 400 IU/ml (elevated). Sweat test is normal. Serum IgG, IgA, and IgM levels are normal, and she has protective antibody titers to diphtheria-tetanus.

This patient with recurrent infiltrates has an allergic diathesis with elevated IgE levels. Reactive airway disease has caused her pulmonary complications, and therapy should appropriately be directed toward her asthma.

Case 3. A 3-year-old boy had fever, vomiting, and diarrhea associated with Pseudomonas *sp. sepsis and ecthyma gangrenosum. He was born at 34 weeks gestation but had an uncomplicated history until 10 months of age, when he developed fever and a pseudomonal perianal ulcer. He was successfully treated with antibiotics and* was discharged home. Other infections included one episode of clinical pneumonia and several episodes of bronchitis, otitis media, and gastroenteritis. No adverse reactions to live vaccines were noted. Physical examination was remarkable for a well-grown 3-year-old boy, growth at the 50th percentile for height and weight, a large perianal ulcer, and poorly developed lymphoid tissue. Laboratory evaluation revealed a white blood count of $14,900/mm^3$ with 67% neutrophils, 10% bands, 18% lymphocytes, and 5% monocytes. Quantitative immunoglobulins were as follows: IgG, 6 mg/dl; IgA, 4 mg/dl; IgM, 18 mg/dl; and IgE, unmeasurable. T- and B-cell enumeration were normal, but the patient did not make antibodies to rubella or measles vaccines. Mitogen stimulation, complement values, and NBT tests were all normal.

Monthly injections of gamma globulin were given, then monthly infusions of gamma globulin were administered without recurrence of serious infection. However, as a teenager the patient developed Crohn disease and Raynaud phenomenon.

This patient has CVID. Replacement therapy has been successful in preventing infections, but he has developed other autoimmune phenomena.

ANNOTATED BIBLIOGRAPHY

Dingle JH, Badger GF, Jordan WS Jr: *Illness in the house*, Cleveland, 1964, The Press of Western Reserve University.

This is a classic, massive study on the incidence of illness in children. It gives important information on the frequency of infections in normal children. Notably this study was performed before the common use of daycare centers.

Stiehm ER: Clinical and laboratory evaluation of the child with suspected immunodeficiency, *Pediatr Rev* 7:53-61, 1985.

This is an excellent review of the simple office evaluation of the child with a suspected immunodeficiency.

Wood RA, Sampson HA: The child with frequent infections, *Curr Probl Pediatr* 19:235-284, 1989.

This is a comprehensive review of the approach to the child with frequent infections.

BIBLIOGRAPHY

Buckley RH: Immunodeficiency diseases. In Primer on allergic and immunologic disorders, *JAMA* 268:2797-2806, 1992.

Falloon J, Eddy J, Wiener L, et al: Human immunodeficiency virus infection in children, *J Pediatr* 114:1-30, 1989.

Gallin JI, Malech HL: Update on chronic granulomatous disease of childhood, *JAMA* 263:1533-1537, 1990.

Goodman RA, Osterholm MT, Granoff DM, et al: Infectious diseases and child daycare, *Pediatrics* 74:134-139, 1984.

Gross S, Blaiss MS, Herrod HG: Role of immunoglobulin subclass and specific antibody determinations in the evaluation of recurrent infection in children, *J Pediatr* 121:516-522, 1992.

Hong R: Recurrent infections, *Pediatr Rev* 11:180-183, 1989.

Smith TF: IgG subclasses, *Adv Pediatr* 39:202-236, 1992.

Stiehm ER: They're back: recurrent infections in pediatric practice, *Contemp Pediatr* 7:20-40, 1990.

Tiller TL, Buckley RH: Transient hypogammaglobulinemia of infancy: review of the literature, clinical and immunologic features of 11 new cases, and long-term follow-up, *J Pediatr* 92:347-353, 1978.

Wald ER, Dashefsky B, Byers C, et al: Frequency and severity of infections in daycare, *J Pediatr* 112:540-546, 1988.

Yocum MW, Kelso JM: Common variable immunodeficiency: the disorder and treatment, *Mayo Clin Proc* 66:83-96, 1991.

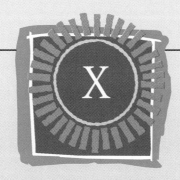

Miscellaneous

27

Fatigue and Chronic Fatigue Syndrome

BASIL J. ZITELLI

 Key Points

- Chronic fatigue syndrome is an increasingly common, poorly understood disorder causing fatigue and withdrawal from daily activities. It affects children and adults.

- Despite extensive investigations into the cause of chronic fatigue syndrome, no convincing link has been established with any infectious agent, including Epstein-Barr virus. Yet, many patients have symptoms suggestive of depression, dysthymia, or adjustment disorder.

- Numerous therapeutic approaches have been attempted with variable results, including a significant placebo effect. A behavioral-cognitive approach has been successful in some adolescents. The long-term outcome generally is good; most patients regain energy and activity.

*F*atigue is a normal consequence of intense physical exertion or mental effort, or it may be a symptom of a variety of specific illnesses. In a survey of primary care practitioners it was the seventh most common complaint, representing 4% of visits to internists and 2.6% of visits to family doctors. In 1984 an estimated $1 billion was expended in the evaluation of fatigue.

Peripheral and Central Fatigue

Fatigue can be divided into peripheral and central causes. Peripheral fatigue occurs as a result of intense muscular action performed either in normal work or recreational activities. It also occurs in disorders, such as myasthenia gravis; my-

opathies; and perhaps postviral infections. In the last condition, muscle deconditioning may occur as a result of bed rest and limited activity or interleukin-1– and prostaglandin E_2–induced proteolysis. In addition a wide variety of organic disorders may have fatigue as part of the symptom complex. A methodologic approach to the differential diagnosis may trace the necessary elements in energy production and use (from respiration and oxygen intake, to hemoglobin and circulation, glucose uptake and use, subcellular energy production, and finally energy expenditure). Virtually every organ system can be involved, and in general a detailed history, meticulous physical examination, and selected screening laboratory tests identify most organic disorders causing persistent fatigue.

Central fatigue normally affects people after periods of intense concentration (e.g., air traffic controlling or studying for a test). It also may be associated with decreased motivation for voluntary motor activity or depressive states. The evaluation of central fatigue presents a major diagnostic dilemma for the clinician because normal peripheral fatigue and fatigue associated with organic disorders also must be considered. A model for the evaluation of chronic fatigue is best exemplified in the holistic approach to the patient with chronic fatigue syndrome (CFS). The following discussion of CFS incorporates essential points in the history, physical examination, differential diagnosis, and approach to the patient that may help the clinician facing any patient with prolonged fatigue.

Chronic Fatigue Syndrome

CFS, an illness that has resurfaced in the 1980s and 1990s, is a major cause of morbidity in industrialized countries. It is characterized by prolonged periods of debilitating fatigue interfering with daily activity levels and often is associated with cognitive deficits and a wide variety of physical complaints, including sore throat, low-grade fever, and lymphadenopathy. In 1990 the Centers for Disease Control (CDC) in Atlanta received nearly 3000 calls per month about CFS and estimated that between 2 and 5 million Americans were affected. Minimum prevalence rates calculated for the 2-year span from 1989 to 1991 ranged from 4.6 to 11.3 per 100,000. More than 80% of the CFS cases affected women, predominantly white. Average age of onset was 30 years.

Although most of the literature deals with CFS in adults, children and adolescents may be affected as well. The studies in children are not as extensive as those in adults, and differences between CFS in children and adults may be noteworthy. The extensive literature on CFS is filled with inconsistencies, contradictions, and differing definitions and denouements, creating confusion and chaos. It is impossible to completely review the entire CFS literature in a brief chapter, but certain consistent trends are reviewed. The history of CFS, particularly as it pertains to Epstein-Barr virus (EBV) infection is summarized to provide a background, and the relationship of CFS to psychobiologic disorders is reviewed. Suspected pathophysiology, differential diagnosis, and evaluation of the patient through routine history and physical examination are presented. An approach to therapy, using holistic methods, is offered.

Pathophysiology

Because the cause of CFS is unknown, the precise pathophysiology is not well understood. Investigators have invoked infections, chronic candidiasis, immune defects, allergies, autoimmune diseases, psychiatric disturbances, sleep disorders, and neurally mediated hypotension as only a few of the possible mechanisms of CFS.

Infection remains one of the favorite theoretical initiating mechanisms of CFS despite the fact that no infectious agent has been isolated. This is in part because of the variety of immune abnormalities found with CFS, reports of elevated levels of interferon-induced 2,5 oligoadenylate synthetase, and the similarity of CFS symptoms to those of injected interferon (fever, fatigue, myalgia, anorexia, dizziness, decreased mental status, depression, confusion, and sleep disturbances). However, elevated interferon levels have not been found.

Disorders of sleep—hypersomnia and insomnia—are common among patients with CFS. Sleep deprivation causes fatigue, irritability, poor mental function, and somatic complaints of musculoskeletal aching, stiffness, nausea, and diarrhea. Sleep and the immune system exhibit bidirectional effects when one is altered, mediated by various cytokines, especially interleukin-1. Investigators found abnormal alpha rhythms during rapid-eye-movement (alpha-delta) sleep in some patients, but this was not a marker for CFS.

Dizziness is a common symptom in CFS, suggesting possible central nervous system (CNS) mechanisms in pathophysiology. Furman found no vestibular abnormality in three adult patients but found nonspecific abnormalities on dynamic posturography suggestive of CNS deficits. Similarly, Rowe and others studied seven pediatric patients with symptoms of chronic fatigue (four satisfied strict criteria for CFS) using upright tilt-table testing (see Fig. 12-1). All seven developed nonsyncopal light-headedness and some degree of hypotension. Four of the patients improved with sodium chloride supplements and beta-blockers or disopyramide (an antidysrhythmic drug). However, both studies were small, had no controls, and could not distinguish between primary pathophysiology and secondary effects of neurally mediated hypotension. In a follow-up study of 23 patients who met the CDC criteria for CFS, all but 1 of the patients had an abnormal response to upright tilt-table testing as compared with 4 of 14 controls. Only nine patients, however, reported complete or nearly complete resolution of symptoms after therapy with fludrocortisone, beta-blockers, or disopyramide. Yet several questions regarding this study and the role of sodium and neurally mediated hypotension in the pathogenesis of CFS remain.

Fatigue is a normal consequence of intensive physical exertion or mental effort, or it may be symptomatic of a variety of specific illnesses. It is a loss of maximal force-generating capacity that develops during muscular activity and persists until the muscle is fully recovered. Fatigue must be distinguished from weakness, which is a diminished ability of the rested muscle to exert maximal force. Fatigue after viral illness may represent deconditioning resulting from bed rest and limited activity. Peripheral fatigue is associated with myasthenia gravis and myopathies. A search for myopathies in CFS has been unrewarding, with most studies revealing no specific muscle pathology. However, CFS patients are deconditioned as evidenced by higher heart rates and blood lactate levels during submaximal exertion, and their perception of the intensity of exercise is distorted. The extent of deconditioning does not explain their fatigue, and investigators suggest that psychologic or psychiatric factors may be of greater importance. Central fatigue may follow lack of motivation, periods of intense concentration, or depressive states. Perhaps the fatigue of CFS begins as postviral deconditioning, progresses to central fatigue, and develops a vicious cycle with progressive deconditioning as well.

Literature Survey

Although a recent resurgence of interest in what is now termed *CFS* has emerged, reports of chronic fatigue date back more than two centuries. In 1750, Manningham published a treatise describing a condition referred to as *febricula*, which bears numerous similarities to CFS. A century later, Beard coined the term *neurasthenia* for a symptom complex thought to reflect an organic weakness of nervous elements occurring in vulnerable people with great potential. At the turn of the century, clustering of cases with symptoms similar to CFS occurred among the upper class in the United Kingdom. A variety of therapeutic approaches, including absolute rest, spas, and mineral baths, were used. No treatment was as effective in restoring activity as encouraging an active and healthy lifestyle. The illness tended to disappear from the ranks of the upper class as more of the middle class began to complain of similar symptoms. Other names used to describe epidemics of fatigue from 1930 to 1950 are listed in Box 27-1, including more modern terminology.

The Role of Epstein-Barr Virus

Persistent fatigue after infectious mononucleosis (IM) was first described by Isaacs in 1948. However, this and other early reports relied on nonspecific tests, such as lymphocytosis and the heterophile antibody test. EBV was not discovered until 1964 and was not linked with IM until 1968. Only after the development of specific EBV serologic testing did investigators begin the quest to link chronic fatigue with EBV infection. Tobi and others were among the first to report a group of patients with prolonged illnesses associated with chronic fatigue, fever, adenopathy, weight loss, malaise, and serologic evidence of EBV infection. In 1984 DuBois reported similar findings in 14 patients, but (as in the study by Tobi) positive EBV serology was required for study entry.

In 1985, 1 year later, two back-to-back articles by Jones and others and Straus and others generated increased interest in the role of EBV in CFS. Jones and others found elevated antibody to viral capsid antigen (VCA) and early antigen (EA) when compared with controls. Five patients with similar symptoms, however, had no antibody to EBV. Immune studies did not differentiate CFS patients from controls when T and B cells were enumerated and lymphocyte function was assessed. These investigators concluded that EBV infection may be responsible for chronic illness.

Straus and others investigated 31 patients referred to the National Institutes of Health (NIH) for symptoms of CFS. Eight patients were found to have other diagnoses, such as Sjögren syndrome, systemic lupus erythematosus, Hodgkin disease, and multiple sclerosis. Similar to Jones, Straus found elevated IgG to VCA and EA when compared with undefined controls. Immune studies showed no expansion of virally transformed lymphocytes and a normal $CD4^+:CD8^+$ ratio. Although interferon levels were not elevated, an enzyme induced by interferon (2,5 oligoadenylate synthetase) was elevated in five patients. Straus concluded that EBV may be associated with chronic illness in adults, but its exact role in causing CFS or continuing symptoms was uncertain.

Despite these reports of a possible association of EBV with CFS, subsequent reports could not show causation. The CDC was called to investigate an epidemic of CFS symptoms in Incline Village, Nevada. Holmes and others interviewed 134 patients. Only 33 patients had symptoms lasting long enough to be considered possible CFS. Of those 33 patients, 18 had other disorders, including parvovirus infection, depression, pregnancy, thyroiditis, Crohn disease, cirrhosis, congestive heart failure, anemia, and other diagnoses, to explain symptoms. Holmes found no difference between patients and controls in

---

BOX 27-1

Terminology Applied to Chronic Fatigue

Older Terminology (1860-1980)	Newer Terminology (1980-1990)
Akureyri disease	Prolonged mononucleosis
Iceland disease	Chronic mononucleosis
Atypical polio	Chronic Epstein-Barr virus
Benign myalgic enceph-	infection
alomyelitis	Chronic fatigue syndrome
Epidemic neuromy-	
asthenia	
Encephalomyelitis	
Postviral syndrome	
Neurasthenia	
Chronic brucellosis	
Postinfluenzal neurasthenia	
Royal Free Hospital disease	

EBV serology. Furthermore, EBV serologic tests were run in three different laboratories, and up to 80% of specimens had fourfold or greater discrepancies in anti-EA(R), and 11% had similar discrepancies in IgG to VCA. These results cast doubt on subjective test interpretation and methodology. In a companion paper, Buchwald surveyed patients in an adult primary care clinic without regard to EBV status and found that CFS symptoms were prevalent (21%) but no differences in EBV serologies were noted between patients and controls.

In a meta-analysis of EBV and CFS, numerous deficiencies plagued the studies advocating EBV as the cause of CFS. Controls were poorly defined, and epidemiologic data were limited. Earlier reports included only patients who were EBV-serology positive, particularly those with persistent anti-EA, which was thought to indicate an ongoing infection. However, Horwitz and others demonstrated that IgG to VCA and antibody to EA can persist normally in high titers for years. Most reports were prevalence studies, which cannot etiologically link causality. Many studies did not measure rheumatoid factor, which may confound and cross-react with IgM to VCA, and different laboratories lacked reproducibility. Often, patients had other diagnoses that were overlooked by physicians. EBV serologies had significant overlap with normal controls, and many investigators did not consider the possibility of nonspecific polyclonal stimulation accounting for elevated EBV titers.

One of the major drawbacks to earlier studies was the lack of consistent case definition for CFS. After the Incline Village outbreak, Holmes and others developed a strict, working case definition (Box 27-2). Because no diagnostic test has been developed for CFS, the definition is based on signs and symptoms. A case of CFS must fulfill both major criteria and certain minor criteria as follows: at least 6 of 11 symptom criteria *and* 2 of 3 physical criteria or

Case Definition of Chronic Fatigue Syndrome

Major Criteria

1. New onset of persisting or relapsing, debilitating fatigue or easy fatigability in a person who has no previous history of similar symptoms that does not resolve with bed rest and is severe enough to reduce or impair average daily activity below 50% of the patient's premorbid activity level for a period of at least 6 months.

2. Other clinical conditions that may produce similar symptoms must be excluded by thorough evaluation based on history, physical examination, and appropriate laboratory findings. These conditions include malignancy; autoimmune disease; chronic or subacute bacterial disease, fungal disease, and parasitic disease; disease related to human immunodeficiency virus (HIV) infection; chronic psychiatric disease, either newly diagnosed or by history; chronic inflammatory disease; neuromuscular disease; endocrine disease; drug dependency or abuse; side effects of a chronic medication or other toxic agent; or other known or defined chronic pulmonary, gastrointestinal, hepatic renal, or hematologic disease.

Minor Criteria

Symptom criteria

To fulfill a symptom criterion, a symptom must have begun at or after the time of onset of increased fatigability and must have persisted or recurred over a period of at least 6 months.

1. Mild fever (oral temperature between 37.5° and 38.6° C, if measured by the patient) or chills

Minor Criteria—cont'd

Symptom criteria—cont'd

2. Sore throat
3. Painful lymph nodes in the anterior or posterior cervical or axillary distribution
4. Unexplained generalized muscle weakness
5. Muscle discomfort or myalgia
6. Prolonged (24 hours or greater) generalized fatigue after levels of exercise that would have been easily tolerated in the patient's premorbid state
7. Generalized headache (different from headache experienced by the patient in the premorbid state)
8. Migratory arthralgia without joint swelling or redness
9. Neuropsychologic complaints (one or more of the following: photophobia, transient visual scotomas, forgetfulness, excessive irritability, confusion, difficulty thinking, inability to concentrate, and depression)
10. Sleep disturbance (hypersomnia or insomnia)
11. Description of the main symptom complex as initially developing over a few hours to a few days

Physical criteria

Physical criteria must be documented by a physician on at least two occasions, at least 1 month apart.

1. Low grade fever (oral temperature between 37.6° and 38.6° C or rectal temperature between 37.8° and 38.8° C)
2. Nonexudative pharyngitis
3. Palpable or tender anterior or posterior cervical or axillary lymph nodes

From Holmes GP, Kaplan JE, Gantz MM, et al: Chronic fatigue syndrome: a working case definition, *Ann Intern Med* 108:387-389, 1988. The patient must have both major criteria and either at least 6 of 11 symptom criteria *and* 2 of 3 physical criteria or at least 8 of 11 symptom criteria.

8 of 11 symptom criteria. The criteria have been criticized for being too strict, excluding many adults who have most of the symptoms; and the criteria may not apply to children and adolescents.

A revised set of diagnostic criteria was suggested by the National Institutes of Health in 1994 (K. Fukuda and others) that requires a complete history, physical and mental status examination, and general laboratory screening tests to exclude other disorders. CFS can be diagnosed if the patient has new onset of fatigue not resulting from ongoing exertion, not alleviated by rest, and causing significant reduction in activities. Patients should have at least four of the following: cognitive dysfunction, sore throat, tender cervical or axillary lymph nodes, myalgias, arthralgia without objective signs, headache of a new pattern, unrefreshing sleep, and postexertional malaise.

The quest for an infectious agent causing CFS continued long after EBV was discarded as the major causative agent because of

numerous immune abnormalities found in patients with CFS. These abnormalities, however, are variable and have not been observed consistently in all groups of patients (Box 27-3). Furthermore the magnitude of the immunologic changes is small and is not related to the severity of the patient's symptoms.

Despite intensive investigation, no infectious agent has been found to consistently cause CFS. Cytomegalovirus (CMV), *Mycoplasma* species, *Toxoplasma* species, herpes simplex virus type 1 (HSV-1), HSV-2, measles, yeast, *Borrelia* species, human herpesvirus 6 (HHV-6), retroviruses, and numerous other agents have been examined without consistent or reproducible results. As of mid-1997, no evidence had been found to implicate any infectious agent.

Psychiatric Implications of Chronic Fatigue

The similarity of CFS symptoms and depression symptoms led numerous investigators to examine the psychiatric implications of the symptom complex. In the 1940s and 1950s, the term *chronic brucellosis* was applied to patients who had persistent nonspecific symptoms after acute *Brucella* organism infection, similar to current-day CFS patients. Although objective clinical and laboratory testing could not distinguish rapidly recovering patients from chronic patients, delay in recovery was found to be largely related to the patient's emotional adjustment rather than ongoing infection. Similarly, patients recovering from an Asian influenza epidemic in 1957 sometimes exhibited delayed recovery. In a group of patients who had psychologic testing before and after the infection, delayed recovery was more frequent in a subset of patients shown to be prone to depression.

Manu and others described 135 patients with debilitating fatigue for more than 6 months who were self-referred to a fatigue clinic. Using the Diagnostic Interview Schedule, evidence of major depression was found in 50% of patients, and other psychiatric diagnoses were found in 31%. Kreusi and others from the NIH assessed the psychiatric status of patients with CFS. Identifiable psychiatric diagnoses were found in 21 of 28 patients (75%), and 19 of 21 had a history of psychiatric disorders (e.g., anxiety disorder, depression, or alcohol abuse) that predated the onset of CFS symptoms. Nearly half of the affected patients had a lifetime prevalence of major depressive episodes greater than a group of patients with a chronic medical illness, diabetes mellitus. Gold and others also found more lifetime episodes of major depression (73% versus 22%) and prevalence of depression in CFS (42% vs 0%) patients compared with controls, and most patients with CFS had onset of depression before symptoms of CFS. Other investigators, however, have concluded that depressive symptoms in CFS patients occur secondary to or share a common pathophysiology with immunologic dysfunction rather than being part of the primary mechanism of illness. It must be emphasized that the strict definition of CFS specifically excludes major psychiatric illness.

Reconciliation of the immune abnormalities with the psychiatric implications of CFS requires examination of the psychobiology of stress. Numerous reports chronicle alterations of the human immune response to life events and psychiatric illnesses. Psychologic stress is associated with an increased risk of acute infectious illnesses. Severe depression and bereavement cause impaired lymphocyte function. "Poor copers" exhibit reduced killer cell activity; loneliness, stress, isolation, and school examinations alter immunoglobulin levels and killer cell activity. Lymphocyte activity, via surface receptors, may be altered by changes in circulating hormone levels associated with changes in emotion. Hence the presence of nonspecific immune abnormalities does not negate the possible contribution of stress to the pathophysiology of CFS.

Children and Chronic Fatigue

Although CFS most commonly affects adults, increasing numbers of children and adolescents are being evaluated for symptoms of chronic fatigue. Jones and others studied 18 children under 15 years of age and concluded that children with CSF were similar to adults in all ways except that children generally had relapsing illness rather than persistent illness. Bell, as noted by Levine and others, studied a cluster of 32 children with similar CSF symptoms to those of adults and found that overt emotional symptoms were less common and somatic symptoms were more common. Although it was difficult to estimate the disability, at least 37% of children missed at least 6 months of school. Interestingly, nearly half (46.9%) had a family member with similar symptoms. In another study by Bell and others in rural upstate New York, 21 children ages 10 to 16 years had symptoms of CFS that were correlated strongly with the following three variables: (1) other family members with symptoms of CFS, (2) recent ingestion of raw milk, and (3) a history of allergy or asthma. Also they found no gender difference. Smith and associates studied 15 adolescents (nine girls and six boys) with CFS and found five subjects with major depression. The other subjects endorsed many secondary symptoms of depression but were less likely to exhibit depressed mood, guilt, and suicidal tendencies. School avoidance related to expectations for high academic performance, overprotection and overindulgence by the family, and difficulties with maternal-child separation may contribute to chronic stress, exacerbating the patient's feelings of depression and fatigue. In addition, adolescent CFS patients had higher scores on measures of somatic complaints, depression, internalizing symptoms, and feeling different than others when compared with a group of matched childhood cancer survivors. In a case-control study of CFS in pediatric patients, significant decline in the quality of life occurred, but CFS patients tended to fall between healthy and depressed controls on measures of affective disturbance.

The diagnosis of depression requires fulfillment of certain diagnostic criteria (Box 27-4). Each of the following criteria is necessary to establish a diagnosis of major depression: (1) a sense of distress and ill-being, (2) self-deprecation, and (3) impaired function. Masked depression may take the guise of somatic complaints, including headache, abdominal pain, dizziness, nausea, and hyperactivity, along with school avoidance, eating disorders, and substance abuse. Dysthymia, a less intense but more chronic form of depression, may be present. Patients diagnosed with dysthymia also must meet diagnostic criteria (Box 27-4). A patient who has no history of a major depressive episode but fulfills five of nine criteria for 2 weeks qualifies for the diagnosis of dysthymia. Note that thoughts of death and suicidal tendencies are not required for dysthymia. Adjustment disorder is even less severe (Box 27-4). The symptoms may manifest themselves as mood alterations, changes in behavior, or physical complaints. Children who are unable to express symptoms accurately or adolescents who do not have major depression may fulfill diagnostic criteria for dysthymia or adjustment disorder.

Follow-Up of Patients With Chronic Fatigue

CFS carries low mortality but high morbidity. Follow-up studies in adults and children emphasize that symptoms may persist for months or even years, but most patients ultimately improve, even without intervention. Over time, many patients have functional improvement but still complain of feeling ill. In a prospective study by Gold and others, at nearly 1 year after initial assessment 19% of 21 adults were completely normal, and another 38% were significantly improved. Two thirds of patients still complained of fatigue. Hellinger found that at follow-up 30 months later approximately half of the patients had resolution of symptoms or were improved, and in a follow-up study to the Incline Village outbreak, Holmes reported that 10 of 15 patients were able to return to work by 18 months. Bell reported that 54% of children had resolved or improved within 6 months. Smith and others followed 15 adolescents for 13 to 32 months and reported 4 were normal, 4 were improved, and 7 were unchanged or worse. With intervention using a joint pediatric-psychiatric approach, all 5 patients accepting therapy were successfully rehabilitated. Variability in clinical improvement is the rule, oftentimes regardless of intervention. If symptoms persist longer than 2 years, recovery rates diminish, and it becomes increasingly difficult to distinguish between effects of illness and lifestyle adaptation to the illness.

Differential Diagnosis

The differential diagnosis of chronic fatigue is large and encompasses disorders affecting virtually every system. Common problems to exclude are listed in Box 27-5. Anemia and its causes should be pursued, and careful history and physical examination should be directed at a search for common infectious agents, such as hepatitis (A, B, or C), EBV, CMV, Lyme disease, tuberculosis, and possibly HIV. Chronic liver disease or renal disease, including chronic urinary tract infection, should be ruled out. Endocrine disorders, such as diabetes mellitus, hyperthyroidism, hypothyroidism, or more uncommonly Addison disease and true hypoglycemia, may

---

BOX 27-4

Diagnosis of Depression, Dysthymia, and Adjustment Disorder

Diagnostic Criteria for Major Depression
Depressive mood
Diminished interest or pleasure
Significant alterations in weight
Sleep disturbances
Psychomotor agitation or retardation
Fatigue
Feelings of self-worthlessness
Lack of concentration
Recurrent thoughts of death or suicide

Diagnostic Criteria for Dysthymia
Depressed or irritable mood for most of the day, persisting for a majority of days for 1 year in children and adolescents
Presence, when depressed, of at least two of the following:
  1. Poor appetite or overeating
  2. Sleep disturbances
  3. Low energy or fatigue
  4. Low self-esteem
  5. Poor concentration or decision-making ability
  6. Feelings of hopelessness
During the 1 year of symptoms, the child or adolescent is not without symptoms for more than 2 months

Diagnostic Criteria for Adjustment Disorder
Reaction within 3 months to identifiable psychologic stressors
Impairment of school or social functioning beyond what would be expected for the stressor
Symptom cluster that is not another instance of a clear pattern of overreaction to stressors
Symptoms lasting no more than 6 months

---

cause fatigue. Cardiopulmonary disorders, especially if associated with chronic hypoxia, and a variety of gastrointestinal diseases, such as Crohn disease, ulcerative colitis, and irritable bowel syndrome, cause fatigue. Autoimmune and collagen disorders, particularly juvenile rheumatoid arthritis, systemic lupus erythematosus, scleroderma, and the CFS rheumatologic equivalent—fibromyalgia—may have associated fatigue. Fibromyalgia shares many common features with CFS. Neurologic disorders, such as seizures (especially frequent absence spells), myasthenia gravis, neuropathies, myopathies, and sleep disorders, should be sought by history and examination. Malignancies, especially leukemia or lymphoma, may initially cause fatigue. Although many investigators doubt the existence of the "tension-allergy-fatigue" syndrome, recurrent allergic disease or sinusitis may have fatigue as part of the symptom complex. Psychiatric disor-

Partial Differential Diagnosis of Chronic Fatigue

Anemia
Infections
  Hepatitis (A, B, C)
  EBV
  CMV
  Lyme disease
  Tuberculosis
  HIV
Liver disease
Renal disease
Endocrine disorders
  Diabetes mellitus
  Hyperthyroidism or
    hypothyroidism
  Addison disease
  True hypoglycemia
Cardiac disease
Pulmonary disease
Gastrointestinal disorders
  Crohn disease
  Ulcerative colitis
  Irritable bowel syndrome
Autoimmune/collagen disorders

Juvenile rheumatoid arthritis
Systemic lupus erythematosus
Scleroderma
Fibromyalgia
Neurologic disorders
  Seizures
  Neuropathies
  Myopathies
  Sleep disorders
Malignancy
Allergy
Psychiatric disorders
  Depression
  Dysthymia
  Adjustment disorder
  Anxiety disorder
Miscellaneous
  Pregnancy
  Medications/drugs/drug abuse
  Toxins
  Changes in lifestyle

Clinical Presentation of Chronic Fatigue Syndrome

Symptom	Percentage
Fatigue	100
Forgetfulness	100
Muscle weakness	93
Headache	86
Inability to concentrate	86
Sleep disturbance	86
Sore throat	78
Tender lymph nodes	64
Myalgia	64
Confusion	57
Feverishness	57
Arthralgia	50
Irritability	43
Depression	43
Allergies	64
Gastrointestinal complaints	64
Dizziness	36

Modified from Dale JK, Straus SE: The chronic fatigue syndrome: considerations relevant to children and adolescents, *Adv Pediatr Infect Dis* 7:63-83, 1992.

ders, particularly depression, dysthymia, adjustment disorders, and anxiety disorders, frequently are found in patients with protracted fatigue. Miscellaneous considerations include pregnancy, medication and drug effects, toxin exposures, and variations in lifestyle, such as excessive or inadequate exercise or work.

History

Because of the complexity of CFS and the broad differential diagnosis, the history is frequently the physician's greatest diagnostic tool. In general the history should be obtained in a quiet, unhurried fashion, with open-ended questions allowing for new leads offered by the patient or family. The parents and the patient should be interviewed together and separately, giving each the opportunity to express fears or concerns that may have been inhibited in the presence of the other. The history frequently is extensive and may take several sessions to complete. A thorough history, however, often is the initial step in therapy, demonstrating that the physician is examining all possibilities and leaving no stone unturned.

Initial history should include the timing of and circumstances surrounding the onset of symptoms (Table 27-1). Frequently, patients relate an abrupt onset of symptoms associated with signs and symptoms of infection. Often the infection disappears, but the symptoms of chronic fatigue persist. Pervasive fatigue does not resolve with bed rest and may be exacerbated by physical activity or emotional stress. Symptoms may be constant or may wax and wane. Feelings of feverishness and possible low-grade fever may be recorded. Straus and others, however, measured body temperature of CFS patients who complained of fever and found none who had documented rectal temperatures above 37.7° C. Patients may complain of sore throat, but on examination little or no hyperemia can be found, and routine throat cultures for common viruses and bacteria are normal. Although tender lymph nodes may be a presenting symptom, truly enlarged lymph nodes are uncommon and may point to another diagnosis. Arthralgias and myalgias commonly affect the extremities and back but are not associated with objective findings. Tenderness at specific trigger points may suggest a diagnosis of fibromyalgia, although this is an uncommon pediatric diagnosis. Headache is common before and after the onset of illness, and the character of the headache should be distinguished from that of headaches that predated CFS symptoms. Gastrointestinal complaints, nonspecific rashes, and genitourinary symptoms also may occur.

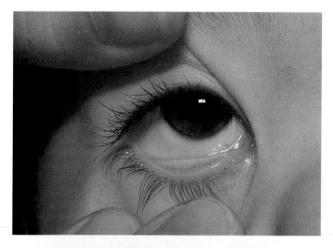

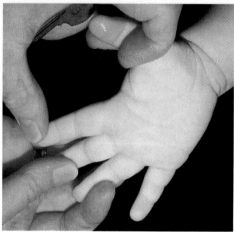

FIG. 27-1   Pale conjunctivae and palmar crease pallor indicating severe anemia, with a hemoglobin level less than 7 g/dl.

Neurocognitive symptoms should be explored. Difficulties with short-term memory, information processing, mild episodic confusion, depression, irritability, anxiety, and sleep disorders may be present.

Searching for other causes of fatigue demands a rigorous review of systems, with questions directed at the common disorders listed in Box 27-5. Pallor (Fig. 27-1) and evidence of blood loss suggests anemia, and fever, adenopathy, rash, cough, or localized pain may point to infection. Jaundice and ascites are linked to liver disorders, and flank pain and a history of urinary tract infections suggest possible renal involvement. Polyuria, polydipsia, changes in weight (see Fig. 28-9), or skin changes (see Fig. 12-5) may implicate endocrine disease. Cyanosis or exercise intolerance points to cardiopulmonary disease, and abdominal pain, vomiting, diarrhea, and linear growth deceleration may suggest gastrointestinal involvement (see Fig. 1-1). Rash, fever, weakness, arthralgia, and arthritis may point to rheumatologic disease. Episodic symptoms, weakness without cognitive changes, and sleep apnea point toward neurologic problems, whereas insidious symptoms of weight loss, fever, organomegaly, and pain may suggest malignancies. Allergy may have a seasonal variation, a positive family history, and other symptoms of atopy, such as eczema, rhinitis, or asthma. Psychiatric disorders may be difficult to separate from pure CFS. A careful, sensitive sexual history may reveal possible sexually transmitted diseases or even early pregnancy. Use of medications or illicit drugs and toxin exposures should be sought. Any changes in lifestyle, such as alteration in family structure; death in the family; moving; and changes in school, peer relations, employment, religious feelings, or a wide variety of other daily activities should be noted.

History of familial or inheritable diseases is important. Also the presence of psychiatric disease within the immediate family may have similar implications for the patient. Similarly, in one study nearly half of the children with protracted fatigue had a parent with similar symptoms.

Physical Examination

The physical examination of patients with chronic fatigue is frequently normal. Particular attention, however, should be paid to growth parameters, noting any plateau of linear growth or excessive changes in weight. Vital signs indicating tachycardia, tachypnea, or hypertension may be important clues to cardiopulmonary or renal disease.

The general examination should be meticulous and preferably done in the presence of the parents to assure them of the completeness of the evaluation. Examination for rash, adenopathy (including accurate measurements), respiratory or cardiac abnormalities, abdominal tenderness or organomegaly, genitourinary abnormalities (including perianal disease and occult blood noted on rectal examination), musculoskeletal tenderness or swelling, and neurologic symptoms is paramount. The neurologic examination should include mental status assessment, a careful retinal examination, and evaluation of motor strength and deep tendon reflexes.

Approach to the Patient

Laboratory evaluation of the patient with protracted fatigue depends largely on the clues the clinician obtains from the history and physical examination. The evaluation may be staged, depending on the expense and invasiveness of the procedures. The clinician must avoid becoming a part of the pathophysiologic process by pursuing a never-ending and increasingly frustrating search for a purely organic cause for symptoms. The following three factors present at diagnosis of CFS predict continuing symptoms 6 months later: (1) the patient's tendency to somatize symptoms; (2) the physician's provision of excuses for school or work; and (3) the physician's uncertainty about the diagnosis. The relentless search for a physical cause emphasizes the inappropriate stigma attached to psychiatric disease and implies that nonorganic disorders have no physical basis. However, some screening laboratory tests may be appropriate and are listed in Box 27-6. Not all of these tests

Some Suggested Screening Laboratory Tests

Complete blood cell count and differential count
Erythrocyte sedimentation rate
Electrolytes, urea nitrogen, creatinine
Liver enzyme panel
Urinalysis
Thyroid function tests
Antinuclear antibodies
Mantoux test with control skin testing
Chest roentgenogram
Pregnancy test
HIV antibodies

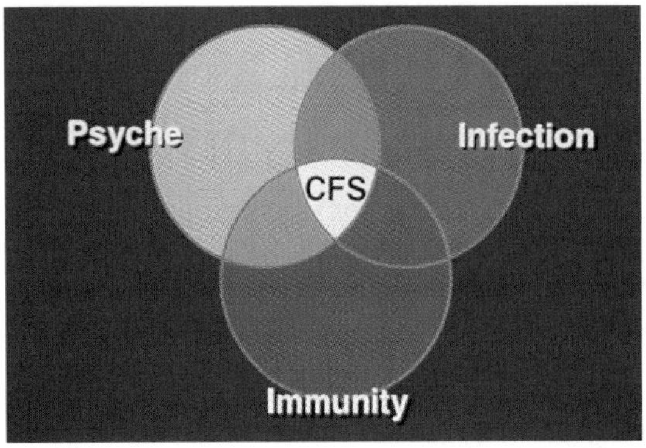

FIG. 27-2 A possible unifying hypothesis. An infection in a psychologically vulnerable patient may set off a vicious cycle of fatigue and lack of energy, leading to alterations of the immune system found in CFS patients.

must be done, and others may be indicated by the clinical assessment. Viral titers to numerous agents may be misleading because nonspecific elevation in humoral responses to a number of antigens may be found without suggesting a specific cause.

It is beyond the scope of this chapter to extensively discuss therapy. Numerous therapies have been applied to patients, including oophorectomy, acyclovir, intramuscular and intravenous gamma globulin, intramuscular liver extract (folic acid), cyanocobalamin, fish oil, licorice, and magnesium sulfate. No single therapy has been shown to be substantially more effective than another, and most studies have demonstrated a significant placebo effect. Tricyclic antidepressants have been beneficial in some patients but not consistently, and other medications, such as fluoxetine or bupropion, also have shown variable results.

Other approaches have used cognitive-behavioral therapy. This program involves recognition and acceptance of an illness that is not well understood and reassurance that serious underlying physical ailments have been excluded. Baseline information about current activity is kept in a daily log or diary. An active rehabilitation program is designed to gradually increase patient activity in school, leisure, social, and physical domains. Home schooling is discouraged after the patient is caught up with current academic activities, and an exercise program, including outings and sports participation, is initiated. Physical therapy may be of benefit as well. Disturbance of sleep cycles is gradually realigned more toward a normal schedule by slowly shifting periods of wakefulness and sleep. In one study by Verecker, using this approach, all children who accepted the therapy exhibited substantial improvement. Other anecdotal reports of success using similar methods have been published.

The clinician should consider referral if he or she is uncertain about the diagnosis of CFS, a psychiatric diagnosis is entertained, or the patient or family is recalcitrant to therapy.

SUMMARY

Chronic fatigue and protracted fatigue are poorly understood, highly emotional clinical syndromes with no mortality but associated with significant morbidity. The clinician is challenged to sort through an extensive differential diagnosis, using all available clinical acumen to arrive at a diagnosis. Conflicting theories of cause and pathogenesis abound. However, one possible unifying hypothesis is represented in Fig. 27-2. A common infectious illness affects a particularly psychosocially vulnerable individual, who frequently is engaged in a busy or frenetic lifestyle. The infection interferes with normal activities and potentially creates abnormal physiologic changes in immune function and cytokine release. The patient's psychologic response may compound these nonspecific changes, and although symptoms of the infection disappear, the changes of chronic fatigue persist. The approach to the patient demands an extensive history, looking for physical and psychosocial causes of fatigue and any possible interplay of the two as well. The physical examination and laboratory studies usually are normal and should reassure the physician and patient so that specific therapeutic interventions, often using a cognitive-behavioral approach, may be employed. Rehabilitation frequently is prolonged, taking weeks to months, but is significantly shorter than the period for improvement without intervention.

ILLUSTRATIVE CASES

Case 1. A 16-year-old white girl was evaluated for complaints of fatigue, headache, and myalgia lasting for 1 year. The illness began with fever, sore throat, and malaise. A Monospot test was normal, but throat culture was positive for Streptococcus pyogenes, *and she was treated with a 10-day course of penicillin. Fever and sore throat resolved, but fatigue, malaise, and myalgia per-*

sisted. She gradually dropped out of extracurricular school activities, such as band and foreign language club, and stopped going to a church youth group. She has required home tutoring over the previous 4 months. She has difficulty falling asleep, sleeps until noon, and is tired on awakening. Headache is constant and bitemporal and occurs daily but is not associated with nausea or vomiting. Difficulty concentrating and forgetfulness developed 9 months ago. Repeated evaluations by her physician have been unrevealing, with repeated normal physical examination and laboratory tests. The physician recommended decreasing activities further and getting more rest. She denied feelings of sadness or hopelessness or having suicidal thoughts.

Family history is positive; her mother was diagnosed as having fibromyalgia and CFS.

Physical examination reveals normal vital signs and no abnormal change in height or weight, and general examination was normal.

Laboratory studies, including complete blood count, electrolytes, thyroid function tests, liver and renal function tests, chest radiograph, and Mantoux test, were all normal.

Rehabilitation began with extensive explanation of the differential diagnosis of CFS and reassurance as to why she did not have any serious organic disease. Initially, her sleep cycle was gradually shifted so she got up at a more usual time, and a graded, gradually increasing exercise program was instituted along with physical therapy. Energy gradually improved, and socialization with friends was encouraged. After 6 weeks she was able to attend school for one half of the day, and after 8 weeks she was in school full time. After 3 months she felt much better and had resumed most of her premorbid activities, although she still said she occasionally felt fatigued.

This case represents a typical adolescent with symptoms of chronic fatigue and successful use of a cognitive-behavioral approach.

Case 2. A 17-year-old boy was seen for a 7-month history of irritability, mood swings, fatigue, difficulty sleeping, and intermittent abdominal pain. The patient had a history of recurrent abdominal pain for 4 years but no diarrhea or weight loss. Irritability and fatigue began insidiously about 7 months previously, and he has missed 3 months of school because of fatigue and difficulty concentrating. Repeated evaluations by his physician, including radiographic gastrointestinal series, blood counts, sedimentation rate, urinalysis, liver tests, and thyroid function tests, were all normal. The patient claimed difficulty falling asleep and fatigue upon arising in the morning. He claimed marked fatigue after minimal exercise. When questioned alone, he said he had feelings of sadness but did not know why and at times cried privately. He saw no end to the illness, and he had entertained thoughts of suicide.

Physical examination was normal except for evidence of a 30-pound weight gain in 5 months.

Screening laboratory tests, including cortisol levels, were normal. He was referred to a child psychiatrist, who diagnosed major depression and began a program of psychotherapy and tricyclic antidepressants resulting in gradual improvement and return to normal activities.

Depression frequently presents as chronic fatigue and may carry many of the same complaints. A careful psychosocial and psychiatric history may reveal warning signs that indicate psychiatric referral may be necessary.

Case 3. A 15-year-old white girl was evaluated for a 5-month history of fatigue and "change of attitude." The patient dated onset of symptoms after an influenza-like illness and complained of progressive fatigue out of proportion to her physical activity. A 10-pound weight loss was noted over the 5-month period. Sleep was unaffected, and she continued to attend school, although her grade average fell. She admitted becoming apathetic about school and usual activities, but she denied decreased concentrating ability or forgetfulness. She also denied feelings of sadness, depression, or suicide. Evaluation by her physician was unremarkable, including blood count, electrolytes, liver and renal function tests, and thyroid function tests. EBV titers indicated distant, past infection, and CMV and Toxoplasma sp. tests were negative. Family history was remarkable for Hodgkin disease in the paternal aunt.

Physical examination was remarkable for a diffuse, even tanning of the skin, including unexposed areas, and darkening of palmar creases. Gingiva demonstrated hyperpigmentation.

Laboratory data revealed the following values: sodium, 135 mEq/L; potassium, 5.8 mEq/L; normal liver tests; urinary electrolytes; sodium, 200 mEq/L; chloride, 238 mEq/L; and low serum cortisol levels, even after stimulation. The patient was diagnosed with Addison disease, and she rapidly improved with glucocorticoid and mineralocorticoid supplementation.

This case emphasizes the value of a careful history and physical examination, looking for any of the myriad of causes of fatigue associated with a primary organic disease.

ANNOTATED BIBLIOGRAPHY

Bock GR, Whelan T, editors: *Chronic fatigue syndrome*, Ciba Foundation Symposium 173, Chichester, 1993, John Wiley & Sons.

This extensive symposium covering virtually all aspects of CFS is detailed, conflicting, and controversial.

Koo D: Chronic fatigue syndrome: a critical appraisal of the role of Epstein-Barr virus, *West J Med* 150:590-596, 1989.

This is an excellent critical review that summarizes data indicating Epstein-Barr virus is not the causative agent of CFS.

Smith MS, Mitchell J, Corey L, et al: Chronic fatigue in adolescents, *Pediatrics* 88:195-202, 1991.

This is a summary of CFS in a small group of adolescents with a fairly typical presentation. It provides excellent discussion with outcome.

BIBLIOGRAPHY

Beard TC: Chronic fatigue syndrome and neurally mediated hypotension, *JAMA* 275:359, 1996.

Bell KM, Cookfair D, Bell DS, et al: Risk factors associated with chronic fatigue syndrome in a cluster of pediatric cases, *Rev Infect Dis* 13(suppl 1):S32-S38, 1991.

Bou-Holaigah I, Rowe PC, Kan J, et al: The relationship between neurally mediated hypotension and the chronic fatigue syndrome, *JAMA* 274:961-967, 1995.

Buchwald D, Sullivan JL, Komoroff AL: Frequency of "chronic active Epstein-Barr virus infection" in a general medical practice, *JAMA* 257:2303-2307, 1987.

Carter BD, Edwards JF, Kronenberger WG, et al: Case control study of chronic fatigue in pediatric patients, *Pediatrics* 95:179-186, 1995.

Cope H, David A, Pelosi A, et al: Predictors of chronic "postviral" fatigue, *Lancet* 344:864-868, 1994.

Dale JK, Straus SE: The chronic fatigue syndrome: considerations relevant to children and adolescents, *Adv Pediatr Infect Dis* 7:63-83, 1992.

DuBois RE, Seeley JK, Brus I, et al: Chronic mononucleosis syndrome, *South Med J* 77:1376-1382, 1984.

Fukuda K, Straus SE, Hickie I, et al: The chronic fatigue syndrome: a comparative approach to its definition and study, *Ann Intern Med* 121:953-959, 1994.

Furman JMR: Testing of vestibular function: an adjunct in the assessment of chronic fatigue syndrome, *Rev Infect Dis* 13(suppl 1):S109-S111, 1991.

Gold D, Bowden R, Sixbey J, et al: Chronic fatigue, *JAMA* 264:48-53, 1990.

Hellinger WC, Smith TF, Van Scoy RE, et al: Chronic fatigue syndrome and the diagnostic utility of antibody to Epstein-Barr virus early antigen, *JAMA* 260:971-973, 1988.

Hickie I, Lloyd A, Wakefield D: Immunological and psychological dysfunction in patients receiving immunotherapy for chronic fatigue syndrome, *Aust N Z J Psychiatry* 26:249-256, 1992.

Holmes GP, Kaplan JE, Gantz NM, et al: Chronic fatigue syndrome: a working case definition, *Ann Intern Med* 108:387-389, 1988.

Holmes GP, Kaplan JE, Stewart JA, et al: A cluster of patients with a mononucleosis-like syndrome, *JAMA* 257:2297-2302, 1987.

Horwitz CA, Henle W, Henle G, et al: Long-term serological follow-up of patients for Epstein-Barr virus after recovery from infectious mononucleosis, *J Infect Dis* 151:1150-1153, 1985.

Imboden JB, Canter A, Cluff LE, et al: Convalescence from influenza: a study of the psychological and clinical determinants, *Arch Intern Med* 108:393-399, 1961.

Isaacs R: Chronic infectious mononucleosis, *Blood* 3:858-861, 1948.

Jones JF, Ray G, Minnick L, et al: Evidence for active Epstein-Barr virus infection with persistent unexplained illness: elevated anti–early antigen antibodies, *Ann Intern Med* 102:1-7, 1985.

Klonoff DC: Chronic fatigue syndrome and neurally mediated hypotension, *JAMA* 275:360, 1996.

Kreusi MJP, Dale J, Straus SE: Psychiatric diagnosis in patients who have chronic fatigue syndrome, *J Clin Psychiatry* 50:53-56, 1989.

Landay AL, Jessop C, Lennette ET, et al: Chronic fatigue syndrome: clinical condition associated with immune activation, *Lancet* 338:707-712, 1991.

Levine PH, Kreuger GRF, Straus SE: The postviral chronic fatigue syndrome: a roundtable, *J Infect Dis* 160:722-724, 1989.

Liang SW, Boyce WT: The psychobiology of childhood stress, *Curr Opin Pediatr* 5:545-551, 1993.

Manu P, Lane TJ, Matthews DA: The frequency of the chronic fatigue syndrome in patients with symptoms of persistent fatigue, *Ann Intern Med* 109:554-556, 1988.

Rowe PC, Bou-Holaigah I, Kan JS, et al: Is neurally mediated hypotension an unrecognized cause of chronic fatigue? *Lancet* 345:623-624, 1995.

Straus SE, Tosato G, Armstrong G, et al: Persisting illness and fatigue in adults with evidence of Epstein-Barr virus infection, *Ann Intern Med* 102:7-16, 1985.

Tobi M, Morag A, Ravid, Z, et al: Prolonged atypical illness associated with serological evidence of persistent Epstein-Barr virus infection, *Lancet* 1:61-64, 1982.

Verecker MI: Chronic fatigue syndrome: a joint pediatric-psychiatric approach, *Arch Dis Child* 57:550-555, 1992.

Wachsmuth JR, MacMillan HL: Effective treatment for an adolescent with chronic fatigue syndrome, *Clin Pediatr* 30:488-490, 1991.

28

Growth Deficiency

BASIL J. ZITELLI

Key Points

- Nonorganic failure to thrive is common in children and may be associated with organic disorders as well. Hypocaloric diets usually are a result of skimpy or erratic meals. Psychosocial short stature results from a severely disturbed parent-child relationship, usually occurring in toddlers older than 2 years of age, and is associated with aberrant endocrine function.

- The differential diagnosis of growth failure is long and complicated. It requires a systematic approach, meticulous history, detailed physical examination, and selected or directed laboratory tests.

- Evaluation of failure to thrive may require a team approach, involving nurses, dieticians, and social workers. Psychosocial short stature also requires a multidisciplinary approach, with primary caretakers, endocrinologists, and behavioral specialists participating in the care of the patient. In each case, prognosis is good with early and aggressive psychosocial and medical intervention.

Growth deficiency is a uniquely pediatric problem that encompasses failure to gain weight and poor linear growth. This chapter addresses three common aspects of poor growth in children as follows: (1) poor weight gain, commonly referred to as *failure to thrive* (FTT); (2) a severe defect of nurturing that primarily affects linear growth and may have associated aberrations of endocrine function, known as *psychosocial short stature* (PSS); and (3) poor linear growth only, called *true short stature*. Although each of these entities is considered separately, they may overlap considerably, thus creating considerable confusion in the differential diagnosis. Together these three entities may account for 10% to 15% of patients seen in a routine pediatric practice;

FTT is the most common, accounting for nearly 10% of patients reported in one community practice; short stature affects 3% of children, and psychosocial dwarfism affects a smaller, yet significant number of toddlers and older children. The clinician must differentiate one disorder from the other, sift through a differential diagnosis, confirm clinical suspicions with appropriate and selective laboratory tests, and appreciate the complexities of psychosocial factors that impact on the child and family before undertaking appropriate therapy.

Failure to Thrive

Poor weight gain is the hallmark of FTT. Numerous clinical definitions abound in the literature, creating confusion when comparing studies. Mitchell and others defined FTT as "inappropriately slow weight gain in infancy without obvious cause." Bithoney and others described it as "children who 'fall across' two or more 'major percentiles' (e.g., 75th to 25th percentile) on the growth chart in 6 months' time" or "children whose weight for height is less than the 5th percentile." Leonard and others defined FTT as an infant "who (1) is full-term at birth, (2) has no demonstrable physical cause for growth failure, and (3) falls progressively below the 3rd percentile in weight and often height according to standard curves." Weight persistently below the 3rd percentile for age or weight less than 80% of ideal weight for age was the standard used by Berwick. These definitions may be inadequate because of the restriction that the child must be below the 3rd percentile or have no obvious cause for the FTT or because they fail to consider that a single assessment of weight may not accurately reflect the changes (gains or losses) in weight over time. Perhaps a more functional definition might be *failure to gain weight at a normal rate in children under 2 years of age*. Several important aspects of this definition should be noted. First, this definition limits the defining parameter to weight. Although growth decelerations in length and head circumference may ultimately occur in FTT, they

TABLE 28-1

Expected Daily Weight and Length Changes

Age Interval (mo)	Mean weight gain (gm/d)		Mean gain in length (mm/d)	
	Boys	Girls	Boys	Girls
0-3	31	26	1.07	0.99
3-6	18	17	0.69	0.67
6-9	13	13	0.52	0.52
9-12	11	11	0.43	0.44
12-15	9	9	0.37	0.38
15-18	8	8	0.33	0.34
18-21	7	8	0.30	0.32
21-24	7	7	0.28	0.29

Modified from Guo S, Roche A, Fomon SJ, et al: Reference data on gains in weight and length during the first two years of life, *J Pediatr* 119:355-362, 1991.

are not a necessary component and may occur only after significant malnutrition has occurred. Second, the standard by which weight gain is measured is known; mean daily weight gain is known for children from birth to 2 years of age and beyond (Table 28-1), and growth charts are readily available for plotting and monitoring growth over time (Fig. 28-1). Children gain almost 1 oz per day in the first 3 months of life and about $^3/_4$ oz per day in the second 3 months. In the last half of the first year of life, infants gain approximately $^1/_2$ oz per day. From 12 months to 18 months, weight gain slows to about $^1/_3$ oz per day, and from 18 months to 2 years, about $^1/_4$ oz is gained daily (Table 28-1). In addition, infants under 6 months of age can be expected to gain about 3.5 g daily for every 100 Kcal consumed. This diminishes to 1.5 g of weight gain daily for the same energy intake between 6 and 12 months of age. Third, at least two measurements of weight must be made to document a deceleration in weight gain. A single point on the growth curve cannot predict whether weight gain is accelerating or decelerating. Last, generally the definition is restricted to young children because children older than 2 years of age with growth deficiency may have psychosocial dwarfism (*vide infra*) rather than FTT. The term *failure to thrive* is purely descriptive and in no way implies an etiology for growth failure.

FTT represents a common problem in pediatrics, accounting for 9.6% of children seen in one primary care setting serving a rural poor community. Although FTT affects all socioeconomic levels, it occurs more frequently among impoverished families. Nearly one in five children in the United States currently lives in poverty. In 1984 a nutrition survey by the state of Massachusetts found that 12% of children receiving Medicaid had evidence on physical examination suggesting chronic malnutrition. In addition, up to 5% of all admissions to tertiary care pediatric hospitals are for FTT.

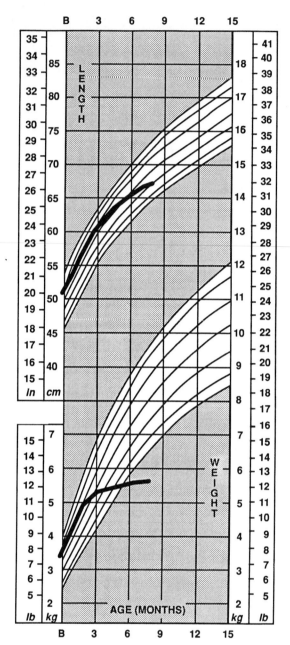

FIG. 28-1 Growth curve of a patient with nonorganic FTT. The growth pattern is not specific and can be seen in hypocaloric diets resulting from a variety of causes, including malabsorption and overuse of energy.

Patients with poor weight gain may fall into several categories of FTT. Depending on the definition and patient source, 15% to 82% of children suffer from environmental deprivation, or nonorganic failure to thrive (NOFTT), or no obvious cause is identified. Organic disease causes FTT in 18% to 85% of cases. However, some patients do not fit neatly into one particular category (Table 28-2). Homer and Ludwig found that of 82 children hospitalized for FTT, 41% had pure psychosocial causes; 26% had organic disorders causing poor weight gain; 4% had iatrogenic causes of poor

TABLE 28-2

Differential Diagnosis of Failure to Thrive

Condition	Clues from the history or physical examination
Poor Caloric Intake	
Breast-feeding mismanagement	Poor nutritional information, preparation
Lactation failure	Maternal stress, poor diet, illness
Eating disorders (older children)	Disturbed body image
Aberrant parental nutritional beliefs	Poor parental education
Iatrogenic causes	Clear liquid or elimination diets
Food faddism	Bizarre dietary habits
Improper formula preparation	Poverty, misinformation
Orofacial anomalies	Micrognathia, cleft lip and palate
Cardiopulmonary disease	Diaphoresis or fatigue while eating
Hypotonia, CNS disease	Poor suck, swallow
Diencephalic syndrome	Vomiting, alert appearance, hyperkinesis, euphoria
Poor Caloric Retention	
Increased ICP	Bulging fontanelle, papilledema, encephalopathy
Labyrinthine disorders	Nystagmus, ataxia
Esophageal obstruction, GER, preampullary obstruction	Frequent nonbilious vomiting
Intestinal obstruction, volvulus, Hirschsprung disease	Abdominal distension, bilious vomiting
Metabolic disorders	Vomiting; hepatic, renal, acid-base disturbances; encephalopathy
Poor Caloric Digestion/Assimilation	
Cystic fibrosis	Recurrent pneumonias, steatorrhea, elevated sweat chloride
Shwachman-Diamond syndrome	Steatorrhea, bone marrow hypoplasia, normal sweat chloride
Fat malabsorption	Abnormal liver/biliary tract function, elevated amylase/lipase
Enteric infections	Diarrhea, dysentery, fever
Poor Caloric Absorption	
Infection	Diarrhea, dysentery, fever
Inflammatory bowel disease	Clubbing, perianal skin tags, diarrhea, short stature
Cancer treatment	History of radiation, chemotherapy
Gluten-sensitive enteropathy	Abdominal distension, diarrhea
Carbohydrate malabsorption	Abdominal bloating, diarrhea
Intestinal lymphangiectasia	Low albumin, lymphopenia
Zinc deficiency	Hypogeusia, anorexia, acrodermatitis enteropathica
Increased Caloric Demands	
Chronic infection	Recurrent/persistent fever
HIV infection	Lymphadenopathy, recurrent infections
Malignancies	Cachexia, mass, fever
Autoimmune disorders	Rash, arthritis, hematologic abnormalities, weakness, abnormal serologic tests
Chronic renal disease	Infection, poor urinary concentration and acidification, hematuria, elevated urea nitrogen and creatinine
Chronic liver disease	Jaundice, hepatomegaly, elevated transaminases
Diabetes mellitus	Polyuria, polydipsia, glucosuria, polyphagia
Adrenal hyperplasia	Ambiguous genitalia, masculinization, electrolyte disturbances
Hypercalcemia	Irritability, constipation
Hypothyroidism	Linear growth affected more than weight
Metabolic errors	Encephalopathy, acidosis, vomiting
Miscellaneous	
CNS impairment	Profound mental retardation, swallowing difficulties
Prenatal growth failure	Small at birth, syndromic appearance
Short stature	Normal weight for height and weight velocity
Lagging-down	Onset midinfancy, shorter midparental height, no weight loss
Normal thinness	Normal history/physical examination, normal weight velocity

CNS, Central nervous system; *GER,* gastroesophageal reflux; *HIV,* human immunodeficiency virus; *ICP,* intracranial pressure.

growth, such as elimination diets for suspected food sensitivity; and 23% had organic disease and overlying psychosocial issues contributing to poor weight gain. The final 6% had no obvious diagnosis. Schmitt and Mauro suggest that 70% of children with poor weight gain have NOFTT. Half of all children with FTT have neglectful FTT, meaning the parent does not spend enough time feeding the infant or is overburdened, psychologically stressed, or depressed. Another 19% of FTT is accidental, caused by errors in formula preparation, faulty feeding techniques, deficient maternal diet with breast feeding, or misguided parental beliefs regarding a healthy diet for a child. Unavailability of food because of poverty, deliberate starvation, or food restriction is rare, each accounting for less than 1% of FTT cases. Experience in most private practice settings and perhaps to a lesser degree in tertiary care settings suggests that the majority of patients evaluated for FTT have no apparent organic basis for poor growth.

Emotional deprivation despite adequate physical care was suspected to contribute to the mortality rates of nearly 90% in orphanages and foundling homes in Baltimore as recently as 1915. At the same time, Chapin, a pediatrician from New York, alerted other physicians about the relationship of failure to grow and poor development to poverty and the institutionalization of infants and children. In 1902 he founded the Speedwell Society, which placed institutionalized marasmic infants with 24 carefully chosen, trained families and reported in 1908 that the mortality was far lower than that of other institutionalized children. Chapin felt that "deficient and inefficient fathers and mothers" were to blame and that both nutrition (nature) and environment (nurture) played important roles in recovery. Nearly 4 decades later, Spitz, of the New York Psychoanalytic Institute, demonstrated that infants in foundling homes consistently showed evidence of anxiety, sadness, retarded physical development, and poor weight gain. Spitz coined the terms *hospitalism* and *anaclitic depression* to describe these infants. In 1949, Bawkin made similar observations about hospitalized infants and called it *loneliness in infants*. These early reports generally concerned hospitalized infants and were associated with marked psychiatric problems within the mother. However, in 1957, Coleman and Provence reported FTT developing at home in the presence of the mother, and marked maternal psychopathology was not present. Since pediatricians became increasingly aware of growth failure, such dramatic and life-threatening instances of FTT are uncommon, and many are now discovered before serious malnutrition occurs.

Pathophysiology

Decreased caloric intake as a cause of NOFTT has been debated through the years since its description in the 1940s. Widdowson, a British nutritionist, concluded that the environment was more instrumental in causing growth failure than was caloric deprivation. She based her conclusions and observations on two orphanages in the British zone of occupation in post–World War II Germany. Both orphanages housed about 50 children who had only official rations to eat, and all were below normal in height and weight. During an initial 6-month period only the rations were given; however, subsequently, one orphanage (A) received supplemental food. The matron of orphanage A was cheerful and nurturing. The matron of orphanage B was stern and strict. At the end of the first 6 months, matron A sought other employment, and matron B was sent to orphanage A. Weight gain in orphanage A with supplemental food before the change in matrons was significantly better than that in orphanage B, as expected. However, after the change in matrons, weight gain of children in orphanage A did not improve any further, whereas children in orphanage B showed rapid gains in weight despite lack of any supplemental food.

The observation that hypocaloric diets may be responsible for poor growth was suggested by Talbot in 1947, when he observed that in a group of 100 children—some with organic disease and some without—all were stunted in height and had significantly hypocaloric diets. He also suggested that growth recovery may require supernormal energy requirements. When monkeys were reared under conditions of total social isolation but were fed an *ad libitum* diet, they all developed gross behavioral disturbances but grew at normal rates. Whitten and others found that parents of children with NOFTT frequently overestimated their child's food intake; actual intake was often inadequate for growth. In addition they found that children gained weight in the hospital when fed 140 Kcal/kg of ideal weight for height despite a poor nurturing environment and that infants continued to grow in a poor home environment when adequate calories were consumed. Pollitt also concluded that inadequate caloric intake was responsible for NOFTT in children when compared with a group of normal infants. When children with organic FTT and NOFTT were provided aggressive intervention, including hypercaloric diets and psychosocial and medical supports, each group grew equally well, indicating that weight gain alone cannot reliably distinguish between the two forms of FTT. Furthermore, when infants who were protected from a poor environment and grew well initially were placed into a poor home situation, no further growth in length or head circumference occurred after 6 months, and weight loss occurred. This implied that early good growth does not protect against FTT, and an adverse environment can easily and readily destroy the advantages of a favorable beginning. Pollitt subsequently demonstrated that growth-retarded children had more feeding difficulties as infants, had skimpier and more irregular meals, and had a lower caloric intake when compared with controls.

Both maternal and infant causes may contribute to breast-fed children with FTT. Infants may have poor intake caused by poor sucking, infrequent feedings, or anatomic impediments, such as a cleft palate. Vomiting, diarrhea, and malabsorption also may contribute. Conversely, high energy requirements, such as chronic pulmonary or heart disease or infection, may use energy at abnormally high rates. Mothers may not produce enough milk because of milk-suppressant drugs, such as pyridoxine, ergotamine, birth control pills, anticholinergics, or excessive alcohol. Maternal illness or fatigue may also lead to poor milk production. A poor let-down reflex can be caused by stress, smoking, and drugs as previously noted. Sore nipples and mastitis may lead to infrequent feedings, with progressively less milk produced. Infants who are more passive than others may not cry because of hunger and therefore may not give adequate feeding clues. These infants can lose from 15% to 25% of body weight by 2 weeks of age. Underlying organic disease also should be suspected. Lukefahr reported that 20% of breast-fed FTT infants had evidence of organic disease (e.g., urinary tract infection, heart disease, central nervous system [CNS] disease); 39% of cases were attributed to maternal misinformation or mismanagement, and 16% were the result of primary lactation failure.

Despite adequate calories given in a controlled hospital environment, 23% to 40% of children still do not demonstrate accelerated weight gain. Krieger demonstrated that energy use in FTT infants was the same as that in normal infants when based on weight for predicted height. However, these infants frequently have decreased body fat and a relatively higher proportion of metabolically active tissue. In addition, increased caloric intake is necessary for active anabolism during recovery. Vigorous activity, especially crying, may increase energy requirements by 100%, and chronic fever increases metabolic activity by 12% per degree centigrade above 38° C. Despite adequate caloric intake via gastrostomy feedings, one third of mentally retarded children with severe neuromotor and orofacial involvement remained underweight for height. No apparent mechanism has been identified.

Literature Survey

In Holt's classic text, *The Diseases of Infancy and Childhood,* published in 1897, he described infantile malnutrition as "a product of modern life." He also claimed,

Many cases are traceable to improper feeding. It is often seen in premature children and in the illegitimate offspring of girls of 16 or 18. In the majority of cases, however, it depends on two factors—food and the surroundings.

Elmer also described social disruption among these families. In a group of 15 children (from 13 families) admitted for FTT, 6 mothers were 17 years old or younger at their first pregnancy, 10 mothers had between 4 and 9 offspring, and the average time between the birth of the preceding sibling and the index child was 17 months. Of 13 sets of parents, 7 were separated, and the location of most fathers was unknown. Only one mother had education beyond the eleventh grade. Many similarly uncontrolled studies reported that mothers of infants with FTT had deprived childhoods, lacked self-esteem, had episodes of acute or chronic depression, and exhibited great dependency needs themselves that inhibited their ability to meet the child's emotional needs. Mitchell and others, however, in their controlled report of

FTT in a primary care clinic found no significant differences in demographic characteristics. Family problems were more evident in FTT cases. In a prospective, controlled study examining antecedents for NOFTT, Altemeier and others found that NOFTT correlated significantly with parental perceptions of poor nurturing during his or her own childhood, including a history of physical abuse of the mother. Maternal life stresses, including more arguments, separations, and reconciliations with the father, were also correlated with NOFTT. Mothers tended to gain less weight and have greater complications during pregnancy. Also, mothers of infants with NOFTT had more difficulties feeding their infants while still in the nursery; nearly half of the mothers did not want to feed or had problems of such a nature that the nurses had to offer most of the feedings. Behaviors indicating inadequate feedings at home, including failure of the mother to respond appropriately to infant cues, poor emotional attachment, inadequate child care knowledge, pressures from sibling rivalry, displaced maternal anger, and undermining of the mother by a grandparent, were identified in 79% of families. Yet other studies report no increased maternal depression, aberrant parent-child attachment, sense of parenting incompetence, social isolation, poor spousal relationships, or other psychopathology in the mother when compared with controls.

Children afflicted with FTT have been portrayed even in the earliest descriptions as showing unusual watchfulness, minimal smiling, decreased socialization, and lack of cuddliness. Fright, apathy, and withdrawn behavior characterize some children. In severe cases the child may assume an infantile posture, with the arms flexed at the elbows, the upper arms abducted and rotated outward, and the hands pronated and held behind the head (which is not normally seen after 4 or 5 months of age).

Other, less severe behavioral and temperamental aberrations also have been noted in these children. The children are described as being in poorer health with more behavioral difficulties than matched controls. In addition they have markedly higher reactivity and distractibility to extraneous stimuli. Parents may have excessive developmental expectations of the child and tend to be frustrated at the child's below-age locomotive skills, more varied tempo of play, and increased fussiness. Children are perceived to be less adaptable, more inconsolable, and more unhappy than a control group. These observations have begun to change the long-accepted, unidirectional concept of maternal deprivation as the sole cause of NOFTT to one of a disturbed maternal-child dyad in which there is a constant action-reaction exchange between the mother and child in an increasingly stressful milieu. The child may also contribute to his or her own disease.

Differential Diagnosis

The major challenge of FTT is to detect which children have organic disease as a cause of poor weight gain and which have NOFTT. Although no single test or observation can accurately distinguish one patient from another, certain clues can lead the clinician in the right direction. A child from a family that has exhibited many of the characteristics previously noted but who was previously healthy and normally grown may be at risk for NOFTT. In addition, infants with NOFTT generally prefer distant social encounters and inanimate objects, whereas patients with medical illnesses respond positively to close personal human interactions, including touching and cuddling. Predictors of organic disease include a history of previous hospitalizations, the presence of symptoms, and the presence of physical findings. However, most children with NOFTT have some physical complaint, such as fever, otitis media, vomiting, diarrhea, feeding problems, or developmental delay. Furthermore the often-accepted standard of usual or catchup weight gain during hospitalization as a diagnostic criteria for NOFTT should not be relied on entirely because patients with organic disease may also gain weight during aggressive nutritional and medical management. The successful discrimination between organic and nonorganic FTT thus requires a comprehensive and meticulous evaluation based on the history and physical examination.

Disorders of any organ system (singly or in combination) can in part result in poor growth. Simplistically, however, the physician can categorize organic disorders as to how they interfere with efficient energy intake or use. Children with FTT frequently have inadequate caloric intake. Breast-fed infants most frequently do not gain weight because of poor feeding technique or lactation failure. Older children may suffer from eating disorders, such as anorexia nervosa, or have an excessive fear of obesity. Altered parental beliefs regarding nutritional requirements may lead to bizarre dietary habits, such as excessive juice intake or hypocaloric diets. Physicians may contribute to poor intake by suggesting hypocaloric (clear liquid) diets that parents inadvertently maintain for prolonged periods of time to treat gastroenteritis, and physicians may recommend elimination diets for suspected food sensitivities or allergies. Food faddism can contribute to inadequate diets as well if not carefully monitored and regulated. Impoverished families may try to "stretch" infant formula to last longer by excessively diluting formula powder or concentrate or may offer infants improper formula, such as whole cow's milk or skim milk. Poor intake can affect patients with orofacial anomalies such as cleft lip and palate, Pierre Robin sequence, fatigue associated with cardiac or pulmonary disease, poor suck and swallow associated with hypotonia, CNS disorders, neuromuscular disease, anorexia, intoxications, drug ingestions, chronic subdural hematoma, and diencephalic syndrome. Children with this last disorder are universally emaciated and have an unusually alert appearance, lid retraction (Collier sign), hyperkinesis, vomiting, and an unusual sense of euphoria about them. Tumors usually are found in the diencephalon, although a small percentage have been located in the optic nerve and fourth ventricle.

Vomiting or regurgitation causing significant caloric loss can be associated with disorders involving the CNS or esophagus, intestinal obstruction, metabolic disorders, and a vari-

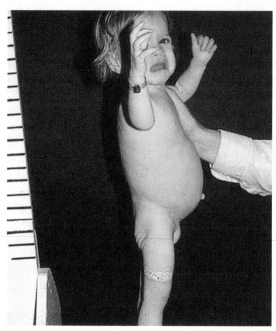

FIG. 28-2 This 2-year-old child had vomiting, weight loss, and abdominal distension. Malabsorption was suspected, and gluten-sensitive enteropathy was diagnosed. The patient improved dramatically on a gluten-free diet.

ety of systemic diseases. Increased intracranial pressure resulting from infection; space-occupying lesions; hydrocephalus; encephalopathies caused by toxins, hypoxia, or metabolic diseases; and labyrinthine disorders can be associated with vomiting and FTT. Anatomic obstruction of the esophagus (stenosis, web, achalasia, or vascular ring), gastroesophageal reflux, and rumination lead to inadequate energy retention and poor growth. Intestinal obstruction at any level of the gastrointestinal tract may have associated vomiting. High-level (preampullary) obstruction usually is not associated with abdominal distension or bile-stained vomitus. Examples include pyloric stenosis, antral web or atresia, and lactobezoars. Obstructions such as duodenal webs, annular pancreas, malrotation, intermittent volvulus, Hirschsprung disease, intussusception, and motility disorders can affect the postampullary gastrointestinal tract. Metabolic disorders, including galactosemia and fructosemia, defects in fatty acid metabolism (acyl-CoA dehydrogenase deficiency), hyperammonemia caused by liver disease or urea cycle defects, and a wide variety of other metabolic defects may have vomiting and poor growth as part of their presentations. Systemic disorders and infections associated with vomiting (e.g., renal disease, pancreatitis, and urinary tract infections) should also be considered.

Poor digestion and assimilation of food despite adequate intake causes poor growth as well. Frequently these patients have abnormal stooling patterns, with diarrhea, constipation, or foul-smelling stools. Prototypes within this category include cystic fibrosis, Shwachman-Diamond syndrome, and any cause of pancreatic exocrine insufficiency. Poor micelle formation, caused by low intraluminal bile acid levels resulting from extrahepatic biliary atresia or intrahepatic disorders, leads to steatorrhea and calorie loss. Enteric infections, particularly with *Salmonella* and *Giardia* organisms, or bacterial overgrowth from a blind loop syndrome also may lead to malabsorption.

Abnormal energy absorption resulting from a wide variety of disorders may be associated with FTT. Abnormal mucosa caused by infection, inflammatory bowel disease, chemotherapeutic drugs, and radiation therapy may not permit adequate gut absorption to allow growth. Gluten-sensitive enteropathy is associated with villous atrophy and decreased surface area for absorption (Fig. 28-2). Primary or secondary carbohydrate malabsorption (e.g., lactose intolerance), disorders of lipid absorption (e.g., abetalipoproteinemia), and intestinal lymphangiectasia with malabsorption produce a classic picture of inadequate energy and FTT. Complications of malabsorption, especially zinc deficiency, may contribute to poor growth, and correction of zinc deficiency in nutritional FTT enhances significant weight gain.

Virtually any chronic illness imposes increased energy needs on the host. Examples include chronic infection (including human immunodeficiency virus [HIV] infection), malignancies, fever, and chronic inflammatory states (autoimmune disorders, chronic lung or heart disease, and hyperthyroidism). Diseases, such as chronic renal disease resulting from chronic renal failure with acidosis, obstructive uropathy, renal cystic disease, and Fanconi syndrome, can also interfere with energy use. Hepatic inflammation and cirrhosis may alter energy metabolism and nutrient use, and a wide variety of endocrine and metabolic disorders profoundly influence energy use and growth. Such disorders include diabetes mellitus, congenital adrenal hyperplasia, disorders of calcium and phosphorus metabolism, and hypothyroidism, which affects linear growth before weight. Metabolic errors of amino acid metabolism, organic acidurias, carbohydrate intolerances (e.g., galactosemia and fructosemia), and disorders of mitochondria interfering with energy use and producing lactic acidosis can all interfere with normal growth.

Prenatal events may have a profound impact on postnatal growth. Exposures to toxins and drugs in utero may affect growth (e.g., maternal ingestion of alcohol produces fetal alcohol syndrome and maternal anticonvulsant use causes postnatal growth deficiency). In addition, some infants who are small for gestational age (SGA) because of a prenatal insult may remain growth retarded postnatally. Over one third of SGA infants remain below the 3rd percentile in height and weight by 4 years of age. Although truly premature, appropriate-for-gestational-age (AGA) infants have a higher incidence of FTT, their prognosis for catchup growth is much better than that for SGA infants. By 3 to 6 months of age, premature AGA infants generally are within 1 standard deviation of the mean normal weight when corrected for gestational age; SGA infants do not achieve that goal until 1 year of age, and even then they may remain below their AGA counterparts in length and head circumference.

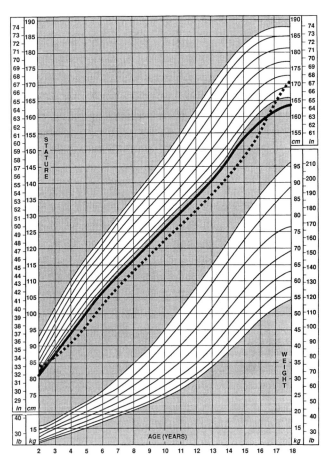

FIG. 28-3 Growth curve of a patient with genetic short stature *(solid line)*. Note normal growth velocity despite short stature. Growth curve of a patient with constitutional delay *(dashed line)*. Note normal initial growth, followed by growth deceleration, resumption of normal height velocity, and prolonged growth to achieve a normal adult height.

Three common variations in growth that can be easily confused with FTT are (1) genetic short stature, (2) growth deceleration that occurs when the patient begins achieving his or her genetic potential, and (3) normal leanness. Genetic short stature usually is associated with an appropriate weight for height and normal growth velocity. The growth curve for height and weight may be parallel to but below the 3rd percentile for age. The family history often reveals close relatives who are also short (Fig. 28-3).

Shifting linear growth occurs frequently in infancy and is not necessarily associated with FTT. During the first year of life, 60% of normal infants shift from their initial growth percentile to another one. Birth length is generally related to maternal size, but by 2 years of age length correlates with mean parental heights, reflecting genetic potential. Infants who are born to taller mothers and are tall at birth experience growth deceleration in midinfancy and achieve their new growth channel at a mean age of 13 months. Children who are small at birth exhibit catchup growth almost immediately and

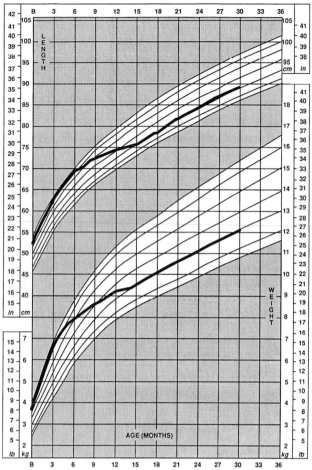

FIG. 28-4 Growth curve of a patient demonstrating normal lagging-down, or achievement of his genetic potential. The child was 8 lb 10 oz at birth, 21.5 inches long, and born to a mother 5 ft 8 inches tall and a father 5 ft 4 inches tall.

achieve their new growth channel by 12 months of age. These children have appropriate weight for height; experience a slow down, or "lag-down," without a period of weight loss or lack of linear growth; and begin to gain at a normal velocity around 1 year of age (Fig. 28-4).

The final common entity confused with FTT is normal thinness. These children may be 10% to 20% below ideal weight for height. The family and social histories generally lack high-risk parent-child interactions, and the child appears well-adjusted and normally developed. Dietary histories reveal normal caloric intake, and physical examinations are normal. Weight velocity is also normal.

History

A meticulous history is the most powerful diagnostic tool available to the clinician attempting to unravel the cause of FTT. The history should begin with a search for a cause of prenatal onset of poor growth, such as maternal illness or use of medications or drugs (including tobacco and alcohol), be-

cause numerous reports suggest that complications of pregnancy may be a risk factor for FTT. Birth weight may indicate whether the infant was SGA and hence has a poorer prognosis for catch-up growth. Children who had even minor perinatal difficulties (jaundice, suspected sepsis, and early feeding difficulties) have a greater incidence of subsequent NOFTT.

The history of the present illness should be thorough and should determine when the parents became concerned about the problems leading to physician consultation. Parents may not have recognized FTT as an issue; vomiting, diarrhea, or acute infection may bring the patient to attention. Recurrent or ongoing symptoms and previous hospitalizations may suggest an organic disorder. Unexplained injuries may indicate a pattern of abuse or neglect.

A detailed nutritional history attempts to verify appropriate caloric intake. Often a dietary calendar kept for several days to 1 week can provide information about the types and amounts of food offered. The caretaker must document how the formula is prepared to ensure proper caloric density. Standard commercial formulas require one 13-oz can of water to one 13-oz can of concentrated formula to give 26 oz of 20-calorie-per-ounce formula. Powdered preparations require two scoops of powder for every 4 oz of water to give the same standard caloric density. Most fruits and vegetables contain 15 calories per ounce, whereas most meats and desserts range from 25 to 30 calories per ounce. A history that suggests a voracious appetite and no associated symptoms of vomiting, diarrhea, polyuria, fever, or excessive crying may cast doubt on the validity of the caregiver's history. Feeding problems may signal organic disease. Vomiting, diarrhea, poor suck and swallow, fatigue during feeding, bizarre eating habits, and constipation all may be significant. (Bizarre eating habits may be seen with food faddism or PSS.) Constipation may be a clue for organic disorders, such as obstructive uropathy, hypothyroidism, hypercalcemia, galactosemia, and diencephalic syndrome (see Chapter 17).

A careful developmental history, examining for clues indicating CNS disorders, may indicate a central cause of poor growth. Usually children with CNS-related FTT have profound mental retardation, cerebral palsy, and feeding difficulties.

A family history of short stature may suggest that the patient is lagging-down and achieving his or her genetic potential. Parental heights and the ages at which the parents achieved puberty may help distinguish genetic short stature from constitutional delay. If other siblings exhibit poor growth, an inherited or metabolic disorder may be present. If siblings or close family relatives have died during early childhood, a lethal metabolic or immunologic disorder may be present. Because HIV infection may present with FTT in infancy, parental high-risk behavior, such as bisexual exposure, intravenous drug abuse, or a history of blood transfusions, may suggest the need for specific HIV testing in the parents and patient.

The social history may be most revealing and should investigate parental issues and the child's behavior. Questions should investigate the issues previously discussed in the Literature Survey section. A review should include parental histories, searching for evidence of neglect or abuse in their childhoods and current stress within the family. Financial difficulties, threat of eviction, unemployment, and marital discord may contribute to social disruption. Inquiries about support from relatives and friends, parental expectations of the child and of themselves as parents, and their perceptions of the child's needs can be enlightening. The degree of enjoyment the family receives from caring for the infant also can be revealing.

The burden of an altered parent-child relationship cannot fall entirely on the parents' shoulders. Neonatal complications may interfere with early bonding, and the child's temperament may lead to parental frustration and anxiety. A colicky infant or an aggressive child may be difficult to handle and may not give the positive feedback that a parent may expect. Yet a passive infant may not provide adequate clues for the parent to provide sufficient feeding. Hence there may be constant dynamic action-reaction within the parent-child dyad that produces a pathologic relationship.

Physical Examination

The physical examination should begin with initial observations of the parent-child interaction as the physician enters the room. Is the mother holding the child close in a comforting, reassuring manner, or is the child held at arm's length? Does the mother talk to the child appropriately, or does she scold or strike the child? Is the mother at the child's side during the examination, or is she sitting passively and acting seemingly uninterested? Similarly the child's reactions are important. A child at risk for NOFTT and neglect may be passive or withdrawn and may not seek comfort from the mother. He or she may be alert and constantly searching the environment with a watchful gaze. In severe cases, children may assume the posture described by Krieger and Sargent with the arms held up and hands behind the head.

Children with NOFTT exhibit certain behaviors with greater frequency than do children with an organic basis to their FTT or a control group of children. Children with NOFTT prefer distant social encounters and play with inanimate objects, whereas children with organic FTT respond more positively to close human interaction, such as touching and holding. In addition, other behaviors tend to set patients with NOFTT apart. These include decreased vocalization; expressionless facies, including infrequent smiling; gaze abnormalities (avoidance and disinterest); increased hand and finger activities, including thumb sucking and rumination; infantile posture; and general motor inactivity.

Careful examination of each organ system may uncover an unrecognized sign pointing to organic disease. In one study, the two areas most frequently neglected by physicians in FTT evaluations were (1) careful auscultation of the heart and (2) a detailed developmental examination. Other important findings among children with FTT that suggest an organic

disorder include cataracts (rubella), heart murmur (patent ductus arteriosus or aortic stenosis), protuberant abdomen (malabsorption or obstructive uropathy), abdominal mass (pyloric stenosis or obstructive uropathy), hepatomegaly (galactosemia), hypospadias (obstructive uropathy), and delayed development (congenital encephalopathy or rubella).

Perhaps the most helpful clues in the physical examination are serial measurements of weight, length, and head circumference. Examination of the growth curves may help distinguish among various causes of growth failure. The child with NOFTT or caloric deprivation has an initial fall-off in weight, followed by a deceleration in length after several months, and finally a plateau of head growth after several more months if no intervention ensues. This is the typical pattern in NOFTT, but it is by no means specific. This pattern is seen in a wide variety of organic disorders as well. In contrast the child with genetic short stature has appropriate weight for height and normal weight velocity. The child who has profound developmental delay and microcephaly may have a CNS basis for poor growth. If all three measurements are below the third percentile, the incidence of organic disease approximates 70%.

Approach to the Patient

The most discriminating diagnostic tools the physician has in the evaluation of FTT are the history and physical examination. Use of laboratory procedures generally is confined to confirmation of suspicions obtained through a meticulous history and physical examination. Ambuel and Harris found that the history and physical examination provided a diagnosis in 91% of children who had an organic disorder. Similarly, Sills summarized the evaluations of 185 children hospitalized for FTT. Of the 34 children who had an organic disease, 17 were diagnosed on the basis of the history alone, one on the basis of the physical examination alone, and 16 on the basis of a combination of the history and physical examination. A total of 2607 laboratory tests were performed on the 185 patients, with an average of 14 tests per patient. Yet, only 10 tests (0.4%) established a diagnosis, and another 26 tests (1%) were supportive of a diagnosis. All 36 tests were indicated by the history or physical examination. Berwick and others found that an average of 40 laboratory tests or radiographs were performed per patient in 122 infants admitted to a teaching hospital for FTT. Yet, only 0.8% of all tests showed an abnormality that contributed to the diagnosis causing poor growth.

Despite the low yield of routine and often cumbersome testing, most physicians perform selected screening tests. Some recommended tests might include a complete blood count and differential to look for anemia, leukocytosis, or leukopenia as evidence of infection or immunodeficiency and examination of the peripheral blood smear for red cell and white cell morphology. A simple urinalysis may indicate glomerular disease with hematuria or proteinuria, the presence of tubular dysfunction with glycosuria, or the inability to concentrate or acidify the urine. A urine culture is important because occult urinary tract infection in young infants may present with only FTT. Examination of the stool for diarrhea, steatorrhea (foul smell and fat droplets on special stain), carbohydrate malabsorption (low pH and positive Clinitest), occult blood, and infection may be helpful. An examination of the patient's biochemical homeostasis with electrolytes, urea nitrogen, creatinine, and total carbon dioxide or venous blood gas may give some clues to silent organic disease. Although these are screening tests, other laboratory examinations, including chest and gastrointestinal radiographs, may be indicated by the history and physical examination.

In most cases the child is in no imminent danger, and the evaluation can be accomplished on an outpatient basis. Because of the complexity of most cases, a multidisciplinary approach is useful. A nutritionist can help evaluate caloric intake and dietary patterns, visiting home nurses can evaluate home conditions and observe feeding patterns, and social workers can provide more detailed psychosocial background of the family and begin intervention when necessary. The physician serves as the medical evaluator and team leader. If the history, physical examination, and selected laboratory tests do not indicate a potential organic disease, a dietary calendar should be kept by the mother for 1 week and average daily caloric intake assessed. Young infants can be fed formula alone for ease of calculation of caloric intake. Infants may require 150 kcal/kg/day, or if the volume permits, 120 kcal/kg of ideal weight for height. This may result in caloric intakes as high as 180 kcal/kg of current weight. While the medical evaluation is proceeding, nursing observations and social service intervention is ongoing. Frequent, close follow-up is necessary to ensure adequate weight gain over a 1-month trial period.

Hospitalization of the infant may be necessary if:
1. The infant does not gain adequate weight during the outpatient evaluation.
2. Evidence of physical abuse or neglect exists or is suspected.
3. Severe protein-calorie malnutrition is present.
4. The mother is severely emotionally disturbed or unable to provide adequate care for the child.

The purpose of hospitalization is to enhance a more detailed medical evaluation if necessary, provide a controlled feeding environment for the child, observe feeding patterns and accurately calculate caloric intake, and provide intensive psychosocial support for the family. Nursing observation of feeding patterns may be useful. A child who has poor swallowing may have a neurologic, orofacial, or metabolic disturbance. The child who eats small amounts and fatigues easily may have cardiopulmonary disease, severe debilitation, chronic infection, or hypothyroidism. If the child eats voraciously but vomits, then rumination, gastroesophageal reflux, esophageal disorders, increased intracranial pressure, or metabolic disturbances may be present.

Most children with NOFTT begin to gain weight in the hospital when given adequate calories. The growth quotient (GQ) can assess whether weight gain is appropriate and whether catchup growth is occurring. The GQ is the patient's mean daily weight divided by the normal mean daily weight gain for age. Normal weight gain achieves a GQ of 1.0, whereas catchup growth has a GQ greater than 1.0.

Hospitalization also provides the opportunity for intensive social service evaluation and intervention. Families with financial needs may be enrolled in the Supplemental Food Program for Women, Infants, and Children (WIC) and may be eligible for food stamps, medical assistance, and Aid to Families with Dependent Children (AFDC). Hospitalization allows social workers and counselors to try to understand the dynamics of the parent-child dyad in NOFTT. For example, one mother remained detached from her child because she feared attachment and the pain she would suffer if the child died. Another mother deliberately fed her child a hypocaloric diet because she misunderstood the normal dietary needs of her infant. Understanding such dynamics allows appropriate counseling and psychologic intervention. In addition, families may receive additional supports through visiting nurse programs, foster grandparents, and parenting and feeding classes. Parental stress centers can provide additional support and counseling. Through intensive medical and psychosocial management, the goal of rehabilitating the family unit often can be achieved.

NOFTT may have significant long-term physical and behavioral sequelae for children. Leonard and others summarized the follow-up of 13 children seen for NOFTT. Five patients had continued good weight gain, five patients had minimal weight gain, and three patients were lost to follow-up. Three children who had developmental impairment achieved normal milestones; however, two of four subsequent children born into these families were later diagnosed with FTT. Elmer and associates reported a grim prognosis for most of 15 children studied. Only two children were functioning "reasonably well" several years after the initial study. Catchup growth occurred in about half of the children, but several children remained below normal for stature. Most disturbing, however, was the observation that over 50% of the children suffered some degree of mental retardation and that behavior problems and poor intellectual performances interfered with school function. Similarly, Hutton and Oates reviewed 21 children 6 years after evaluation of NOFTT. Five children remained below the 10th percentile for weight, and only one child was below the 10th percentile for height. Three children had Wechsler Intelligence Scale for Children (WISC) full-scale IQ quotients below 90. Ten children were described by teachers as functioning below normal, and two thirds had significantly delayed reading ages. Parental perceptions of their child's behavior were disturbing; parents complained of lying, stealing, temper tantrums, enuresis, and hyperactivity. Of great concern were two children's deaths under suspicious circumstances. In contrast, although weight measurements of children followed in a primary care setting remained significantly below those of control children at 3 to 5 years of age, no differences were found in behavior or intellect. Oates, in a subsequent series of reports on children with NOFTT, noted that one child later died as a result of physical abuse, and two other children sustained injuries from suspected abuse. In studying 14 children seen 12 years after initial evaluation, all weights were above the 3rd percentile, but verbal scale scores on the WISC-R averaged 90, which is significantly below a control group's mean score of 102. Language scores also were significantly lower. Social maturity factors related to ego strength and emotional stability were lower than those of controls, and personality disorders in seven children placed them at higher risk for educational and social dysfunction.

In a classic report, Evans and others studied 40 children and their families and found that prognosis was closely associated with three patterns of family dysfunction. In the group with the best prognosis the mother suffered a recent loss, resulting in depression and a strained maternal-child relationship. The mother perceived the children as being ill. Living conditions and physical care of the child were good. Children had excellent ultimate growth, and no significant behavioral problems emerged. In the second group, living conditions were deprived, and physical care of the child was poor. The mother had suffered chronic losses and stresses, leading to depression. She considered her child ill or retarded. Prognosis in this group was guarded, with family problems continuing. School difficulties and behavioral problems affected most of the children, although most gained weight above the 3rd percentile. Two of eight children required foster care, and two children were evaluated for suspected abuse. The third group had the poorest prognosis and was characterized by a mother who was angry and hostile, undergoing chronic losses. These mothers saw their children as "bad," and despite good living conditions, childcare was neglectful. Most children still were above the 3rd percentile for weight and height, but developmental and school problems were prevalent. Three of seven children required foster care, and two children were evaluated for suspected abuse. Notably, two children demonstrated no abnormalities. In both of these families, intensive intervention occurred and resulted in dramatic improvement in home conditions. Despite this seemingly grim overall prognosis, Reinhart reported a 50-year follow-up study of a single patient who was at birth weight at 7 months of age. Once removed from the caretaker, "whose name still gives . . . an unhappy feeling," the patient thrived, gained weight, and went on to higher education without behavioral problems, evidence of learning disabilities, or serious illness.

Numerous similarities exist between NOFTT and child abuse. Environmental conditions are similar in both groups when assessments of the mother's childhood home, supports, living conditions, and attitude toward the child and the child's characteristics are studied. The abusive families tend to be even more impoverished and live in more crowded conditions. Abusive mothers tend to be more isolated, have lower self-esteem, have higher expectations of their children, and are more demanding and suspicious than mothers of the NOFTT group. Growth patterns in NOFTT children are similar to those in abused children, and both groups have long-standing developmental deficits in language, reading, and verbal intelligence. In addition, what seemingly may present as NOFTT may be an unusual manifestation of child abuse, Munchausen syndrome by proxy, a particularly malignant form of abuse perpetrated on the child in the guise of a true medical illness.

What role early malnutrition plays in intellectual development remains controversial; yet numerous follow-up studies emphasize generally lower intelligence scores among children with FTT. Most studies are confounded by other coexisting environmental factors known to impact on development, such as poverty, alcoholism, child abuse, neglect, emotional deprivation, and family disruption. Hertzig found lower IQ scores in boys hospitalized for severe malnutrition during the first 2 years of life when compared with siblings and classmates. Supplemental feedings given to children at risk for malnutrition were associated with significantly higher IQ scores when compared with malnourished siblings or non-supplemented siblings, indicating that aggressive intervention may be successful. The damage caused by malnutrition may not be permanent, and the child has greater potential for recovery from early malnutrition as long as good nutrition and a nurturing environment are maintained. The positive effects, however, may be lost if the rehabilitative programs are stopped.

Generally the family that was involved with accidental FTT or had acute family disruption responds well to psychosocial supportive intervention and has a good prognosis. Close follow-up may be all that is necessary. Involvement of children's protective services may be necessary for the welfare of the children when physicians are faced with angry or hostile, intellectually limited parents who cannot provide proper care or neglectful and abusive parents. In these cases, careful documentation of growth (both in and out of the hospital) and observations by impartial observers, such as nursing staff, social workers, and developmental specialists may be important courtroom evidence should custody hearings be necessary. The ultimate goal, however, is to rehabilitate the family and child and maintain the family unit.

Psychosocial Short Stature

PSS is a variant of growth deficiency in children characterized by short stature in association with psychologic disturbances, emotional deprivation, or both. It frequently is associated with endocrine abnormalities, particularly growth hormone (GH) deficiency. A poor nutritional state may or may not be present. PSS should not be confused with NOFTT, which may not have linear growth failure as part of its presentation and has few if any endocrine disturbances. The only endocrine disturbances sometimes found with NOFTT are elevated cortisol secretion rates and low thyroxine levels (usually related to low thyroxine-binding globulin levels). GH is not decreased in NOFTT. Although the etiologies of NOFTT and PSS may be similar, significant differences allow clinical discrimination and individual therapeutic approaches.

PSS can be divided into two subtypes. The infantile form (PSS-I) occurs in children younger than 2 years of age and is associated with short stature. Malnutrition without endocrine disturbance is the primary cause of PSS-I, which may be considered an extension of NOFTT when associated with short stature. PSS-II, however, occurs in children older than 2 years of age and has an underproduction of GH as a major hormonal abnormality.

The true incidence of PSS is unknown, relating in part to underrecognition and difficulty in diagnosis. Only nine children were recognized as having PSS over a 4-year period in one pediatric program, whereas 50 children were diagnosed with PSS in a large endocrine clinic over a 5-year period.

Literature Survey

It had been suggested as early as 1947 that severe psychologic disturbances in children may effect hormonal imbalances, leading to growth failure. Lack of sensitive hormonal assays prevented further elucidation of the mechanisms involved. Descriptions of maternal deprivation in children with short stature lead to hypothetical descriptive terms, such as *transient hypopituitarism*, *reversible hyposomatotrophism*, *"garbage can" syndrome*, and *psychosocial short stature*.

In 1967, Silver and Finkelstein reported nine children who were afflicted with what they termed *deprivational dwarfism*. All children were well-grown at birth and grew normally for a variable period of time ranging from several months to 6 years before short stature was noted. Each child was extremely short (height age–chronological age, range 0.23 to 0.55), had a voracious appetite, had delayed skeletal maturation, and had experienced emotional and psychologic deprivation. Feeding difficulties dating back to infancy were common, and infants were frequently described as irritable and fussy. The patients' eating patterns were unusual; they consumed abnormally large quantities of food, stole and hid food, and sometimes ate from garbage cans. Grossly disturbed family relationships were present in all families, with mothers being described as depressed and withdrawn or aggressive and rejecting. The mothers may have had neglectful childhoods themselves. Some children had physical evidence suggestive of abuse. Bone age was uniformly delayed, but GH testing was not performed.

Shortly after this report, Powell and others published their classic description of the syndrome, including GH levels. They emphasized family disruption caused by marital strife, separation or divorce, alcoholism, and poor maternal attachment. Bizarre eating behaviors, including gorging, eating entire jars of condiments, eating pet food, and unusual polydipsia (drinking from toilet bowels, puddles, and old, rusty beer cans) were similarly described. Endocrinologic evaluation generally revealed normal thyroid function but deficient adrenocorticotropic hormone (ACTH) and GH levels. Remarkably, after treatment and a period of growth, endocrine abnormalities normalized. These levels improve as rapidly as within 24 hours after hospitalization, suggesting that immediate testing is important for accurate diagnosis.

The psychiatric profile of the child with PSS includes severe depression, personality disorder, and shared deviant behaviors. Depression often exists for months; the personality disorder frequently is characterized by immature motivations, disturbed self-esteem, and poor foundations for relationships. Abnormal behaviors as previously described frequently disappear when the child is not in the home. Behavioral aberrations, such as enuresis, encopresis, social apathy or inertia, defiant aggressiveness, temper tantrums, sleep disorders, pain agnosia, and self-injury, are prevalent as well. In addition, many children exhibit retarded motor development and intellectual delays.

Retarded intellectual development has long been recognized as a component of chronic child abuse or neglect and was specifically described in association with PSS in 1977. The mean baseline IQ of 23 children at the time they were diagnosed with PSS was 66 (SD 16). However, among children who were rescued from the abusive environment, IQ improved by 24 points; children who were younger than $5\frac{1}{2}$ years of age when they were rescued had the most significant IQ increase. IQ scores tended to continue to increase with longer follow-up.

History

In PSS the history may be difficult to elicit from a guarded parent. Besides the time of onset of growth failure and a complete review of systems looking for potential organic causes of short stature, behavioral abnormalities and parent-child relationships should be emphasized. Behavioral questions should examine the wide range of bizarre eating habits previously noted, as well as motor and intellectual delays. Family history and psychodynamics may include maternal depression, marital conflict, an unsupportive father, and a history of physical abuse and deprivation in the parental background. Common social stresses include financial difficulties, unemployment, illness, and substance abuse. Other children in the family may have been evaluated for FTT, and the family may already have a history with child protective services.

Physical Examination

The hallmark of PSS is short stature; most children are under the 3rd percentile when they come to medical attention. Weight may be proportionate to height or more often slightly below mean weight for height (Fig. 28-5). Overt malnutrition, however, is rare. Body proportions tend to be immature, and signs of physical abuse may be present and are manifested by unusual bruises or burns. Generally the remainder of the physical examination is normal.

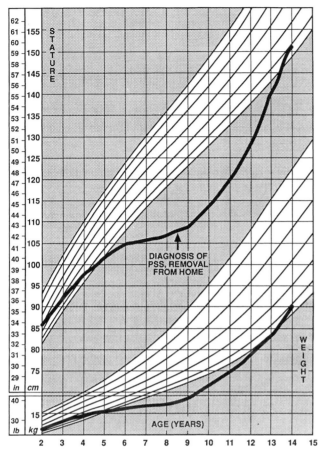

FIG. 28-5 Growth curve of a patient with PSS. Note growth deceleration affecting height and marked growth after removal from the home environment.

Approach to the Patient

When PSS is entertained as a diagnosis, hospitalization is necessary to allow a thorough multidisciplinary evaluation. Laboratory investigations should be directed toward specific disorders suggested by the history and physical examination. Routine hematologic and biochemical screening tests are usually normal, or if mildly abnormal, they often rapidly correct during catchup growth.

Endocrine abnormalities have been the most intensively studied area in PSS. Generally, thyroid functions are normal or rapidly normalize with growth, and steroid hormone response to metyrapone stimulation may be normal or low. Approximately half of the patients have a blunted serum GH response to provocative stimulation. These tests should be done within 24 hours of hospitalization because some patients may rapidly correct this abnormality. Insulin-like growth factor I (IGF-I) levels are often subnormal and variably return to normal levels after growth occurs. Insulin secretion is depressed, and gonadotropin levels are appropriate for the stage of sexual maturity. Skeletal age is retarded and usually equal to or slightly advanced when compared with

height age. Growth arrest lines in the distal radius or knee are found in 87% of patients with PSS as compared with only 8% of idiopathic GH-deficient patients. Also, temporary widening of the cranial sutures during growth recovery has been observed radiographically.

Approach to the patient involves a multidisciplinary team consisting of the primary physician; consultants in endocrinology, psychiatry, and developmental medicine; social service workers; and nutritionists. The only effective therapy is to change the child's environment and psychologic milieu. Hospitalization affords the opportunity for evaluation, testing, and observation of behavior. Because of long-standing psychologic abuse, immediate rehabilitation of the family is difficult, and removal of the child from the home and placement in a nurturing environment is often necessary. During hospitalization, counseling may begin for both the parents and the child, and frequently the marked behavioral aberrations disappear. Laboratory abnormalities frequently spontaneously normalize when growth begins.

Prognosis generally is good for patients who are diagnosed early. Growth potential is excellent, and developmental and intellectual recovery can be complete. Emotional development parallels physical growth, and close monitoring of the child while in foster care is essential. If the family is recalcitrant to counseling, permanent separation and adoption may provide the best alternative.

Short Stature

Failure of linear growth is defined as length or height under the 3rd percentile for age or an abnormally low height velocity. Approximately 5% of children in a longitudinal study conducted in Newcastle upon Tyne were under the 3rd percentile for height; 84% had normal variants of short stature, and less than 20% had organic disease causing linear growth failure. Serial height measurements plotted on standard curves developed by the National Center for Health Statistics allow longitudinal observations of growth. These curves are based on cross-sectional data for each gender from two age groups—birth to 3 years and 2 to 18 years of age. The data do not include Hispanic or Asian children, although the curves are useful in monitoring growth trends in these racial groups. Infants can be measured best in a recumbent position, using an infantometer. The stadiometer provides an accurate upright height measurement, especially after 3 years of age.

Linear growth is greatest during intrauterine life and is generally determined by maternal size, nutrition, and placental function. After birth there is constant growth deceleration; linear growth rate at birth is approximately 18 cm/yr, and it decreases to 5 to 7.5 cm/yr by 2 years of age. Two thirds of children experience a shifting of linear growth during infancy; upward shifts begin in early infancy, and downward shifts begin in midinfancy (Fig. 28-4). Generally, shifting is completed and infants track along their new curve by 12 to

TABLE 28-3

Summary of Normal Linear Growth Data

Age	Mean height (cm)		Height velocity (cm/yr, mean; [3%]‡)		U/L*		Span minus height† (cm)	
	Girls	Boys	Girls	Boys	Girls	Boys	Girls	Boys
Birth	50.8	50.8	41	47.0	1.70	1.70	−2.5	−2.5
12 mo	74.2	76.2	14.7 (10.6)	13.4 (9.4)	1.52	1.54	−3.3	−2.5
24 mo	86.1	87.4	9.3 (6.1)	9.0 (5.9)	1.41	1.42	−3.5	−3.0
10 yr	141.0	141.0	5.5 (3.9)	5.2 (3.8)	1.00	0.99	−1.0	0
12 yr	154.2	151.4	8.3§ (6.3)	5.0 (3.6)	0.99	0.98	0	+2
15 yr	164.8	171.2	0.6 (0.1)	5.9‖ (3.6)	1.01	0.98	+1.2	+4.3

*U/L, upper body/lower body segment ratio.
†Arm span minus height in centimeters.
‡Height velocity at the 3rd percentile.
§Peak velocity at age 12 years.
‖Peak velocity is 9.45 cm at age 14 years.

BOX 28-1

Differential Diagnosis of Short Stature

Disproportionate Short Stature
Osteochondrodysplasia
Rickets

Proportionate Short Stature
Genetic short stature
Constitutional delay
Intrauterine growth retardation
Dysmorphic syndromes
Growth hormone deficiency or unresponsiveness
Hypothyroidism
Systemic disease
  Inflammatory bowel disease
  Cystic fibrosis
  Cardiac insufficiency
  Pulmonary disease
  Renal failure
  Renal tubular acidosis
  Immunodeficiency
  Metabolic disorders
  Central nervous system impairment
Psychosocial short stature

18 months of age. Growth remains relatively constant at a minimum of 5 cm/yr until the adolescent growth spurt, which lasts about 4 years and peaks 2 years after the onset of puberty. A constant growth deceleration continues for another 2 years. Because the onset of puberty in girls is at about 10 years, they attain 98.5% of their adult height by age 16. Boys, with a mean age of onset of puberty at age 12, reach 98.5% of adult height by 18 years. Normal growth rates are summarized in Table 28-3. Estimates of adult height can be made using different equations. The simplest method is the use of the Bailey-Pinneau tables published in Greulich and Pyle's *Radiographic Atlas of Skeletal Development of the Hand and Wrist.* This method uses the patient's current height, bone age, and chronologic age and is reliable to within 4 to 6 cm. The Roche, Wainer, and Thissen (RWT) method is more complex, using chronologic age, recumbent length, weight, and parental heights. A simple estimation in patients with normal variant growth patterns follows:

$$\text{Boys: } \frac{\text{Mother's height (cm)} + 13 \text{ cm} + \text{father's height (cm)}}{2}$$

$$\text{Girls: } \frac{\text{Father's height (cm)} - 13 \text{ cm} + \text{mother's height (cm)}}{2}$$

These midparental height projections are generally accurate within 8 cm or 2 standard deviations. In contrast to prenatal growth, GH and thyroxine are important determinants in postnatal linear growth, with gonadotropins exercising their influence during puberty.

Differential Diagnosis

Similar to FTT, the differential diagnosis of short stature is complex. Generally it can be separated into conditions causing proportionate short stature and those causing disproportionate short stature (Box 28-1). Useful indices of body proportions are the upper body/lower body segment ratio (U/L) and the arm span minus height measurement. The U/L is obtained by subtracting the length of the lower segment from the patient's height to obtain the upper segment value. The lower segment is measured from the symphysis pubis to the floor. The arm span is measured from the tip of the third finger to the tip of the other third finger with the arms held out to the sides, parallel to the floor, and fingers extended.

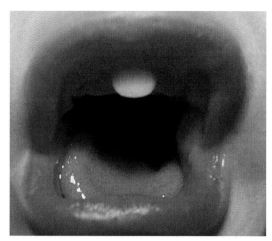

FIG. 28-6 A single central maxillary incisor should alert the clinician to search for GH deficiency. (Courtesy Dr. P. Lee.)

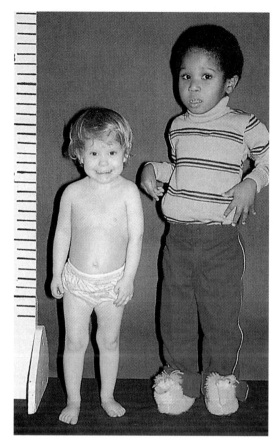

FIG. 28-7 The normal 3½-year-old boy (dressed) is in the 50th percentile for height. The short 3-year-old girl has a characteristic Kewpie doll appearance, suggesting GH deficiency.

Normal age-related values are summarized in Table 28-3. Children with disproportionate short stature often have one of a variety of osteochondrodysplasias, with either short-limbed dwarfism or short-trunk dwarfism. Rickets, with its associated poor osseous development, also causes disproportionate body proportions, usually a disparately short lower body segment.

Causes of proportionate short stature are summarized in Box 28-1. Genetic short stature and constitutional delay are the most common causes of short stature. Criteria for genetic short stature include projected height falling within 10 cm of midparental height, short stature in parents or close relatives, normal bone age, normal growth velocity, and the absence of a syndrome or systemic disease. Constitutional delay represents the lower end of normal skeletal and pubertal maturational timing. Children usually have normal birth size and grow normally for several months before growth deceleration occurs between 6 and 36 months of age. Normal growth velocity resumes, but puberty is delayed and is associated with a later-than-average pubertal growth spurt. Growth continues for a longer-than-normal period of time, and ultimate adult height is normal. Usually a family history of a similar growth pattern or delayed onset of puberty can be obtained. Bone age is delayed consistent with height age.

Prenatal onset of poor growth may include the multitude of causes of intrauterine growth retardation (IUGR). Fetal infections and maternal consumption of alcohol, heroin, tobacco, anticonvulsants, and other drugs may produce small infants. Restriction of intrauterine space caused by multiple births, tumors, or placental insufficiency can cause either temporary or permanent growth failure. Prognosis for growth of IUGR infants is variable and depends on the original cause. Dysmorphic syndromes (with or without chromosomal abnormalities) are often identified by small birth size and the presence of anomalies. Specific identification may require

specialist consultation or review in a compendium of recognizable syndromes. The most common chromosomal abnormalities causing short stature are Down syndrome and Turner syndrome. Turner syndrome may be difficult to diagnose when chromosomal mosaicism exists. The classic features of pterygium, low hairline, shield chest, typical facies, micrognathia, cubitus valgus, lymphedema, and hyperconvex nails may not be present (see Fig. 29-11). Growth failure may be the only presenting sign.

Endocrine disorders leading to short stature are numerous but usually are not difficult to diagnose. Idiopathic GH deficiency is probably the most common cause of GH deficiency, although tumors, such as craniopharyngioma, histiocytosis X, and cranial irradiation should be considered. Hypopituitarism may be present along with other midline defects, such as cleft lip or palate; single, central incisor (Fig. 28-6); or septo-optic dysplasia. Birth weight is usually normal, and growth proceeds normally until growth failure is noted at 12 to 18 months of age. Children have a cherubic appearance with a round face and delayed development of the naso-orbital bridge. Truncal and buttocks obesity contributes to the "Kewpie doll" appearance (Fig. 28-7). GH levels are low on provocative stimulation, although variants may exist where somatomedin-C levels are low or a GH-receptor defect exists, such as in Laron dwarfism. Bone age

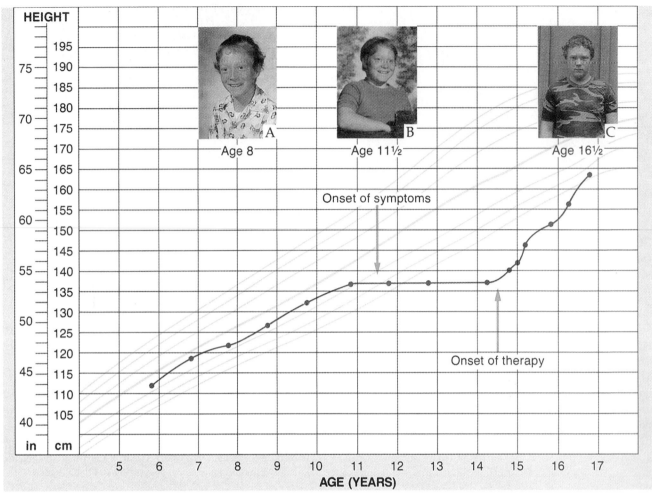

FIG. 28-8 Growth of a child with acquired hypothyroidism, showing marked plateau of growth with resumption and catchup growth after the onset of therapy. Note the change in body habitus associated with hypothyroidism and its resolution with therapy.

is significantly delayed. Hypothyroidism is frequently associated with linear growth failure; other symptoms of weight gain, skin and hair changes, constipation, and cold intolerance may be variable or of such an insidious onset that they are unrecognized (Fig. 28-8). Autoimmune thyroiditis is the most common cause of acquired hypothyroidism. Low thyroxine levels, elevated thyroid stimulating hormone levels, and a delayed bone age are classic diagnostic laboratory tests. Glucocorticoid excess, either from Cushing syndrome or excessive intake, produces a characteristic appearance of moon facies, plethoric complexion, truncal obesity, acneiform rash, striae, and linear growth failure (Fig. 28-9). Occasionally, growth failure is the only manifestation.

Systemic diseases affecting any organ system may be associated with poor growth. Most disorders are apparent by the time growth failure occurs, although a few disorders may be silent. Inflammatory bowel disease may have growth deceleration as its only presenting sign. Of patients with Crohn disease and patients with ulcerative colitis, 15% to 30% and 5% to 10% respectively have associated growth failure (see Fig. 1-1).

In addition, gluten-sensitive enteropathy may not cause classic features of diarrhea and cramps but only present with short stature. Renal disease also can be a silent cause of growth failure, either with unrecognized chronic renal failure or renal tubular acidosis. Gastrointestinal imaging studies and tissue samples may help diagnose inflammatory bowel disease, and antigliadin and antiendomysial antibodies frequently are present in gluten-sensitive enteropathy. Renal function tests, urinalysis, urine culture and assessment of acid-base status may lead to the diagnosis of chronic renal disease.

History

The medical history should begin with a summary of prenatal events, including growth parameters at birth. Complications of pregnancy, perinatal events, and unusual events in the nursery may help elucidate the cause of short stature. If growth failure was postnatal in onset, consideration should be given to genetic short stature, with confirmation of short stature within the family. Patients with constitutional delay frequently have a

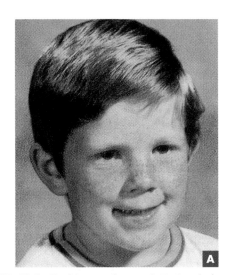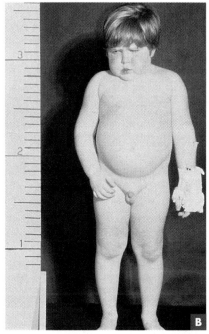

FIG. 28-9 Cushing syndrome. *A,* Patient before onset of illness. *B,* Same patient 4 months later, showing truncal obesity and moon facies.

family history of delayed puberty or delayed growth spurt. Delayed puberty with anosmia (absent sense of smell) may indicate the diagnosis of Kallmann syndrome (anosmia and gonadotropin deficiency). A detailed review of systems is necessary to examine for symptoms of systemic disease. A history of drug intake, including topical or systemic steroids, methylphenidate, or other medications that may suppress growth, may provide important clues. Perhaps most helpful is the plotting of sequential growth points to determine the onset of growth deceleration and the growth velocity.

Physical Examination

The physical examination should be meticulous; the examiner should initially obtain growth measurements of height, weight, head circumference, U/L, and arm span minus height. These measurements help determine whether short stature is proportionate and lead to specific differential diagnoses. Anomalies may suggest a particular syndrome, and midline defects may indicate hypopituitarism. Careful examination of all organ systems, including a funduscopic and neurologic evaluation, is particularly important.

Approach to the Patient

The history and physical examination should suggest an appropriate laboratory approach to the patient. Some screening tests may include a complete blood count, differential count, and sedimentation rate; biochemical profile, including renal function tests and assessment of acid-base status; urinalysis and urine culture; total thyroxine, free thyroxine, and thyroid-stimulating hormone levels; and consideration of a karyotype in the case of a girl with short stature. Bone age determination by radiograph of the left hand and wrist may be helpful. A bone age less than 60% of chronologic age or less than the height age is suggestive of long-standing GH deficiency or hypothyroidism. Bone age equivalent to height age suggests constitutional delay. In addition, some skeletal dysplasias and evidence of rickets may be noted on the radiograph, or the radiograph may show a shortened fourth metacarpal, suggesting Turner syndrome, pseudohypoparathyroidism, or pseudo-pseudohypoparathyroidism. Most importantly, although bone age delay is not specific for any disorder, it may help with prognosis. Children with delayed bone age have greater potential for further growth than those with more advanced epiphyseal maturation. Specific endocrine evaluation, including provocative GH testing and assessment of the hypothalamic-pituitary-adrenal axis often is best accomplished via endocrine consultation.

Treatment is specific to the underlying cause of short stature. Genetic short stature requires no therapy. Therapy for constitutional delay is controversial because generally it is a benign condition associated with ultimate normal height and pubertal development. However, the delay in achieving those goals may cause significant psychologic turmoil, and therapy may be undertaken after psychologic and endocrine consultation.

SUMMARY

Growth deficiency in children may affect weight or length and can indicate psychologic stresses, organic disease, or both. The hallmark of the evaluation is a careful and thorough history and a meticulous physical examination. Most diagnoses can be derived from this basic evaluation, with selected laboratory tests confirming clinical suspicions. Therapy must be specific and directed to the cause of growth failure. Generally, early intervention carries the best prognosis for growth and psychologic and emotional recovery.

ILLUSTRATIVE CASES

Case 1. J.B., a 5-month-old white boy, presented to the local emergency room with fever and irritability. Physical examination revealed a right otitis media, but weight was below the 3rd percentile for age. (He was at the 50th percentile for a 2-month-old infant 3 months ago.) The child had an uncomplicated prenatal and perinatal course, and birth weight was 7 lb 5 oz. The mother appeared disheveled and fatigued. Further history revealed the infant was fed formula, which was properly prepared from concentrate, and took four 8-oz bottles daily. The father recently separated from the family, and the mother was the sole caretaker for three other preschool-age children.

Physical examination showed only the otitis media and decreased subcutaneous fat. The mother appeared distant from the child, and the infant did not exhibit stranger anxiety. The child was managed as an outpatient with social service evaluation and visiting nurse consultation. Screening laboratory tests showed a hemoglobin of 8.7 g/dl and a mean cell volume of 87 fl. Electrolytes were normal, but the blood urea nitrogen was 72 mg/dl, and creatinine was 4.3 mg/dl. Urine culture was sterile, but renal ultrasound was consistent with bilateral dysplastic kidneys.

This case exemplifies the complexity of FTT. Although the profile of the mother and child suggested significant stress and NOFTT would be a strong diagnostic consideration, screening tests revealed coexisting renal insufficiency. The approach to the family concentrated on the renal disease and on providing adequate parenting skills and emotional, psychologic, and financial support.

Case 2. S.R., a 6-year-old boy, was evaluated for short stature. His height age was 3.5 years, and he was mildly underweight for height. The mother described foul-smelling stools and intermittent abdominal distension. Initial evaluation for cystic fibrosis and other malabsorption syndromes was unremarkable. After extensive social service evaluation, it was learned the patient ate dog food and garbage and drank from toilet bowls. He had recurrent temper tantrums and exhibited self-abusive behavior with head-banging. The mother was depressed and ultimately claimed she hated the patient. Physical examination was normal except for small stature. Laboratory examination revealed a bone age of 3.5 years and a blunted GH response to provocative testing. During hospitalization his

eating pattern normalized, and abnormal behaviors almost immediately ceased. The child was placed in foster care, and his growth improved, reaching the 50th percentile by 12 years of age.

This child presented with typical findings of PSS, although the history of aberrant behaviors was initially difficult to elicit from the mother. The child rapidly improved in a changed environment, and growth and development normalized when he was placed in a nurturing environment.

Case 3. M.W. was noted by his parents to be the shortest boy in his third-grade class. At 9 years of age he had the height age of a 7-year-old boy. M.W. always seemed healthy and normally developed without a significant history of illness or hospitalization. Birth weight was 8 lb 7 oz, and length was 21 inches. Both parents are healthy; the mother is 5 ft 8 inches tall, and menarche was at age 12; the father is 5 ft 11 inches tall, and puberty as marked by shaving began at age 17 with attainment of final adult height at age 21. Physical examination, including neurologic and funduscopic examination, was normal except for short stature. Plotting of sequential growth data revealed normal growth until 8 months of age, and then a gradual deceleration until 24 months of age, with resumption of normal growth thereafter. Screening laboratory data were all normal; bone age was 7.3 years, and thyroid functions were normal. The patient appeared to be well-adjusted and accepted by his peers in school.

M.W. represents one of the most common causes of short stature, constitutional delay. The normal birth weight and initial growth suggested postnatal onset of growth delay, and the history of the father's pubertal and growth spurt delay strongly support the diagnosis. Laboratory tests confirm the clinical suspicion, with normal screening tests and a bone age equivalent to height age. Because the patient did not seem disturbed by the short stature, the parents elected not to intervene therapeutically at this time.

ANNOTATED BIBLIOGRAPHY

Berwick DM: Nonorganic failure-to-thrive, *Pediatr Rev* 1:265-270, 1980.

This is an excellent overall review of nonorganic failure to thrive.

Powell GF, Brasel JA, Blizzard RM: Emotional deprivation and growth retardation simulating idiopathic hypopituitarism. I. Clinical evaluation of the syndrome, *N Engl J Med* 276:1271-1278, 1967.

This is a classical description of psychosocial dwarfism that with its companion paper describes clinical and endocrinologic aberrations.

Sills RH: Failure to thrive: the role of clinical and laboratory examination, *Am J Dis Child* 132:967-969, 1978.

This study demonstrates that careful history and physical examination rather than laboratory tests are the clinician's most powerful diagnostic tools.

BIBLIOGRAPHY

Altemeier WA, O'Connor SM, Sherrod KB, et al: Prospective study of antecedents for nonorganic failure to thrive, *J Pediatr* 106:360-365, 1985.

Ambuel JP, Harris B: Failure to thrive, *Ohio Med J* 59:997-1001, 1963.

Berwick DM, Levy JC, Kleinerman R: Failure to thrive: diagnostic yield of hospitalization, *Arch Dis Child* 57:347-351, 1982.

Bithoney WG, Dubowitz H, Egan H: Failure to thrive/growth deficiency, *Pediatr Rev* 13:453-460, 1992.

Elmer E, Gregg GS, Ellison P: Late results of the "failure to thrive" syndrome, *Clin Pediatr* 8:84-589, 1969.

Evans SL, Reinhart JB, Succop RA: Failure to thrive: a study of 45 children and their families, *J Am Acad Child Adolesc Psychiatry* 11:440-457, 1972.

Gardner LI: Deprivation dwarfism, *Sci Am* 227:76-82, 1972.

Guo S, Roche A, Fomon SJ, et al: Reference data on gains in weight and length during the first two years of life, *J Pediatr* 119:355-362, 1991.

Hertzig ME, Birch HG, Richardson SA, et al: Intellectual levels of school children severely malnourished during the first two years of life, *Pediatrics* 49:814-824, 1972.

Homer C, Ludwig S: Categorization of etiology of failure to thrive, *Am J Dis Child* 135:848-851, 1981.

Hutton IW, Oates RK: Nonorganic failure to thrive: a long-term follow-up, *Pediatrics* 59:73-77, 1977.

Krieger I: The energy metabolism in infants with growth failure due to maternal deprivation, undernutrition, or causes unknown: metabolic rate calculated from the insensible loss of weight, *Pediatrics* 38:63-76, 1966.

Lacey KA, Parkin JM: Causes of short stature, *Lancet* 1:42-45, 1974.

Leonard MF, Rhymes JP, Solnit AJ: Failure to thrive in infants, *Am J Dis Child* 111:600-612, 1966.

Lukefahr JL: Underlying illness associated with failure to thrive in breastfed infants, *Clin Pediatr* 29:468-470, 1990.

Mitchell WG, Gorrell RW, Greenberg RA: Failure-to-thrive: a study in a primary care setting—epidemiology and follow-up, *Pediatrics* 65:971-977, 1980.

Money J, Annecillo C, Kelley JF: Growth of intelligence: failure and catch-up associated retrospectively with abuse and rescue in the syndrome of abuse dwarfism, *Psychoneuroendocrinology* 8:309-319, 1983.

Oates RK, Peacock A, Forrest D: Long-term effects of nonorganic failure to thrive, *Pediatrics* 75:36-40, 1985.

Pollitt E: Failure to thrive: socioeconomic, dietary intake, and mother-child interaction data, *Federation Proceedings* 34:1593-1597, 1975.

Pollitt E, Eichler A: Behavioral disturbances among failure-to-thrive children, *Am J Dis Child* 130:24-29, 1976.

Powell GF, Brasel JA, Raiti S, et al: Emotional deprivation and growth retardation simulating idiopathic hypopituitarism. II. Endocrinologic evaluation of the syndrome, *N Engl J Med* 276:1279-1283, 1967.

Reinhart JB: Failure to thrive: 50 year follow-up, *J Pediatr* 81:1218-1219, 1972.

Roche AF, Wainer H, Thissen D: The RWT method for the prediction of adult stature, *Pediatrics* 56:1026-1033, 1975.

Schmitt BD, Mauro RD: Nonorganic failure to thrive: an outpatient approach, *Child Abuse Negl* 13:235-248, 1989.

Silver HK, Finkelstein M: Deprivation dwarfism, *J Pediatr* 70:317-324, 1967.

Smith DW, Truog W, Rogers JE, et al: Shifting linear growth during infancy: illustration of genetic factors from fetal life through infancy, *J Pediatr* 89:225-230, 1976.

Whitten CF, Fischoff J, Pettit M, et al: Evidence that growth retardation in the maternal deprivation syndrome is secondary to an inadequate intake of calories (undereating), *J Pediatr* 72:563-565, 1968 (abstract)

29

Congenital Anomalies

ANDREW H. URBACH

 Key Points

- Despite major technical developments in the field of genetics, meticulous history and physical examination remain the foundation of accurate diagnosis.

- The four major morphologic pathogenic mechanisms in humans are deformation, disruption, dysplasia, and malformation. Familiarity with these concepts can facilitate diagnosis.

- When assessing a child with multiple congenital anomalies, the most uncommon of these anomalies is the pivotal feature, or diagnostic handle. This feature is often the key to diagnosis.

My friend is not perfect—nor am I—and so we suit each other admirably.

ALEXANDER POPE

Few events in a parent's life are filled with as much import and implication as the birth of a child with a congenital anomaly. The shock, fear, anger, and guilt that a distraught parent might feel can be overwhelming. The parent's fantasy of having the "perfect child" gives way rapidly to questions about intellectual status, cosmetic appearance, and future level of function. The primary care physician is the focal point for the care of many such children. This chapter presents the terms and concepts necessary to critically evaluate children with congenital anomalies and provides the practitioner with a logical approach to assessing the child with birth defects.

A congenital anomaly is a deviation from the body's normal architecture. These abnormalities may be major or minor. Major anomalies occur in approximately 3% of live births, and minor anomalies occur in about 3% to 15%. Major anomalies raise more than purely cosmetic concerns and may necessitate surgery, intense medical management, and perhaps a change in lifestyle and life expectancy. Examples of these types of anomalies include cleft lip and palate (Fig. 29-1), duodenal atresia (see Fig. 20-2), and spina bifida (Fig. 29-2). On the other end of the spectrum, minor anomalies, such as pilonidal dimples, clinodactyly (Fig. 29-3), and eartags (Fig. 29-4), are of minimal consequence. Should a deviation from "normal" be part of a family trait or common in a particular ethnic group, the term *normal variant* is used. Note that some minor variants may be classified as minor anomalies when the finding is recognized as part of an underlying syndrome.

With experience and a trained eye, the practitioner generally can recognize variations from normal. The task that at first may appear overwhelming, however, is the integration of these often minor findings into an accurate, unifying diagnosis. The rarity of congenital anomalies precludes memorization or even gestalt recognition but rather necessitates a methodical, step-wise approach. Furthermore, the fact that each of the individual 5000 genetic disorders currently described is rare does not mean that they are rare as a group. Studies estimate that 11% to 27% of pediatric inpatients have a condition with significant genetic impact. Chromosome disorders occur in approximately 1 in 150 to 200 live births, and half of all girls with primary amenorrhea have an abnormality of the X chromosome. Of spontaneous first-trimester miscarriages, 60% are a result of a chromosomal aberration. All of this is sobering to clinicians who thought they could "elude" these complex and difficult-to-recognize entities on the basis of their rarity. Additionally the argument that most of these entities are not treatable contradicts the fact that approximately 50% of congenital anomalies can be surgically corrected. Also, many metabolic disorders can be effectively managed through dietary enhancement or restriction, and gene transfer as a therapeutic modality is advancing rapidly. Even in the case of a child with an "irreversible" problem, such as Down syndrome, the benefits of accurate diagnosis can be enormous.

In the newborn period, recognition of the child with trisomy 13 or trisomy 18 syndrome allows the clinician and family to choose a nonaggressive approach to life-threatening anomalies, such as heart disease. Less dramatic but of equal importance is the child with Beckwith-Wiedemann syndrome and neonatal hypoglycemia. Failure to recognize this disorder

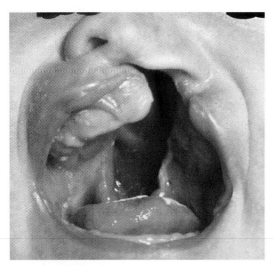

FIG. 29-1 Major anomalies present at birth. Note the cleft lip and palate.

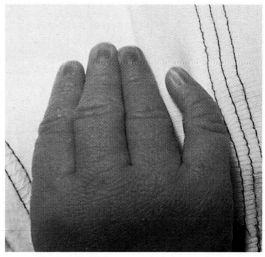

FIG. 29-3 Minor anomalies present at birth. Note the clinodactyly of the fifth finger. (Courtesy Dr. Christine L. Williams, New York Medical College.)

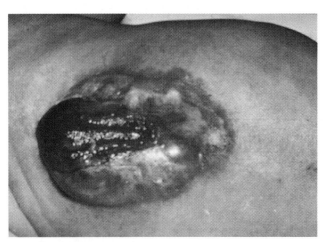

FIG. 29-2 Major anomalies present at birth. Note the meningomyelocele. (Courtesy Dr. Christine L. Williams, New York Medical College.)

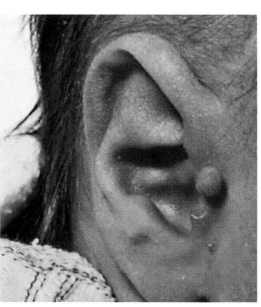

FIG. 29-4 Minor anomalies present at birth. Note the preauricular skin tag.

early may result in hypoglycemic seizures and brain injury. In the older child with Down syndrome, correct diagnosis directs the practitioner to timely evaluation of atlantoaxial instability, myopia, strabismus, and potential thyroid abnormalities. Additionally, assigning a child a definitive diagnosis provides insight into future intellectual function. The knowledge that Down syndrome is invariably associated with intellectual handicap and that Treacher Collins syndrome generally is not can have profound implications for the families and physicians of these children. Although precise diagnosis cannot predict the future, it does provide a framework within which

the physician and family can operate. Inability to provide a diagnosis may leave the family with the impression that their child's anomalies are so unique that no one can assist them. Even when a diagnosis carries negative implications, often the vagueness of "not knowing" is harder on families than dealing with the reality of a diagnosis. Genetic counseling is also facilitated by accurate diagnosis. The risk of recurrence in future children may be as low as zero or as high as 100% (Table 29-1). The ability to provide an accurate prediction of risk is vital to informed decision-making on the part of the family and is dependent on making the correct diagnosis.

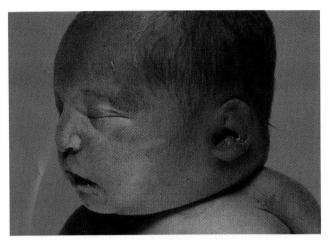

FIG. 29-5 Potter facies. This infant with bilateral multicystic dysplasia died at 12 hours of age with pulmonary insufficiency. The altered facies produced by the fetal compression syndrome of oligohydramnios includes small, posteriorly rotated ears; micrognathia; a beaked nose; and wide-set eyes. (Courtesy Dr. Elizabeth MacPherson, Magee-Women's Hospital, Pittsburgh.)

TABLE 29-1

Recurrence Risk in Siblings of Dysmorphic Children

Risk in siblings (%)	Condition
1-2	Trisomy 21, trisomy 13, trisomy 18
3-7	Spina bifida, cleft palate and lip, hypospadias
25	Autosomal recessive disease, Smith-Lemli-Opitz syndrome; X-linked recessive disease, X-linked hydrocephalus
50	Autosomal dominant disease, neurofibromatosis and tuberous sclerosis
100	Chromosomal disorder, 21/21 translocation Down syndrome with carrier parent

Modified from Keele DK: A diagnostic approach to the dysmorphic child, *Contemp Pediatr* 2:63-84, 1985.

The last decade has witnessed such dramatic technologic expansion in the field of clinical genetics that the practitioner may find it impossible to have up-to-date information. Fortunately, despite these advances the field of dysmorphology largely remains a visual specialty. Without a careful history and meticulous physical examination, the efficacy of these advanced genetic tools is diminished, and they lack focus. The clinician must develop a sense for size, proportion, position, and symmetry. These cost-effective observational skills offer the quickest possible route to diagnosis. The clinician with a passion for problem-solving therefore remains the key to dysmorphology.

Pathophysiology

Dysmorphologists, as is true of other subspecialists, have developed their own language and style of communication. To the uninitiated these terms may seem cumbersome, but with a small amount of effort they can be used easily and serve as descriptive tools that facilitate communication and diagnosis.

The terms *major anomaly, minor anomaly,* and *normal variant* were defined earlier. Leppig reports that of 4305 newborns, 28.2% had one minor anomaly, 8.65% had two minor anomalies, and only 3.67% had three or more minor anomalies. Major anomalies were seen in 3.74% of infants. The newborn with three or more minor anomalies has an approximately 20% risk of having a major anomaly and hence is at very high risk for the eventual diagnosis of a syndrome. Although each minor anomaly alone may seem insignificant, it is the constellation of anomalies that defines a syndrome. This is particularly true because few if any individual anomalies are truly pathognomonic for a given syndrome. A minor anomaly carries as much weight as a major anomaly in the eventual diagnosis of a syndrome. For example, in Down syndrome, about 80% of the anomalies found on clinical examination are minor ones. Over 70% of minor anomalies occur on the face and hands, reflecting the complexity of these structures.

Once identified, these anomalies must be incorporated into a pathogenic mechanism. There are four major morphologic pathogenic mechanisms in humans—*deformation, disruption, dysplasia,* and *malformation.* Although each of these terms has a distinct meaning, real-life situations occasionally reflect some overlap between various pathogenic processes.

Deformations represent external compression and eventual distortion of a normally formed and intact body part. As the fetus grows a relative crowding occurs as a result of a small or abnormal uterus or a large fetus relative to the space available (Fig. 29-5). Oligohydramnios or a lack of fetal movement can also result in mechanical compression of bodily structures (Box 29-1). These "deformities" tend to occur late in pregnancy (early deformations also occur and can be quite severe), tend to be multiple, and are often associated with breech,

BOX 29-2

Common Deformation Anomalies

Head and Neck
Synostosis of one or
    more sutures
Vertex birth molding
Plagiocephaly-torticollis
    sequence
Micrognathia
Mandibular asymmetry
Nose compression (down-
    ward deviation)
Ear deformities
    Overfolding of helix
    Flattening against head
    Crumpling between
        head and shoulder
    Uplifted auricle by
        shoulder constraint

Thorax
Pectus carinatum
Pectus excavatum
Pulmonary hypoplasia
    caused by oligohy-
    dramnios

Back
Scoliosis

Limbs
Dorsiflexion of foot
    (calcaneovalgus)
Metatarsus adductus
    (pigeon-toe)
Talipes equinovarus
    (clubfoot)
Deformed toes (crowd-
    ing, overlapping)
Tibial torsion
Joint dislocations (hip,
    knee, radial head)

Nerve Compression
Facial nerve palsies
Erb palsy
Leg weakness

Modified from Keele DK: A diagnostic approach to the dysmorphic child, *Contemp Pediatr* 2:63-84, 1985.

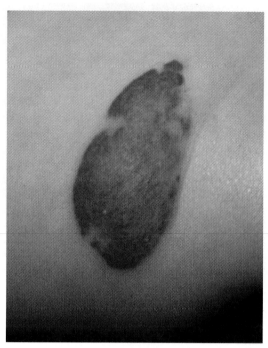

FIG. 29-6   Capillary (strawberry) hemangioma.

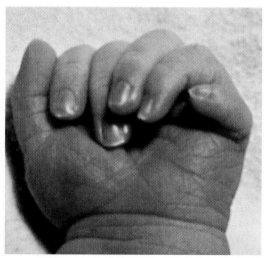

FIG. 29-7 Major anomalies present at birth. Note the polydactyly (postaxial).

transverse, or another uncommon presentation. Frequently, reassurance is in order because the affected fetus was "destined" to be normal but encountered external forces because of an altered uterine environment. Intellectual function is generally unaffected, but some anomalies, such as craniosynostosis and clubfoot deformity, may require significant attention. Most deformities, such as tibial bowing, positional clubfoot, and unilateral micrognathia, improve after removal of the offending pressure. The recurrence risk for deformation syndromes is low unless an intrinsic abnormality of the uterine environment exists. A list of common deformations is provided in Box 29-2.

Disruptions represent an actual destruction of tissue rather than simply a deformation of tissue. Disruption occurs in a fetus that is "programmed" to be normal, but outside forces intervene, resulting in tissue and cell death. Disruptive agents include amniotic bands, mechanical forces, vascular insufficiency, and viral infections. Injuries follow geographic patterns rather than embryologic patterns. Entire structures or tissues adjacent to the affected tissue may be completely normal, whereas the disrupted area has all embryologic cell lines affected. Intellectual prognosis is usually excellent, and therapy focuses on reconstruction and rehabilitation of damaged structures.

Dysplasias are intrinsic abnormalities of underlying cells and their function (see Fig. 9-4). Typically, one tissue type is

affected, but when a metabolic pathway common to several cell types is affected (e.g., mucopolysaccharidosis), various body systems are involved. Rarely does effective therapy exist, and commonly these entities evolve over time, causing more severe involvement with age. Marfan syndrome and neurofibromatosis are examples of generalized dysplasias, and the superficial ("strawberry") hemangioma is a good example of a localized dysplasia (Fig. 29-6).

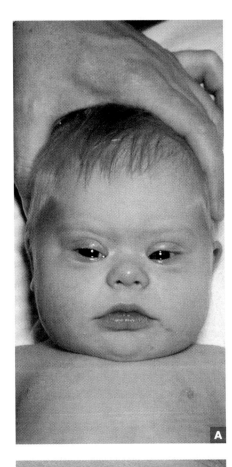

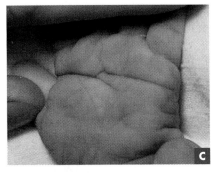

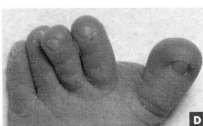

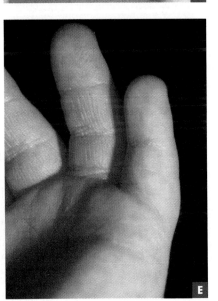

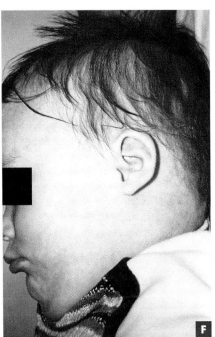

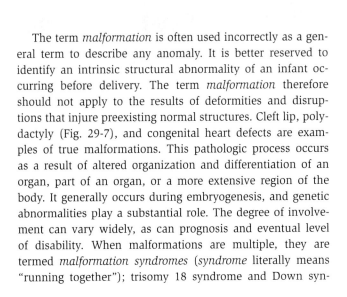

FIG. 29-8 Several minor anomalies associated with Down syndrome. *A,* Typical facies (note epicanthal folds). *B,* Brushfield spots. *C,* Simian crease. *D,* Wide space between first and second toes. *E,* Short fifth finger. *F,* Small ears.

The term *malformation* is often used incorrectly as a general term to describe any anomaly. It is better reserved to identify an intrinsic structural abnormality of an infant occurring before delivery. The term *malformation* therefore should not apply to the results of deformities and disruptions that injure preexisting normal structures. Cleft lip, polydactyly (Fig. 29-7), and congenital heart defects are examples of true malformations. This pathologic process occurs as a result of altered organization and differentiation of an organ, part of an organ, or a more extensive region of the body. It generally occurs during embryogenesis, and genetic abnormalities play a substantial role. The degree of involvement can vary widely, as can prognosis and eventual level of disability. When malformations are multiple, they are termed *malformation syndromes* (*syndrome* literally means "running together"); trisomy 18 syndrome and Down syndrome (Fig. 29-8) are examples. On occasion a malformation by nature of its size or shape also leads to intrauterine constraint, and the problem is compounded by a deformation process as well. Hence overlap between two very different pathophysiologic processes may occur.

With these underlying mechanisms identified, the clinician can conceptualize how structural anomalies can occur; the surprise is that they do not occur more often. At times, anomalies occur in a seemingly random pattern, but at other times, order can be brought to this chaos and a label assigned to a collection of anomalies. The following section identifies various patterns and types of birth defects; again, "genetic jargon" and its significant functional use are reviewed. Minor anomalies and variants that are isolated or affect only a localized body area are most common and generally carry an excellent overall prognosis. At times, examination of other

---

BOX 29-3

Examples of Common Minor Anomalies

Skull
Parietal foramina
Parietal bossing
Prominent forehead

Ears
Preauricular pits
Preauricular tags
Anomalies of auricular
  cartilage

Eyes
Heterochromia of the iris
Coloboma of the iris

Nose
Short columella
Bulbous nasal tip

Perioral Zone
Smooth philtrum
Narrow vermilion
Angular lip pits

Mouth
Palatal pits
Torus palatinus
Hypoplastic lateral
  incisors
Short lingual frenulum

Neck
Branchial arch remnants

Chest
Supernumerary nipples

Abdomen
Single umbilical artery
Umbilical hernia

Genitalia
Labial adhesions
Hydrocele
Mild hypospadias
Undescended testis

Anus and Perineum
Anal tags
Anal stenosis

Back
Sacral dimples

Skin
Isolated pigmented nevi
Small vascular nevi
Skin dimples overlying
  bony prominences

Hair
Upswept posterior hair-
  line
Supernumerary scalp hair
  whorl
"Electric" hair
White forelock

Nails
"Spooned" nails
Nail grooves

Joints
Infantile bowleg
Camptodactyly of fifth
  fingers

Hands
Clinodactyly of fifth
  fingers

Feet
Syndactyly of second and
  third toes
Short fourth metatarsal

Modified from Aase JM: Dysmorphology diagnosis for the pediatric practitioner, *Pediatr Clin North Am* 39:135-156, 1992.

family members reveals variants, supplying further support for optimism. An extensive list of minor anomalies is provided in Box 29-3. Major anomalies occur in isolation about two thirds of the time and are believed to result from multifactorial inheritance. When multiple anomalies are encountered in the same individual, it is incumbent on the clinician to attempt further classification. For this purpose, the terms *association, developmental field complex, sequence,* and *syndrome* are useful.

Associations are nonrandom, statistically significant collections of anomalies with no defined underlying cause. At the core of associations are six to eight anomalies. Each patient rarely displays all of these features but must have several features noted before such a diagnosis can be comfortably entertained. An example of this type of genetic category is VACTERRL (or VATER) association (Fig. 29-9). *V*ertebral anomalies, *a*nal atresia, *c*ardiac defects, *t*racheoesophageal fistula, *r*adial anomalies, *r*enal anomalies, and *l*iver anomalies make up the acronym. Patients with associations do not display these anomalies exclusively but may have many other anomalies in conjunction with the core findings.

The term *developmental field complex,* described by Opitz, suggests that disparate types of embryologic tissues located in the same body area may all be affected by a common agent or event. Many of these field defects may be caused by vascular insufficiency or total absence of arteries. The final result is an absence, hypoplasia, or defect of the involved structures. Because the defect occurs early in gestation and is permanent, outlook for reconstruction is generally poor. Sacral agenesis with its extreme counterpart, sirenomelia, displays the impact of a field complex on the distal spine, pelvis, and lower extremities.

In contrast to associations, *sequences* and *syndromes* occur in a more uniform and consistent pattern from child to child. Although variations certainly exist, to the experienced eye the similarities of anomalies and presentations dominate the clinical picture. As opposed to patients with developmental field complexes, these patients often have distant bodily structures affected in a pattern consistent in many patients affected by the process. For example, children with Down syndrome frequently have Brushfield spots, a simian crease, congenital heart disease, and hypogonadism. Despite some variability in presentation, the cause of a syndrome is believed to be the same for all affected children. A sequence is a cascade of malformations or deformities that begins with an isolated anomaly. For example, Pierre Robin sequence begins with the development of a hypoplastic mandible very early in gestation. The chin at birth is small, but perhaps more important, upward and posterior displacement of the tongue during embryogenesis leads to cleft palate. Glossoptosis (downward displacement or retraction of the tongue) at birth may lead to airway obstruction, anoxia, and central nervous system injury (see Fig. 16-1).

Literature Survey

The list of recognized dysmorphic syndromes is vast and is expanding rapidly. Even skilled dysmorphologists do not have a working knowledge of all known syndromes. Fortu-

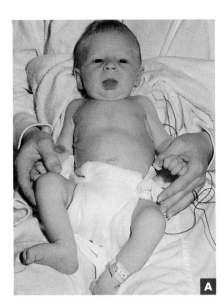

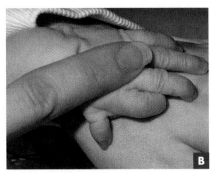

FIG. 29-9 This child with VATER association has a relatively normal facial appearance, *(A);* radial dysplasia and an abnormal thumb are present *(B).*

nately, wonderful tools are available in the form of dysmorphology compendiums, textbooks, and computer programs that provide minutiae on even the rarest of described syndromes. Perhaps the best known to the generalist is *Smith's Recognizable Patterns of Human Malformation.* Other sources are listed in the reference section. One look at these voluminous resources and the point made earlier about developing an approach to dysmorphology rather than memorizing becomes clear.

Differential Diagnosis

The differential diagnosis of congenital anomalies is quite extensive, and several key principles should be followed. As any successful clinician will attest, establishing a rapid and correct diagnosis is grounded in the detail and accuracy of the history and physical examination (see following section). A meticulous review of this information, and preexisting laboratory studies is critical. With these data in hand, the clinician should attempt to develop a theory about the pathogenic mechanism—deformation, disruption, dysplasia, malformation, or some combination of these four. An attempt should then be made to determine the pattern of dysmorphic features (i.e., association, complex, sequence, or syndrome). At this point, if the diagnosis is still not apparent, the most unusual features noted in the child should be identified. The indices of reference texts provide lists of syndromes displaying these features. By choosing the rarest finding, the list of potential syndromes is the narrowest. For example, in a dysmorphic child with heart disease, cleft lip, cryptorchidism, single umbilical artery, and posterior midline scalp defects, the scalp defect is the rarest and can be defined specifically. *Smith's Recognizable Patterns of Human Malformation* lists four syndromes with midline

posterior scalp defects—Adams-Oliver, Johanson-Blizzard, trisomy 13, and trisomy 4p-. On comparing these syndromes with the patient, only trisomies 13 and 4p- fit the description. Further evaluation of the patient might reveal holoprosencephaly, hemangiomata, and polydactyly, adding weight into the eventual diagnosis of trisomy 13 (Fig. 29-10). The scalp defect might be referred to as a *pivotal feature* or *diagnostic handle.* The laboratory might then be used to reveal increased frequency of nuclear projections in neutrophils (a distinctive feature of trisomy 13), and eventually definitive diagnosis can be made based on chromosomal analysis. It is worth noting that the evaluation of neutrophils for typical projections is a very focused laboratory evaluation clearly based on careful history and physical examination.

As the clinician proceeds through the differential diagnosis, an evolutionary process, a number of points warrant attention. Often wide variation exists within a given syndrome. This concept is known as *phenotypic variation.* Although a given syndrome has a core of definitive features, they may be obvious or quite subtle. Additionally, common features may be absent, and more unusual features may be present. Adding to the challenge is the concept known as *changing phenotype.* With age, facial features can appear or disappear. Examples include Down syndrome, in which abnormal facies are less obvious in the immediate neonatal period, and Noonan syndrome, in which abnormal facies may mature into a more subtle or nondiagnosable form as an adult.

Lastly, the temptation to "force" a diagnosis is great. An incorrect diagnosis is certainly more damaging than no diagnosis. In fact, 30% to 50% of patients cannot be diagnosed even by experienced dysmorphologists. Time, however, is on the side of the clinician because 10% of undiagnosed patients eventually will be diagnosed as new data become available and time passes.

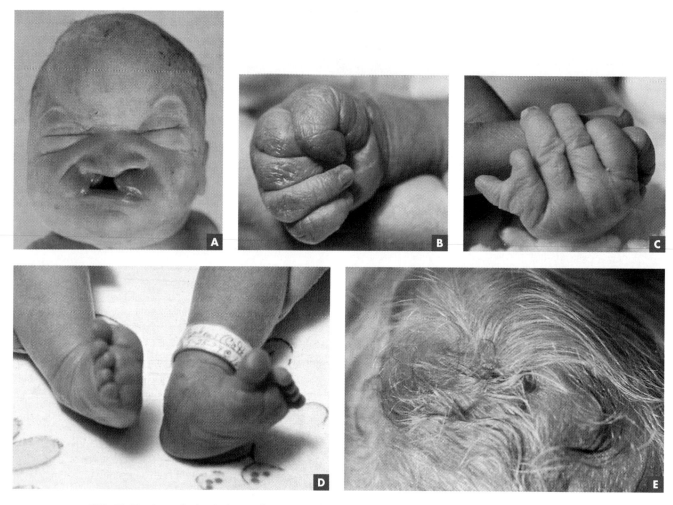

FIG. 29-10 Several physical manifestations of trisomy 13. *A,* Facies showing a midline defect. *B,* Clenched hand with overlapping fingers. *C,* Preaxial polydactyly. *D,* Equinovarus deformity. *E,* Typical punched-out posterior scalp lesions. (*A* courtesy Dr. T. Kelly, University of Virginia Medical Center, Charlottesville; *B* to *E* courtesy Dr. Kenneth Garver, Pittsburgh.)

History

Medical History

The process of obtaining a dysmorphology history is complex and challenging. In addition to the many details required to complete the "story," families may be anxious, defensive, or angry and feel a strong sense of guilt for having knowingly or unknowingly contributed to their child's condition. This heightens the need for a quiet setting and an unhurried, caring approach. A nonjudgmental, supportive style is most effective. Eliciting free-flowing narrative from the family with open-ended questions and balancing this with direct questions is likely to be most successful. The history should be very detailed and verified carefully to assure that all pertinent issues are revealed. Active listening, avoidance of medical jargon, gentleness, and compassion go a long way toward building trust and confidence. As put quite succinctly by Aase, in the process of solving the mystery the parents are "expert witnesses not defendants."

The first step in developing a historic record is a review of all preexisting records (Box 29-4). This review should include prenatal information, birth history, growth curves, development, laboratory studies, and radiologic procedures. In all cases, hard copies of imaging studies should be reviewed with a pediatric radiologist. This assures that the test quality and interpretation are proper and also provides the clinician with a depth of understanding that is invaluable.

Personal style dictates where the history should begin. It is useful to initiate the data-gathering at the time when parents first learned of the pregnancy. Was this pregnancy planned, and have there been other pregnancies, live births, miscarriages, abortions, premature infants, or previous pregnancy complications? Prenatal diagnosis, ultrasound studies, fetal growth records, and fetal activity (onset, strength, and frequency) can be helpful data on fetal development. Was there prenatal care, and what was the maternal weight gain and nutrition during pregnancy? Is there a history of hypertension, diabetes mellitus, trauma, vaginal bleeding, illness, or hyper-

Medical and Family History Often Needed for Diagnosing Genetic Diseases

Pedigree
Similar problems in the family
Age of onset of the problem in other family members
Clinical expression of the problem in other family members
Other significant problems in the family (e.g., mental retardation, birth defects, or early deaths)
Paternity
Consanguinity

Maternal Medical History
Diabetes mellitus or phenylketonuria, etc.
Immunization status
Uterine anomalies

Maternal Pregnancy History
Recurrent miscarriages
Parity
Chemical, radiation, and cigarette smoke exposures
Complications (e.g., preeclampsia, placenta previa, or amniotic fluid leak)
Polyhydramnios or oligohydramnios
Fetal movements
Fetal growth assessments
Prenatal screening results

Neonatal History
Fetal presentation
Complications during labor and delivery
Gestational age
Feeding problems
Results of newborn screening tests

Dietary History
Feeding behavior
Formula or food intolerance
Temporal relation of signs and symptoms to meals
Relation of signs and symptoms to types of food eaten

Developmental History
Temporal progression of development
Regression of development
School performance

Modified from Fong CT: Clinical diagnosis of genetic diseases, *Pediatr Ann* 22:277-281, 1993.

Known Teratogens

Environmental
Infections—TORCH syndrome, viruses, varicella
Radiation
Hyperthermia
Tobacco

Maternal
Metabolic—diabetes mellitus, phenylketonuria, hypothroidism, galactosemia
Endocrine—virilizing tumors, hyperthyroidism
Disease-related—systemic lupus erythematosus, myotonic dystrophy, myasthenia gravis

Drugs
Alcohol
Alkylating agents
Androgens
Anticonvulsants
Antithyroid agents
Cocaine
Diethylstilbestrol
Folic acid antagonists
Lithium
Mercury
Polychlorinated biphenyl
Penicillamine
Tetracycline
Thalidomide
Vitamin A
Warfarin

Modified from Hall JG: When a child is born with congenital anomalies, *Contemp Pediatr* 5:78-87, 1988.

emesis during this pregnancy? Careful assessment of medication use (including over-the-counter and topical medications) and exposure to chemicals, fumes, radiation, heat (hot tubs and saunas), alcohol, drugs, and tobacco is important. A list of known teratogens is supplied in Box 29-5. Was there evidence of viral infection or infectious illnesses during pregnancy (including *t*oxoplasmosis, *o*ther agents, *r*ubella, *c*ytomegalovirus, *h*erpes simplex [TORCH] syndrome and human immunodeficiency virus [HIV])? A history of animal exposure and travel should be addressed. As this history progresses, accurate dates should allow the questioner to time events and exposures during embryologic development. Salient milestones of embryologic life are presented in Table 29-2.

Evaluation of the uterine environment should include size and shape of the uterus (any anomalies, such as bicornuate uterus), placental evaluation (prenatal and postdelivery), polyhydramnios (suggesting increased urine output or decreased swallowing), and oligohydramnios (suggesting poor renal function).

Birth history should include whether labor was spontaneous or induced and the duration of and any complications during labor. During labor, was there fetal monitoring, and what was the timing of rupture of membranes? How did the baby present (breech, transverse, etc.)? What was the birth weight, length, head circumference, and Apgar score? Was

TABLE 29-2

Major Events in Human Embryonic Development

Age	Event
Day 5	Implantation
Day 16	Three germ layers distinct
Day 19	Neural plate formed
Day 27	Neural tube closed
Day 30	Limb buds appear
Weeks 4-5	Branchial arches, clefts, and pouches formed; optic vesicle formed
Weeks 5-7	"Mature" heart formed, kidneys formed
Week 7	Hard palate fuses, upper lip formed, physiologic herniation of intestines
Week 8	Mature limb architecture achieved
Weeks 7-10	Sex differentiation of internal and external genitalia
Week 10	Return and rotation of intestines into abdominal cavity
Weeks 10-16	Hair patterning established
Weeks 13-19	Dermal ridges and creases formed

Modified from Hall JG: When a child is born with congenital anomalies, *Contemp Pediatr* 5:78-87, 1988.

there a need for oxygen or resuscitation, and was any special care provided? Note that breech delivery occurs in 3% to 4% of individuals but is associated with a higher incidence of anomalies. (Perhaps a neurologic handicap limited the ability of the baby to turn itself.) Difficult deliveries as well may be the result of an intrinsic problem with the baby rather than the cause of a child's problem. In general, was there any feature about this delivery that may have caused trauma, hypoxia, or bleeding?

Neonatal status should be assessed next. What form of nutrition did the infant receive, and was feeding uncomplicated? How did the infant suck, and was there vomiting, diarrhea, or poor growth? Other issues to touch on include evidence of jaundice, seizures, abnormal tone, or fever. Developmental delay alone warrants a thorough examination for anomalies (see Chapter 9). Of patients with idiopathic mental retardation, 42% have three or more anomalies (mostly minor). All information should be compared with other pregnancies and siblings. The child's history after this period also should be addressed and specific attention given to growth, development, behavior, and any cognitive or sensory testing. Photographs of the child at various ages should be scrutinized.

Family History

Family history should be obtained next. The framework of the family's genetic features is best formatted with a pedigree.

Special attention should be paid to any condition of genetic significance. When possible, similarly affected individuals should be examined and when appropriate photographed. Parental ages, occupations, ethnic origins, consanguinity, and medical conditions, including intellectual function, should be addressed. Special attention should be paid to mode of inheritance. Autosomal dominant disorders often have variable expressivity with some family members being asymptomatic and not yet diagnosed. Autosomal recessive and X-linked recessive disorders may not be clinically evident because heterozygote carriers and females are unaffected. Autosomal dominant and X-linked disorders display a vertical mode of inheritance. Affected females and a male-to-male inheritance pattern are unlikely for an X-linked disorder. Horizontal inheritance, with normal parents but varying numbers of affected siblings, is typical of autosomal recessive disorders. Should no obvious pattern come to light, chromosomal or polygenic inheritance is a possibility. It is important to recognize that a pedigree may not always be helpful. The high rate of mutations of some conditions and the multiple factors that may play a role in transmission often result in isolated cases. A summary of various modes of inheritance is provided (Table 29-3). A review of the dysmorphology history is provided in Box 29-4.

Physical Examination

Perhaps nowhere else in pediatrics is the meticulous observation of minute details more central to diagnosis than in the child with congenital anomalies. The expression "head-to-toe" evaluation may more appropriately read "scalp-to-soles." Dysmorphologists have trained themselves in the style of Sherlock Holmes and base diagnoses on "the observation of trifles." Careful description and documentation is essential for personal record review and for use by others. Using the description of "short stature" is inadequate. Rather, upper/lower segment ratios should be noted; proportionality must be assessed and limb length judged, and if short, location of the abnormality—proximal, middle, or distal (rhizomelic, mesomelic, or acromelic) must be described. The answers to each of these questions may lead to completely different diagnoses and hence a different prognosis and genetic counseling. Obviously the dysmorphology evaluation is not the place for a cursory physical examination. Even when gestalt recognition serves to bring a syndrome to mind, an analytical, detail-focused confirmation is indicated. Because of the concept of changing phenotype (discussed earlier), documentation by words, diagrams, or photographs can be most helpful. An example of this is provided by the child with Turner syndrome and associated transient congenital edema (Fig. 29-11). With time these findings abate, eliminating an excellent clue to timely diagnosis. Should the evaluator overlook this finding or improperly document it, diagnosis may be delayed. Any attempt on the child's part to negotiate a less-than-complete skin examination because of modesty should be countered. Often a

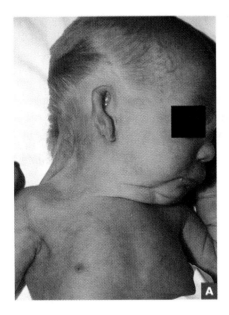
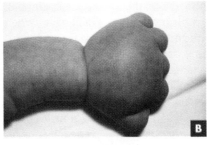
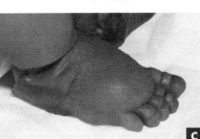

FIG. 29-11 Physical manifestations associated with Turner syndrome. *A*, Webbed neck, widespread nipples, abnormal ears, and micrognathia. *B* and *C*, Lymphedema of the hands and feet.

TABLE 29-3

Categories of Congenital Anomalies

Mode of transmission	Typical presentation	Example
Chromosomal abnormalities	1st trimester spontaneous abortion, history of recurrent abortions, multiple major and minor anomalies, mental handicap, poor growth (prenatal and postnatal), advanced maternal age *	Down syndrome
Single gene abnormalities (mendelian inheritance)	Positive family history, consanguinity, advanced paternal age leads to autosomal dominant disorders with new mutation, able to map on specific chromosomes, prenatal diagnosis often possible	Cystic fibrosis, Zellweger syndrome
Multifactorial disorders	Single defects, genetic and environmental factors combine to create defect anomaly, recurrence risk 2% to 5%, never cause multiple anomalies	Cleft lip
Environmental effects	TORCH, radiation, drugs, chemicals, alcohol	Congenital rubella, fetal alcohol syndrome

Modified from Hall JG: When a child is born with congenital anomalies, *Contemp Pediatr,* 5:78-87, 1988; and Witt DR, Hall JG: Multiple congenital anomaly syndromes. In Rudolph AM, Hoffman JIE, Rudolph CD, editors: *Rudolph's textbook of pediatrics,* Norwalk, Conn, 1991, Appleton and Lange.
*Absence of these findings does not eliminate a chromosomal abnormality as a possibility.

subtle but diagnostic feature is uncovered by a thorough examination. Identifying the hidden café au lait spot or hypopigmented macule and the accurate assessment of bodily symmetry depend on a full inspection of the unclothed child.

Normal variants form a continuum with minor anomalies, and where the line is drawn in the examiner's mind is vital. Careful evaluation of parents and other family members is an excellent reference point. Certainly a shared feature may be a familial, inherited variant; however, it is also possible that both affected family members may have varying degrees of expression of the same autosomal dominant entity. Although the gestalt or qualitative approach is excellent for the experienced clinician, this subjective method may not serve all

equally. A photograph allows subsequent physicians to come to their own conclusions. It should be noted that the child with prominent eyes may have large globes, shallow orbits, or retracted eyelids, all creating a similar phenotypic appearance. Using measurement and applying a child's values to normal tables may be of great assistance. Many texts provide useful norms for height, weight, head circumference, and the size of a child's chest, anterior fontanelle, hands, feet, inner canthal and interpupillary distance, palpebral fissure length, and ear length. These tools allow for a more objective and presumably accurate assessment. In the same way that a clinician would not be comfortable judging growth without a growth curve, a child should not be labeled as having small ears without plotting ear length on a curve. Furthermore, the clinician should recognize that adjacent bodily structures can serve as clues to the evaluation of a given structure or can mislead the examiner because they alter correct assessment of the structure in question. For example, a child may appear to have hypertelorism, when in fact the interpupillary distance may be normal. The appearance of hypertelorism may be created by lateral displacement of the medial canthi. In addition to observing structures, palpation, auscultation, range of motion, smell (unusual odors), sound (unusual cry), and the other standard techniques of examination should be employed.

Hall focuses on a number of specific physical examination features, including placement (e.g., low-set umbilicus), contour (e.g., brachycephaly or flat occiput), proportion (e.g., finger length) and mass (e.g., fat obscuring lack of muscle mass). Each of these features should be applied to various bodily regions. Again, whenever possible, measurements should be taken and compared with age-related norms. Any abnormalities should be assessed for underlying causes. The child who has an increased head circumference may have familial macrocephaly, hydrocephalus, or Proteus syndrome, all of which have very different implications. In this setting of macrocephaly, examining family members, checking fontanelle size, and looking for other anomalies may lead the diagnostician to the clue that provides a diagnosis. Once the database has been collected, the process of integration and assessment can begin. What follows is an overview of various bodily regions and their salient features. A detailed discussion of individual parts of the examination is beyond the scope of this text but is nicely reviewed in a variety of sources.

The general examination of the child with anomalies should include height, weight, and head circumference. These measurements should be plotted on a growth curve for comparison against previous points. Upper versus lower segment and arm span measurements can be useful in many settings. The child's state of alertness, paying attention to developmental stage, overall behavior, and interaction with the examiner, should be assessed. Does the child look proportional? Is he or she symmetric from side-to-side? How well-nourished does the child appear?

The head should be examined for shape, symmetry, and ridging (craniosynostosis; see Chapter 8). In children with Crouzon syndrome, frontal bossing, coronal suture craniosynostosis, and short anteroposterior dimension (brachycephaly) assist in diagnosis. While the head is being examined, attention should also be directed to hair whorls. Scalp hair pattern is a reflection of underlying brain formation. Hair can be abnormal in a variety of conditions. Alopecia is seen in progeria, hirsutism in Cornelia de Lange syndrome, and kinky hair in Menkes syndrome.

The eyes are complex, and a multitude of anomalies are possible. For example, lens dislocation is seen in Marfan and homocystinuria syndromes. Detection is central to diagnosis, but the ability to distinguish between downward dislocation (homocystinuria) and upward dislocation (Marfan) is also important. When examining the ears, attention should be given to position on the head ("set"), size, shape, definition, and preauricular pits and tags.

Nasal appearance is very variable and has strong familial similarities. It may be bulbous, anteverted, or hypoplastic with atretic choanae or a flat nasal bridge. Choanal atresia is a cardinal feature of CHARGE association, as are the anteverted nostrils of Williams syndrome.

The lips and oropharynx should be examined for philtrum appearance (smooth in fetal alcohol syndrome), lip pits, lip appearance (full in Hunter syndrome), and mouth shape (downturned in Russell-Silver syndrome). A small mouth is seen in trisomy 18, and a large mouth is seen on occasion in Beckwith-Wiedemann syndrome. A detailed palatal examination by visual inspection and palpation is important. A bifid uvula may be a hint to the presence of a submucous cleft palate. A large tongue may indicate athyrotic hypothyroidism sequence, and a small tongue is seen in Moebius sequence. The timing of the eruption of dentition and the color, shape, and condition of the teeth are also features to note (enamel hypoplasia is a common feature of Prader-Willi syndrome).

The neck should be evaluated for remnants of branchial cleft structures, webbing (seen in Turner and Noonan syndromes), torticollis (part of plagiocephaly-torticollis sequence), and any evidence of a short neck (Down syndrome).

The chest should be auscultated for evidence of heart disease. Some syndromes are so typically linked with specific types of heart diseases that an accurate cardiac evaluation provides the best clues for diagnosis (e.g., Kartagener syndrome and situs inversus, Williams syndrome and supravalvular aortic stenosis). Chest shape, muscle symmetry, nipple appearance and number, pectus deformities, and bony abnormalities should be evaluated.

The abdomen should be palpated for evidence of organomegaly. The umbilicus and its vessels are clues to diagnosis. Distinguishing between umbilical hernia, omphalocele, and gastroschisis can be central to diagnosis. The last is an isolated defect, whereas omphalocele and umbilical hernia are associated with many syndromes (trisomy 18 can have both). The length of the umbilical cord is believed to correlate with fetal movement. An inactive baby has a short cord as a result of limited traction.

The spine and back should be assessed for any deviation from the normal linear appearance with normal lumbar lordosis and convexity of the thoracic spine. The sacral region should be carefully assessed for evidence of a lipoma, hair tuft, hemangioma, or any evidence of a dysraphic state (see Fig. 2-4). (Fetal valproate effects are associated with meningomyelocele.)

Genitalia require a full assessment as well. Penile size, scrotal appearance, urethral opening, and testes should be examined. In a girl, labia majora, labia minora, and vaginal introitus should be examined. If the genitalia are ambiguous, gender assignment should be delayed and a detailed evaluation initiated. Particular concern should focus on the possibility of salt-losing congenital adrenal hyperplasia and its potentially lethal nature. Tanner staging should be performed.

The extremities are evaluated in detail, with particular attention given to the hands, where 25% of minor bodily anomalies occur. The hands should be evaluated for size (small in Prader-Willi syndrome), palmar creases, and finger markings and details (fusion, length, straightness, overlap, nails, and placement [especially thumb]). As alluded to earlier, limb size, symmetry, and proportion are valuable clues to a wide range of syndromes. (Patients with Marfan syndrome have long, slim limbs.)

Lastly, the skin may have pigmentary changes, as with the phakomatoses (tuberous sclerosis and neurofibromatosis). A Woods lamp can be of value in this assessment by enhancing the hypopigmented lesions of tuberous sclerosis. Skin may be lax, thick, or thin or display increased elasticity (Ehlers-Danlos syndrome).

Approach to the Patient

Laboratory and Radiographic Procedures

The explosion of genetic technology may leave the clinician overwhelmed by its sheer volume and complexity. It is therefore worth reinforcing the fact that most dysmorphology diagnoses rest on the basic clinical tools of history and physical examination. The use of the laboratory is confined to supporting or disproving theories or potential diagnoses. The specifically and judiciously ordered evaluation that confirms a diagnosis is the quickest and cheapest way to use the laboratory. For example, a child with mild prenatal growth deficiency, medial eyebrow flare, depressed nasal bridge, stellate pattern in the iris, anteverted nares, long philtrum, hypoplastic nails, and a murmur may have Williams syndrome. The clinician might consider a serum calcium test and an echocardiogram. Should the calcium level be high or the echocardiogram reveal supravalvular aortic stenosis, the diagnosis is solidified. Further genetic testing with *fluorescent in situ hybridization* (FISH) may then be suggested by the consulting geneticist to confirm the diagnosis. Future expectations can then be delineated and special attention focused on behavior, intellectual function, hypertension, and a variety of other problems that beset children and adults with Williams syndrome. Also of major benefit to the family is the fact that cases are sporadic, with little risk of subsequent children being affected.

Specific evaluations that may be of help in confirming a diagnosis include magnetic resonance imaging, computed tomography, skeletal survey, echocardiogram, abdominal sonogram, and countless other technical tools. Use of these aids without clear indications in a "shotgun" fashion should be discouraged. The discomfort to the child and the expense and inconvenience to the family all mitigate against indiscriminate testing.

Cytogenetics

It was not until 1956 that geneticists were able to accurately analyze and count chromosomes. Within several years, trisomy 21 was the first recognized chromosomal disorder. Shortly thereafter, Turner syndrome was defined as the first known sex chromosome abnormality. Various staining techniques performed on metaphase cell preparations allow for the now familiar bands seen in the human karyotype. The geneticists can evaluate these preparations for any deletions, additions, or rearrangements. The use of cells in prometaphase has allowed for higher band resolution because the chromosomes are "stretched out" during this phase of mitosis. FISH technology allows for detection of genetic material abnormalities of even higher resolution than prometaphase banding techniques. A specific deoxyribonucleic acid (DNA) probe is hybridized to a desired section of a metaphase chromosome. A fluorochrome stain then detects the presence of the DNA target on the patient's DNA, hence confirming the presence of the genetic material in question. This technique therefore can pinpoint suspected minute fragments of DNA. The technique is also used to uncover aneuploidy (any deviation from the exact multiple of the haploid number of chromosomes) and therefore enhances "routine" cytogenetic diagnosis. FISH has also been used effectively to detect microdeletions seen in conditions such as DiGeorge syndrome. The microdeletion on chromosome 22 can be detected by this method, whereas high-resolution banding appears normal.

Another useful diagnostic technique is folate-sensitive fragile site testing, a technique that can be used to diagnose fragile X syndrome. This syndrome is the most common cause of inherited mental deficiency. Boys with this disorder display a prominent jaw, thickened nasal bridge, large ears with soft cartilage, and large testes. Specific DNA testing is also available to look for FMR-1 (the fragile X gene).

With time and the help of technology, many new syndromes are being defined, and the underlying causes for previously described syndromes are being established. For example, Smith-Lemli-Opitz syndrome, which displays anteverted nostrils, eyelid ptosis, syndactyly of the second and third toes, hypospadias, and cryptorchidism in boys, is now recognized as a disorder of cholesterol metabolism. The rapid advances in genetics therefore require that the clinician consult closely with the dysmorphologist, clinical geneticist, metabolic specialist, and a wide range of other specialists. In treating the child with Sturge-Weber syndrome, a neurologist is important in evaluating associated neurologic findings. A child with Pierre Robin sequence often requires the services of an otolaryngologist, as do children with CHARGE association and choanal atresia. Each syndrome has its own set of unique associated findings. The complexity of medical problems and the enormous psychosocial and economic needs of these children and their families place the primary care physician in a central position. The practitioner can act as a conductor, who carefully and sensibly orchestrates the input of various skilled specialists into an overall cohesive plan for the patient.

Protocol for Evaluating Abortuses and Stillbirths

Complete internal and external examination, including measurements and weights
Histologic investigations
Examination of placenta, umbilical cord, membranes
Photography
X-ray, xeroradiography
Cultures—amniotic fluid/membranes, tissues
Karyotype—blood, skin fibroblasts, other tissues
Biopsy and storage of skin and representative tissues
Metabolic studies
DNA (analysis or storage)

Modified from Witt DR, Hall JG: Multiple congenital anomaly syndromes. In Rudolph AM, Hoffman JIE, Rudolph CD, editors: *Rudolph's textbook of pediatrics,* Norwalk, Conn, 1991, Appleton and Lange.

At this point, it is imperative to reinforce the importance of establishing a diagnosis in each and every child if at all possible. This includes children who have already succumbed to their condition. When a child with deformities appears *in extremis,* the clinician should ensure that a variety of studies are obtained. These studies include full chromosome evaluation, photographs, total body radiographs, definition of visceral organ and central nervous system anomalies, and metabolic studies (serum and urine amino acids, organic acids, etc.). Whenever possible, an autopsy should be performed, and tissue should be frozen for future evaluation. A protocol for abortuses and stillbirths is provided in Box 29-6.

Management

The rarity of individual dysmorphic or genetic conditions precludes a meaningful discussion of the management of any single condition. This is, however, an opportunity to briefly outline an approach that can be applied to any child with congenital anomalies. Families of these children require consistent, coordinated, organized, and empathetic care. Without a central "clearinghouse" for all subspecialty input, families are caught in a web of confusion, and their frustration and the lack of focused care may impact the overall quality of life for the child. The primary care physician can assume this role by addressing three main aspects of care—medical, psychosocial, and developmental.

Medical

At birth a detailed search for abnormalities in each organ system should be conducted and an underlying unifying diagnosis sought. Occasionally, major anomalies distract the clinician from a thorough review of other, less obvious findings. A definitive diagnosis can direct this workup but should not necessarily discourage an investigation into other organs not usually affected by a given disorder. Specialists are invaluable in this search, but their focus may be solely on their particular area of expertise.

Psychosocial

The impact of the birth of an abnormal child ripples through the family in an intense fashion. The exact nature of a family's needs changes with time. An objective and supportive style facilitates the discussion of these issues and increases the likelihood that they are addressed and effectively worked through. The clinician may handle this form of support but should not hesitate to rely on the skill of behavioralist colleagues.

Developmental

The developmental aspect of care should focus on a child's sensory and intellectual function, in addition to growth and nutrition. A full exploration of hearing, vision, and possible explanations of other handicaps is in order. The underlying evaluation for any of these problems may be related to a given syndrome, but environment, psychosocial, and other medical factors should not be overlooked. Further exploration of the issues of management are beyond the scope of this text.

SUMMARY

The process of arriving at a diagnosis in the child with possible dysmorphology is complex. To aid the clinician in an approach to this problem an algorithm may help (Fig. 29-12). The process usually begins with parental concern about unusual physical features, developmental delay, or growth anomalies. The astute physician may also note these findings during the process of history taking and detailed physical examination. Figs. 29-12, *A, B, C,* and *D,* provide a logical approach and summary of many of the issues raised in this chapter.

ILLUSTRATIVE CASES

Case 1. R.T. was the 10-lb, 2-oz product of a full-term gestation to a 21-year-old gravida I para I woman. The delivery was vaginal vertex without complications. In the delivery room the examining pediatrician noted minimal micrognathia, pectus excavatum, talipes equinovarus (clubfoot), and bilateral dislocable hips. No other abnormalities were noted on examination. Because of the large size of this infant and a pattern consistent with deformation, an excellent prognosis was predicted. After orthopedic management of the talipes equinovarus and dislocable hips, R.T. had minimal cosmetic deformities, and he functioned normally developmentally and intellectually. This case illustrates a classic deformation in a primigravida with a large fetus. Deformities either correct over time or after surgical intervention.

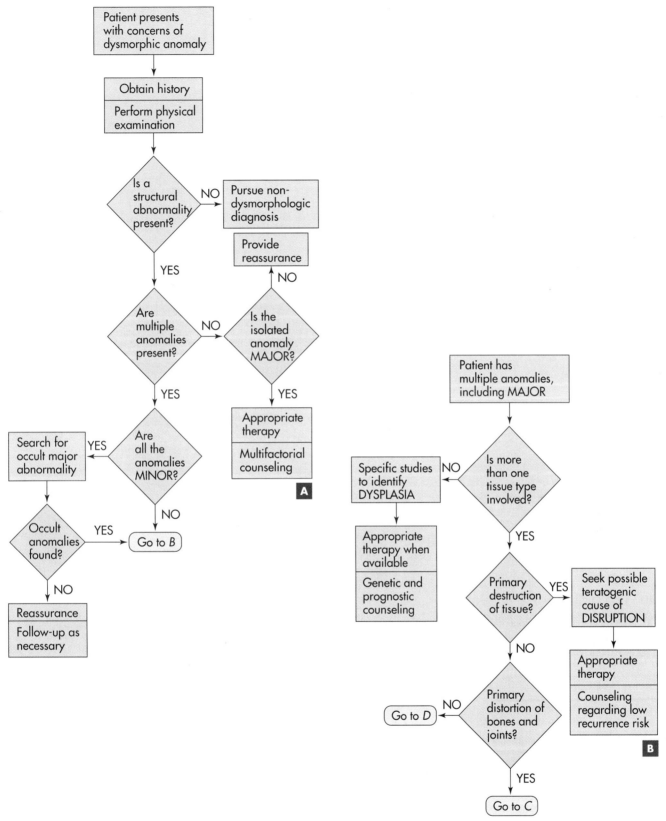

FIG. 29-12 *A,* An algorithm for dysmorphic evaluation. Initial evaluation and categorization of general class of abnormalities. *B,* Evaluation of dysplasia and disruptions. (**A** to **D** Modified from Aase JM: dysmorphic diagnosis for the pediatric practitioner, *Pediatr Clin North Am* 39:135-156, 1992.)

Continued

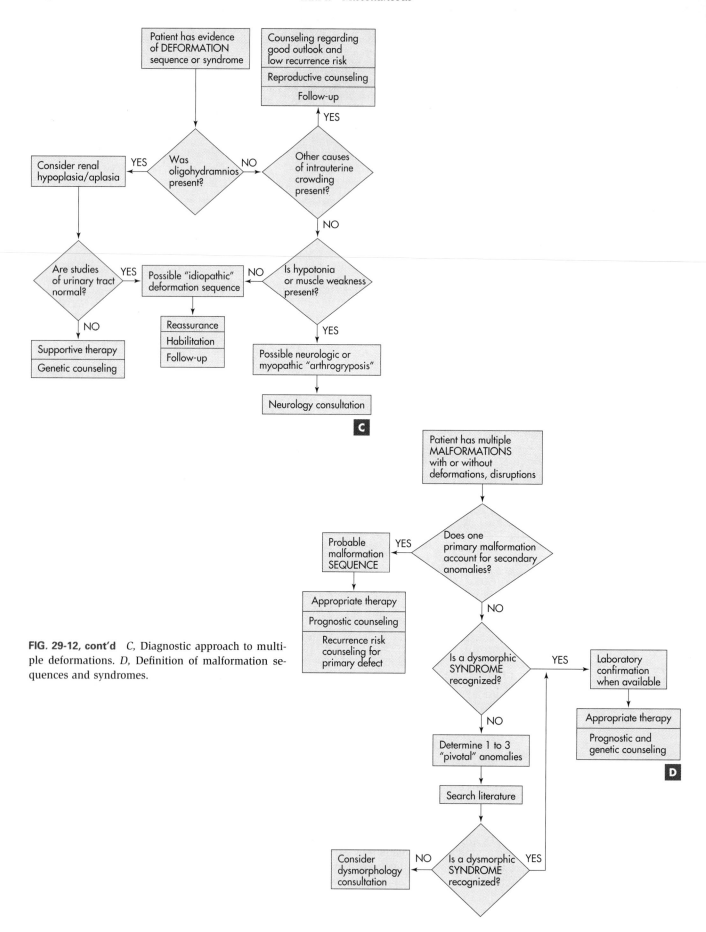

FIG. 29-12, cont'd   *C,* Diagnostic approach to multiple deformations. *D,* Definition of malformation sequences and syndromes.

Case 2. S.L. was born weighing 5 lb at 36 weeks gestation to a 31-year-old gravida II para I woman. The mother reported decreased fetal activity as compared with her first child, and at birth the infant was noted to have a weak cry. Polyhydramnios was noted by the obstetrician, and the placenta was smaller than expected.

Physical examination revealed a prominent occiput with low-set, malformed ears and micrognathia. Examination of the hands and feet revealed overlapping fingers. The sternum was quite short, and the nipples were small. There was an umbilical hernia and diastasis recti. A prominent murmur consistent with a patent ductus arteriosus was noted. Further evaluation by a pediatric cardiologist revealed evidence of transposition of the great vessels. Sonogram of the abdomen revealed a horseshoe kidney with hydronephrosis.

Because of the presence of many major and minor anomalies, a chromosomal abnormality was suspected, specifically trisomy 18 syndrome. Bone marrow chromosomes were obtained, and several hours later a preliminary diagnosis of trisomy 18 syndrome was confirmed. Because of the extremely poor long-term prognosis, a decision to provide limited medical care was made by the parents and medical staff. At 3 weeks of age, S.L. suffered a cardiorespiratory arrest, and based on the family's wishes resuscitation was not performed. This case illustrates the value of rapid diagnosis and the significant impact that correct diagnosis can have on clinical care.

Case 3. C.H. was the 7-lb, 8-oz product of a full-term gestation to a gravida III para II 27-year-old woman. Delivery was vaginal vertex without complications. At birth this infant was noted to have bilateral syndactyly of the second and third toes, a right-sided eartag, and a supernumerary nipple on the left side. On careful questioning it was learned that two other family members also had syndactyly of the second and third toes bilaterally. Because of the lack of other anomalies, this infant was observed without further intervention or evaluation. At age 5 years, the child was growing and developing normally with no evidence of any medical problems. This case illustrates that several minor anomalies can be present in an infant who is otherwise completely normal.

ANNOTATED BIBLIOGRAPHY

Hall JG: When a child is born with congenital anomalies, *Contemp Pediatr* 5:78-87, 1988.
This outstanding overview article on the approach to a child with congenital anomalies provides excellent definitions and a practical clinical approach.

Jones KL: *Smith's recognizable patterns of human malformation*, Philadelphia, 1997, WB Saunders.

This is the classic text on malformations. This resource is extremely easy to use and is filled with photographs of each syndrome, lists of salient features, and tables of anomalies and the syndromes in which they are found. This text is a necessity for the clinician.

Keele DK: A diagnostic approach to the dysmorphic child, *Contemp Pediatr* 2:63-84, 1985.
This is an excellent review of the four major morphologic, pathogenic mechanisms. Very useful tables of these mechanisms and specific correlations to clinical findings are provided. The focus on the physical examination is quite useful.

BIBLIOGRAPHY

Aase JM: Dysmorphologic diagnosis for the pediatric practitioner, *Pediatr Clin North Am* 39:135-156, 1992.

Aase JM: The dysmorphology detective, *Pediatr Ann* 10:38-43, 1981.

Aase JM: *Diagnostic dysmorphology*, New York, 1990, Plenum Medical.

Buyse ML: *Birth defects encyclopedia*, Cambridge, 1990, Blackwell Scientific.

Davenport SLH: The child with multiple congenital anomalies, *Pediatr Ann* 19:23-33, 1990.

Fong CT: Clinical diagnosis of genetic diseases, *Pediatr Ann* 22:277-281, 1993.

Friedman JM: A practical approach to dysmorphology, *Pediatr Ann* 19:95-101, 1990.

Gorlin RJ, Cohen MM, Jr, Levin S: *Syndromes of the head and neck*, New York, 1989, Oxford University Press.

Graham JM: *Recognizable patterns of human deformation*, Philadelphia, 1988, WB Saunders.

Hall BD: The state of the art of dysmorphology, *Am J Dis Child* 147:1184-1189, 1993.

Leppig KA, Werler MM, Cann CI, et al: Predictive value of minor anomalies. I. Association with major malformations, *J Pediatr* 110:531-537, 1987.

Ludman MD: Assessing the child with congenital anomalies. In Goldbloom RB, editor: *Pediatric clinical skills*, New York, 1992, Churchill Livingstone.

McKusick VA: *Mendelian inheritance in man*, ed 1, Baltimore, 1990, Johns Hopkins University Press.

Opitz JM: The developmental field concept in clinical genetics, *J Pediatr* 101:805-809, 1982.

Shapiro LR, Wilmot PL: Cytogenetic diagnosis of genetic diseases, *Pediatr Ann* 22:298-303, 1993.

Taybi H, Lachman RS: *Radiology of syndromes, metabolic disorders, and skeletal dysplasias*, Chicago, 1993, Mosby–Year Book.

Tint GS, Irons M, Elias ER, et al: Defective cholesterol biosynthesis associated with the Smith-Lemli-Opitz syndrome, *N Engl J Med* 330:107-113, 1994.

Wilson GN: Office approach to the genetics patient, *Pediatr Ann* 19:79-91, 1990.

Winter RM, Baraitser M: *Multiple congenital anomalies: a diagnostic compendium*, London, 1991, Chapman & Hall Medical.

Witt DR, Hall JG: Multiple congenital anomaly syndromes. In Rudolph AM, Hoffman JIE, Rudolph CD, editors: *Rudolph's textbook of pediatrics*, Norwalk, Conn, 1991, Appleton and Lange.

Index

Coagulation—cont'd
　description of, 331–332
Coagulation cascade, disorders of, 343–346
Cocaine, congenital anomaly diagnosis and maternal exposure to, 441
Coccidioidomycosis
　fever associated with, 84
　lymphadenopathy caused by, 367
　lymphadenopathy diagnosis and, 375
Coccidiomycosis
　hemoptysis caused by, 196
　hepatosplenomegaly associated with, 358
Codeine, chronic cough treated with, 197
Cognitive skills, development of, 113
Cognitive-behavioral therapy, chronic fatigue syndrome treated with, 409
Coin rubbing, bruising as result of, 348
Colic, 41–50
　recurrent infection indicated by, 382
Colitis
　causes of, in infant, 279
　pseudomembranous, 251
　ulcerative
　　jaundice associated with, 265
　　vomiting associated with, 283
Collagen disorder, chronic fatigue syndrome diagnosis and, 406
Collagen fiber, coagulation process and, 331
Collagen vascular disease
　blood vessel inflammation and, 348
　chronic weakness associated with, 148
　fever associated with, 84
　signs of, 352
Complement disorder, treatment of, 395
Complete blood count
　airway obstruction diagnosis and, 227
　chronic cough diagnosis and, 197
　chronic diarrhea diagnosis and, 256
　chronic nasal obstruction diagnosis and, 212
　edema diagnosis and, 325
　excessive bleeding diagnosis and, 352
　hepatosplenomegaly diagnosis and, 362
　jaundice diagnosis and, 269
　lymphadenopathy diagnosis and, 377
　recurrent abdominal pain diagnosis and, 11
　recurrent infection diagnosis and, 392
　thrombocytopenia diagnosis and, 335
Compulsive drinking, description of, 298
Computed tomography
　airway obstruction diagnosis and, 228
　ascites diagnosis and, 320
　chest, chronic cough diagnosis and, 197
　chronic nasal obstruction diagnosis and, 212
　congenital anomaly diagnosis and, 445

Computed tomography—cont'd
　developmental disorders diagnosis and, 128–129
　diagnosis of spells and, 140
　lymphadenopathy diagnosis and, 377
Computer-assisted tomography, headache diagnosis and, 60
Concentration, lack of, chronic fatigue syndrome associated with, 407t
Confusion
　chronic fatigue syndrome associated with, 407t
　hydrocephalus associated with, 56
　migraine and, 53
Congenital adrenal hyperplasia
　chronic diarrhea diagnosis and, 251
　congenital anomaly diagnosis and, 445
　vomiting associated with, 279
Congenital anomaly, 433–449
Congenital anterior nasal occlusion, 208
Congenital berry aneurysm, migraine and, 53
Congenital central hypoventilation syndrome, 179
Congenital chloride diarrhea, chronic diarrhea diagnosis and, 250
Congenital heart defect, as example of malformation, 437
Congenital heart disease, microcephaly associated with, 101
Congenital hepatic fibrosis
　ascites and, 320
　diagnosis of, 271
　jaundice associated with, 265
Congenital infection, description of, 119
Congenital villous atrophy, chronic diarrhea diagnosis and, 250
Congestive heart failure
　edema in child associated with, 313
　hepatomegaly associated with, 357
　hepatosplenomegaly associated with, 358
　macrocephaly associated with, 105
　periorbital edema associated with, 316
　persistent infant crying caused by, 44
　portal, fetal hydrops associated with, 313
Conjunctivitis
　allergic rhinitis as cause of, 203
　chlamydial, 374
　lymphadenopathy diagnosis and, 376
　periorbital edema associated with, 317
　recurrent infection diagnosis and, 392
　Reiter syndrome and, 24, 72
Connective tissue disease
　constipation and, 241
　hepatosplenomegaly associated with, 358
Constipation, 233–246
　illustrative cases of, 245–246
　persistent infant crying caused by, 44

Constipation—cont'd
　recurrent abdominal pain associated with, 5
　recurrent abdominal pain caused by, 4
　recurrent vomiting diagnosis and, 285
Continence, fecal, pathophysiology of, 234
Conversion disorder
　gait affected by, 64
　syncope associated with, 163
Conversion reaction, nonpainful limp associated with, 75
Coombs test
　excessive bleeding diagnosis and, 352
　jaundice diagnosis and, 269
Copper, liver tissue content of, 272
Cornea
　clouding of, developmental delay diagnosis and, 126
　infection of, periorbital edema associated with, 318
Corneal abrasion, persistent infant crying caused by, 44
Cornelia de Lange syndrome
　congenital anomaly diagnosis and, 444
　developmental delay associated with, 115t
　hoarseness associated with, 219
Coronal synostosis, abnormal head shape associated with, 102
Coronary artery, anomalies of, syncope associated with, 165
Corticosteroid drug(s)
　blood vessels affected by, 347
　neonatal immune thrombocytopenia treated with, 337
　neonatal thrombocytopenia treated with, 337
　thrombic thrombocytopenia purpura treated with, 340
Costochondritis, chest pain associated with, 34
Cough
　chronic, 189–200
　　recurrent infection indicated by, 382
　complications of, 190
　fever diagnosis and, 87
　importance of, 189
　paroxysmal, 196
　pathophysiology of, 189–190
　psychogenic
　　adolescent and, 195
　　illustrative case of, 199
Cough mechanism, description of, 189–190
Cough receptor, location of, 189
Cough reflex, description of, 189
Cough suppressant, chronic cough treated with, 197

Erythema nodosum
   chronic diarrhea diagnosis and, 255
   jaundice diagnosis and, 268
Erythrocyte sedimentation rate
   chronic weakness diagnosis and, 154
   lymphadenopathy diagnosis and, 377
   recurrent infection diagnosis and, 392
Erythromycin
   sinusitis treated with, 198
   vomiting treated with, 287
Esophageal atresia, diagnosis of, 278
Esophagitis
   chest pain associated with, 34, 36
   recurrent vomiting associated with, 287
Esophagogram, apnea diagnosis and, 183
Esophagus
   cough receptor in, 189
   disorder of, chest pain associated with, 36
   obstruction of, failure to thrive and, 418
Ethanol, fetal alcohol syndrome associated with, 101
Ethyl alcohol, diabetes insipidus caused by, 299
Ewing sarcoma
   back pain associated with, 24
   painful limp associated with, 72
Exaggerated startle syndrome, 134
Exercise, repetitive
   knee pain associated with, 66
   microtrauma caused by, 65
Exercise intolerance
   excessive bleeding diagnosis and, 351
   recurrent infection indicated by, 382
Extracellular fluid, percentage of, in body, 311
Extremity
   inflammation of, inguinal adenopathy associated with, 374
   swollen, diagnosis of, 323
Eye
   disorders of, chronic nonprogressive headache associated with, 54
   examination of, hepatosplenomegaly diagnosis and, 359
   inflammation of, back pain diagnosis and, 27
   size and shape of, developmental delay diagnosis and, 125
Eye contact, avoidance of, autism and, 122
Eyelid, edema involving, 311

F

FABERE maneuver, back pain diagnosis and, 28
Face, long, fragile X syndrome associated with, 115
Facial nerve palsy, congenital anomaly and, 436

Factor IX, coagulation deficiency and, 344
Factor VIII, coagulation deficiency and, 344
FAE; *see* Fetal alcohol effect
Failure to thrive, 413–423
   child abuse associated with, 423
   chronic airway obstruction and, 217
   chronic intestinal pseudoobstruction syndrome and, 241
   chronic nonimmunologic disease indicated by, 382
   constipation diagnosis and, 242
   definition of, 413
   differential diagnosis of, 415*t*, 417–420
   DiGeorge syndrome associated with, 388
   emotional deprivation as cause of, 416
   generalized edema in child associated with, 316
   Hirschsprung disease associated with, 238
   hospitalization for treatment of, 422
   human immunodeficiency virus associated with, 383
   literature survey of, 417
   maternal deprivation as cause of, 417
   mental retardation associated with, 422
   neglectful, 416
   nervous vomiting and, 277
   nonorganic, 414
      psychosocial short stature and, 423
   pathophysiology of, 416–417
   patient approach and diagnosis of, 421–422
   patient history and, 420–421
   physical examination and diagnosis of, 421
   recurrent vomiting associated with, 287
   severe combined immunodeficiency and, 389
Familial intrahepatic cholestasis, bilirubin production affected by, 260
Familial periodic paralysis, description of, 147
Family, disruption in, psychosocial short stature and, 424
Family history
   apnea diagnosis and, 182
   chronic cough diagnosis and, 195–196
   chronic diarrhea diagnosis and, 255
   chronic fatigue syndrome incidence and, 405
   chronic weakness diagnosis and, 150
   congenital anomaly diagnosis and, 440–442, 442
   developmental delay and, 124
   edema diagnosis and, 323
   failure to thrive diagnosis and, 420
   fever diagnosis and, 87

Family history—cont'd
   hepatosplenomegaly diagnosis and, 359
   jaundice diagnosis and, 266
   macrocephaly or microcephaly and, 104–106
   recurrent infection diagnosis and, 390
Fanconi anemia, 341–342
Fanconi syndrome, osmotic diuresis and, 300
Farber disease, hoarseness associated with, 219
FAS; *see* Fetal alcohol syndrome
Fat
   decreased, recurrent infection diagnosis and, 392
   fecal, chronic diarrhea diagnosis and, 257
   malabsorption of, chronic diarrhea diagnosis and, 256
Fatigue, 401–411; *see also* Chronic fatigue syndrome
   acquired aplastic anemia associated with, 342
   back pain diagnosis and, 27
   bone marrow evaluation and diagnosis of, 341
   causes of, 401, 407–408
   central, 401
   chronic fatigue syndrome associated with, 407*t*
   migraine associated with, 52
   myopericardial disease and, 35
   peripheral, 401
   poor food intake caused by, failure to thrive associated with, 418
   recurrent abdominal pain associated with, 8
   tension-type headache associated with, 54
Fatty acid, intestinal absorption and, 247
Fatty acid metabolism, failure to thrive and, 418
Fearfulness, recurrent abdominal pain associated with, 4
Feature(s), dysmorphic, developmental delay diagnosis and, 125
FEBERE maneuver, 28
Febricula, 402
Fecal incontinence, encopresis and, 298
Feeding, poor, cervical adenopathy associated with, 371
Feeding history, apnea diagnosis and, 182
Fetal alcohol effect, 117
Fetal alcohol syndrome
   congenital anomaly diagnosis and, 444
   congenital nasal obstruction associated with, 208
   mental retardation associated with, 116
Fetal hydantoin syndrome, 118
Fetal-maternal blood group incompatibility, 259

Myxedema, edema differentiated
from, 312

N

NAIT; *see* Thrombocytopenia, neonatal
alloimmune
Narcolepsy, description of, 137
NARES; *see* Nonallergic rhinitis with
eosinophilia syndrome
Nasal cycle, description of, 201
Nasal obstruction
chronic, 210–214
congenital abnormalities as cause of,
207–208
Nasal secretion, apnea diagnosis and, 183
Nasopharyngitis
apnea associated with, 181
streptococcosis as cause of, 206
Nasopharynx
examination of, lymphadenopathy
diagnosis and, 376
obstruction in, 215
tumor in, 373
tumor of, nasal obstruction caused
by, 208
Nausea
depression diagnosis and, 406
description of, 275
diskitis associated with, 23
function of, 275
hydrocephalus associated with, 56
migraine associated with, 52
testis torsion and, 321
NEC; *see* Necrotizing enterocolitis
Neck
anatomy of, 368*f*
congenital masses in, 369
deformations of, 436
edema of, 319
enlarged lymph nodes in, 368–374
examination of, lymphadenopathy
diagnosis and, 376
lymph nodes in, 370*f*
malignant tumors in, 372–373
mass in, evaluation of, 378*f*
neuroblastoma in, 374
Necrosis
avascular, limp caused by, 65–66
fat, scrotal swelling associated
with, 322
Necrotizing enterocolitis
constipation associated with, 236
vomiting associated with, 278
Necrotizing lymphadenitis, 372
Neimann-Pick disease,
hepatosplenomegaly associated
with, 358
Neonate
constipation in, causes of, 236
hoarseness in, 218–219
jaundice in, 260–262

Neonate—cont'd
palpable lymph nodes in, 365
persistent crying in, 49
thrombocytopenia in, 335–337
Neoplasia, urinary incontinence
and, 298
Neoplasm
cerebellar, 55*f*
swollen extremity and, 323
Nephritis, Henoch-Schonlein purpura
associated with, 349
Nephrolithiasis, 297
Nephronophthisis
juvenile, osmotic diuresis and, 300
polyuria and, 300
Nephropathy, Henoch-Schonlein purpura
associated with, 349
Nephrotic syndrome
causes of, 315
illustrative case of, 326
periorbital edema associated with, 316
plasma oncotic pressure and, 312
scrotal swelling associated with, 322
Nerve, deformations of, 436
Nerve conduction velocity test, chronic
weakness diagnosis and, 154
Nervous system
autonomic, urinary control and, 293
headache diagnosis and examination
of, 59
Neural tube, failure of closure of, 119
Neurasthenia, 402
Neuroblastoma
back pain associated with, 24
chronic diarrhea diagnosis and, 252
edema associated with, 316
fever associated with, 84
in head and neck, 373
hepatomegaly associated with, 358
jaundice associated with, 265
lymphadenopathy caused by, 367
myoclonic encephalopathy associated
with, 134
periorbital edema associated with, 318
urinary incontinence and, 298
Neurocutaneous disorder,
megalencephaly associated with, 104
Neurocutaneous syndrome,
developmental delay and, 116
Neurodegenerative disorder,
developmental delay associated with,
120–121
Neurofibroma, intraspinal, back pain
associated with, 25
Neurofibromatosis
congenital anomaly diagnosis and, 445
constipation and, 241
constipation diagnosis and, 242
developmental delay and, 116
as example of generalized dysplasia, 436
headache diagnosis and, 59

Neurofibromatosis—cont'd
illustration of, 118*f*
nonneurologic manifestations of, 99
periorbital edema associated with, 318
Neurofibrosarcoma, frequency of, 374
Neuroimaging, developmental disorders
diagnosis and, 128–129
Neurologic deficit, migraine and, 53
Neurologic examination, developmental
delay diagnosis and, 126
Neuromuscular disease, poor food intake
caused by, failure to thrive associated
with, 418
Neuromuscular disorder, peripheral, 123
Neuromuscular junction, disease in
chronic weakness associated with, 147
weakness associated with, 144
Neuromyasthenia, epidemic, 403
Neurosarcoidosis, thirst center defect
and, 298
Neutropenia
common variable immunodeficiency
and, 385
cyclic, 86
Newborn
generalized edema in, 313
hemorrhagic disease of, 346
jaundice in, 259
Nezelof syndrome, 388
Niemann-Pick disease, lymphadenopathy
caused by, 367
Night sweats
back pain diagnosis and, 27
fever diagnosis and, 87
lymphadenopathy diagnosis and, 375
Night terrors, 137
persistent infant crying caused by, 44
Nil disease, 315
NITP; *see* Thrombocytopenia, neonatal
immune
Nitric oxide, vascular tone and, 331
Nitroblue tetrazolium test, phagocytic
defect and, 390
NOFTT; *see* Failure to thrive, nonorganic
Nonallergic rhinitis with eosinophilia
syndrome, 204
Nonepileptic neurologic disorder,
134–136
Nonneuropathic dyssynergia, 302
Noonan syndrome
congenital anomaly diagnosis and, 444
developmental delay associated
with, 115*t*
edema associated with, 316
swollen extremity and, 323
Normal variant, definition of, in
congenital anomaly diagnosis, 433
Norwalk virus, chronic diarrhea
diagnosis and, 252
Nose
anatomy and physiology of, 201